Venous Embolization of the Liver

David C. Madoff • Masatoshi Makuuchi
Masato Nagino • Jean-Nicolas Vauthey
Editors

Venous Embolization of the Liver

Radiologic and Surgical Practice

Springer

Editors
David C. Madoff, M.D., F.S.I.R
Professor of Radiology
Chief, Division of Interventional Radiology
Department of Radiology
New York-Presbyterian Hospital/Weill
Cornell Medical Center
New York, NY, USA

Masato Nagino, M.D., Ph.D.
Professor and Chairman
Division of Surgical Oncology
Department of Surgery
Nagoya University Graduate
School of Medicine
Nagoya, Japan

Masatoshi Makuuchi, M.D., Ph.D.
President
Japanese Red Cross Medical Center
Tokyo, Japan

Jean-Nicolas Vauthey, M.D.
Professor and Chief, Liver Service
Department of Surgical Oncology
The University of Texas M.D. Anderson
Cancer Center
Houston, TX, USA

ISBN 978-1-4471-5950-6 ISBN 978-1-84882-122-4 (eBook)
DOI 10.1007/978-1-84882-122-4
Springer London Dordrecht Heidelberg New York

Cover design: eStudioCalamar, Figueres/Berlin

Printed on acid-free paper

Springer Science+Business Media (www.springer.com)

Foreword

The past two decades have seen remarkable advances in the understanding of hepatobiliary anatomy and in hepatobiliary surgery. Precise anatomical description of the liver has transformed our understanding of this organ and revealed a detailed network of vessels and bile ducts delineating well-defined territories. Improved imaging techniques, including CT, MRI, and intraoperative ultrasonography, have also facilitated localization of all the avenues and streets by which the liver can be accessed along Couinaud's segmental anatomy. These remarkable developments have improved the information available regarding tumor extent and characteristics, contributing to better surgical planning.

Today, new resection techniques and improved vascular control enable surgeons to perform an increasing variety of resections, ranging from partial segmentectomy to complex resections involving removal of six segments with reconstruction of the bile ducts, portal veins, and inferior vena cava. Not only do these techniques allow surgeons to perform a wide range of resections with increasing confidence, they are also safe, associated with mortality rates of less than 1–2% at centers with expertise. Currently, resection remains the only option to offer a chance of cure to patients with liver tumors, and curative resection is the main indication for liver resection. Recently, procedures have been developed to reduce the size of tumors or increase the size of the liver that will remain after resection (the "remnant liver") and thereby broaden the population of patients considered candidates for liver resection, which now includes some patients with very large tumors or multiple tumors.

Reduction in tumor size may be achieved by chemoembolization in patients with hepatocellular carcinoma and by neoadjuvant chemotherapy in patients with colorectal liver metastases, the most frequent indication for liver resection in Western countries. However, in some patients, tumor size reduction is not sufficient to allow resection because of the small volume of the remnant liver. To address this problem, procedures have been developed to increase the remnant liver volume. The first of these was reported by Professor Masatoshi Makuuchi in 1990 for patients scheduled to undergo liver resection for hilar cholangiocarcinoma. Embolization of portal vein branches induces atrophy of the deprived portal territory but also, more importantly, distributes the functional portal blood flow completely to the remaining liver, leading to hypertrophy of the anticipated future liver remnant. This book describes in detail all aspects of this strategy of venous embolization of the liver: preoperative imaging to study the liver territories; functional studies of the parenchyma; techniques for portal and hepatic vein embolization, whether percutaneous or ileocolic; indications and contraindications; clinical outcomes and complications; and associated procedures, including chemotherapy and arterial embolization.

For all those involved in the modern era of treatment of liver tumors – hepatologists, radiologists, oncologists, and surgeons – this book is an outstanding tool, and the editors should be congratulated for gathering a wealth of knowledge in a treatise that updates the fascinating new field of hepatobiliary surgery and liver regeneration. The techniques described herein may help physicians to alter the disease course and allow the possibility of curative resection for many patients who were not previously considered candidates for major hepatobiliary surgery.

Paul Brousse Hospital
Villejuif, France

Henri Bismuth, M.D., FACS (Hon)

Preface

Until recently, patients with primary and metastatic liver cancer had dismal prognoses. However, with improvements in screening, detection, and therapeutics, the paradigms for managing these patients have shifted dramatically. Nowadays, the management algorithms require a multidisciplinary effort which includes medical oncologists, surgeons, radiologists, radiation oncologists, hepatologists, gastroenterologists, and many other physicians and health care professionals. Interestingly, one of the major changes has been the increased utilization, safety, and survival benefit of surgical options for patients previously considered unresectable.

Although tremendous advances in hepatobiliary surgical techniques have been made over the years, substantial perioperative morbidity and mortality still occurs. For this reason, many investigators have attempted to understand the basic mechanisms of postoperative hepatobiliary physiology and the limits for performing safe resection. One method for improving perioperative outcomes, and ultimately survival, has been to increase the size and function of the anticipated future liver remnant before surgery by utilizing hepatic venous embolotherapy techniques such as portal vein embolization. Not only does this reduce complication rates, it also enables patients previously considered unresectable due to limited hepatic reserve to undergo major hepatic resection.

For this book, we invited Eastern and Western authors who specialize in the diagnosis and treatment of patients with hepatobiliary malignancy to give the reader a global perspective on its management. A multitude of pertinent topics have been addressed including the history of hepatic resection, vascular and surgical anatomy, liver regeneration, factors affecting hypertrophy, pathophysiology of embolization and resection, embolization techniques, the indications for embolization and resection, potential complications, outcomes data for different diseases, novel strategies, and future perspectives. The editors thank all of the authors for their contributions to this book. We hope this work will spur the interest of clinicians and basic scientists with a focus in hepatobiliary malignancy and liver regeneration physiology so that we can continue to improve the lives of patients with these diseases.

David C. Madoff, M.D.
Masatoshi Makuuchi, M.D., Ph.D.
Masato Nagino, M.D., Ph.D.
Jean-Nicolas Vauthey, M.D.

Contents

Part III Embolization Techniques

Part IV Clinical Outcomes

Part V Additional Strategies for Resection and Embolization

Contributors

Eddie K. Abdalla, M.D. Department of Surgical Oncology, The University of Texas M.D. Anderson Cancer Center, Houston, TX, USA

Taku Aoki, M.D., Ph.D. Division of Hepato-Biliary-Pancreatic and Transplantation Surgery, Department of Surgery, Graduate School of Medicine, The University of Tokyo, Tokyo, Japan

Mathew M. Augustine, M.D. Department of Surgery, The Johns Hopkins Hospital, Baltimore, MD, USA

Béatrice Aussilhou, M.D. Department of Hepato-Pancreato-Biliary Surgery and Liver Transplantation, Beaujon Hospital, Clichy, France

Philippe Bachellier, M.D., Ph.D. Centre de Chirurgie Viscérale et de Transplantation, Hôpital de Hautepierre, Université Louis Pasteur, Hôpitaux Universitaires de Strasbourg, Strasbourg, France

Kevin E. Behrns, M.D. Department of Surgery, Division of General and GI Surgery, University of Florida, Gainesville, FL, USA

Jacques Belghiti, M.D. Department of Hepato-Pancreato-Biliary Surgery and Liver Transplantation, Beaujon Hospital, Clichy, France

Roelof J. Bennink, Ph.D. Department of Nuclear Medicine, Academic Medical Center, University of Amsterdam, Amsterdam, The Netherlands

Pierre Bize, M.D. Department of Radiology, Bâtiment Hospitalier CHUV, University of Lausanne, Lausanne, Switzerland

Chusilp Charnsangavej, M.D. Department of Diagnostic Radiology, The University of Texas M.D. Anderson Cancer Center, Houston, TX, USA

Byung Ihn Choi, M.D. Department of Radiology, Seoul National University Hospital, Seoul, South Korea

Yun Shin Chun, M.D. Department of Surgical Oncology, Fox Chase Cancer Center, Philadelphia, PA, USA

Anne M. Covey, M.D. Department of Diagnostic Radiology, Memorial Sloan-Kettering Cancer Center, New York, NY, USA

Thierry de Baere, M.D. Department of Interventional Radiology, Institut Gustave Roussy, Villejuif, France

Wilmar de Graaf, M.D., Ph.D Department of Surgery, Academic Medical Center, University of Amsterdam, Amsterdam, The Netherlands

Nicolas Demartines, M.D. Department of Surgery, University Hospital (CHUV), Lausanne, Switzerland

Alban Denys, M.D. Department of Radiology and Interventional Radiology, CHUV, University of Lausanne, Lausanne, Switzerland

Richard K.G. Do, M.D., Ph.D. Department of Radiology, Memorial Sloan-Kettering Cancer Center, New York, NY, USA

Takumi Fukumoto, M.D. Department of Surgery, Kobe University Graduate School of Medicine, Kobe, Japan

Günter Fürst, M.D. Department of Diagnostic and Interventional Radiology, University Hospital and Heinrich-Heine-University of Düesseldorf, Düesseldorf, Germany

Takuya Hashimoto, M.D., Ph.D. Hepato-Biliary-Pancreatic Surgery, Japanese Red Cross Medical Center, Tokyo, Japan

Yuky Hayashi, M.D., Ph.D. Department of Gastrointestinal Medical Oncology, The University of Texas M.D. Anderson Cancer Center, Houston, TX, USA

Shin Hwang, M.D., Ph.D. Division of Hepatobiliary Surgery and Liver Transplantation, Department of Surgery, Asan Medical Center, University of Ulsan College of Medicine, Seoul, South Korea

Hiroshi Imamura, M.D., Ph.D. Department of Hepatobiliary-Pancreatic Surgery, Juntendo School of Medicine, Tokyo, Japan

Daniel Jaeck, M.D., Ph.D., F.R.C.S. Centre de Chirurgie Viscérale et de Transplantation, Hôpital de Hautepierre, Université Louis Pasteur, Hôpitaux Universitaires de Strasbourg, Strasbourg, France

William R. Jarnagin, M.D., F.A.C.S. Department of Surgery, Memorial Sloan-Kettering Cancer Center, New York, NY, USA and Department of Surgery, Weill Medical College of Cornell University, New York, NY, USA

Ihab R. Kamel, M.D., Ph.D. Department of Radiology, The Johns Hopkins Hospital, Baltimore, MD, USA

Harmeet Kaur, M.D. Department of Diagnostic Radiology, The University of Texas M.D. Anderson Cancer Center, Houston, TX, USA

Yoji Kishi, M.D., Ph.D. Hepato-Biliary-Pancreatic Surgery, University of Tokyo, Tokyo, Japan

Jae-Sung Kim, Ph.D. Department of Surgery, Division of General and GI Surgery, University of Florida, Gainesville, FL, USA

Robin D. Kim, M.D. Department of Surgery, Division of General and GI Surgery, University of Florida, Gainesville, FL, USA

Wolfram T. Knoefel, M.D., F.A.C.S. Department of Surgery, University Hospital Duesseldorf and Heinrich-Heine-University of Duesseldorf, Duesseldorf, Germany

Yoshihisa Kodama, M.D., Ph.D. Department of Radiology, Teine Keijinkai Medical Center, Sapporo, Japan

Norihiro Kokudo, M.D., Ph.D. Division of Hepato-Biliary-Pancreatic and Transplantation Surgery, Department of Surgery, Graduate School of Medicine, The University of Tokyo, Tokyo, Japan

Yonson Ku, M.D., Ph.D. Department of Surgery, Kobe University Graduate School of Medicine, Kobe, Japan

Keiichi Kubota, M.D., Ph.D. Department of Gastroenterological Surgery, Dokkyo Medical University, Tochigi, Japan

Jeong Min Lee, M.D., Ph.D. Department of Radiology, Seoul National University Hospital, Seoul, South Korea

Evelyne M. Loyer, M.D. Department of Diagnostic Radiology, The University of Texas M.D. Anderson Cancer Center, Houston, TX, USA

David C. Madoff, M.D., F.S.I.R. Division of Interventional Radiology, Department of Radiology, New York-Presbyterian Hospital/Weill Cornell Medical Center, New York, NY, USA

Ajay V. Maker, M.D. Department of Surgery, Division of Surgical Oncology, University of Illinois at Chicago, Chicago, IL, USA

Masatoshi Makuuchi, M.D., Ph.D. Japanese Red Cross Medical Center, Tokyo, Japan

Masato Nagino, M.D., Ph.D. Division of Surgical Oncology, Department of Surgery, Nagoya University Graduate School of Medicine, Nagoya, Japan

Yuji Nimura, M.D. Aichi Cancer Center, Nagoya, Japan

Elie Oussoultzoglou, M.D. Centre de Chirurgie Viscérale et de Transplantation, Hôpital de Hautepierre, Université Louis Pasteur, Hôpitaux Universitaires de Strasbourg, Avenue Molière, Strasbourg, France

Timothy M. Pawlik, M.D., M.P.H. Division of Surgical Oncology, Department of Surgery, Johns Hopkins Hospital, Baltimore, MD, USA

Edoardo Rosso, M.D. Center for Visceral Surgery and Transplantation, Hospital Hautepierre, Université Louis Pasteur, Strasbourg University Hospitals, Strasbourg, France

Jan Schulte am Esch, M.D. Department of General Surgery, Heinrich-Heine-University of Duesseldorf, Duesseldorf, Germany

Yasuji Seyama, M.D., Ph.D. Department of Hepato-Biliary-Pancreatic and Transplant Surgery, Graduate School of Medicine, University of Tokyo, Tokyo, Japan

Colette M. Shaw, M.D. Interventional Radiology Section, Division of Diagnostic Imaging, The University of Texas M.D. Anderson Cancer Center, Houston, TX, USA

Ken Takasaki, M.D., Ph.D. Department of Surgery, Institute of Gastroenterology, Tokyo Women's Medical University, Tokyo, Japan

Bachir Taouli, M.D., M.S. Department of Radiology, Mount Sinai Medical Center, New York, NY, USA

Raymond H. Thornton, M.D. Department of Radiology, Memorial Sloan-Kettering Cancer Center, New York, NY, USA

Thomas M. van Gulik, M.D. Department of Surgery, Academic Medical Center, University of Amsterdam, Amsterdam, The Netherlands

Jean-Nicolas Vauthey, M.D. Liver Service, Department of Surgical Oncology, The University of Texas M.D. Anderson Cancer Center, Houston, TX, USA

Masakazu Yamamoto, M.D., Ph.D. Department of Surgery, Institute of Gastroenterology, Tokyo Women's Medical University, Tokyo, Japan

Yukihiro Yokoyama, M.D., Ph.D. Division of Surgical Oncology, Department of Surgery, Nagoya University Graduate School of Medicine, Nagoya, Japan

Stéphane Zalinski, M.D. Department of Digestive and Hepatobiliary Surgery, Hôpital Saint-Antoine, Assistance Publique,
Hôpitaux de Paris, Université Pierre et Marie Curie, Paris, France

Daria Zorzi, M.D. Department of Surgical Oncology, The University of Texas M.D. Anderson Cancer Center, Houston, TX, USA

Part I

History and Anatomy

History of Major Liver Resections

1

Yun Shin Chun and Jean-Nicolas Vauthey

Abstract

The history of major liver resection has evolved from primitive amputations for trauma to extended hepatectomies performed with minimal blood loss and morbidity. An understanding of hepatic segmental anatomy through the works of Glisson, Couinaud, and others has led to the modern era of hepatobiliary surgery. In addition, advances in methods of hepatic parenchymal transection, vascular control, and studies on liver regeneration have increased the safety of major hepatectomy.

Keywords

Major liver resection • Hepatic anatomy • Couinaud • Segmental anatomy • Brisbane terminology • Hepatobiliary surgery • Liver resection history

The history of liver resection dates back to the ancient Greek myth of Prometheus, who angered Zeus and was chained to a mountain, where an eagle fed on his liver daily. Each night, his liver regenerated, and in the morning, the eagle returned for its feed. The first surgical resection of the liver was reported in 1716 when Berta of Italy amputated a portion of the liver protruding from a patient with a self-inflicted knife wound.[1] True hepatobiliary surgery was not possible until the development of anesthesia and antisepsis in the 1800s.[2] In 1886, Lius of Italy removed a pedicled mass hanging off the left liver of a 67-year-old woman.[3] He tried ineffectively to suture the stump of the severed pedicle to the abdominal wall, but the woman hemorrhaged from the pedicle and died 6 h postoperatively.

The first successful elective hepatectomy was reported in 1887 by Langenbuch of Germany.[4] He removed a pedicled tumor hanging from the left liver of a 30-year-old woman by transfixing the pedicle with sutures. Postoperatively, the patient required reexploration for bleeding from a hilar vessel but survived. Tiffany is credited with the first liver resection in the United States in 1890.[5] He reported debridement of a walnut-sized mass of biliary calculi and debris from the edge of the left liver but did not document how much liver parenchyma was resected.[6] In 1892, Keen of Philadelphia reported enucleation of a biliary adenoma using cautery and his thumbnail.[7] In 1897, he resected a hemangioma by a technique he termed extraperitoneal elastic constriction, by which a rubber elastic was tied around the pedicle of the hemangioma which was exteriorized out of the peritoneal cavity; 6 days later, he transected the pedicle and removed the

J.-N. Vauthey (✉)
Liver Service, Department of Surgical Oncology,
The University of Texas M.D. Anderson Cancer Center,
1515 Holcombe Boulevard, Unit 444, Houston,
TX 77030, USA
e-mail: jvauthey@mdanderson.org

D.C. Madoff et al. (eds.), *Venous Embolization of the Liver*,
DOI 10.1007/978-1-84882-122-4_1, © Springer-Verlag London Limited 2011

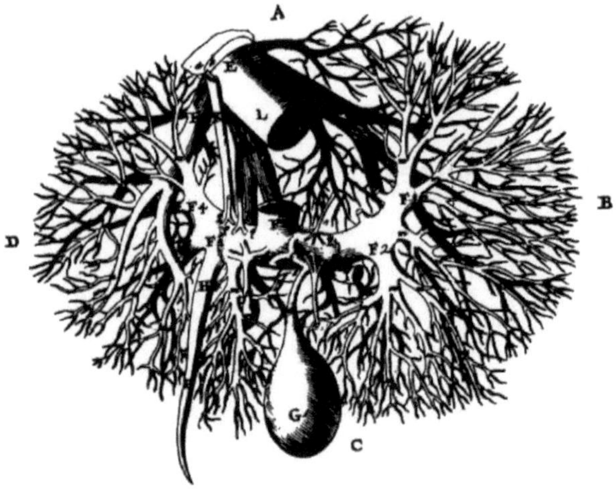

Fig. 1.1 Drawing of intrahepatic vasculature from Glisson's *Anatomia Hepatis*, London, 1654

necrotic tumor.[8] In 1899, he completed the first true left lateral sectionectomy, which he termed left lobectomy.[9] The parenchyma was transected with cautery, and bleeding was controlled with five catgut ligatures.

These first liver resections were performed without a true understanding of liver anatomy, and most surgeons believed the right and left livers were divided along the line of the falciform ligament. In 1654, Glisson of England first depicted a segmental anatomy of the liver in his book *Anatomia Hepatis* (Fig. 1.1).[10] He performed cast and injection studies that detailed the fibrous framework of the liver and intrahepatic vascular anatomy. Rex in Germany (1888) and Cantlie in England (1897) described a plane from the gallbladder bed to the right of the inferior vena cava, separating the right and left halves of the liver.[11,12] Recognizing and following this plane, Wendel in 1911 achieved the first successful right hepatectomy using hilar ligation.[13] He ligated the right hepatic artery and bile duct but not the right portal vein for fear of thrombosis, and instead, ligated its branches.

The modern era of hepatobiliary surgery began in 1949, when Ichio Honjo of Japan performed an extended right hepatectomy for a 22-year-old patient with metastatic rectal cancer via a bilateral subcostal incision with vertical midline extension (Fig. 1.2).[14,15] After complete mobilization of the right liver, the right hepatic artery and portal vein were ligated. The liver was divided after three mass ligations of the parenchyma to the right of the falciform ligament. Three years later in France, Lortat-Jacob also completed an extended right hepatectomy by obtaining extraparenchymal control of vascular inflow and outflow before parenchymal transection in a 42-year-old woman with metastastatic colon cancer (Fig. 1.3).[16] For exposure,

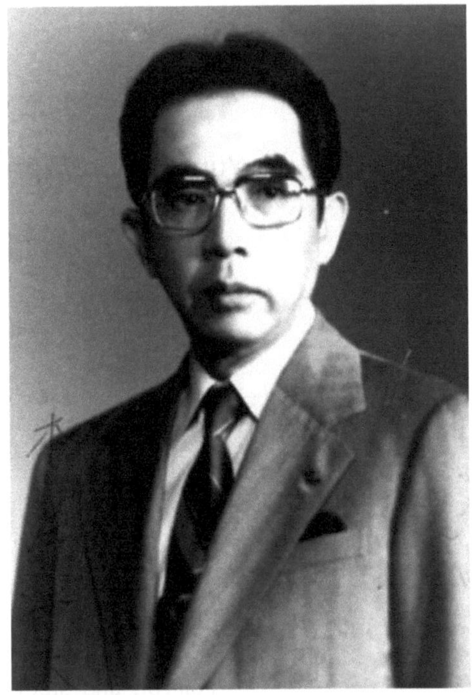

Fig. 1.2 Ichio Honjo (Courtesy of Dr. M. Makuuchi)

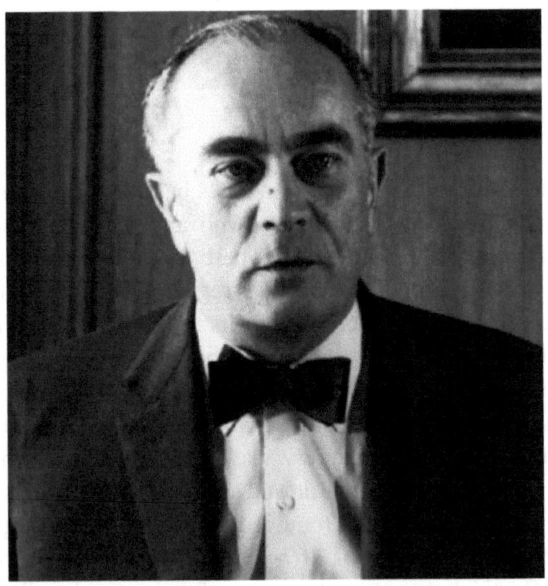

Fig. 1.3 Jean-Louis Lortat-Jacob (From Naef AP[54] with permission. http://icvts.ctsnetjouirnals.org. Copyright ICVTS)

he used a right thoracoabdominal approach, which became the standard incision for major hepatectomies at the time. Later, the introduction of costal arch retractors improved exposure and obviated the need for thoracotomy.[17] In the United States, several months after Lortat-Jacob's resection, Quattlebaum of Georgia performed an extended right hepatectomy in a woman with hepatocellular carcinoma, which was presented at the Southern Surgical Association meeting.[18] Later in the year 1952, Pack at Memorial Sloan-Kettering Cancer Center in New York also completed an extended right hepatectomy in a 40-year-old man who presented with a palpable mass arising from the right liver; surgical pathology revealed a granulomatous lesion.[19] Unlike Honjo and Lortat-Jacob, who obtained vascular control before parenchymal transection, Ton That Tung in 1939 described hepatectomy by primary parenchymal transection and ligation of portal pedicles and hepatic veins within the liver.[20] This technique was further developed by Ken Takasaki, who in 1986 first described obtaining vascular control by following the sheathlike extension of Glisson's capsule around portal pedicles from the hepatic hilum into the liver.[21,22] Launois[23] and Lazorthes[24] also used this method to perform major resections and segmentectomies.

The ability to perform major hepatic resections is predicated on the capacity of the liver to regenerate. Lortat-Jacob recognized the work of Ponfick de Breslau, who at the end of the nineteenth century in Germany, demonstrated that ablation of 70% of the liver in dogs was well-tolerated and that the liver regenerated within 6–8 weeks.[17] Additional animal studies by Tillmans (1879) and Gluck (1883) demonstrated that up to 75% of the liver could be resected followed by nearly full restitution of liver mass by regeneration.[25,26] In 1962, Pack studied liver regeneration in human beings and suggested that complete regeneration occurs over a period of 3–6 months.[27] In 1971, Blumgart analyzed liver weights and serial radioisotope scans and found that liver regeneration begins soon after major hepatectomy and progresses rapidly during the ensuing 10 days.[28] In 1972, Weinbren described the proliferative pathologic response in murine liver parenchyma after portal vein ligation.[29]

A significant deterrent to major hepatectomy was massive, uncontrollable hemorrhage from hepatic veins and the transected edge of the liver. In 1908, Pringle of Scotland reported eight patients with fatal liver hemorrhage from trauma.[30] He recognized that digital occlusion of the portal vein and hepatic artery at the hilum could temporarily arrest hemorrhage. He confirmed this observation with animal experiments, in which clamping the portal vessels with forceps covered in rubber tubing prevented bleeding from cut liver edges. Thus, temporary vascular inflow occlusion is named the Pringle maneuver.

In addition to vascular inflow occlusion, various methods of parenchymal transection have been employed to reduce bleeding from the liver. In 1954, Lin of Taiwan proposed finger fracture dissection with intrahepatic ligation of vascular and ductal structures.[31] Forebearers of this technique include Keen (1882), who used his thumbnail, and Ogilvie (1953), who used the blunt end of a hemostat.[7,32] In 1952, Quattlebaum accomplished parenchymal transection with the handle of a scalpel to expose larger vessels and ducts without cutting them, which were then divided between clamps and ligated.[18] In 1979, Hodgson developed an ultrasonic scalpel that fragments tissue with high water content such as the liver parenchyma, while sparing collagen-rich blood vessels and bile ducts.[33] More recently, Voyles (1989) and McEntee (1991) introduced vascular staplers to divide hepatic and portal veins.[34,35]

In parallel with milestones in surgical technique, a deeper understanding of anatomy led to further refinements in major liver resection. In 1951, Hjortsjo studied corrosion specimens and cholangiograms and found that bile ducts and hepatic arteries were oriented in a segmental pattern.[36] In 1953, Healy and Schroy also examined intrahepatic biliary architecture and divided the left liver into medial and lateral segments based on the falciform ligament, and the right liver into anterior and posterior segments.[37] Couinaud's seminal work in 1954 simplified segmental anatomy by dividing the liver into eight segments, based on the intrahepatic distribution of the portal vein (Fig. 1.4).[38] Using this anatomical classification, Prof H. Bismuth (Fig. 1.5) described in the early 1980s the principles of modern hepatic surgery with resection along the anatomical resection planes defined by Couinaud;[39] Goldsmith and Woodburne also advocated division of the liver based on the portal vein, but instead of numbering the liver segments, they assigned medial and lateral divisions of the left liver, and anterior and posterior divisions of the right liver.[40] To unify nomenclature of hepatic anatomy and resections, the International Hepato-Pancreato-Biliary Association convened in Brisbane, Australia in 2000 and based on the recommendation of Steven Strasberg,

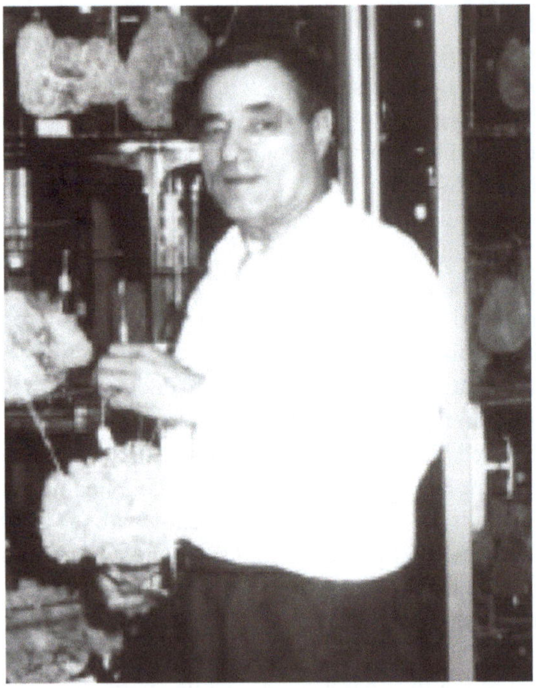

Fig. 1.4 Claude Couinaud (Courtesy of Patrice Couinaud)

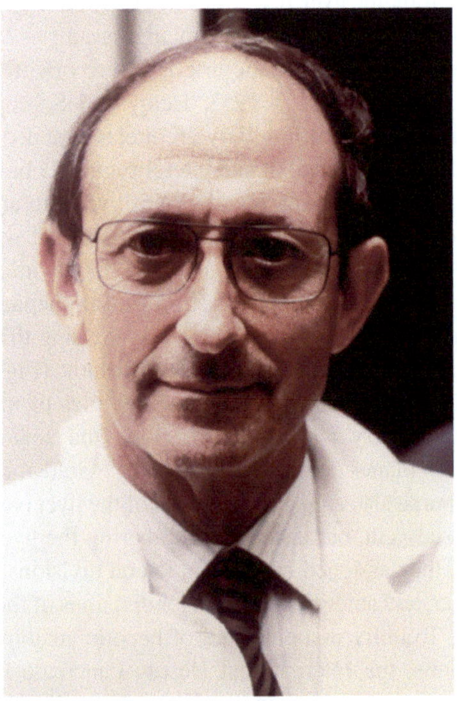

Fig. 1.5 Henri Bismuth (Courtesy of Dr. H. Bismuth)

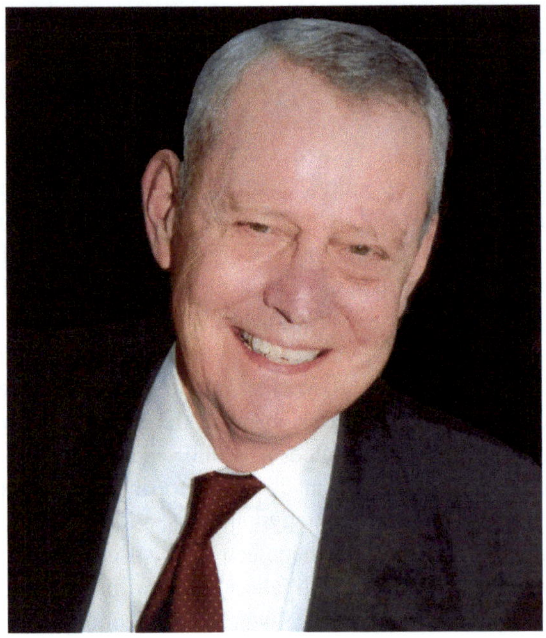

Fig. 1.6 Thomas Starzl (Courtesy of Dr. J.W. Marsh)

established consensus terminology of hepatic anatomy and resections.[41] According to the Brisbane 2000 system, a right hepatectomy or hemihepatectomy is resection of Couinaud segments 5–8, while a right trisectionectomy or extended right hepatectomy includes resection of segment 4. A left hepatectomy or hemihepatectomy is resection of Couinaud segments 2–4, while a left trisectionectomy or extended left hepatectomy includes resection of segments 5 and 8.

In the past several decades, hepatobiliary surgery has progressed rapidly, and extended hepatectomies are now achieved with morbidity and mortality rates as low as 31% and 1%, respectively.[42] These advances are credited to pioneering surgeons including Martin Adson at the Mayo Clinic, Thomas Starzl (Fig. 1.6) at the University of Pittsburgh, and Joseph Fortner at Memorial Sloan-Kettering Cancer Center.[43-45] Leslie Blumgart (Fig. 1.7) pioneered major resection for the treatment of hilar cholangiocarcinoma[46]; his textbook, *Surgery of the Liver, Biliary Tract, and Pancreas*, is read by generations of fledgling young surgeons, as well as seasoned veterans.[47] Modern hepatobiliary surgery would not be possible without advances in radiology, low central venous pressure anesthesia, and the use of intraoperative ultrasound to define anatomy and identify occult lesions, as exemplified by Prof M. Makuuchi (Fig. 1.8).[48] A 1993 study on an aggressive

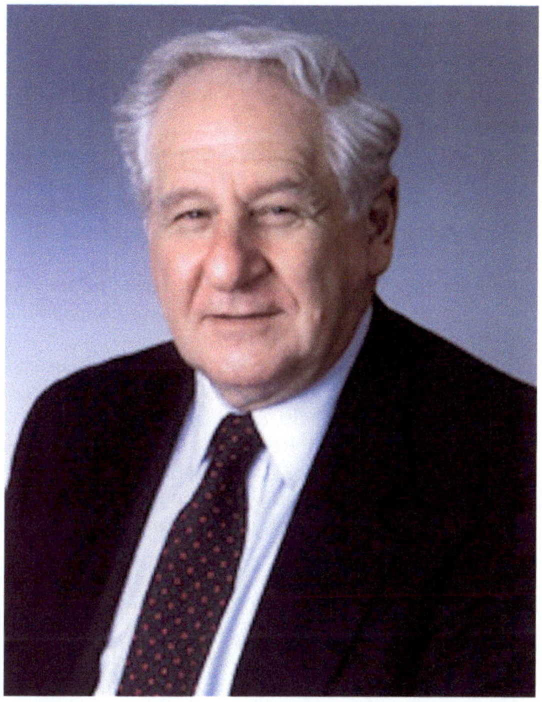

Fig. 1.7 Leslie Blumgart (Courtesy of Dr. L. H. Blumgart)

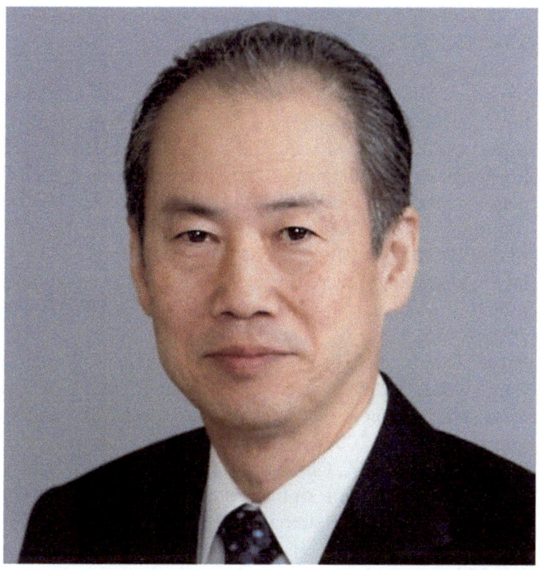

Fig. 1.8 Masatoshi Makuuchi (Courtesy of Dr. M. Makuuchi)

approach to hepatic neoplasms demonstrated that extensive liver resections were accomplished with low morbidity and mortality rates, and with short-term survival comparable to that in patients undergoing lesser resections.[49] These results were expanded in a more recent study, demonstrating a median survival of 42 months among 127 patients who underwent extended hepatectomy for hepatobiliary malignancies.[42]

Preoperative portal vein embolization was first performed in 1982 by Makuuchi et al. to induce atrophy of the liver to be resected and compensatory hypertrophy of the contralateral future liver remnant before extended hepatectomy for bile duct carcinoma.[50,51] As detailed in subsequent chapters of this book, portal vein embolization[52,53] has allowed major liver resections to be performed more safely, despite the increasing prevalence of liver disease in today's patient population due to various factors, including preoperative chemotherapy, hepatic steatosis, and cirrhosis.

References

1. Berta G. Cited in Di Valmaggiore P. L'epatectomie. *Proceedings of 16th Congress of the International Society of Surgery (Copenhagen): Imprimerie Medicale et Scientifique*. 1955 (1716), p. 1009.
2. Fortner JG, Blumgart LH. A historic perspective of liver surgery for tumors at the end of the millennium. *J Am Coll Surg*. 2001;193(2):210-222.
3. Lius A. Di un adenoma del fegato. *Gazz Clini*. 1886;23:225.
4. Langenbuch C. Ein fall von resektion eines linksseitigen schnurlappens der leber. *Berl Klin Wochenschr*. 1888;25:37-39.
5. Tiffany LM. The removal of a solid tumor from the liver by laparotomy. *Md Med J*. 1890;23:531.
6. Foster JH. History of liver surgery. *Arch Surg*. 1991;126(3):381-387.
7. Keen WW. On resection of the liver, especially for hepatic tumors. *Boston Med Surg J*. 1892;126:405.
8. Keen WW. Removal of an angioma of the liver by elastic constriction external to the abdominal cavity, with a table of 59 cases of operations for hepatic tumors. *Pa Med J*. 1897;1:193.
9. Keen WW. IV. Report of a case of resection of the liver for the removal of a neoplasm, with a table of seventy-six cases of resection of the liver for hepatic Tumors. *Ann Surg*. 1899;30(3):267-283.
10. Glisson F. *Anatomia Hepatis*. London: O. Pullein; 1654.
11. Rex H. Beitrage zur morphologie der saugerleber. *Morphol Jahrb*. 1888;14:517.
12. Cantlie J. On a new arrangement of the right and left lobes of the liver. *J Anat Physiol*. 1898;32:4.
13. Wendel W. Beitrage zur chirurgie der leber. *Arch Klin Chir*. 1911;95:887.
14. Honjo I. Total resection of the right lobe of the liver. *Shujutsu*. 1950;4:345-349.
15. Honjo I, Araki C. Total resection of the right lobe of the liver: report of a successful case. *J Int Coll Surg*. 1955;23:23-28.
16. Lortat-Jacob JL, Robert HG. Hepatectomie droite reglee. *Presse Méd*. 1952;60:549-551.
17. Belghiti J. The first anatomical right resection announcing liver donation. *J Hepatol*. 2003;39(4):475-479.

18. Quattlebaum JK. Massive resection of the liver. *Ann Surg.* 1953;137(6):787-796.
19. Pack GT, Baker HW. Total right hepatic lobectomy; report of a case. *Ann Surg.* 1953;138(2):253-258.
20. Tung TT. *La vascularisation veineuse du foie et ses applications aux resections hepatiques.* Vietnam: Theses Hanoi; 1939.
21. Takasaki K, Kobayashi S, Tanaka S, et al. New developed systematized hepatectomy by Glissonean pedicle transection method. *Shujutsu.* 1986;40:7-14.
22. Takasaki K, Kobayashi S, Tanaka S, Saito A, Yamamoto M, Hanyu F. Highly anatomically systematized hepatic resection with Glissonean sheath code transection at the hepatic hilus. *Int Surg.* 1990;75(2):73-77.
23. Launois B, Jamieson GG. The importance of Glisson's capsule and its sheaths in the intrahepatic approach to resection of the liver. *Surg Gynecol Obstet.* 1992;174(1):7-10.
24. Lazorthes F, Chiotasso P, Chevreau P, Materre JP, Roques J. Hepatectomy with initial suprahilar control of intrahepatic portal pedicles. *Surgery.* 1993;113(1):103-108.
25. Tillmans H. Experimentelle und anatomische untersuchungen ueber wunden der leber und der niere. *Virchows Arch.* 1879;78:437-465.
26. Gluck T. Ueber die bedeutung physiologisch-chirurgischer experimente an der leber. *Arch Klin Chir (Berl).* 1883;29: 139-143.
27. Pack GT, Islami AH, Hubbard JC, Brasfield RD. Regeneration of human liver after major hepatectomy. *Surgery.* 1962;52: 617-623.
28. Blumgart LH, Leach KG, Karran SJ. Observations on liver regeneration after right hepatic lobectomy. *Gut.* 1971;12(11): 922-928.
29. Weinbren K, Stirling GA, Washington SL. The development of a proliferative response in liver parenchyma deprived of portal blood flow. *Br J Exp Pathol.* 1972;53(1):54-58.
30. Pringle JH. V. Notes on the arrest of hepatic hemorrhage due to trauma. *Ann Surg.* 1908;48(4):541-549.
31. Lin TY, Tsu KY, Mien C, Chen CS. Study on lobectomy of the liver. *J Formosa Med Assoc.* 1958;57:742-759.
32. Ogilvie H. Partial hepatectomy; observations on an illustrative case. *Br Med J.* 1953;2(4846):1136-1138.
33. Hodgson WJ, Poddar PK, Mencer EJ, Williams J, Drew M, McElhinney AJ. Evaluation of ultrasonically powered instruments in the laboratory and in the clinical setting. *Am J Gastroenterol.* 1979;72(2):133-140.
34. Voyles CR, Vogel SB. Hepatic resection using stapling devices to control the hepatic veins. *Am J Surg.* 1989;158(5): 459-460.
35. McEntee GP, Nagorney DM. Use of vascular staplers in major hepatic resections. *Br J Surg.* 1991;78(1):40-41.
36. Hjortsjo CH. The topography of the intrahepatic duct systems. *Acta Anat (Basel).* 1951;11(4):599-615.
37. Healey JE Jr, Schroy PC. Anatomy of the biliary ducts within the human liver; analysis of the prevailing pattern of branchings and the major variations of the biliary ducts. *AMA Arch Surg.* 1953;66(5):599-616.
38. Couinaud C. Lobes et segments hepatiques: notes sur architecture anatomique et chirurgicale du foie. *Presse Méd.* 1954;62:709-712.
39. Bismuth H. Surgical anatomy and anatomical surgery of the liver. *World J Surg.* 1982;6(1):3-9.
40. Goldsmith NA, Woodburne RT. The surgical anatomy pertaining to liver resection. *Surg Gynecol Obstet.* 1957;105(3): 310-318.
41. Strasberg SM. Nomenclature of hepatic anatomy and resections: a review of the Brisbane 2000 system. *J Hepatobiliary Pancreat Surg.* 2005;12(5):351-355.
42. Vauthey JN, Pawlik TM, Abdalla EK, et al. Is extended hepatectomy for hepatobiliary malignancy justified? *Ann Surg.* 2004;239(5):722-730. discussion 30–2.
43. Adson MA, Weiland LH. Resection of primary solid hepatic tumors. *Am J Surg.* 1981;141(1):18-21.
44. Starzl TE, Bell RH, Beart RW, Putnam CW. Hepatic trisegmentectomy and other liver resections. *Surg Gynecol Obstet.* 1975;141(3):429-437.
45. Fortner JG, Fong Y. Twenty-five-year follow-up for liver resection: the personal series of Dr. Joseph G. Fortner. *Ann Surg.* 2009;250(6):908-913.
46. Blumgart LH, Hadjis NS, Benjamin IS, Beazley R. Surgical approaches to cholangiocarcinoma at confluence of hepatic ducts. *Lancet.* 1984;1(8368):66-70.
47. Blumgart L. *Surgery of the Liver, Biliary Tract, and Pancreas.* 4th ed. Philadelphia: Saunders-Elsevier; 2007.
48. Makuuchi M, Hasegawa H, Yamazaki S. Ultrasonically guided subsegmentectomy. *Surg Gynecol Obstet.* 1985;161(4): 346-350.
49. Vauthey JN, Baer HU, Guastella T, Blumgart LH. Comparison of outcome between extended and nonextended liver resections for neoplasms. *Surgery.* 1993;114(5):968-975.
50. Makuuchi M, Takayasu K, Takuma T, et al. Preoperative transcatheter embolization of the portal venous branch for patients receiving extended lobectomy due to the bile duct carcinoma. *J Jpn Soc Clin Surg.* 1984;45:14-20.
51. Makuuchi M, Thai BL, Takayasu K, et al. Preoperative portal embolization to increase safety of major hepatectomy for hilar bile duct carcinoma: a preliminary report. *Surgery.* 1990;107(5):521-527.
52. Ribero D, Abdalla EK, Madoff DC, Donadon M, Loyer EM, Vauthey JN. Portal vein embolization before major hepatectomy and its effects on regeneration, resectability and outcome. *Br J Surg.* 2007;94(11):1386-1394.
53. Kishi Y, Abdalla EK, Chun YS, et al. Three hundred and one consecutive extended right hepatectomies: evaluation of outcome based on systematic liver volumetry. *Ann Surg.* 2009;250(4):540-548.
54. Naef AP. The mid-century revolution in thoracic and cardiovascular surgery: part 3. *Interact Cardiovasc Thorac Surg.* 2004;3:3-10.

2 Microcirculation of the Liver

Shin Hwang

Abstract

The microcirculation of the liver has important roles in maintenance of liver function. It guarantees the supply of the parenchymal tissue with oxygen and nutrients, serves as the gate for leukocyte entrance in hepatic inflammation, and is responsible for the clearance of toxic materials and foreign bodies from the bloodstream. The morphology and physiology of the hepatic microcirculation are described in this chapter to help the understanding of the physiology of the hepatic microcirculation.

Keywords

Microcirculation of the liver • Liver microcirculation • Liver function • Hepatic microcirculation • Physiology of hepatic microcirculation

The microcirculation of the liver has important roles in maintenance of liver function. It guarantees the supply of the parenchymal tissue with oxygen and nutrients, serves as the gate for leukocyte entrance in hepatic inflammation, and is responsible for the clearance of toxic materials and foreign bodies from the bloodstream. The morphology and physiology of the hepatic microcirculation are described to help the understanding of the physiology of the hepatic microcirculation.

S. Hwang
Division of Hepatobiliary Surgery and Liver Transplantation, Department of Surgery, Asan Medical Center, University of Ulsan College of Medicine, 388-1 Poongnap-dong, Songpa-gu, Seoul 138-736, South Korea
e-mail: shwang@amc.seoul.kr

2.1 Dual Blood Perfusion of the Liver and Hepatic Arterial Buffer Response

The liver constitutes about 2% of the body weight in adults, thus being the largest organ in the body. It receives 25% of the cardiac output via two inflows, the portal vein and the hepatic artery. Total amount of hepatic perfusion is about 1 mL/min per 1 g liver tissue, and oxygen consumption by the liver accounts for 20% of total body oxygen consumption.

The portal vein is a valveless afferent vessel that drains the splanchnic blood flow from the capillary system of the intestine, spleen, pancreas, omentum, and gallbladder. Portal blood flow occupies about 75% of total hepatic inflow, or 90 mL/min per 100 g liver, and the remaining 20–25% is supplied by the hepatic arterial flow. The hepatic circulation drains into the hepatic venous system. The hepatic artery is a vessel of

D.C. Madoff et al. (eds.), *Venous Embolization of the Liver*,
DOI 10.1007/978-1-84882-122-4_2, © Springer-Verlag London Limited 2011

resistance, whereas the portal and hepatic veins are vessels of capacitance. The resistance in the hepatic arterial bed is 3–40 times that in the portal venous bed.

The hepatic arterial blood is well-oxygenated, whereas the portal vein carries partly deoxygenated, but nutrient-rich blood after passing the splanchnic system. Since half of the hepatic oxygen requirements are supplied by portal venous blood due to its high flow rate, both hepatic artery and portal vein nearly equally provide hepatic oxygenation.

The dual blood supply of the liver is a unique feature of the hepatic vasculature and distinctly determines the regulation and distribution of blood flow. There is an intimate relationship between the two vascular systems, named the "hepatic arterial buffer response," representing the ability of the hepatic artery to produce compensatory flow changes in response to changes in portal venous flow.[1,2] The artery usually has an intrinsic regulatory mechanism showing the myogenic constrictive response of the hepatic artery on rise of arterial pressure. In addition to this intrinsic autoregulation of arterial flow, the hepatic artery has another intrinsic mechanism showing regulatory responses on the change of portal flow. If the portal flow decreases, the hepatic artery dilates to increase its flow, whereas it constricts to decrease arterial flow on increase of portal flow.[3] This increase in hepatic arterial blood flow is capable of buffering 25–60% of the decreased portal flow. The hepatic arterial buffering mechanism makes the liver being perfused by a steady rate in order to cope with the wide fluctuation of splanchnic blood flow. The hepatic arterial flow also serves the hepatic role as a regulator of blood levels of nutrients and hormones by maintaining blood flow, by which hepatic clearance becomes steady.[4,5] In contrast, the portal vein cannot control its blood flow, not showing reciprocity of the hepatic arterial buffer response.[2,6] Changes in the hepatic arterial flow do not induce compensatory changes of the portal vascular flow or resistance.

The underlying mechanism of the hepatic arterial buffer response is not associated with the neural or myogenic control. Instead, adenosine is known as the putative mediator in the space of Mall driving the communication between the hepatic artery and the portal vein. The space of Mall surrounds the hepatic arterial resistance vessels and portal venules and is contained within a limiting plate that separates this space from other fluid compartments. According to the wash-out hypothesis of adenosine, adenosine accumulates in or less adenosine is washed away from the space of Mall, if portal blood flow is reduced. Elevated adenosine concentrations lead to a dilation of the hepatic artery with a subsequent increase of hepatic arterial flow.[1,7,8] In addition to adenosine, other vasoactive substances such as nitric oxide, carbon monoxide, and hydrogen sulfide, might contribute to this regulatory mechanism.[9,10]

The intrinsic arterial buffer response of the liver is preserved in cirrhotic livers.[11-13] Decreased portal venous inflow to the liver leads to a decrease in oxygen supply and thus induces a compensatory increase of hepatic arterial blood flow. This arterial buffer mechanism is maintained even after liver transplantation.[14,15] After implantation of a small-for-size liver graft, increased portal flow and pressure usually lead to reduction of the hepatic arterial flow, leading to functional dearterialization, ischemic cholangitis, and parenchymal infarcts. Reduction of portal inflow through various inflow modulation methods such as hemi-portocaval shunt or splenic artery embolization appears to be beneficial for amelioration of the overactive hepatic arterial buffer response.[15,16]

2.2 Anatomy of the Hepatic Microvascular Bed

The microcirculation is the most active part of the hepatic circulation because it regulates nutrition and function of the hepatic parenchyma and its supporting tissues. The anatomy of the hepatic microvascular bed is illustrated at Fig. 2.1.[17] Communicating networks are developed between the portal venous and the hepatic arterial circulation.[18,19] After repeated branching, the terminal hepatic arterioles and terminal portal venules supply the blood to the hepatic sinusoids. The inlet sphincters are located at the transition of the terminal portal venule to the sinusoid. The hepatic arterioles wind themselves around the portal venules sending short branches to the portal venules as arteriolo-portal anastomoses and also to the capillaries of the peribiliary plexus, which nourish the bile duct and drain into the sinusoids via arteriosinus twigs. Within the periportal tissue at the periphery of the lobule, these twigs have a complete basement membrane and unfenestrated endothelium, still resembling capillaries. A short distance downstream into the parenchyma they lose their basement membrane, become fenestrated, and

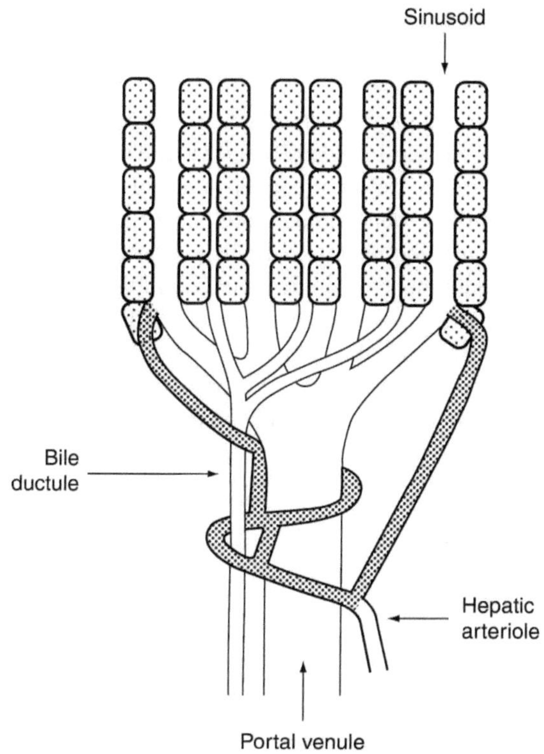

Fig. 2.1 Illustrative presentation of the microvascular bed of the liver. The hepatic arterioles, portal venules, and bile ductules are anatomically associated. The shaded area at the hepatic arterioles indicated the probable site of action responsive to vasoactive agents on the hepatic arterial circulation (From Mathie[17] with permission of Elsevier)

are true sinusoids. The terminal hepatic arteriole-derived capillaries further supply the portal venular wall as vasa vasorum and the connective tissue including the nerves of the portal tract.[19,20]

The hepatic sinusoids correspond to the capillary bed of the liver and represent the segment of the microcirculation in which supply of nutrients and removal of metabolic products take place. Main sinusoids run straight between the liver cell cords and communicate with each other through shorter interconnecting sinusoids running across the liver cell cords. Sinusoids are invested with a unique type of lining consisting of endothelial cells with flattened processes perforated by small fenestrae. These open fenestrations are arranged in clusters of 10–50 pores forming so-called "sieve plates" and represent, apart from the absence of a basement membrane, the structural peculiarity of hepatic sinusoids.[1,21,22] There is a decrease in diameter but an increase of frequency from periportal to centrilobular zones, which results in higher centrilobular porosity.

A unique cellular component of the hepatic sinusoids is the fat- and vitamin A-storing perisinusoidal cell, known as stellate cell.[23,24] External to the endothelium stellate cells are located in the space of Disse, which is the space between the basal microvilli-rich surfaces of the hepatocytes and the sinusoidal lining cells. The stellate cells not only involve in retinol metabolism and hepatic fibrogenic response to injury but also play a central role in the regulation of blood flow through hepatic sinusoids.

After flowing through the sinusoids, blood passes through outlet or efferent sphincters composed of sinusoidal endothelial cells and collected in the terminal central veins. Several of these terminal central veins may combine, increasing in diameter and reaching the sublobular vein and hepatic veins, which leave the liver on the dorsal surface and extend to the extrahepatic inferior vena cava.[18] Thus, the hepatic microcirculatory unit consists of the two terminal afferent vessels, the network of sinusoids running between the liver cords and the efferent terminal hepatic venule. The classic lobule, comprising several cone-shaped primary lobules, is a polygonal structure featured by placing the terminal central vein in the center with portal tracts distributed along its periphery. Primary lobules were renamed as hepatic microvascular subunits, consisting of a group of sinusoids supplied by a single inlet venule and its associated termination of a branch of the hepatic arteriole, finally draining into a central venule.

2.3 Regulation of the Hepatic Microvascular Blood Flow

The liver is morphologically and structurally multifaceted and has been considered second only to the brain in its complexity. All vascular segments of the hepatic microvascular subunit represent potential sites of regulation of blood flow. Regulation of portal flow by the terminal portal venule is nearly absent because its wall has no smooth muscles, but it can adjust its width to the volume flow that is determined by constriction or dilatation of the splanchnic arterioles. The hepatic arterioles are highly sensitive to metabolites, electrolytes, and vasoactive substances. These make the arterial microcirculation be adjusted to the local requirements. Various endothelial mediators, including thromboxane A2, prostaglandin I2, angiotensin II, nitric oxide, endothelin-1, carbon monoxide, and hydrogen sulfide, are known to delicately control vascular tone under both physiological and pathological conditions.[1,2,9,10]

In addition to the presence of smooth muscle cells restricted to the afferent and efferent vessels and its branches, the sinusoids contain contractile cells, such as stellate cells, sinusoidal endothelial cells, and Kupffer cells, which all are involved in the regulation of blood flow through sinusoids. The hepatic microvascular blood flow is regulated and redistributed at the level of the microcirculation, in which both stellate cells and endothelial cells can actively control various functions of the microvasculature.

There is adjustment of microcirculation for bile secretion through a direct link between food ingestion and absorption and increased hepatic arterial flow mediated by the dilated arterioles of the peribiliary plexus. Increase in the arterial supply further leads to maintain the ratio of arterial to portal flow that is augmented during digestion.[25]

Sinusoidal perfusion failure is critically associated with the pathogenesis of tissue injury from warm ischemia-reperfusion, cold preservation and transplantation, acute liver failure, and drug-induced hepatotoxicity.[26-29] Several mechanisms are well established to contribute to sinusoidal perfusion failure, including sinusoidal narrowing caused by sinusoidal endothelial cell edema or stellate cell-mediated vasoconstriction. These cause a gradient of perfusion failure, which is most pronounced in the periportal segment of the sinusoids.[30] Upon entrapment of activated leukocytes, sinusoidal flow velocity decreases due to increased hindrance, further inducing perfusion heterogeneity and perfusion deficits. In addition, inflammation- and injury-associated adherence of leukocytes in outflow venules may alter sinusoidal perfusion due to an increase of blood viscosity and vascular resistance. Perfusion failure in sinusoids is thought to be caused by sluggish blood flow, intravascular hemoconcentration, and procoagulant conditions.[31,32]

Vascular remodeling is an important component contributing to increased intrahepatic resistance in portal hypertension in addition to alterations in vasoreactivity. Different anatomic lesions are apparent as important structural changes to the vascular compartment, including fibrosis, sinusoidal collapse, defenestration of sinusoidal cells (capillarization), hepatocyte enlargement, and formation of a basement membrane in the space of Disse, all narrowing the sinusoid.[33,34] These changes result in a reduced access of plasma and plasma-dissolved substances to hepatocytes due to their limited diffusion in the extravascular space. Capillarization of hepatic sinusoids is known to occur only in very limited regions of the cirrhotic parenchyma and seems to be less relevant for functional consequences in cirrhotic livers than the markedly smaller areas occupied by sinusoids per unit of parenchyma and the sinusoid/hepatocyte interfaces disposable for metabolic exchanges.[35] Sinusoids of cirrhotic livers further lack features of zonation, thereby contributing to the development and progression of liver failure.

References

1. Vollmar B, Menger MD. The hepatic microcirculation: mechanistic contributions and therapeutic targets in liver injury and repair. *Physiol Rev*. 2009;89:1269-1339.
2. Lautt WW. Role and control of the hepatic artery. In: Lautt WW, ed. *Hepatic Circulation in Health and Disease*. New York: Raven; 1981:203-226.
3. Lautt WW et al. Quantitation of the hepatic arterial buffer response to graded changes in portal blood flow. *Gastroenterology*. 1990;98:1024-1028.
4. Lautt WW. Control of hepatic arterial blood flow: independence from liver metabolic activity. *Am J Physiol Heart Circ Physiol*. 1980;239:H559-H564.
5. Lautt WW. The hepatic artery: subservient to hepatic metabolism or guardian of normal hepatic clearance rates of humoral substances. *Gen Pharmacol*. 1977;8:73-78. Minireview.
6. Legare DJ, Lautt WW. Hepatic venous resistance site in the dog: localization and validation of intrahepatic pressure measurements. *Can J Physiol Pharmacol*. 1987;65:352-359.
7. Lautt WW et al. Adenosine as putative regulator of hepatic arterial flow (the buffer response). *Am J Physiol Heart Circ Physiol*. 1985;248:H331-H338.
8. Lautt WW, Legare DJ. The use of 8-phenyltheophylline as a competitive antagonist of adenosine and inhibitor of the intrinsic regulatory mechanism of the hepatic artery. *Can J Physiol Pharmacol*. 1985;63:717-722.
9. Cantré D et al. Nitric oxide reduces organ injury and enhances regeneration of reduced-size livers by increasing hepatic arterial flow. *Br J Surg*. 2008;95:785-792.
10. Hoetzel A et al. Nitric oxide-deficiency regulates hepatic heme oxygenase-1. *Nitric Oxide*. 2008;18:61-69.
11. Aoki T et al. Intraoperative direct measurement of hepatic arterial buffer response in patients with or without cirrhosis. *Liver Transpl*. 2005;11:684-691.
12. Mücke I et al. Significance of hepatic arterial responsiveness for adequate tissue oxygenation upon portal vein occlusion in cirrhotic livers. *Int J Colorectal Dis*. 2000;15:335-341.

13. Richter S et al. Impact of intrinsic blood flow regulation in cirrhosis: maintenance of hepatic arterial buffer response. *Am J Physiol Gastrointest Liver Physiol*. 2000;279:G454-G462.
14. Demetris AJ et al. Pathophysiologic observations and histopathologic recognition of the portal hyperperfusion or small-for-size syndrome. *Am J Surg Pathol*. 2006;30:986-993.
15. Henderson JM et al. Hemodynamics during liver transplantation: the interactions between cardiac output and portal venous and hepatic arterial flows. *Hepatology*. 1992;16:715-718.
16. Smyrniotis V et al. Hemodynamic interaction between portal vein and hepatic artery flow in small-for-size split liver transplantation. *Transpl Int*. 2002;15:355-360.
17. Mathie RT et al. Liver blood flow: physiology, measurement and clinical relevance. In: Blumgart LH, ed. *Surgery of the Liver and Biliary Tract*. 2nd ed. New York: Churchill Livingstone; 1994:95-110.
18. McCuskey RS. Morphological mechanisms for regulating blood flow through hepatic sinusoids. *Liver*. 2000;20:3-7.
19. Oda M et al. Regulatory mechanisms of hepatic microcirculatory hemodynamics: hepatic arterial system. *Clin Hemorheol Microcirc*. 2006;34:11-26.
20. Oda M et al. Regulatory mechanisms of hepatic microcirculation. *Clin Hemorheol Microcirc*. 2003;29:167-182.
21. Wisse E. An electron microscopic study of fenestrated endothelium lining of rat liver sinusoids. *J Ultrastruct Res*. 1970;31:125-150.
22. Wisse E et al. The liver sieve: considerations concerning the structure and function of endothelial fenestrae, the sinusoidal wall and the space of Disse. *Hepatology*. 1985;5:683-692.
23. Friedman SL. Hepatic stellate cells: protean, multifunctional, and enigmatic cells of the liver. *Physiol Rev*. 2008;88: 125-172.
24. Rockey DC. Hepatic blood flow regulation by stellate cells in normal and injured liver. *Semin Liver Dis*. 2001;21:337-349.
25. Rappaport AM, Wanless IR. Physioanatomic considerations. In: Schiff L, Schiff ER, eds. *Diseases of the Liver*. 6th ed. Philadelphia: JBLippincott Company; 1993:1-41.
26. Rentsch M et al. Benefit of Kupffer cell modulation with glycine versus Kupffer cell depletion after liver transplantation in the rat: effects on postischemic reperfusion injury, apoptotic cell death graft regeneration and survival. *Transpl Int*. 2005;18:1079-1089.
27. Vollmar B et al. Hepatic microcirculatory perfusion failure is a determinant of liver dysfunction in warm ischemia-reperfusion. *Am J Pathol*. 1994;145:1421-1431.
28. Le Minh K et al. Attenuation of inflammation and apoptosis by pre- and posttreatment of darbepoetin- in acute liver failure of mice. *Am J Pathol*. 2007;170:1954-1963.
29. Burkhardt M et al. The effect of estrogen on hepatic microcirculation after ischemia/reperfusion. *Int J Colorectal Dis*. 2008;23:113-119.
30. Brock RW et al. Microcirculatory perfusion deficits are not essential for remote parenchymal injury within the liver. *Am J Physiol Gastrointest Liver Physiol*. 1999;277:G55-G60.
31. Braide M et al. Quantitative studies on the influence of leukocytes on the vascular resistance in a skeletal muscle preparation. *Microvasc Res*. 1984;27:331-352.
32. Menger MD et al. Role of microcirculation in hepatic ischemia/reperfusion injury. *Hepatogastroenterology*. 1999;46(suppl 2): 1452-1457.
33. Oda M et al. Endothelial cell dysfunction in microvasculature: relevance to disease processes. *Clin Hemorheol Microcirc*. 2000;23:199-211.
34. Villeneuve JP et al. The hepatic microcirculation in the isolated perfused human liver. *Hepatology*. 1996;23:24-31.
35. Onori P et al. Hepatic microvascular features in experimental cirrhosis: a structural and morphometrical study in CCl4-treated rats. *J Hepatol*. 2000;33:555-563.

Portal and Hepatic Vein Anatomy

3

Yoji Kishi, Takuya Hashimoto,
and Masatoshi Makuuchi

Abstract

Assessment of portal vein anatomy is mandatory to evaluate the indication or strategy of portal vein embolization. Recent advances in radiological imaging facilitate the precise assessment of intrahepatic tertiary or more peripheral tributaries of the intrahepatic vascular system. Not only the portal vein anatomy itself, but also the hepatic vein anatomy and anatomical relationship between the portal vein and hepatic vein should be accurately evaluated for the following reasons: First, sacrifice of hepatic vein tributaries may result in the congestion of large part of remnant liver after hepatic resection. Second, the intersegmental plane after major hepatectomy may not necessarily be straight but curved.

Keywords

Anatomy of the liver • Portal and hepatic vein anatomy • Hepatic vein anatomy • Portal vein embolization • Radiology of portal and hepatic vein anatomy

Evaluation of the vascular anatomy is mandatory in order to perform portal vein embolization (PVE) safely, which is followed by major hepatic resection. Recent advances in radiologic imaging allow for more precise evaluation of the intrahepatic vascular anatomy, including the tertiary and much peripheral branches. Anatomic liver resection is defined as a resection of the region perfused by specific portal vein branch(es). Both the portal vein and the hepatic vein anatomy indicate the hepatectomy procedures that may be achieved.

M. Makuuchi (✉)
Japanese Red Cross Medical Center,
4-1-22 Hiroo, Shibuya-ku, Tokyo 150-8935, Japan
e-mail: makuuchi_masatoshi@med.jrc.or.jp

In this section, the following points are discussed:

1. General knowledge of the portal vein and the hepatic vein anatomy necessary for assessing the indications for PVE and the safety of PVE.
2. Variations of portal and hepatic veins.

3.1 Relationship Between the Portal Vein and the Hepatic Vein

Liver segmentation is determined accordingly to the portal and the hepatic vein anatomy, and two types of liver segmentation have generally been used. Healey et al.[1] proposed a segmentation under which each segment is bordered by the middle and the right hepatic veins and the umbilical portion of the left portal vein. Whereas Couinaud[2] proposed a

D.C. Madoff et al. (eds.), *Venous Embolization of the Liver*,
DOI 10.1007/978-1-84882-122-4_3, © Springer-Verlag London Limited 2011

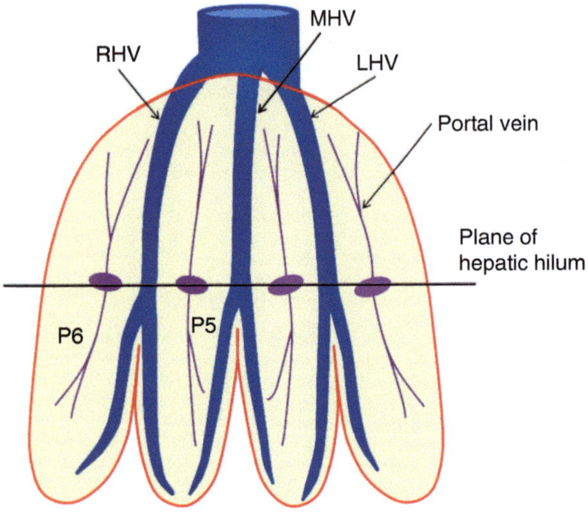

Fig. 3.1 Liver of mammals with lobulation. The portal vein runs parallel to the RHV tributaries in segment 6

segmentation defined by the anatomy of the portal vein, and sectors are separated by three major hepatic veins. In this chapter, Couinaud's nomenclature will be used.

Some authors have described that the sectors bordered by the three major hepatic veins do not necessarily coincide with the sectors defined as the regions perfused by portal vein branches. Hata et al.[3] has recently reported that the right hepatic vein (RHV) tributaries and portal vein branches of segment (S) 6 frequently run parallel rather than perpendicular to each other. Another example is a well-developed middle hepatic vein (MHV) tributary draining S6 found in as many as 23% of examined cases.[4] In this type of variation, an extended left hepatectomy including the MHV[5], and right paramedian sectoriectomy[6] result in the congestion of a large part of the remnant right liver. These fact do not conflict with the conventional liver anatomy when the lobulated mammalian liver is considered[7] (Fig. 3.1). Cho et al.[8] reported that the dorsal branch of the S8 portal vein distributes perfusion over the entire dorsal and cranial area of the right liver posterior to the RHV in 90% of cases. However, the location of the intersectorial lines on the surface of the liver varies. Imagine the cut surface of a solid pineapple. As shown in Fig. 3.2, the intersectorial line on the surface differ by patients. This is easily perceived

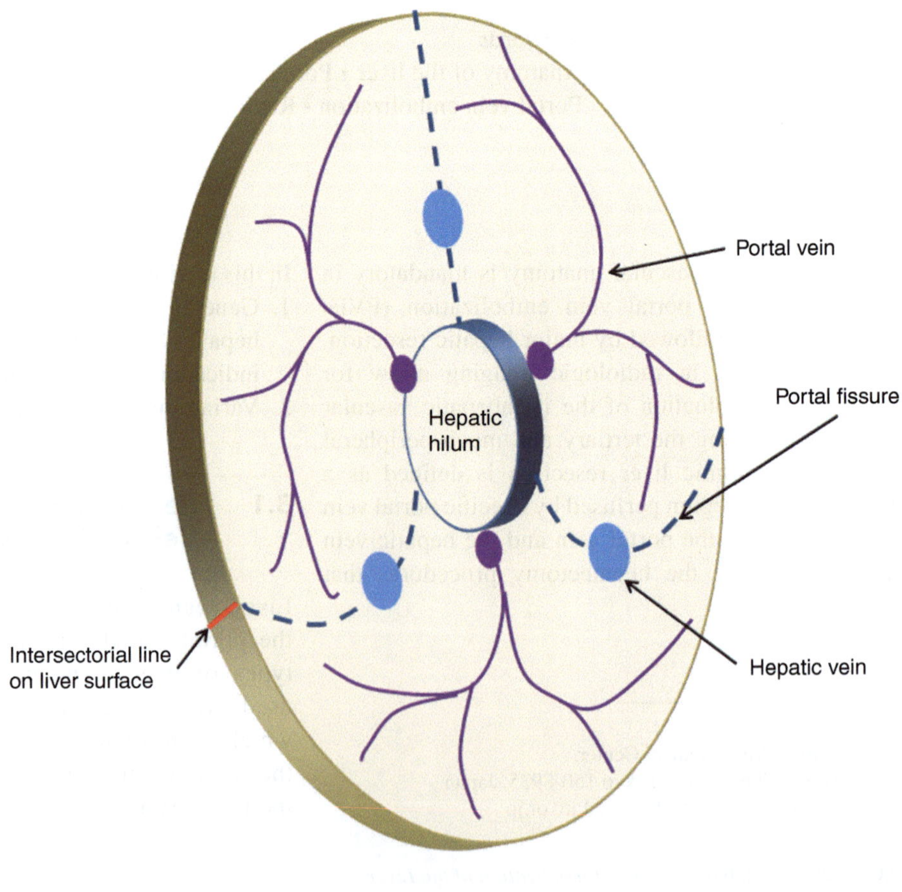

Fig. 3.2 Scheme of intersectorial line defined as the border of portal vein branches in each sector

by observing where the falciform ligament is attached on the liver surface under CT scan.

Evaluation of the hepatic vascular anatomy based only on thick-slice axial CT images can result in an underestimation of variations. Atasoy and Ozyurek[9] suggested that multi-row detector CT may reveal a higher incidence of variations compared to conventional axial thick-slice CT, whereas Savier et al.[10] suggested that ultrasonography is more sensitive compared to CT for detecting the right-sided round ligament and emphasized the importance of evaluating the liver anatomy three-dimensionally.

3.2 Necessary Knowledge for Volumetric Analysis

Because the indication for PVE is determined based on the remnant liver volume, volumetry is mandatory before and after PVE. The recent advances in imaging techniques have allowed for the use of the volume-rendering method to precisely evaluate the volume of each segment of the liver based on calculations of the volume of the region fed by a selected portal vein branch. Among the several softwares, recently released SYNAPSE VINCENT® (FUJIFILM, Co., Ltd., Tokyo, Japan) is a 3D volume analyzer easy to manipulate and enables quick assessment of intrahepatic vascular structures and segmental volumes.[11] The border between any two adjacent segments is not a two-dimensional flat plane, as can be seen by the demarcation line that appears after inflow occlusion of the branches of the liver to be resected (Fig. 3.3). Fischer et al.[12] compared the results of volumetry performed by a volume-rendering method based on the portal vein branching pattern and by calculating each segment delineated by two-dimensional plane. The results showed a large dissociation, especially of S5, S7, and S8. Unfortunately, there is limited availability of such special software for volumetry based on volume-rendering method, and a more popular method resently progressed based on manual delineation of each sector is employed. Usually, the border along the plane of the umbilical fissure, main portal fissure, and the right portal fissure indicate the border of each sector. Basically, the umbilical fissure is the plane in which the umbilical portion of the left portal vein and the cranial portion of the fissural vein (Fig. 3.4) run. And the left, the main and the right portal fissure are the planes in which the left, the middle and the right hepatic veins, run, respectively. These vascular structures, however, may not be recognized in all CT slices. Ideally, the borderline between the portal vein branches on both sides of the sectors recognized in each slice of CT images should be delineated. However, the borderline between S3 and S4 is sometimes difficult to define because the portal vein branches originate from the umbilical portion and usually run along the umbilical fissures, which are often defined as S3 branches.

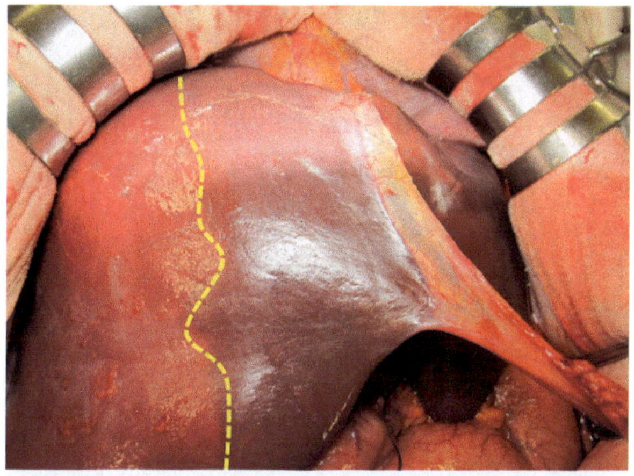

Fig. 3.3 Demarcation line that appeared after ligation of the left hepatic artery and portal vein. Although this line approximately coincides with Rex's line, it is not straight

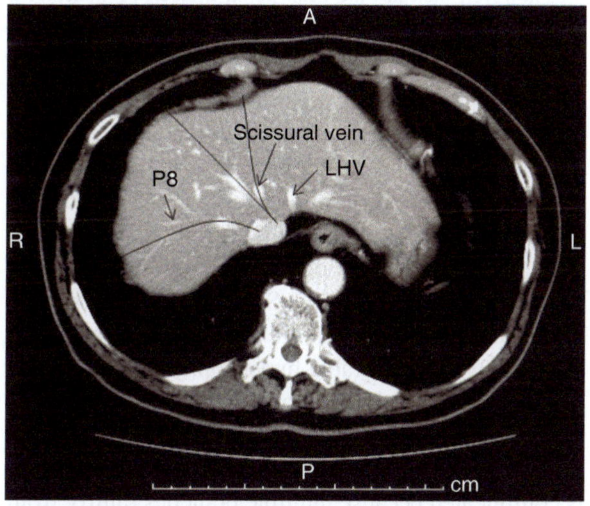

Fig. 3.4 Scissural vein that drains the cranial part of segment 4 and conjugates into the root of the middle hepatic vein is indicated by an *arrow*. This vein usually runs along or left to the same plane as the umbilical fissure and indicates the border between segments 3 and 4. Further, if this vein is preserved during an extended right hepatectomy, a large area of congestion of segment 4 can be prevented. P8 indicates a portal vein branch of segment 8

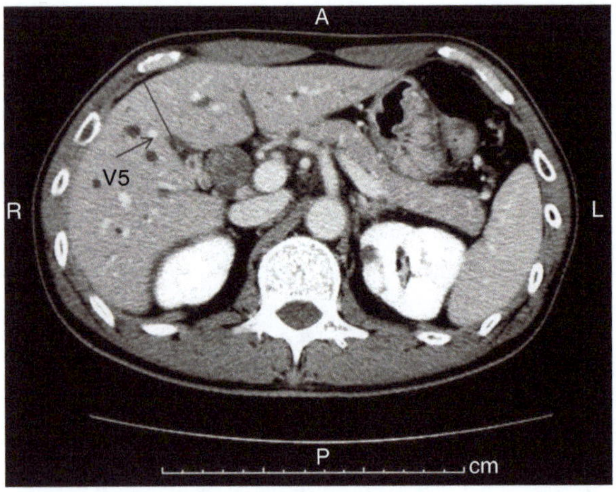

Fig. 3.5 In the caudal portion of the liver, the middle hepatic vein does not consist of one intersegmental branch, but only the branches running within segments 4 and 5 are recognized. The gallbladder bed, however, indicates the main portal fissure. V5 indicates a tributary of the middle hepatic vein that drains segment 5

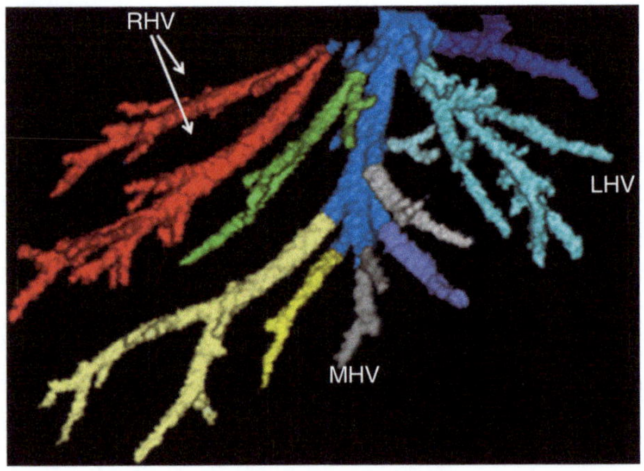

Fig. 3.6 Short common trunk of the right hepatic vein (RHV). The RHV does not run along the plane of the right portal fissure, even in the cranial portion

This becomes an issue when embolization of the S4 portal veins is indicated. It is still controversial as to whether the portal vein branches of S4 should be embolized before a right lobectomy (S4-8 resection). Nagino et al.[13] first reported the PVE technique for the right liver and S4, and observed a significant degree of hypertrophy of S2 and S3. Similar results have been reported by Kishi et al.[14] In contrast, Capussotti et al. showed comparable hypertrophy of S2/S3 after right PVE with or without additional embolization of the S4 branches.[15] In practice, embolization of the S4 branches with preservation of the S2 and S3 branches is complicated because multiple branches ramify from the umbilical portion, and it is difficult to completely embolize all of these branches. However, this may be overcome by evaluating several different projections using C-arm CT.[16] However, it is enough to embolize the major branches (superior and inferior branches of S4), actually.

The main trunk of the left, the middle and the right hepatic veins usually runs along the intersectorial plane in the cranial portion of the liver. Under caudal CT slices, however, they are not observed as one main trunk running along the same plane, but rather as several peripheral branches running within each sector. The border between S4 and the right paramedian sector is easily recognized because the gallbladder bed is a good indicator (Fig. 3.5). The border between S5 and S6 on the other hand is sometimes difficult to define because there is no definitive indicator; therefore, the peripheral portal vein branches of these two segments should be recognized in order to determine the border for the preoperative evaluation and the ultrasound guided staining technique should be used during hepatectomy. Even in the cranial portion, the RHV does not indicate an unequivocal plane between the right paramedian and the lateral sectors (right portal fissure). In 10–60% of cases, the common trunk of the RHV is short and the confluence of two to three branches of equal sizes is located near the root of the RHV (Fig. 3.6).[2,17,18]

3.3 Portal Vein Variations

Incidence of portal vein anatomic variations at the level of the hepatic hilum is much lower than that at the bile duct or hepatic artery. A common portal vein variation is the lack of the main trunk of the right portal vein, that is, trifurcation of the right paramedian branch, right lateral branch, and left main trunk, or the right lateral branch independently originating from the main portal vein. These types of variations are not contraindications for PVE. However, close attention must be paid so that coils or embolization materials do not protrude or migrate into the left portal vein during the right PVE.

Rare but important variations associated with the indication for PVE and hepatectomy are the right-sided round ligament or the complete absence of the right or the left main trunk (horizontal portion) of the portal vein.

The right-sided round ligament was first described by Matsumoto[19] in 1986. The incidence is reported to be 0.1–0.7%.[20] Intrahepatic portal vein anatomy with a right-sided round ligament is divided into two types. In the first type, the right lateral branch ramifies first, with the left main trunk extending to the left side giving rise to S2 and S3 branches. From the umbilical portion, ramifies the right paramedian branches. No apparent branch of S4 is observed at the left side of MHV. In the second type, the left portal vein (S2 and S3 branches) ramifies first, with the right main trunk giving rise to the right lateral branch ending at the umbilical portion, where the right paramedian branches ramify.[21] Special attention must be paid to associated variations, such as the absence of the umbilical portion of the left portal vein or the horizontal part of the left hepatic duct.

Complete absence of the left main trunk (horizontal portion) or the right main trunk of the portal vein is another rare variation that would usually be a contraindication for hemihepatectomy. However, using the transparenchymal division technique or the portal pedicle preserving the main arcade of the portal vein and transection of the liver parenchyma along the MHV under inflow occlusion, right or left hemihepatectomy is possible. But in our vast experiences of hepatic resections, we have never encountered the anomaly. Absence of the left portal vein was initially observed by Couinaud[2] in 1 out of 103 specimens and recently by Fraser-Hill et al.[22] in 7 out of 18,550 patients (0.04%) who had undergone abdominal ultrasonography. In Couinaud's case, after the ramification of S6 and S7 branches, the main portal vein entered the hepatic parenchyma and extended as usual into the right anterior branch. Then, it headed for the left liver, curving toward the cranial side and running along the umbilical fissure in the opposite direction after the ramification of S3 and S4 branches, and ended up as an S2 branch. Complete absence of the right portal vein is rarer, and was observed by Fraser-Hill et al.[22] in 4 out of 18,550 (0.02%) ultrasonography studies. In these four cases, the right liver was atrophic and was supplied only by small branches arising from the main and the left portal veins, although anatomy of RHV of MHV was not described in this report.[22]

3.4 Hepatic Vein Variations

3.4.1 Left Hepatic Vein

The main trunk of the left hepatic vein (LHV) runs along the intersegmental plane of S2 and S3, draining these two segments. However, there usually exists a fissural vein that runs along the umbilical fissure and conjugates into the root of the LHV. This vein drains the cranial portion of S4. This means that an extended right hepatectomy including the MHV will at least not result in the congestion of the cranial portion of S4 if the vein can be preserved.

3.4.2 Middle Hepatic Vein

The MHV runs along the main portal fissure and is the drainage vein for S4 and the right paramedian sector. The volume of S4 that drains via the tributaries of the MHV is usually small due to the scissural vein that joins with the left hepatic vein. Even if the drainage vein of the cranial part of S4 joins with the MHV near its confluence to the inferior vena cava, the cranial part of S4 may be preserved in most cases because an extended right hepatectomy is most frequently indicated in cases with tumor invading the hepatic hilum or MHV. Therefore, this S4 drainage vein can be preserved and complete resection of S4 (right lobectomy) rarely becomes necessary.

A large portion of the right paramedian sector on the other hand, is drained via the tributaries of the MHV, and in some cases, there is a long and thick MHV tributary draining a portion of S6 (Fig. 3.7).[5,6] Therefore, sacrifice of the MHV in an extended left hepatectomy may result in the congestion of a large part of the right anterior sector and S6. The volumes of the areas congested after sacrificing the MHV must be pre-estimated because intrahepatic venous communication (in the peripheral MHV and right hepatic vein and/or IRHV) exists in only about 20% of the cases,[23] and these congested area would not function normally without the MHV.

If the volume of the remnant liver without congestion is estimated to be small, reconstruction of the MHV should be considered. Ideally, an accurate evaluation of the volumes of the areas expected to be congested should be performed using the volume-rendering method (the volume of liver parenchyma fed by a specific portal vein branch or drained by a specific hepatic vein branch estimated). Approximate estimation is also possible by using standard CT axial images, as reported by Hwang et al.[24] In brief, the tributaries of the MHV and RHV draining the right paramedian sector are identified in each slice, and an imaginary line is drawn midway between the MHV tributaries and the RHV tributaries. The area confined between this imaginary line and the main portal fissure is defined as the area of congestion,

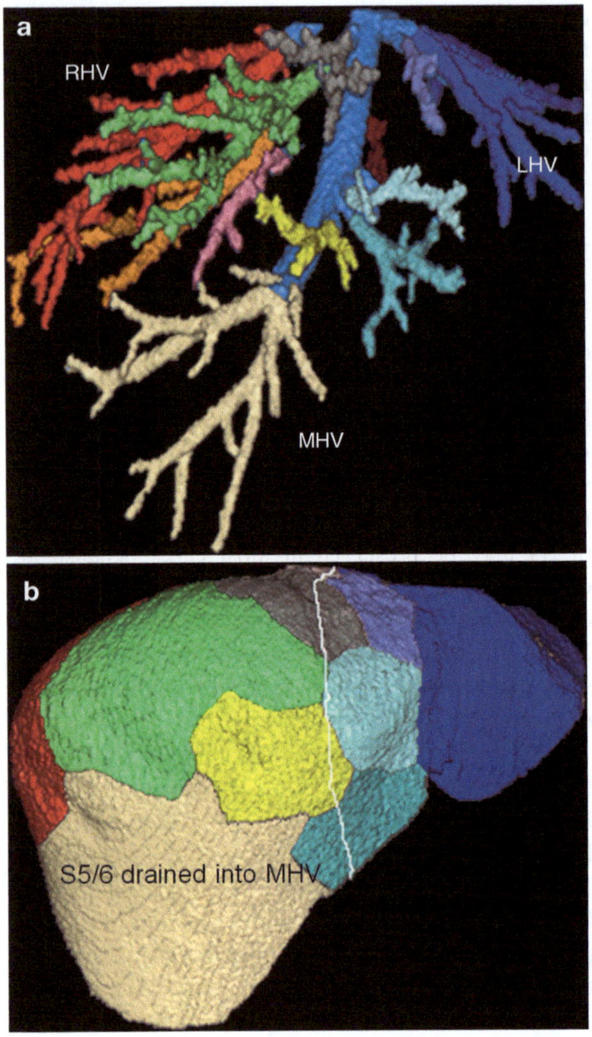

Fig. 3.7 (**a**) Middle hepatic vein (MHV) tributary draining segments 5 and 6. The region drained by each tributary is calculated by volume rendering software. (**b**) Area drained by this MHV tributary is shown

and stacked images of congestion areas are used to calculate the expected congestion volume.

An approximate assessment of the congestion area may be much easier intraoperatively using Doppler ultrasonography. Under this method, the MHV trunk or tributaries are clamped during transection of the liver parenchyma which is then followed by clamping of the hepatic artery. This results in surface discoloration of the congested region, and Doppler ultrasonography would show no signal of the MHV tributaries or hepatofugal flow of the portal vein branches in the congested region. If the congested region shown by this technique is large, reconstruction of the MHV or its tributaries must be considered.[23]

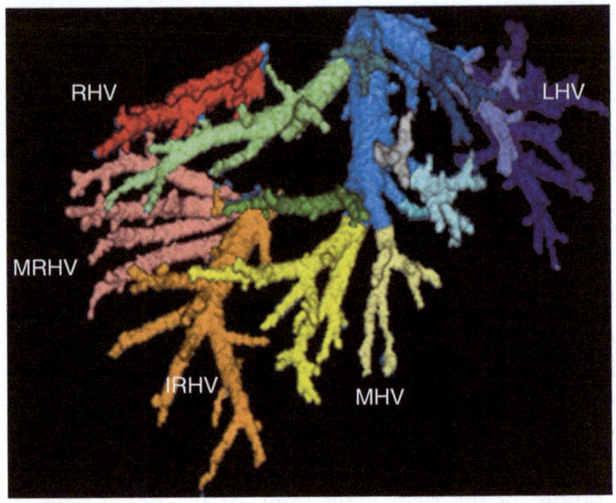

Fig. 3.8 Three-dimensional hepatic vein anatomy with well-developed middle right hepatic vein (MRHV) and inferior right hepatic vein (IRHV). Note that the right hepatic vein (RHV) does not descend in the caudal direction and drains only the cranial portion of the right liver

3.4.3 Right Hepatic Vein

It should be noted that the RHV is the main drainage vein of the right lateral sector. As mentioned previously, the RHV does not always mark an unequivocal distinction between the paramedian and the lateral sectors of the right hemiliver,[25] especially in cases with thick IRHV or MRHV. IRHV or MRHV is reported to exist in approximately 60–70% of cases.[2,26] and in 20–25% of these cases, they are thick and easily recognized by ultrasonography[27], and the RHV is relatively less developed.[13] Depending on the location of the tumor (e.g., tumor invading the root of three major hepatic veins) and remnant liver volume, an extended left trisectionectomy with resection of the RHV may be an option.[28]

3.4.4 Inferior and Middle Right Hepatic Vein

In cases with a well-developed inferior right hepatic vein (IRHV) or middle right hepatic vein (MRHV), the main RHV does not descend in the caudal direction but just drains the cranial portion of the right liver (Fig. 3.8).[26] In addition, the IRHV or MRHV runs within the dorsal part of S6 or S7, respectively, which is different from the plane in which the ordinal RHV runs.[25]

3.4.5 Caudate Vein Branches (S7/S1 Border)

In cases when resection of the caudate lobe is required, it is usually difficult to recognize the border between the right liver and the caudate lobe. A recent study aiming to identify the hepatic veins draining the caudate lobe in cadaveric livers showed that the caudate process hepatic vein that appears without exception by opening the space between the paracaval portion and IVC runs along the boundary between the regions fed by the portal vein branches of the caudate process and the right liver.[29]

3.5 Conclusion

Indications for hepatic resection vary with the type of the tumor. For example, hepatocellular carcinoma is usually encapsulated, and therefore tumors compressing the major hepatic vein or IVC may easily be dissected, whereas adenocarcinoma such as metastatic cancer from the colon and rectum or intrahepatic cholangiocarcinoma may not be dissected from the adjacent hepatic veins, and the vein must usually be sacrificed. In the latter cases, the volume of the would be congested area must be considered. Therefore, not only the portal vein anatomy but also the hepatic vein anatomy should be evaluated.

Furthermore, major hepatic resection is frequently required in cases with tumor invasion into the hepatic hilum such as hilar cholangiocarcinoma or intrahepatic cholangiocarcinoma, or a large tumor compressing major vascular structures. The branches to be preserved should be evaluated precisely in each case according to the pattern and location of tumor infiltration, in order to determine and carry out safe hepatic resection.

References

1. Healey JE Jr, Schroy PC. Anatomy of the biliary ducts within the human liver; analysis of the prevailing pattern of branchings and the major variations of the biliary ducts. *AMA Arch Surg*. 1953;66:599-616.
2. Couinaud C. *Le foie: études anatomiques et chirugicales*. Paris: Masson; 1957.
3. Hata F, Hirata K, Murakami G, Mukaiya M. Identification of segments VI and VII of the liver based on the ramification patterns of the intrahepatic portal and hepatic veins. *Clin Anat*. 1999;12:229-244.
4. Masselot RL, Leborgne J. Anatomical study of the hepatic veins. *Anat Clin*. 1978;1:109-125.
5. Hui AM, Makuuchi M, Takayama T, et al. Left hemihepatectomy in living donors with a thick middle hepatic vein draining the caudal half of the right liver. *Transplantation*. 2000;69:1499-1501.
6. Kakazu T, Makuuchi M, Kawasaki S, et al. Reconstruction of the middle hepatic vein tributary during right anterior segmentectomy. *Surgery*. 1995;117:238-240.
7. Rex H. Beitrage zur Morphologie der Säugerleber. *Morph. Jb*. 1888;14:517-616.
8. Cho A, Okazumi S, Takayama W, et al. Anatomy of the right anterosuperior area (segment 8) of the liver: evaluation with helical CT during arterial portography. *Radiology*. 2000;214:491-495.
9. Atasoy C, Ozyurek E. Prevalence and types of main and right portal vein branching variations on MDCT. *AJR Am J Roentgenol*. 2006;187:676-681.
10. Savier E, Taboury J, Lucidarme O, et al. Fusion of the planes of the liver: an anatomic entity merging the midplane and the left intersectional plane. *J Am Coll Surg*. 2005;200:711-719.
11. FUJIFILM Annual Report 2009. http://www.fujifilmholdings.com/en/pdf/investors/annual_report/ff_ar_2009_part_012.pdf. Accessed 26 May 2011.
12. Fischer L, Cardenas C, Thorn M, et al. Limits of Couinaud's liver segment classification: a quantitative computer-based three-dimensional analysis. *J Comput Assist Tomogr*. 2002;26:962-967.
13. Nagino M, Kamiya J, Kanai M, et al. Right trisegment portal vein embolization for biliary tract carcinoma: technique and clinical utility. *Surgery*. 2000;127:155-160.
14. Kishi Y, Madoff DC, Abdalla EK, et al. Is embolization of segment 4 portal veins before extended right hepatectomy justified? *Surgery*. 2008;144:744-751.
15. Capussotti L, Muratore A, Ferrero A, Anselmetti GC, Corgnier A, Regge D. Extension of right portal vein embolization to segment IV portal branches. *Arch Surg*. 2005;140:1100-1103.
16. Wallace MJ. C-arm computed tomography for guiding hepatic vascular interventions. *Tech Vasc Interv Radiol*. 2007;10:79-86.
17. Soyer P, Bluemke DA, Choti MA, Fishman EK. Variations in the intrahepatic portions of the hepatic and portal veins: findings on helical CT scans during arterial portography. *AJR Am J Roentgenol*. 1995;164:103-108.
18. Orguc S, Tercan M, Bozoklar A, et al. Variations of hepatic veins: helical computerized tomography experience in 100 consecutive living liver donors with emphasis on right lobe. *Transplant Proc*. 2004;36:2727-2732.
19. Matsumoto H. A newer concept of the segments of the liver. *Jpn J Med Ultrason*. 1986;13:551-552.
20. Nakanishi S, Shiraki K, Yamamoto K, Koyama M, Nakano T. An anomaly in persistent right umbilical vein of portal vein diagnosed by ultrasonography. *World J Gastroenterol*. 2005;11:1179-1181.
21. Nagai M, Kubota K, Kawasaki S, Takayama T, Bandai Y, Makuuchi M. Are left-sided gallbladders really located on the left side? *Ann Surg*. 1997;225:274-280.
22. Fraser-Hill MA, Atri M, Bret PM, Aldis AE, Illescas FF, Herschorn SD. Intrahepatic portal venous system: variations demonstrated with duplex and color Doppler US. *Radiology*. 1990;177:523-526.

23. Sano K, Makuuchi M, Miki K, et al. Evaluation of hepatic venous congestion: proposed indication criteria for hepatic vein reconstruction. *Ann Surg*. 2002;236:241-247.
24. Hwang S, Lee SG, Park KM, et al. Hepatic venous congestion in living donor liver transplantation: preoperative quantitative prediction and follow-up using computed tomography. *Liver Transpl*. 2004;10:763-770.
25. van Leeuwen MS, Noordzij J, Fernandez MA, Hennipman A, Feldberg MA, Dillon EH. Portal venous and segmental anatomy of the right hemiliver: observations based on three-dimensional spiral CT renderings. *Am J Roentgenol*. 1994; 163:1395-1404.
26. Nakamura S, Tsuzuki T. Surgical anatomy of the hepatic veins and the inferior vena cava. *Surg Gynecol Obstet*. 1981; 152:43-50.
27. Makuuchi M, Hasegawa H, Yamazaki S, Bandai Y, Watanabe G, Ito T. The inferior right hepatic veinb: ultrasonic demonstration. *Radiology* 1983;148:213-217.
28. Makuuchi M, Hasegawa H, Yamazaki S, Takayasu K. Four new hepatectomy procedures for resection of the right hepatic vein and preservation of the inferior right hepatic vein. *Surg Gynecol Obstet*. 1987;164:68-72.
29. Kogure K, Kuwano H, Yorifuji H, Ishikawa H, Takata K, Makuuchi M. The caudate processus hepatic vein: a boundary hepatic vein between the caudate lobe and the right liver. *Ann Surg*. 2008;247:288-293.

Surgical Anatomy of the Liver in the Glissonean Pedicle Approach: What We Need to Know

4

Ken Takasaki and Masakazu Yamamoto

Abstract

The Glissonean pedicle approach in liver surgery provides new knowledge of the surgical anatomy and progresses the technique of liver surgery. The Glissonean pedicle is wrapped by the connective tissue referred to as the Walaeus sheath and includes the hepatic artery, the portal vein, the bile duct, the nerves, and the lymphatic vessels. This approach provides extrafascial access to the hepatic hilus, and the secondary Glissonean pedicles are taped and ligated at the hepatic hilus without liver dissection. The approaching point must be over the hilar plate; therefore, surgeons do not have to consider any variation of the artery or bile ducts. The tertiary branches can be approached through the hepatic hilus or in the liver on the borderlines between the segments. Any anatomical hepatectomy can be done using this technique which allows simple, safe, and easy liver surgery. Liver surgeons should, therefore, know the fundamental concept of the Glissonean pedicle approach.

Keywords

Anatomy of the liver • Glissonean pedicle approach • Liver surgery with Glissonean pedicle approach • Walaeus sheath

In liver surgery, surgical techniques have advanced with increased knowledge of the surgical anatomy of the liver. Many cases of small hepatocellular carcinoma have been detected by ultrasonography (US) or computed tomography scan (CT) in the cirrhotic liver since the 1980s. Two important surgical procedures in liver surgery were introduced around 1985 in Japan. One of these is Makuuchi's US-guided hepatectomy[1], and the other is Takasaki's Glissonean pedicle approach.[2-6] These two procedures have provided knowledge of the surgical anatomy and allow small anatomical liver resection, such as Couinaud's segmentectomy, in the cirrhotic liver. In this section, we describe the surgical anatomy of the liver that surgeons should know to use the Glissonean pedicle approach.

4.1 Walaeus Sheath and the Plate System

Couinaud referred to the Walaeus sheath as the most important component of the liver in his book entitled *Surgical Anatomy of the Liver Revisited.*[7] This sheath

K. Takasaki (✉)
Department of Surgery, Institute of Gastroenterology, Tokyo Women's Medical University, 8-1, Kawada-cho, Shinjuku-ku, Tokyo 162-8666, Japan
e-mail: kentakasaki@ige.twmu.ac.jp

D.C. Madoff et al. (eds.), *Venous Embolization of the Liver*,
DOI 10.1007/978-1-84882-122-4_4, © Springer-Verlag London Limited 2011

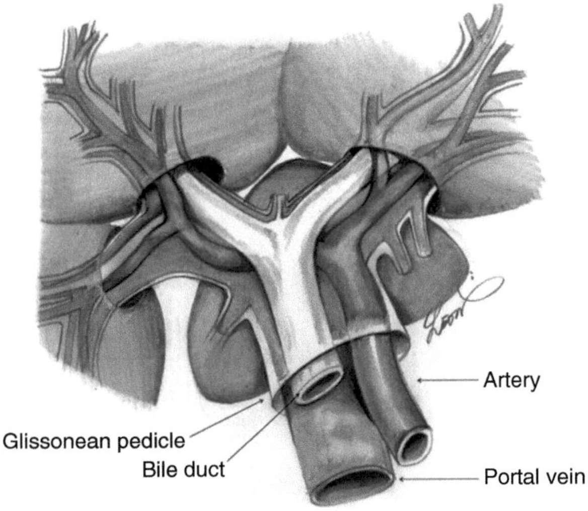

Fig. 4.1 Components of the Glissonean pedicle (From Takasaki[6] with kind permission of Springer Science+Business Media)

was discovered by Johannes Walaeus in 1640. The connective tissue wraps the portal vein, the hepatic artery, the bile duct, the lymphatic duct, and the nerves in the liver and connects to the capsule of the liver and the hepatoduodenal ligament (Fig. 4.1). However, the Walaeus sheath originates from the vasculo-biliary sheath and is not derived from the peritoneum or the capsule of the liver (Laennec's capsule). Therefore, the separation between Laennec's capsule and the Walaeus sheath can be seen microscopically at the hepatic hilum.[7]

The Walaeus sheath forms a thick plate at the inferior part of the liver referred to as the hilar plate. The hilar plate connects to the cystic plate, the umbilical plate, and the Arantian plate. The hilar plate can be detached from the quadrate lobe because no branch originates from along the anterior margin or the upper surface of the hilar plate. The small caudate branches originate from along the posterior margin of the hilar plate. When the hilar plate is pulled down after detaching the liver parenchyma of the quadrate lobe, the right and the left Glissonean pedicles are easily approached.

The portal pedicle (the portal vein, the hepatic artery, and the bile duct) enters the liver wrapped by the Walaeus sheath which is attached to the parenchymal plates, whereas the hepatic veins are directly in contact with the liver parenchyma. The most important point is that any variation, in particular in the arteries and the bile ducts, occurs under the plates. Therefore, dissection under the plates is difficult and dangerous. The elements of the segmental pedicle or sectional pedicle must supply the segment or section into which the pedicles enter. We do not need to consider any injury to the elements that supply the remaining liver when we interrupt the pedicles above the plates.

4.2 Ramification of the Glissonean Pedicles and Liver Segmentation

The classification of the liver anatomy and resections was defined in the IHPBA Brisbane 2000 terminology.[8] The second-order division in the classification in the IHPBA Brisbane 2000 terminology is based on the ramification of the artery and the bile duct. The classification according to the Glissonean pedicles is different from that in the IHPBA Brisbane 2000 terminology (Table 4.1). The secondary Glissonean pedicles are divided into three at the hepatic hilus (Fig. 4.2). These pedicles can be approached outside of the liver without liver dissection (Fig. 4.3). Therefore, the liver can be divided into three segments according to the ramification of the Glissonean pedicles (Fig. 4.2). The left segment corresponds to the left medial section and the left lateral section in the Brisbane 2000 system. Couinaud had already mentioned that the left pedicle could be approached at the left end of the hilar plate in *Surgery* in 1985.[9] There are hepatic veins between Takasaki's

Table 4.1 Comparison of classification systems of liver anatomy and resection

Healey	Couinaud		Takasaki	Brisbane 2000
Right lobe				Right liver
Posterior segment	Right lateral sector	S6S7	Right segment	Right posterior section
Anterior segment	Right paramedian sector	S5S8	Middle segment	Right anterior section
Left lobe			Left segment	Left liver
Medial segment	Left paramedian sector	S3S4		Left medial section
Lateral segment	Left lateral sector	S2		Left lateral section
Caudate lobe		S1	Caudate area	

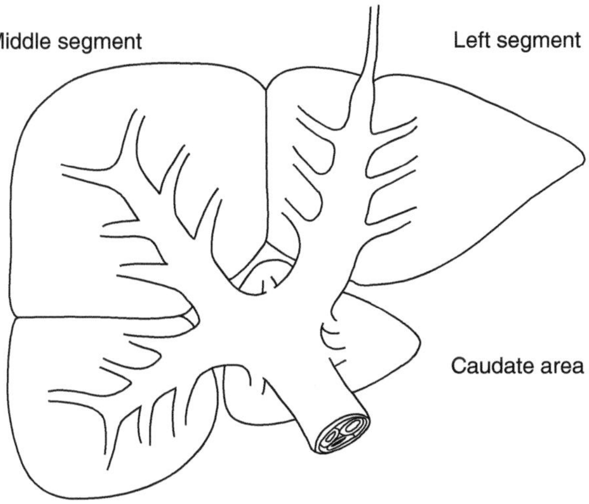

Fig. 4.2 The liver is divided into three segments and a caudate area according to the ramification of the Glissonean pedicles (From Takasaki[6] with kind permission of Springer Science+Business Media)

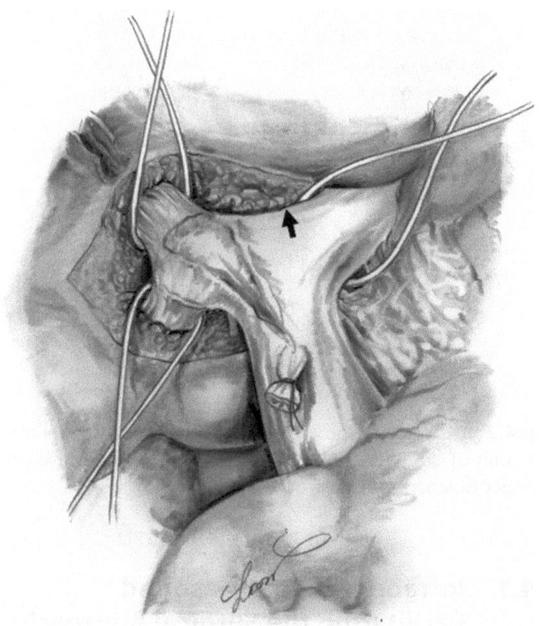

Fig. 4.3 The hilar plate (*arrow*) is detached from the quadrate lobe. The three secondary Glissonean pedicles are taped without liver dissection (From Takasaki[6] with kind permission of Springer Science+Business Media)

segments (Figs. 4.4 and 4.5). For example, the middle hepatic vein is situated between the left and the middle segments. The right hepatic vein is situated between the middle and the right segments.

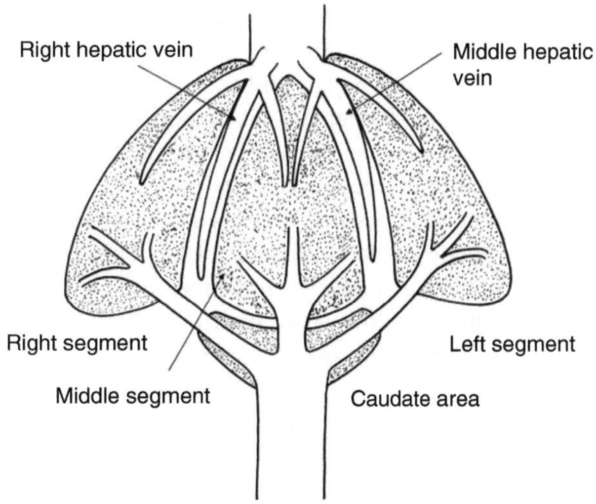

Fig. 4.4 Relation between the segments and the hepatic veins (From Takasaki[6] with kind permission of Springer Science+Business Media)

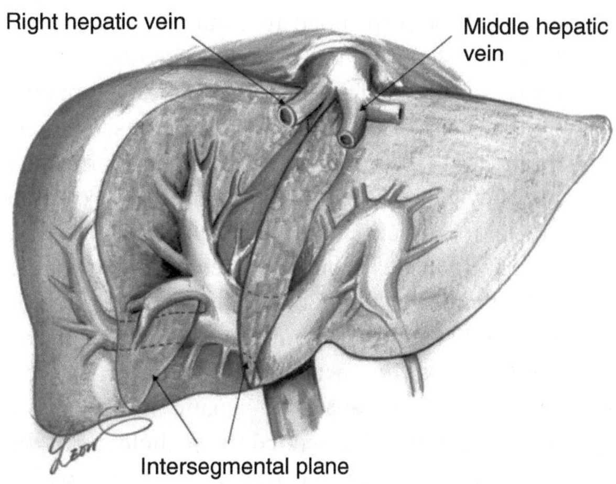

Fig. 4.5 The intersegmental planes between the segments (From Takasaki[6] with kind permission of Springer Science+Business Media)

4.3 Approach to the Glissonean Pedicles at the Hepatic Hilus

Couinaud described three approaches to the hepatic hilus.[7] The conventional dissection at the hilus or within the sheath is referred to as the hilar access (intrafascial approach). The dissection is performed under the hilar plate; therefore, this procedure is dangerous and surgeons have to consider variations of the hepatic artery and the bile ducts. The extrafascial approach is referred to as Takasaki's procedure. The Glissonean pedicle is dissected from the liver parenchyma at the hepatic hilus. Only the pedicle which belongs to the territory is ligated and cut. The main portal fissure or the left supra-hepatic fissure is opened after dissecting the liver parenchyma, and the surgeon confirms the pedicles which arise from the hilar plate or the umbilical plate. This procedure is referred to as the fissural approach. Okamoto demonstrated that the right anterior pedicle at the hepatic hilus could be approached after dissection of the parenchyma of the quadrant segment. He named this procedure an unroofing method in his text.[10]

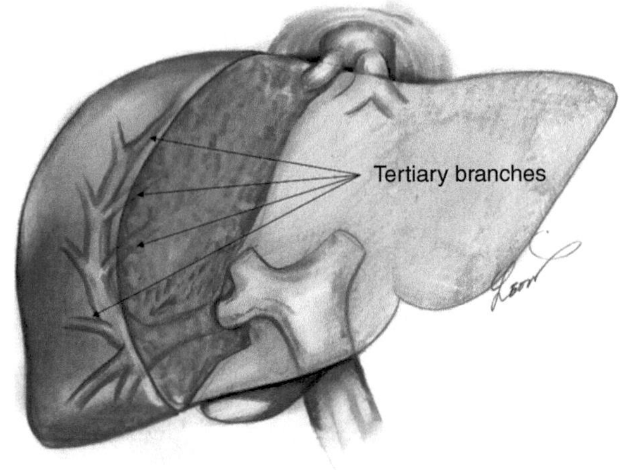

Fig. 4.6 One secondary pedicle has six to eight tertiary branches (From Takasaki[6] with kind permission of Springer Science+Business Media)

4.4 Approach to the Tertiary Branches

One secondary pedicle has six to eight tertiary branches (Fig. 4.6). The territory of a single tertiary branch does not correspond to Couinaud's segment. We therefore refer to the area fed by one tertiary branch as a cone unit of the liver[5] (Fig. 4.7). Couinaud's segments consist of three or four cone units. The tertiary branches in the left liver can easily be approached because they can be seen along the umbilical portion without liver dissection. However, in the right liver, the tertiary branches cannot be seen at the hepatic hilus. We therefore should clamp the secondary pedicle of the right anterior section at the hepatic hilus and confirm the borderline between the sections. The tertiary branches from near the hepatic hilus can be approached around the secondary pedicle near the hepatic hilus. However, the tertiary branches which originate from deep portions of the secondary branches cannot be approached from the hepatic hilus. Such deep branches can be approached after first dissecting the liver parenchyma on the borderline between the sections. The borderline between the sections can be confirmed by clamping the secondary pedicle at the hepatic hilus. If the tertiary branch, which might feed the territory including the tumor, is found, the tertiary branch is clamped and the territory is confirmed. After the procedure, we are able to check the tumor located in the territory on intraoperative US. We have performed over 2,000 anatomical liver resections at our institute since 1986. About a quarter of these were anatomical liver resections smaller than Couinaud's segment.

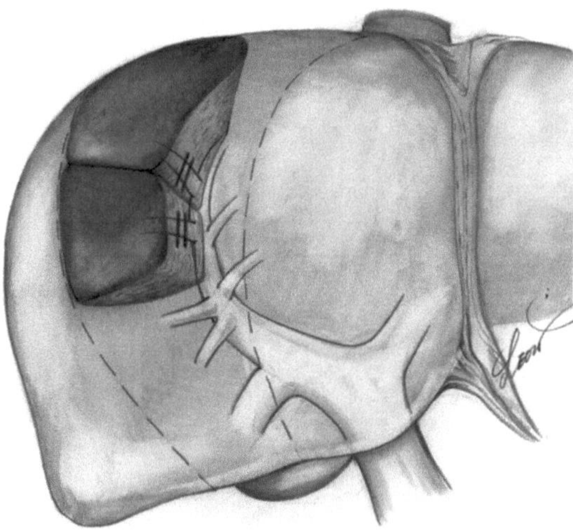

Fig. 4.7 We refer to the area fed by one tertiary branch as a cone unit of the liver (From Takasaki[6] with kind permission of Springer Science+Business Media)

4.4.1 Intraoperative Ultrasound Facilitating the Surgical Approach

Intraoperative ultrasound (US) greatly facilitates the surgical approach. Makuuchi's US-guided hepatectomy is a renowned procedure which enables identification of branches which feed the tumor and confirmation of the area including the tumor by injection of dyes. However, the procedure requires skillful technique, and it is sometimes difficult to obtain the precise staining area. In Takasaki's Glissonean pedicle approach, intraoperative US shows the relation between the tumor and cone units or segments identified by the clamping of the tertiary branches or the secondary Glissonean pedicles. In all cases, it is important to detect any other lesions and to confirm the major intrahepatic vessels on the dissecting plane. Intraoperative US facilitates a safe and appropriate surgical approach.

4.5 Summary

Any type of anatomical hepatectomy can be achieved safely by the Glissonean pedicle approach. Therefore, liver surgeons should know the concept and the surgical anatomy of the approach.

References

1. Makuuchi M, Hasegawa H, Yamazaki S. Ultrasonically guided subsegmentectomy. *Surg Gynecol Obstet*. 1985;161:346-350.
2. Takasaki K, Kobayashi S, Tanaka S, et al. Highly selected hepatic resection by Glissonean sheath-binding method. *Dig Surg*. 1986;3:121.
3. Takasaki K, Kobayashi S, Tanaka S, et al. New developed systematized hepatectomy by Glissonean pedicle transection method (in Japanese). *Shujutsu*. 1986;40:7-14.
4. Takasaki K, Kobayashi S, Tanaka S, et al. Highly anatomically systematized hepatic resection with Glissonean sheath cord transection at the hepatic hilus. *Int Surg*. 1990;75: 73-77.
5. Takasaki K. Glissonean pedicle transection method for hepatic resection: a new concept of liver segmentation. *J Hepatobiliary Pancreat Surg*. 1998;5:286-291.
6. Takasaki K. *Glissonean Pedicle Transection Method for Hepatic Resection*. Tokyo: Springer; 2007.
7. Couinaud C. *Surgical Anatomy of the Liver Revisited*. Paris (self-printed); 1989.
8. Strasberg SM. Nomenclature of hepatic anatomy and resections: a review of the Brisbane 2000 system. *J Hepatobiliary Pancreat Surg*. 2005;12:351-355.
9. Couinaud C. A simplified method for controlled left hepatectomy. *Surgery*. 1985;97:358-361.
10. Okamoto E. *Hepatic Resection for Primary Hepatocellular Carcinoma: New Trial for Controlled Anatomic Subsegmentectomies by an Initial Suprahilar Glissonian Pedicular Ligation Method* (in Japanese). Shoukaki geka [seminar] 23, Health Shyuppan, Tokyo, pp. 230-241, 1986.

Liver Anatomy: Variant Venous Anatomy and Implications for Resection

5

Ajay V. Maker, William R. Jarnagin, and Anne M. Covey

Abstract

The complexity of radiologic and surgical interventions on the liver has increased in the last decade. Knowledge of anatomical variants is crucial for safe hepatic resection and for preservation of adequate inflow and outflow to the functional remnant liver tissue. There are many congenital and acquired anomalies of the portal vein that need to be identified preoperatively, and their presence may indicate concomitant variations in biliary ductal anatomy.

Keywords

Congenital anomalies of the liver • Hepatic anatomy variants • Hepatic vein variations • Liver anatomy • Venous anatomy variants

Surgical resection remains the most effective therapy for patients with primary and metastatic liver tumors. All techniques for partial hepatectomy ultimately rely on control and transection of the vascular inflow and the biliary and venous outflow of the segments to be resected. Variations in portal venous anatomy are not uncommon and have important implications for both hepatic resection and for interventional procedures including preoperative portal vein embolization and TIPS. With an increase in complex surgical resections and percutaneous hepatobiliary interventions, a thorough understanding of variant hepatic venous anatomy is critical. This chapter addresses the congenital and acquired anomalies of the portal vein, the implications these have on biliary ductal anatomy and portal vein embolization, and the variations of the hepatic veins.

5.1 Congenital Anomalies of the Portal Vein

The splenic and superior mesenteric veins join to form the main portal vein posterior to the head of the pancreas. The main portal vein typically divides at the hilum into the left and right portal branches. The right portal vein typically has a short extrahepatic course and then divides into the right anterior sectoral trunk, which feeds segments V and VIII, and the right posterior sectoral trunk, which supplies segments VI and VII. The left portal vein has a longer extrahepatic course along the dorsocaudal aspect of segment IV before it curves ventrally into the umbilical fissure to supply the caudate and segments II, III, and IV (Fig. 5.1).

Embryologically, the portal vein is formed between the 4th and 10th weeks of gestation.[1-3] By the fourth

A.M. Covey (✉)
Department of Diagnostic Radiology, Memorial Sloan-Kettering Cancer Center,
1275 York Avenue, New York, NY 10021, USA
e-mail: coveya@mskcc.org

D.C. Madoff et al. (eds.), *Venous Embolization of the Liver*,
DOI 10.1007/978-1-84882-122-4_5,

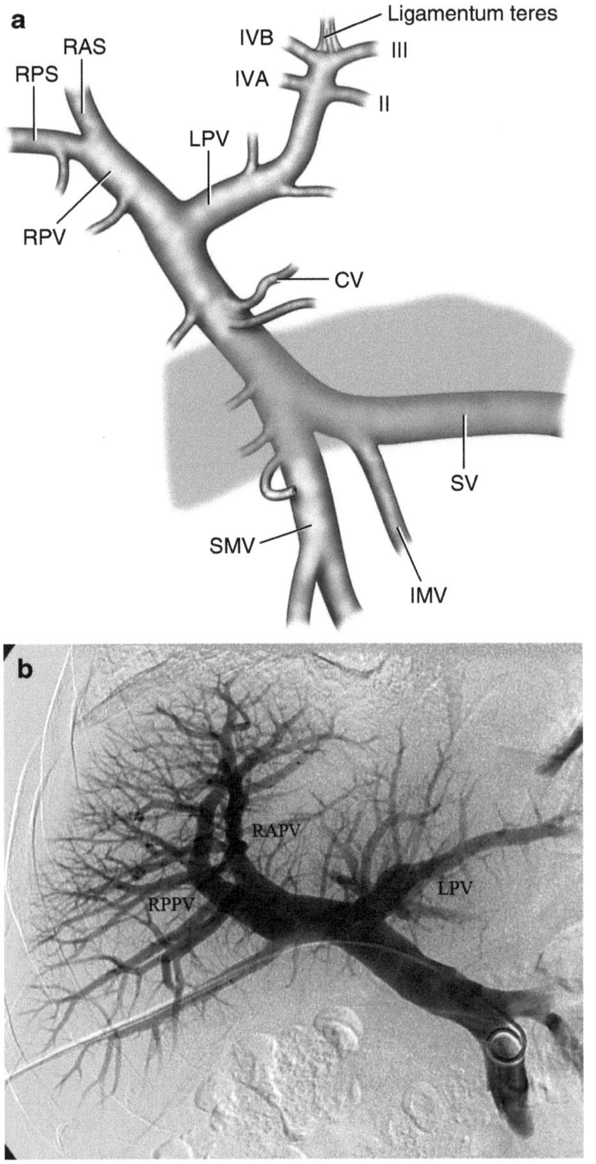

Fig. 5.1 (**a, b**) In standard anatomy, the portal vein is formed by the confluence of the splenic vein (SV) and the superior mesenteric vein (SMV). The inferior mesenteric vein (IMV) ends in the splenic vein. The main portal vein typically divides at the hilum into the left and right portal branches. The right portal vein (RPV) typically has a short extrahepatic course and then divides into the right anterior sectoral trunk (RAS), which feeds segments V and VIII, and the right posterior sectoral trunk (RPS), which supplies segments VI and VII. The left portal vein (LPV) has a longer extrahepatic course along the inferior aspect of segment IV before it curves cranially into the umbilical fissure to supply the caudate and segments II, III, and IV

week, there are three paired venous systems: the cardinal veins, the vitelline veins from the yolk sac, and the umbilical veins from the chorion. By the end of the fourth week, the right and left vitelline veins are cross-linked, with the superior anastomoses forming the intrahepatic portal veins. The extrahepatic portal veins are formed by selective involution of the right and left vitelline veins.[3] Alterations in the pattern of obliteration of these anastomoses can result in several variants, and failure to form these anastomoses results in complete or partial absence of the portal system.[4]

Major congenital portal vein variants include total or partial agenesis, duplication, a single main portal vein, and venous malposition, including a prepancreatic portal vein.[5-8] These variants are often accompanied by cardiac and other congenital malformations.[9] With modern preoperative cross-sectional imaging, these anomalies are often obvious, and surgical and interventional planning can be tailored based on the specific anatomy. For patients with congenital absence of the portal vein, the treatment of liver tumors, such as in hepatocellular carcinoma, remains radical resection,[10] and patients who have undergone resection have had uncomplicated postoperative courses despite a lack of portal blood and the associated hepatotropic factors.[1,11-14]

Far more common variations, however, involve the branching pattern of the portal vein. These can range from anomalies at the main portal vein bifurcation, to far more subtle intrahepatic variations, all of which can have significant clinical consequences during hepatic resection. Failure to properly identify the origin of the portal inflow to the remaining functional liver remnant and inadvertent ligation can result in a necrotic liver segment, or even hepatic failure and death.

5.1.1 Branching Patterns of the Portal Vein

In our experience, there are five major branching patterns of the portal vein. The most common, *type 1*, is the standard portal venous anatomy in which the main portal vein divides into the right and left portal branches. The right portal vein then gives rise to anterior and posterior sectoral branches that supply Couinaud segments V/VIII and segments VI/VII, respectively (Fig. 5.1). We found this pattern present in 65% of 200 patients studied with CT portography.[15]

Trifurcation of the main portal vein into the right anterior, right posterior, and left portal vein branches, or *type 2* anatomy, occurred in 9% of our patients (Fig. 5.2). This is important to recognize in right-sided resections where instead of controlling inflow via the main right portal vein, both the anterior and posterior sectoral branches would need to be separately controlled.

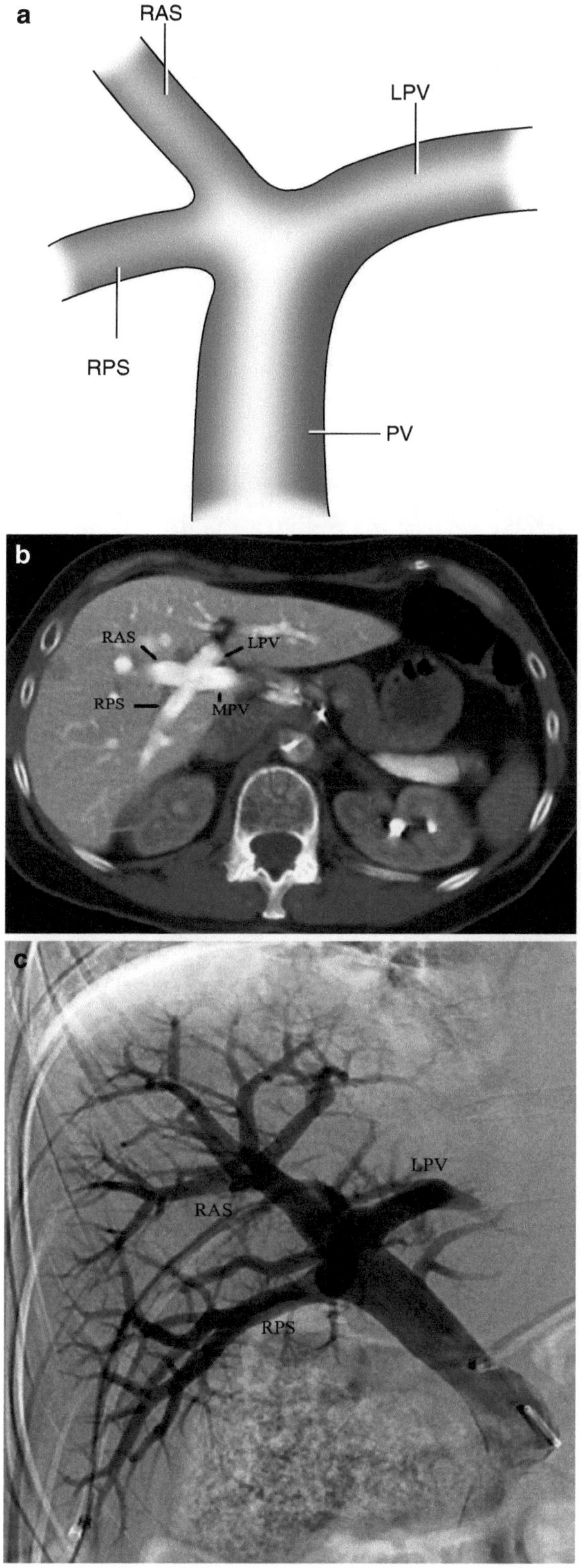

Fig. 5.2 (**a–c**) *Type 2* portal vein anatomy: trifurcation of the main portal vein (MPV) into the right anterior sector (RAS), right posterior sector (RPS), and left portal vein (LPV) branches

Likewise, preoperative portal vein embolization, which is performed most commonly on the right side, would require separate embolization of both branches.

The most common variation on the standard anatomy is the "Z-type" anatomy, *type 3*, seen in 13% of patients in our study and in 6–11.4% by others.[16-18] It is referred to as "the portal vein variation" by Kitani and colleagues, who encountered it almost 10% of the time in 478 consecutive patients.[19] In this variation, the first branch of the main portal vein is the right posterior portal vein, and the right anterior portal vein and the left portal vein bifurcate (Fig. 5.3). In right hepatectomy, the right portal vein is often controlled extrahepatically. However, in this anatomic configuration, ligation of what may appear to be the right branch of the main portal vein for the right-sided resections may actually be the right posterior portal vein or the trunk to the right anterior sector and the left lobe. Similarly, for left-sided resections, the approach to the left portal vein will not be in its standard position. Thus, ligation of this venous trunk of the right anterior and the left portal veins would leave a wide nonperfused liver remnant, and risk of hepatic failure and death.

In less than 10% of patients, we found that the segment VII or VI branch was the first branch of the right portal vein (*types 4* and *5*, respectively) and that the right anterior portal vein trifurcated to supply the anterior sector and one segment of the posterior sector (Fig. 5.4). This is important to note in extended left hepatic resection, where if the right anterior sectorial branch with one segmental branch of the posterior sector is ligated, a large portion of the remnant liver would be without portal flow, possibly resulting in hepatic failure. Similarly, for any resection of the posterior sector, each individual pedicle would need to be identified and ligated since there is no common posterior sectorial pedicle. It is well known that intrahepatic vessel ramification of the right posterior sector is extremely variable, and careful planning with preoperative imaging and intraoperative ultrasound is critical in these patients.[20,21]

In addition to the five main types of portal vein branching patterns described, "other" portal vein variants were identified in 6% of patients. Half of these had trifurcation of the right portal vein into the right anterior sectorial portal trunk, segment VI, and segment VII branches. One patient each had the following anomalies: quadrification of the main portal vein into segment VI, segment VII, the right anterior portal vein, and the left portal vein; trifurcation of the right portal vein into branches supplying segment V, segment VIII, and the right posterior sectoral trunk; trifurcation of

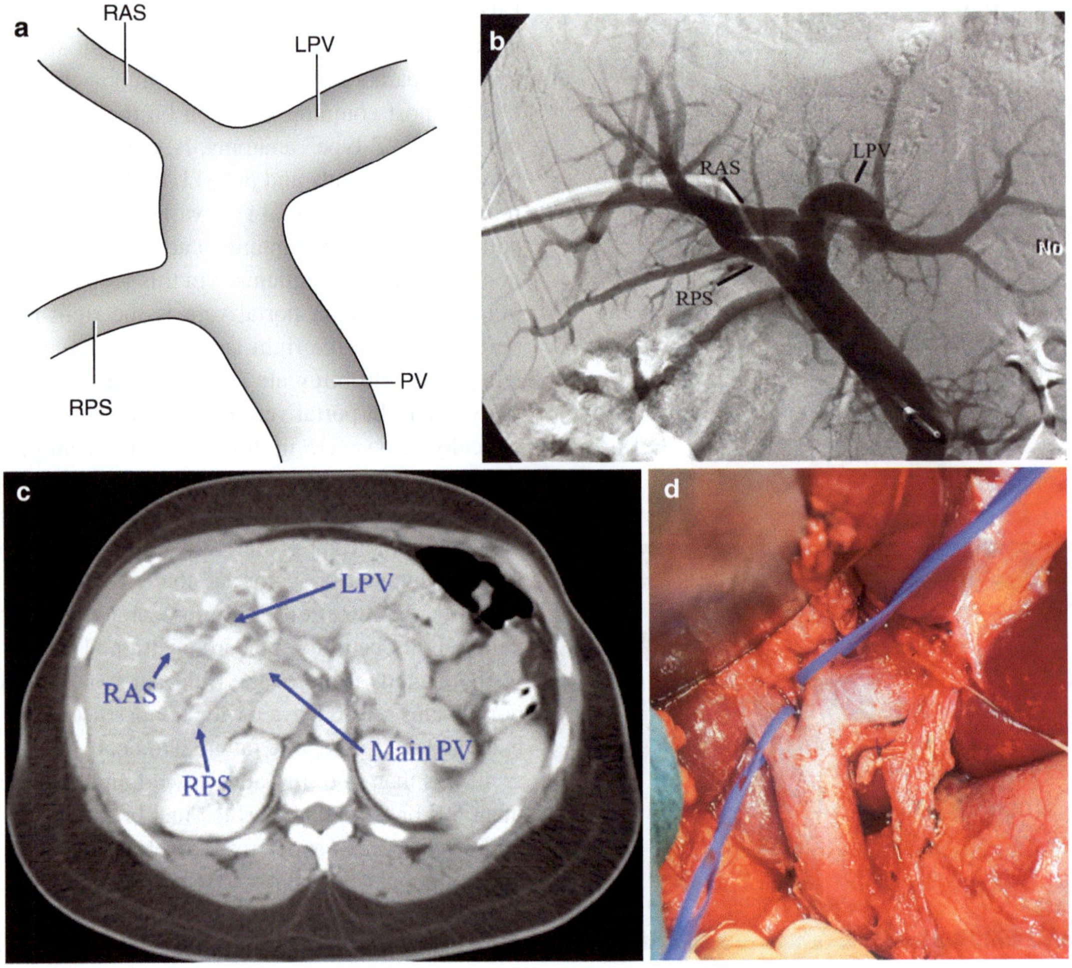

Fig. 5.3 (**a–d**) *Type 3* anatomy: the most common variation on the standard anatomy. The first branch of the main portal vein is the right posterior sector portal vein (RPS) leaving a common trunk that divides into the right anterior sector portal vein (RAS) and the left portal vein (LPV)

the main portal vein into segment VI, segment VII, and the left main and right anterior sectoral branch; the segment IV and VII branches originating from the right anterior portal vein; and an accessory segment VI branch from the right portal vein in a patient with *type 5* portal vein branching.

Older sonographic literature identifies variant portal vein anatomy in 10–15% of patients; however, in recent studies utilizing portography, the incidence is closer to one-third of the patients studied.[15,22-24] Variants of the left portal vein are rare, but, when variations of the right portal vein exist and the main portal branching pattern is anomalous, the left vein may not be found in its standard position, and it must be clearly identified and controlled prior to left-sided resections.

5.2 Acquired Anomalies

Acquired portal vein anomalies of clinical significance to the interventionalist arise from venous collaterals. These collaterals can be secondary to portal hypertension, splenic or splenomesenteric venous stenosis, or portal vein obstruction due to pancreatitis, tumor, or surgery. Multiple patterns of venous collaterals are described, the most common being gastroesophageal, paraumbilical, splenorenal, and inferior mesenteric. Gastric collateral veins most often present on imaging in patients with portal hypertension, and associated esophageal varices are a clinically important source of upper gastrointestinal hemorrhage. Obliteration of the splenic vein is also the source of gastric collaterals.

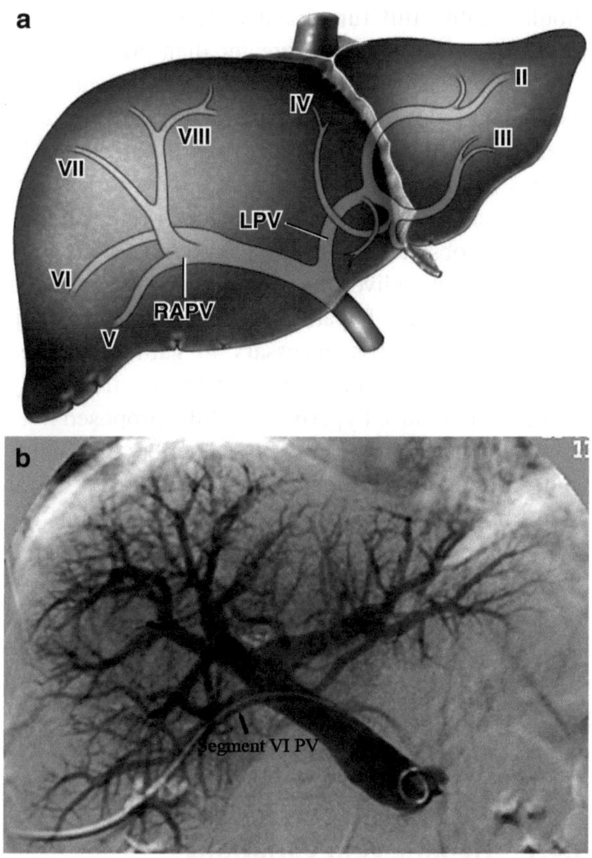

Fig. 5.4 (**a**, **b**) An uncommon but surgically relevant anomaly occurs when the first branch of the portal vein is the segment VI (type 5) or VII branch (type 4). In this situation, the segment VI or VII branch, respectively, and the right anterior portal vein (RAPV) share a common trunk. Inadvertent ligation of the RAPV during left trisegmentectomy can result in hepatic failure due to insufficient portal flow to the remnant

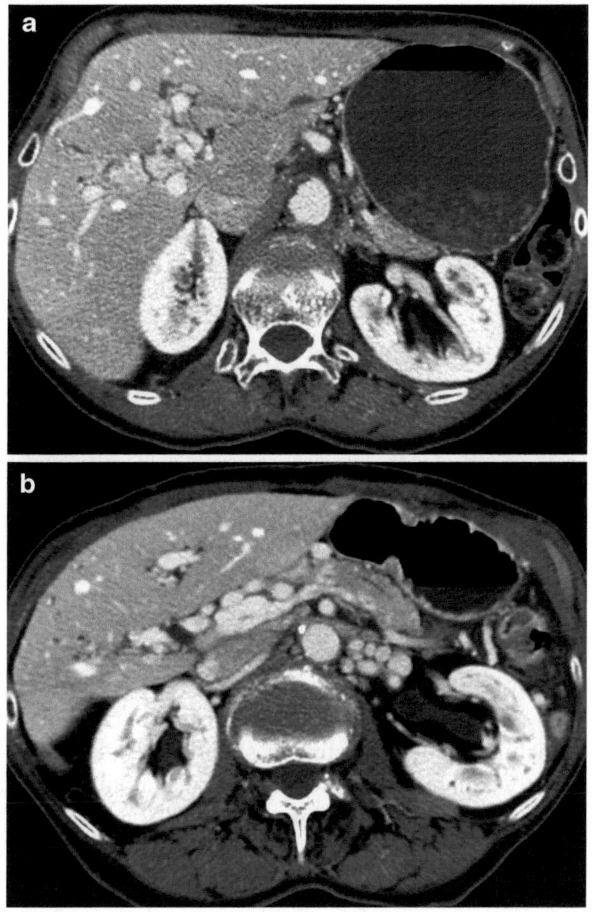

Fig. 5.5 (**a**, **b**) Contrast-enhanced CT images from a patient with cavernous transformation of the portal vein. There are extensive varices as a result and a large splenorenal shunt

Paraumbilical varices arise from the left portal vein via the umbilical vein. Although this vein is obliterated in patients with normal portal pressure, it has the potential to recanalize and serve as a conduit via the epigastric veins to the external iliac veins[25] or course subcutaneously, forming a caput medusa.[26,27] It is for this reason that the ligamentum teres must be securely ligated during mobilization of the liver. Similarly, care must be taken when dividing the triangular ligaments of the liver, as small vessels within these structures can become prominent with venous congestion. Sharp dissection without ligation or diathermy will result in hemorrhage from these vessels. Furthermore, in a stenosed or occluded portal vein, cavernous transformation can occur within 1 week of the event.[28] This results in the formation of venous channels within and around the affected portal vein (Fig. 5.5).

Major resection in the setting of portal hypertension is hazardous and predisposes the liver to even higher portal pressures postoperatively, thereby inhibiting normal liver regeneration and increasing the risk of life-threatening bleeding. Evidence of varices on preoperative radiography and endoscopy may be the only findings to alert the surgeon of hepatic dysfunction in the absence ICG testing or other hepatic function tests.

5.3 Implications on Ductal Anatomy

Of interest to the surgeon and interventionalist, especially when biliary cannulation or reconstruction is necessary, is the fact that portal vein variations are

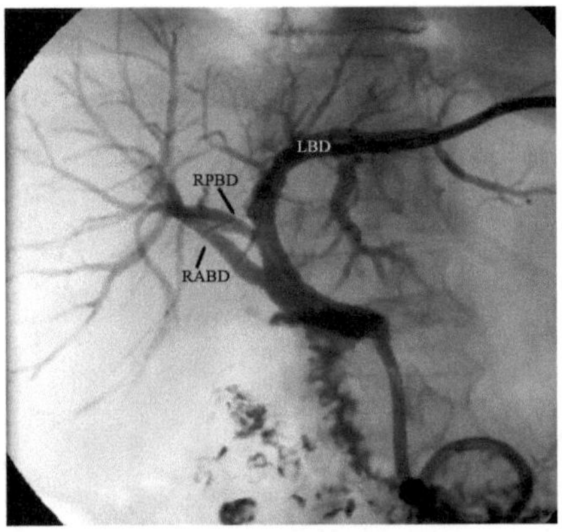

Fig. 5.6 Catheter cholangiogram shows the most common anatomic variant of the bile ducts associated with variant portal vein anatomy in which the right posterior bile duct (RPBD) drains into the left bile duct (LBD).

associated with distinct bile duct variations. This has been identified in studies of liver cast specimens and by conventional cholangiography.[16,29,30] In patients with *type 3* portal vein anatomy, a classic bile duct branching pattern is found significantly less frequently than in patients with standard anatomy. These patients often have a right posterior sectoral duct draining into the left hepatic duct with a supraportal course, or into the common bile duct with an infraportal course (Fig. 5.6). Furthermore, these patients have a higher incidence of left lateral segment ducts coursing caudal to the umbilical portion of the left portal vein.[19] As in cases of variant portal anatomy, variant biliary anatomy must be investigated prior to ligation, as biliary congestion of the functional remnant can lead to liver dysfunction. Evidence of portal vein anomalies should alert the surgeon to possible biliary variation and careful dissection during liver resection. The safest course of action in these patients is to address the biliary radicals during parenchymal transection and to avoid extrahepatic dissection of the ducts. Other ways to avoid biliary complications are to perform magnetic resonance cholangiopancreatography (MRCP) or intraoperative cholangiography.

5.4 Implications for Portal Vein Embolization

A healthy, non-cirrhotic individual requires a functional hepatic reserve of at least approximately 20% the original liver volume. The regenerative capacity of the liver should enable full functional compensation within weeks of resection. Once greater than 50% of liver volume is resected, the risk of clinically significant liver insufficiency does exist, and particular care must be taken, especially with extended right hepatectomy. In patients who are otherwise candidates for hepatic resection, the lack of adequate functional liver remnant may be the only obstacle to curative resection.

In cases where liver function may be impaired due to steatohepatitis, hepatitis, or cirrhosis, or when extended resection is necessary to gain tumor-free margins, portal vein embolization is frequently employed to induce hypertrophy of the proposed liver remnant in an effort to increase the number of patients who are candidates for hepatic resection.[31,32] Portal vein embolization was described in humans in the 1980s,[33,34] more than 50 years after it was discovered that rabbit portal vein ligation induced contralateral lobar hypertrophy.[35,36] Knowledge of the portal venous anatomy for each patient determines the success of the forced liver hypertrophy, and more importantly, spares the functional liver remnant from inadvertent embolization.

5.4.1 Hepatic Vein Variations

Although there are multiple small veins that drain the right lobe and segment I directly into the retrohepatic vena cava, the majority of hepatic blood flow drains into the inferior vena cava (IVC) via the left, middle, and right hepatic veins. In major hepatectomy, extrahepatic control of these vessels is preferred, especially when the tumor is large and near the confluence of the hepatic veins, or is attached to the IVC or the diaphragm. Standard anatomy consists of a single right hepatic vein entering the vena cava, and left and middle hepatic veins that join the vena cava as a single trunk. Autopsy studies of the left and middle hepatic venous trunk have elucidated at least five types of middle and hepatic vein trunk variants[37] (Fig. 5.7). Type I has no branching within 1 cm of the IVC, type II has two branches within 1 cm of IVC (most common), type III is a trifurcation, type IV is a quadrification, and type V has independent middle and left hepatic veins draining into the IVC. When the left and middle hepatic veins form a common trunk, control of the left hepatic vein alone is often not possible extrahepatically. Complete exposure generally requires full mobilization of the left liver, and division of the

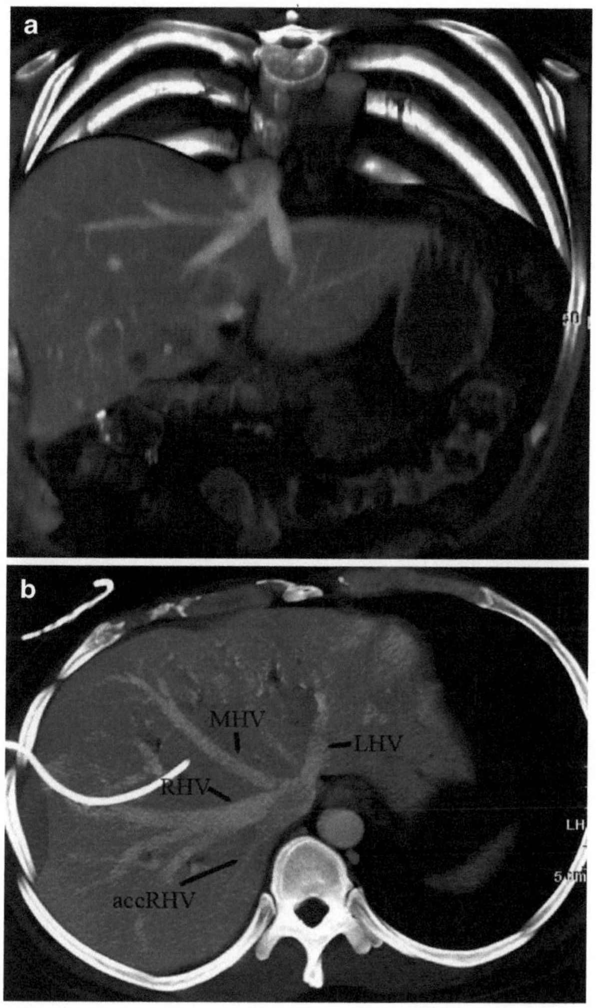

Fig. 5.7 (**a**) Coronal oblique reformatted CT demonstrates type II hepatic vein anatomy. (**b**) Axial contrast-enhanced CT showing type III hepatic vein anatomy in which the right (RHV), middle (MHV), and left (LHV) hepatic veins trifurcate from the IVC. Incidental note is made of a small accessory RHV

ligamentum venosum allows a tunnel to be dissected between the IVC and the middle and left hepatic veins. It is important to identify the hepatic venous anatomy preoperatively and realize if there are variations in the branching patterns since bleeding in this area can be difficult to control.

5.5 Conclusion

The complexity of radiologic and surgical interventions on the liver has increased in the last decade. Knowledge of anatomical variants is crucial for safe hepatic resection and for preservation of adequate inflow and outflow to the functional remnant liver tissue. There are many congenital and acquired anomalies of the portal vein that need to be identified preoperatively, and their presence may indicate concomitant variations in biliary ductal anatomy.

References

1. Joyce AD, Howard ER. Rare congenital anomaly of the portal vein. *Br J Surg*. 1988;75(10):1038-1039.
2. Marks C. Developmental basis of the portal venous system. *Am J Surg*. 1969;117(5):671-681.
3. Massin M, Verloes A, Jamblin P. Cardiac anomalies associated with congenital absence of the portal vein. *Cardiol Young*. 1999;9(5):522-525.
4. Walsh G, Williams MP. Congenital anomalies of the portal venous system – CT appearances with embryological considerations. *Clin Radiol*. 1995;50(3):174-176.
5. Gallego C, Velasco M, Marcuello P, Tejedor D, De Campo L, Friera A. Congenital and acquired anomalies of the portal venous system. *Radiographics*. 2002;22(1):141-159.
6. Hu GH, Shen LG, Yang J, Mei JH, Zhu YF. Insight into congenital absence of the portal vein: Is it rare? *World J Gastroenterol*. 2008;14(39):5969-5979.
7. Laverdiere JT, Laor T, Benacerraf B. Congenital absence of the portal vein: case report and MR demonstration. *Pediatr Radiol*. 1995;25(1):52-53.
8. Zhang JS, Wang YP, Wang MQ, et al. Diagnosis of an accessory portal vein and its clinical implications for portosystemic shunts. *Cardiovasc Interv Radiol*. 1996;19(4):239-241.
9. Parisato FO, Pataro EF. Anomalous portal vein. Vena porta anomalia. *Angiologia*. 1965;17(3):119-123.
10. Lundstedt C, Lindell G, Tranberg KG, Svartholm E. Congenital absence of the intrahepatic portion of the portal vein in an adult male resected for hepatocellular carcinoma. *Eur Radiol*. 2001;11(11):2228-2231.
11. Guariso G, Fiorio S, Altavilla G, et al. Congenital absence of the portal vein associated with focal nodular hyperplasia of the liver and cystic dysplasia of the kidney. *Eur J Pediatr*. 1998;157(4):287-290.
12. Marois D, van Heerden JA, Carpenter HA, Sheedy PF 2nd. Congenital absence of the portal vein. *Mayo Clin Proc*. 1979;54(1):55-59.
13. Matsuoka Y, Ohtomo K, Okubo T, Nishikawa J, Mine T, Ohno S. Congenital absence of the portal vein. *Gastrointest Radiol*. 1992;17(1):31-33.
14. Nakasaki H, Tanaka Y, Ohta M, et al. Congenital absence of the portal vein. *Ann Surg*. 1989;210(2):190-193.
15. Covey AM, Brody LA, Getrajdman GI, Sofocleous CT, Brown KT. Incidence, patterns, and clinical relevance of variant portal vein anatomy. *AJR Am J Roentgenol*. 2004; 183(4):1055-1064.
16. Cheng YF, Huang TL, Chen CL, et al. Anatomic dissociation between the intrahepatic bile duct and portal vein: risk factors for left hepatectomy. *World J Surg*. 1997;21(3):297-300.
17. Ko S, Murakami G, Kanamura T, Sato TJ, Nakajima Y. Cantlie's plane in major variations of the primary portal vein ramification at the porta hepatitis: cutting experiment using cadaveric livers. *World J Surg*. 2004;28(1):13-18.

18. Yamane T, Mori K, Sakamoto K, Ikei S, Akagi M. Intrahepatic ramification of the portal vein in the right and caudate lobes of the liver. *Acta Anat.* 1988;133(2):162-172.
19. Kitami M, Takase K, Murakami G, et al. Types and frequencies of biliary tract variations associated with a major portal venous anomaly: analysis with multi-detector row CT cholangiography. *Radiology.* 2006;238(1):156-166.
20. Goldsmith NA, Woodburne RT. The surgical anatomy pertaining to liver resection. *Surg Gynecol Obstet.* 1957;105:310-318.
21. Hata F, Hirata K, Murakami G, Mukaiya M. Identification of segments VI and VII of the liver based on the ramification patterns of the intrahepatic portal and hepatic veins. *Clin Anat.* 1999;12(4):229-244.
22. Atri M, Bret PM, Fraser-Hill MA. Intrahepatic portal venous variations: prevalence with ultrasound. *Radiology.* 1992;184: 523-526.
23. Cheng YF, Huang TL, Chen CL, Chen YS, Lee TY. Variations of the intrahepatic bile ducts: application in living related liver transplantation and splitting liver transplantation. *Clin Transplant.* 1997;11(4):337-340.
24. Filly RA, Laing FC. Anatomic variation of portal venous anatomy in the porta hepatitis: ultrasonographic evaluation. *J Clin Ultrasound.* 1978;6(2):83-89.
25. Williams PL. Veins of the abdomen and pelvis: hepatic portal system. In: Williams PL, ed. *Gray's Anatomy.* 38th ed. New York: Churchill Livingstone; 1999:1602-1604.
26. Cho KC, Patel YD, Wachsberg RH, Seeff J. Varices in portal hypertension: evaluation with CT. *Radiographics.* 1995;15(3):609-622. A review publication of the Radiological Society of North America, Inc.
27. Ito K, Higuchi M, Kada T, et al. CT of acquired abnormalities of the portal venous system. *Radiographics.* 1997;17(4):897-917.
28. De Gaetano AM, Lafortune M, Patriquin H, De Franco A, Aubin B, Paradis K. Cavernous transformation of the portal vein: patterns of intrahepatic and splanchnic collateral circulation detected with Doppler sonography. *Am J Roentgenol.* 1995;165(5):1151-1155.
29. Ishiyama S, Yamada Y, Narishima Y, Yamaki T, Kunii Y, Yamauchi H. Surgical anatomy of the hilar bile duct. *Tan Sui J Biliary Tract Pancreas.* 1999;20:811-820.
30. Kumon M, Matsuhima M, Itahara T. Gross anatomy of the liver hilus and caudate lobe using corrosion casts of the liver. *Tan Sui Biliary Tract Pancreas.* 1989;10:1417-1422.
31. Abulkhir A, Limongelli P, Healey AJ, et al. Preoperative portal vein embolization for major liver resection: a meta-analysis. *Ann Surg.* 2008;247(1):49-57.
32. Covey AM, Brown KT, Jarnagin WR, et al. Combined portal vein embolization and neoadjuvant chemotherapy as a treatment strategy for resectable hepatic colorectal metastases. *Ann Surg.* 2008;247(3):451-455.
33. Kinoshita H, Sakai K, Hirohashi K. Preoperative portal vein embolization for hepatocellular carcinoma. *World J Surg.* 1986;10(5):803-808.
34. Makuuchi M, Thai BL, Takayasu K, et al. Preoperative portal embolization to increase safety of major hepatectomy for hilar bile duct carcinoma: a preliminary report. *Surgery.* 1990;107(5):521-527.
35. Bax HR, Mansens BJ, Schalm L. Atrophy of the liver after occlusion of the bile ducts or portal vein and compensatory hypertrophy of the unoccluded portion and its clinical importance. *Gastroenterology.* 1956;31(2):131-155.
36. Makuuchi M et al. Preoperative transcatheter embolization of the portal venous branch for patients receiving extended lobectomy due to the bile duct carcinoma. *J Jpn Soc Clin Surg.* 1984;45:1558.
37. Nakamura S, Tsuzuki T. Surgical anatomy of the hepatic veins and the inferior vena cava. *Surg Gynecol Obstet.* 1981; 152(1):43-50.

Liver Regeneration and the Atrophy–Hypertrophy Complex

6

Robin D. Kim, Jae-Sung Kim, and Kevin E. Behrns

Abstract

The Atrophy–Hypertrophy Complex (AHC) refers to the liver's response to hepatocellular loss by the controlled restoration of liver parenchyma. Although atrophy can be due to various types of injury (e.g., toxins, ischemia, biliary obstruction, and partial hepatectomy), hypertrophy is relatively constant when there is a minimum amount of functional liver remnant. The AHC requires complex anatomic, histologic, cellular, and molecular processes, some of which have been defined. In patients in whom extended liver resection would result in liver insufficiency, preoperative portal vein embolization may increase the remnant liver sufficiently to permit aggressive resection. Continued basic science research may increase our understanding of the AHC to prevent or treat liver insufficiency.

Keywords

Atrophy-hypertrophy complex in liver • Liver ischemia and atrophy • Liver parenchyma • Regeneration • Liver regeneration • Portal vein embolization

Abbreviations

PVE	Portal Vein Embolization
BCS	Budd-Chiari Syndrome
I/R	Ischemia/Reperfusion
MPT	Mitochondrial Permeability Transition
TNFα	Tumor Necrosis Factor Alpha
NO	Nitric Oxide
iNOS	Inducible Nitric Oxide Synthetase
MAPK	Mitogen Activated Protein Kinase
HGF	Hepatocytes Growth Factor
TGF-α	Transforming Growth Factor Alpha
EGFR	Epidermal Growth Factor Receptor
PI3K	Phosphoinositide-3 Kinase
PVL	Portal Vein Ligation
TGF-β	Transforming Growth Factor Beta
ECM	Extracellular Matrix
uPA	Urokinase-like Plasminogen Activator

The Atrophy–Hypertrophy Complex (AHC) refers to the liver's response to hepatocellular loss by the controlled restoration of liver parenchyma. Although atrophy can be due to various types of injury (e.g., toxins, ischemia, biliary obstruction, and partial hepatectomy (PH)), hypertrophy is relatively constant when there is a minimum amount of functional liver remnant.

The AHC may be elicited by injury from obstructed biliary, portal venous, or hepatic venous flow to a

K.E. Behrns (✉)
Department of Surgery, Division of General and GI Surgery, University of Florida, 1600 SW Archer Road, P.O. Box 100118, 32610 Gainesville, FL, USA
e-mail: kevin.behrns@surgery.ufl.edu

D.C. Madoff et al. (eds.), *Venous Embolization of the Liver*,
DOI 10.1007/978-1-84882-122-4_6,

part of the liver. The resulting atrophy induces restorative hyperplasia through liver regeneration. The AHC is defined histologically by a decrease in hepatocellular mass relative to biliary composition.[1] The ability to induce the AHC through portal vein embolization (PVE) to grow the future remnant liver allows aggressive liver resections while minimizing liver insufficiency.

In this chapter, the cellular and molecular mechanisms of the AHC are discussed. The roles of apoptosis and necrosis during atrophy and liver regeneration during hypertrophy will be described, especially as they relate to PVE. Differences in these mechanisms in the healthy and diseased liver will be examined, and strategies to increase these restorative mechanisms will be outlined.

6.1 The Atrophy–Hypertrophy Complex in Liver Disease

6.1.1 Biliary Obstruction and the AHC

In unilateral biliary obstruction, atrophy of the obstructed side results in hypertrophy of the contralateral side. In this scenario, the AHC possesses not only the three characteristics of AHC, but also ductal inflammation and injury, periductal venous injury, ductal proliferation, sinusoidal widening, and a late progressive septal fibrosis and nodular changes (Table 6.1).[13,14] These findings, along with animal studies, suggest that bile duct obstruction alone is insufficient to cause the AHC.[15]

Various causes of biliary obstruction are associated with the AHC. The AHC has been associated with hilar cholangiocarcinoma,[3] postcholecystectomy biliary strictures,[4] primary sclerosing cholangitis,[5] hepatolithiasis in recurrent pyogenic cholangitis,[6] benign bile duct tumors (e.g., papillomas, cystadenomas, and granular cell tumors), and infestations of the biliary tree (e.g., *Clonorchis sinensis* and *Ascaris lumbricoides*).[7] In large liver lesions causing compression, combined biliary and portal venous obstruction may induce the AHC.[2]

6.1.2 Portal Vein Inflow Obstruction and the AHC

Portal vein occlusion may induce the AHC when disease blocks a lobar or segmental portal vein, causing atrophy through ischemia and hypertrophy of the uninvolved liver. Portal vein obstruction is the most important factor in AHC associated with malignancy.[8] Portal vein embolization achieves the AHC through the same mechanisms and hence shares the same histological characteristics.

Liver malignancies have been implicated as the cause of portal vein occlusion including hilar cholangiocarcinoma, hepatocellular carcinoma, colon cancer metastases, and pancreatic cancer.[16] Other causes of AHC from portal vein occlusion include hydatid cysts near the hilum,[2] hepatolithiasis,[9] and portal vein occlusion from hypercoagulable states.[10]

Table 6.1 The atrophy–hypertrophy complex in liver disease

Anatomic compromise	Mechanism	Diseases	Reference
Biliary obstruction	Ductal inflammation, hepatocyte injury, fibrosis	Large liver tumors (hepatoma)	2
–	–	Cholangiocarcinoma	3
–	–	Bile duct injury	4
–	–	Primary sclerosing cholangitis	5
–	–	Recurrent pyogenic cholangitis	6
–	–	Benign bile duct tumors (cystadenoma)	7
–	–	Bile duct infestations (Chlonorchis)	7
–	–	–	–
Portal vein occlusion	Ischemic cell death	Malignancy (cholangiocarcinoma, hepatoma)	8
–	–	Infestations (echinococcus)	2
–	–	Hepatolithiasis	9
–	–	Thrombosis from hypercoagulability	10
–	–	–	–
Hepatic vein occlusion	Sinusoidal portal hypertension, ischemic necrosis, fibrosis	Budd-Chiari (thrombosis)	11
–	–	Large liver tumors	12

6.1.3 Hepatic Vein Outflow Obstruction and the AHC

The AHC may occur with hepatic vein obstruction from Budd-Chiari Syndrome (BCS) in which at least two of three hepatic veins are occluded.[11] Hepatic vein obstruction is due to hypercoagulable states such as primary myeloproliferative disorders, factor V Leiden mutations, anticardiolipin antibodies, and Behcet's disease. Compression of hepatic veins from liver lesions is the cause in 5% of cases.[12] Outflow obstruction causes sinusoidal pressure, sinusoidal portal hypertension, ischemic necrosis of centrilobular areas, and later fibrosis.[11] Because the caudate lobe drains separately into the inferior vena cava, it hypertrophies in 80% of patients.[17]

6.2 Liver Ischemia and Atrophy

Portal vein occlusion or embolization decreases blood supply with resultant hypoxia, especially in the pericentral area of the liver lobule.[18,19] The features of tissue ischemia are the loss of energy substrate and acidosis.[20] Hepatocytes can maintain their functionality and viability during extended periods of ischemia. One mechanism allowing for this survival is the acidosis that results from hydrolysis of high energy phosphates, accumulation of lactate, and the release of protons from acidic organelles.[21-23] Although reperfusion of tissue restores oxygenation and normal pH, it paradoxically aggravates cell death.[20] The mechanisms causing this ischemia/reperfusion (I/R) injury are multifactorial, and they include reactive oxygen species (ROS), elevation of calcium, activation of injurious catabolic enzymes, and mitochondrial dysfunction. Moreover, the restoration of normal pH without reoxygenation is by itself a major cause of cell death, whereas reoxygenation at acidic pH prevents I/R injury.[20,22-24] In this paradoxical cell death after reperfusion, mitochondrial permeability transition (MPT), a process by which mitochondria lose the integrity of their inner membrane, is a major cause of both necrosis and apoptosis after I/R.[20,22,25]

6.2.1 Mitochondrial Permeability Transition (MPT) and Ischemia/Reperfusion

The MPT was first characterized by Hunter and Haworth in the mid-1970s.[26] This pathological process starts with the opening of high-conductance pores in the mitochondrial inner membranes.[20] Under normal conditions, the mitochondrial membranes are virtually impermeable to all solutes except for those having specific transporters. However, when cells are exposed to insults such as I/R, oxidative stress, and hepatocellular toxins, permeability transition pores in the mitochondria open. Solutes with a molecular mass of up to 1,500 Da can then nonselectively diffuse into the mitochondria,[27] resulting in mitochondrial depolarization, uncoupling of oxidative phosphorylation, and large amplitude swelling leading to ATP depletion and cell death. The MPT can be directly assessed in live cells using confocal microscopy with calcein, a green fluorescing fluorophore.[22,28,29]

Conditions that promote the MPT include calcium loading, inorganic phosphate, alkaline pH, ROS, and nitrogen radicals, whereas those that decrease the MPT include cyclosporin A, magnesium, acidic pH, and phospholipase. Inhibition of the MPT by cyclosporin A or its derivatives prevents I/R injury to cells such as hepatocytes[22] and myocytes.[28]

6.2.2 Hepatocellular Necrosis and Apoptosis After Ischemia/Reperfusion

In hepatocellular necrosis, the plasma membrane blebs are an early sign of ischemic injury and result from cytoskeletal changes from ATP depletion (Fig. 6.1). Although surface blebs protruding into the sinusoidal lumen can impair microcirculation, they are often reversible. However, ruptured blebs cause irreversible cell injury.[31,32] After reperfusion and before cell death, hepatocytes develop a metastable state characterized by mitochondrial permeabilization, loss of lysosomal membrane integrity, coalescence and growth of surface blebs, and cell swelling. After rupture of the plasma membranes, cells release cytosolic enzymes and cofactors needed for cell survival. Furthermore, loss of the permeability barrier in the plasma membranes causes disruption of ion homeostasis and electrical gradient. The resulting cell necrosis can be detected by the uptake of trypan blue or propidium iodide, which are normally excluded by healthy cells.

Reperfusion of ischemic livers can cause apoptosis, characterized by cell shrinkage, caspase activation, chromatin condensation, and nuclear fragmentation.[33,34]

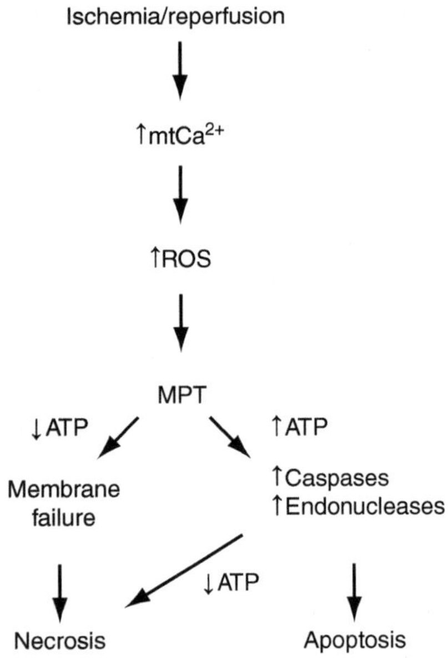

Fig. 6.1 Events leading to hepatocytes death following ischemia/reperfusion. *ATP*, adenosine triphosphate; *MPT*, mitochondrial permeability transition; *mtCa*$^{2+}$, mitochondrial calcium; *ROS*, reactive oxygen species (From Kim et al.[30] With permission)

In contrast to necrosis, apoptotic cell death is associated with inflammation, scarring, and release of intracellular contents and requires ATP (or dATP).[35,36]

Mitochondria are essential to apoptosis as they contain pro-apoptotic proteins such as cytochrome *c*, apoptosis-inducing factor, and Smac/Diablo, which promote apoptosis when released.[37] However, pathological conditions such as I/R, overproduction of tumor necrosis factor alpha (TNF-α), and Fas ligand induce apoptosis by either a mitochondrial or non-mitochondrial pathway.[38,39] In the mitochondrial pathway, release of cytochrome *c* from the mitochondrial intermembrane space to the cytosol forms a complex with apoptosis protease activating factor-1 and ATP (or dATP), leading to activation of caspases 9 and 3.[40] The mechanisms of release of pro-apoptotic proteins remain controversial. In one proposed mechanism, specific mitochondrial channels with Bcl-2 family contribute to their release.[41] In another mechanism, the MPT induces mitochondrial swelling, rupture of mitochondrial outer membranes, and release of cytochrome *c*.[42]

Although necrosis is the predominant mode of cell death after I/R, apoptosis often coexists.[43,44] Pathways to necrosis and apoptosis can be shared, and the MPT is a common initiating mechanism following I/R.[25] If the MPT is widespread and glycolytic energy substrates are unavailable, cells become depleted of ATP, leading to loss of plasma membrane integrity and necrosis. However, if the MPT is limited and cells maintain 15–20% of normal ATP levels, ATP-dependent apoptosis predominates. Over time, cells depleted of ATP may undergo a secondary necrosis that is often observed in pathological conditions. Thus, necrosis and apoptosis can alternate.

6.3 Portal Vein Embolization and Liver Hypertrophy

6.3.1 Anatomical and Histologic Changes During Hypertrophy

The liver undergoes anatomic and histologic changes due to the AHC to varying degrees following PVE or partial hepatectomy. The liver initially rotates about its hilar axis and toward the atrophic side. This rotation can change the relative locations of the bile duct (posterior), hepatic artery (anterolateral), and portal vein (anteromedial) within the hepatoduodenal ligament,[45] which may be important for surgical planning.

Higher rates of hepatocellular proliferation occur in the periportal regions (zone 1), with a decrease toward the central veins (zone 3),[45] and may reflect the concentration gradient of growth factors across the liver lobule.[15] The concept of hepatotrophic factors carried in portal venous blood is further corroborated by the occurrence of (1) atrophy that occurs when portal blood flow is absent[15] and (2) circadian variations in DNA synthesis related to postprandial increases in portal venous blood flow.[46]

6.3.2 Liver Regeneration: Compensatory Hypertrophy and Hyperplasia in Response to Injury

Although 0.0012–0.01% of hepatocytes in the uninjured adult liver replicate at any given time, this percentage increases significantly following two-thirds hepatectomy such that the lost volume is restored within weeks.[45] Although loosely termed hypertrophy, regeneration involves mainly hyperplasia, or an increase in cell number, with some hypertrophy, or increased cell size.[47]

6.3.3 Proliferative Signaling in the Liver Following PVE

Although little is known about the connection between hepatocyte hypertrophy and proliferation after PVE, the early proliferative signals have been defined in animal models of partial hepatectomy. The proliferation of the non-occluded liver appears to precede the loss of liver mass because compensatory hyperplasia begins before atrophy of the occluded liver.[48]

Hemodynamic changes within the portal vein may initiate liver regeneration, as increased portal pressure (shear stress) causes endothelial cells and/or hepatocytes to produce nitric oxide (NO) within 4–6 h after partial hepatectomy. Nitric oxide promotes DNA synthesis in hepatocytes,[49] and conversely, iNOS (inhibitor of nitric oxide synthase) knockout mice show impaired liver regeneration and hepatocyte apoptosis.[50] In addition, NO mediates the inactivation of methionine adenosyltransferase and consequently extracellular signal-regulated kinase (ERK 1/2) activation in vitro.[51]

Hepatocyte swelling from increased portal venous flow in the non-occluded liver may be another initiating mechanism of liver regeneration following hepatectomy or PVE. Swelling activates signaling pathways such as mitogen activated protein kinases (MAPKs), jun N-terminal kinases, and ERK.[47]

Several growth factors and cytokines are important for hepatocyte replication and modulate subsequent transcription factors during liver regeneration. In contrast to liver regeneration after hepatectomy, little is known about the contribution of growth factors, cytokines, or transcription factors after PVE.

Hepatocyte Growth Factor (HGF) binds the HGF receptor, c-met, to induce DNA synthesis in hepatocytes and is produced by nonparenchymal cells in the liver. In animal studies, HGF mRNA in the nonligated lobes increases at 6–24 h, followed by increased DNA synthesis.[52] In contrast, DNA was not increased in the ligated lobe although there was a slight elevation in HGF mRNA expression. Elevated serum HGF may also be important as the liver lobes of rats with continuous HGF infusion after portal vein ligation showed increased weight and DNA synthesis compared to that of untreated rats.[53] *Transforming growth factor alpha* (TGF-α) is an autocrine factor produced by hepatocytes. TGF-α binds the epidermal growth factor receptor (EGFR) to stimulate hepatocyte replication in vitro and regeneration after partial hepatectomy. TGF-α is increased in hepatocytes in both the embolized and non-embolized parts of the human liver.[54] The c-met and EGF receptors are members of the receptor tyrosine kinase family and activate intracellular signaling pathways. Two of these pathways, the phosphoinositide-3 kinase (PI3K)-Akt-mTOR (mammalian target of rapamycin) and the Ras-Raf-MEK cascades, activate several transcription factors such as Ccaat enhancing binding protein (C/EBP) and c-jun, a protein transcription factor, to induce proliferation.

Activin is a growth and differentiation factor of the TGF-β family, which transduces signals to Smads (homologues of *Caenorhabditis elegans* protein *S*MA and *Drosophila* protein, *m*others *a*gainst *d*ecapentaplegic). Activin A, a dimeric protein of two β_A subunits, is expressed primarily in hepatocytes and promotes the termination of liver regeneration.[55] Animal studies show that the pattern of β_A mRNA expression in the ligated and nonligated lobes are similar; the levels increase initially at 12 h after portal vein occlusion, return to baseline, and then increase maximally at 120 h.[56]

TNF-α is a cytokine that primes hepatocytes for replication. TNF-α is produced primarily by Kupffer cells during liver regeneration and activates NF-κB (nuclear factor kappa B) in nonparenchymal cells to promote IL-6 (interleukin-6) production. Liver regeneration is inhibited by anti-TNF-α antibody[57] and in TNF-α receptor type I knockout mice.[58] TNF-α mRNA in the nonligated lobe by cDNA expression array is increased fourfold over controls.[59] In contrast, others have questioned the importance of TNF-α as normal liver regeneration after partial hepatectomy has been observed in TNF-α knockout mice.[60]

IL-6 activates STAT3 (signal transducer and activator of transcription 3) and is released by hepatic stellate and Kupffer cells upon stimulation by TNF-α. Activated STAT3 enters to the nucleus and induces the transcription of immediate-early genes for liver regeneration. IL-6 mRNA is induced in both ligated and nonligated liver lobes in the first hour after portal vein ligation (PVL).[61] Serum IL-6 peaks at 6 h after PVL. An in situ hybridization study showed that IL-6 mRNA in the nonligated lobe was predominantly expressed in sinusoidal endothelial cells around the periportal area (zone 1) 3 h after PVL.[62]

In mouse studies, the transcription factors NF-κB, STAT3, c-fos, c-myc, and c-jun are upregulated after PVL.[61] Increased mRNA of c-fos, c-myc, and c-jun

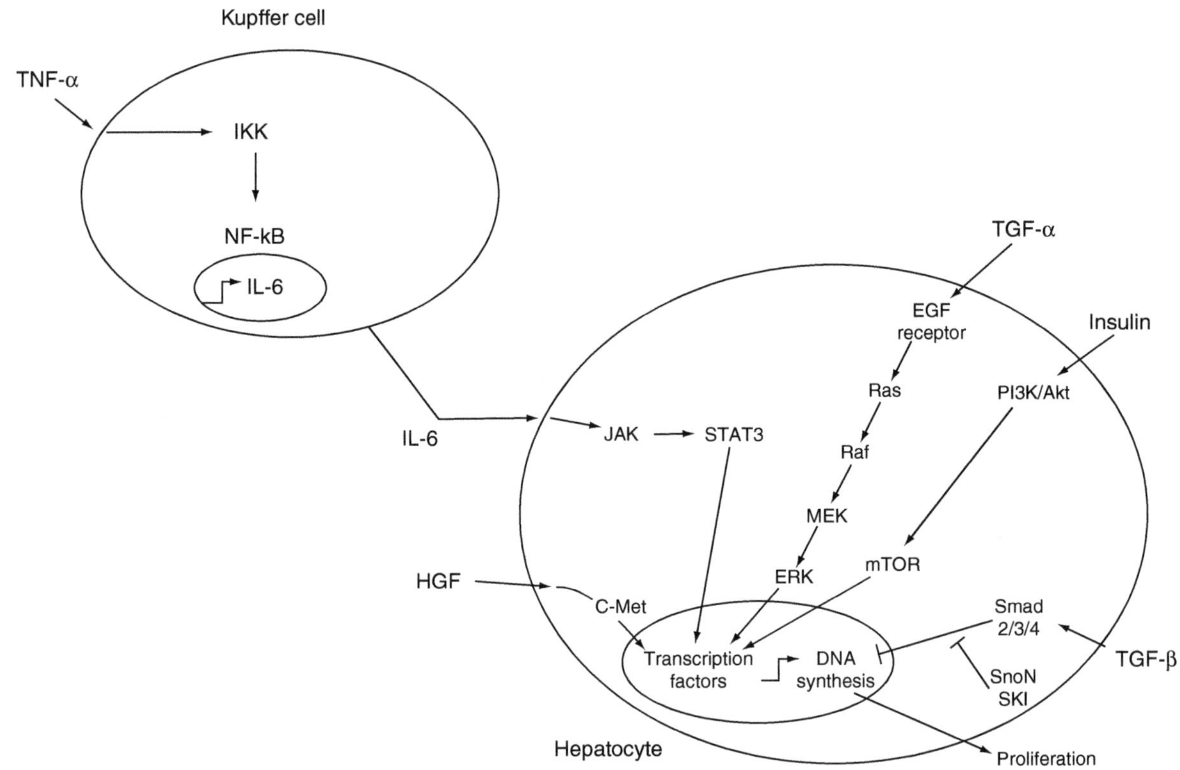

Fig. 6.2 Signaling pathways that modulate the atrophy–hypertrophy complex. *HGF*, hepatocytes growth factor; *IL-6*, interleukin-6; *TGF-α*, transforming growth factor alpha; *TGF-β*, transforming growth factor beta; *TNF-α*, tumor necrosis factor alpha (From Kim et al.[30] With permission)

during the first 2 h are observed in both the ligated and nonligated lobes. However, such findings are of unknown significance as STAT3 levels also increased with sham operations. Recently, a non-stress-PVL rat model which minimizes the effects of surgical stress was established and has been used to examine the signals after PVL.[59] The patterns of NF-κB p65, phosphorylated STAT3, c-fos, and c-jun levels differed. Nonligated lobes demonstrated biphasic activation of these transcription factors with peaks at 1 and 3–6 h after PVL. However, ligated lobes showed decreased levels of activation which reached maximum concentrations 2 h after PVL.

6.3.4 Growth Arrest Following the Hypertrophic Response

Transforming growth factor beta (TGF-β) plays an important growth regulatory role in epithelial cells (Fig. 6.2). TGF-β binds to the type II TGF-β serine/threonine kinase receptor, which then forms a dimer with the type I receptor.[63] Through adaptors, Smads 2 and 3 are recruited to the TGF-β receptor complex and phosphorylated by the type I receptor. This releases Smad 2 or 3 from the transmembrane complex and allows formation of a heterotrimeric complex with the common mediator, Smad 4.[64] The Smad complex then translocates to the nucleus where it activates TGF-β-responsive genes through cooperative interactions with DNA and other DNA-binding proteins. These events activate the Smad pathway with resultant growth arrest and/or apoptosis.

TGF-β signaling is modulated by several different mechanisms. Smad 7, a target gene of TGF-β, acts at the membrane receptor to inhibit Smads 2 and 3. Smurf1 and Smurf2 associate with the nuclear Smad 7 after stimulation by TGF-β. The Smurfs regulate ubiquitination of embryonic liver fodrin (ELF), which can become displaced from the signaling pathway and degraded by proteasomes. Smad activity is modulated by adaptors such as Smad anchor for receptor activation (SARA), filamin, ELF, as well as by functional interactions with other signal transduction pathways.[65-67] Other intracellular regulators of Smad include microtubules that serve as cytoplasmic sequesters, controlling Smad 2 phosphorylation by TGF-β receptor.[68] In the nucleus, gene transactivation can be blocked by binding of the Smad complex to nuclear corepressors such as Ski, SnoN, or TGIF. Additionally, p53 has been shown to modulate TGF-β signaling through the independent binding of the Smads.

Although TGF-β mRNA is increased in the regenerating liver after partial hepatectomy, the proliferating hepatocytes are resistant to its growth inhibitory effects. A recent study provided indirect evidence of active TGF-β signaling by observing an increase in Smad 2 phosphorylation during the first 5 days after hepatectomy.[69] However, concomitant increases in protein levels of SnoN (2–48 h) and Ski (24–72 h) and increased activity of TGF-β repressors also occurred. A complex was formed between SnoN (ski-related novel protein N), Ski (*S*loan *K*ettering oncogene), phosphorylated-Smad 2, Smad 3, and Smad 4 during the 5 days following partial hepatectomy, thus explaining the resistance to TGF-β growth arrest. TGF-β signaling causes early ubiquitination and proteasome-mediated degradation of Ski and SnoN to allow Smad-induced gene activation. The up-regulation of SnoN mRNA can serve as negative feedback to return TGF-β signaling to basal levels.[70]

Inhibition of growth may also involve the cyclin-dependent kinase (CDK)-inhibitory proteins (CDKIs). The p21WAF has bimodal up-regulation as an immediate-early gene within 30 min and at 48–72 h after partial hepatectomy. CDKIs bind cyclin/CDK complexes and p21 to regulate CDK1, CDK2, CDK4, and CDK6. The early expression of p21 may synchronize entry into the G1 phase, while the latter expression may limit growth. The expression of p21 is also modulated by the growth inhibitory cytokines, TGF-β 27and activin.[71]

6.3.5 Hypertrophy in the Injured Liver

Patients with compromised liver function may benefit from preoperative PVE to increase the size of the future liver remnant before extended liver resections.[72] However, the injured liver regenerates less efficiently following both PVE and hepatectomy. In one study, the regeneration rate of the non-embolized lobes in cirrhosis (9.3 cm^3/day) was slower than that of the normal liver (11.8 cm^3/day).[73] Others have found an insignificant difference in the final volume of the non-embolized lobe between (a) cirrhotic versus normal livers,[72] (b) between livers with cirrhosis versus those with mild or moderate fibrosis,[74] and (c) between normal and injured livers due to viral hepatitis.[75]

The metabolic function of the regenerating liver may also impact its ability to grow. Hypertrophy of the non-embolized lobe was shown to be impaired in patients with high serum bilirubin at PVE[76] while biliary decompression before PVE resulted in a normal regenerative rate of 12 cm^3/day.[77] A more direct link between hepatocellular bile acid clearance and regeneration has been established in studies of *Farnesoid X receptor*, a bile acid-regulated nuclear receptor that promotes bile acid metabolism and liver regeneration.[78]

Other clinical factors found to negatively impact liver hypertrophy include diabetes mellitus and male gender.[77] Although the mechanisms underlying these associations remain unclear, one group has found that the fat-secreted plasma protein *adiponectin* decreases fibrosis and promotes regeneration in mouse livers following PH.[79] The fact that adiponectin is found in lower levels in diabetic and obese patients may be one reason for the blunted hypertrophic response found in diabetics.

Others have used animal models to demonstrate the resilience of liver regeneration to injury. In one study using PVL in a rat model, both cirrhotic and noncirrhotic hepatocytes had comparable elevations in mitotic index at 3 days. However, DNA synthesis was delayed in the cirrhotic livers.[73] In another study, the common bile duct was ligated 5 days before PVL in a rat model, and then DNA polymerase α expression, a marker of hepatocyte replication, was measured. These studies showed that the induction of liver hypertrophy in the cholestatic rats was similar to that of the noncholestatic rats following PVL.[80]

6.3.6 The Roles of Non-hepatocytes During Liver Regeneration

After PH, mature hepatocytes proliferate maximally at 24 h, followed by biliary ductal cells, Kupffer cells, stellate cells, and lastly, endothelial cells.[81] One important component of liver regeneration is the *extracellular matrix (ECM)*. Urokinase-like plasminogen activator (uPA) initiates the degradation of the ECM through activation of the matrix metalloproteinase (MMP) cascade.[82]

Within 5 min of partial hepatectomy, increased uPA activity correlates with the conversion of inactive pro-MMP-2 and pro-MMP-9 to their active forms, and initiates disruption of the ECM.[83] This uPA-dependent degradation of the ECM causes release of bound HGF with a subsequent increase in serum HGF concentration.[84] In uPA mice treated with monoclonal anti-Fas antibody (a stimulator of apoptosis), serum HGF concentrations increased later than in controls, but delayed HGF release was reversed upon transfection with the uPA gene.[85] Collectively, these studies suggest that uPA is an important initiator of free HGF and that ECM remodeling is needed in the early phase of liver regeneration.

Oval cells are dormant hepatic stem cells that possess oval nuclei and scant cytoplasm and reside in the bile ductules and canals of Hering. These cells can differentiate into cholangiocytes or hepatocytes. Hepatocyte differentiation leads to the formation of intermediate hepatocyte-like cells, which are defined as polygonal cells with a size between that of oval cells and hepatocytes. Some have shown that repopulation of the liver occurs following drug-induced injury that normally precludes mature hepatocyte replication, suggesting that regeneration occurs through the stem/oval cell compartment.[86]

Stellate cells are pericytes in the perisinusoidal space which, when active during liver injury, contribute to fibrosis. Recently, studies have shown that stellate cells may be involved in regenerative paracrine signaling following the binding of Lymphotoxin-beta (LT-beta), a member of the tumor necrosis factor family.[87]

Bone marrow or *hematopoietic stem cells* have been shown to enter the liver through the portal vasculature. During and after episodes of severe liver injury, a large proportion of mature hepatocytes and cholangiocytes are derived from hematopoietic stem cells.[88] Severely injured livers regenerate after transplantation of bone marrow-derived stem cells which fuse with hepatocytes.[89] Further studies are needed to define the potential uses of stem cell transplantation as a therapy for end-stage liver disease.

6.4 Other Factors and Potential Strategies to Improve the Hypertrophic Response

Many factors have been identified that may be used to modulate hepatocytes proliferation. *Bone morphogenic protein-7* (BMP-7), a protein involved in liver organogenesis, has been shown to enhance liver regeneration following PH in an animal model.[90] *Prostaglandin E(1) in lipid microspheres* (Lipo PGE(1)) has been shown to increase DNA synthesis and survival following 90% PH in rats.[91] *Hepatopoietin* (HPO) has been shown to stimulate proliferation in cultured hepatocytes and hepatoma cells and liver regeneration in animal studies.[92] In a *Cdc42* knockout mouse model, decreased DNA synthesis following partial hepatecomty was observed suggesting that Cdc42 played an important role in liver regeneration.[93]

Ischemic preconditioning, whereby a measured duration of ischemia is delivered to the liver prior to a surgical intervention, may take advantage of some of these proliferative factors. Ischemic preconditioning promotes liver regeneration in animal models by up-regulating growth-promoting factors, suppressing growth-inhibitory factors, and preserving energy levels.[94]

Regeneration may also be potentiated by changing the liver cell population itself. In one prospective study of patients undergoing preoperative PVE for the resection of liver malignancies, those patients receiving preoperative stem cells showed significantly increased remnant liver growth as compared to controls.[95] Others have found that transplanted bone marrow cells can generate hepatocytes and help in liver repair and regeneration.[96] Although preliminary, these strategies may someday be used in conjunction with preoperative PVE to maximize the growth of the future liver remnant.

In summary, the atrophy–hypertrophy complex is a regulated compensatory response to liver injury which reestablishes adequate liver function for survival. The AHC involves anatomic, histologic, cellular, and molecular processes that result in partial liver loss and its restoration. The mechanisms involved are both intrinsic and extrinsic to the liver and involve both physical forces and biochemical interactions. These mechanisms may be compromised in the injured liver. When used in conjunction to portal vein embolization, the AHC may someday be exploited to permit curative resections in patients with marginal liver function.

References

1. Bellentani S, Hardison WG, Manenti F. Mechanisms of liver adaptation to prolonged selective biliary obstruction (SBO) in the rat. *J Hepatol.* 1985;1:525-535.

2. Rozanes I, Acunas B, Celik L, et al. CT in lobar atrophy of the liver caused by alveolar echinococcosis. *J Comput Assist Tomogr*. 1992;16:216-218.
3. Hadjis NS, Adam A, Gibson R, et al. Nonoperative approach to hilar cancer determined by the atrophy-hypertrophy complex. *Am J Surg*. 1989;157:395-399.
4. Hadjis NS, Blumgart LH. Role of liver atrophy, hepatic resection and hepatocyte hyperplasia in the development of portal hypertension in biliary disease. *Gut*. 1987;28: 1022-1028.
5. Hadjis NS, Adam A, Blenkharn I, et al. Primary sclerosing cholangitis associated with liver atrophy. *Am J Surg*. 1989;158:43-47.
6. Jeyarajah DR. Recurrent pyogenic cholangitis. *Curr Treat Options Gastroenterol*. 2004;7:91-98.
7. Rana SS, Bhasin DK, Nanda M, et al. Parasitic infestations of the biliary tract. *Curr Gastroenterol Rep*. 2007;9:156-164.
8. Lorigan JG, Charnsangavej C, Carrasco CH, et al. Atrophy with compensatory hypertrophy of the liver in hepatic neoplasms: radiographic findings. *AJR Am J Roentgenol*. 1988; 150:1291-1295.
9. Ishida H, Naganuma H, Konno K, et al. Lobar atrophy of the liver. *Abdom Imaging*. 1998;23:150-153.
10. Vilgrain V, Condat B, Bureau C, et al. Atrophy-hypertrophy complex in patients with cavernous transformation of the portal vein: CT evaluation. *Radiology*. 2006;241:149-155.
11. Valla DC. The diagnosis and management of the Budd-Chiari syndrome: consensus and controversies. *Hepatology*. 2003;38:793-803.
12. Denninger MH, Chait Y, Casadevall N, et al. Cause of portal or hepatic venous thrombosis in adults: the role of multiple concurrent factors. *Hepatology*. 2000;31:587-591.
13. Schaffner F, Bacchin PG, Hutterer F, et al. Mechanism of cholestasis. 4. Structural and biochemical changes in the liver and serum in rats after bile duct ligation. *Gastroenterology*. 1971;60:888-897.
14. Gall JA, Bhathal PS. Origin and involution of hyperplastic bile ductules following total biliary obstruction. *Liver*. 1990;10:106-115.
15. Schweizer W, Duda P, Tanner S, et al. Experimental atrophy/hypertrophy complex (AHC) of the liver: portal vein, but not bile duct obstruction, is the main driving force for the development of AHC in the rat. *J Hepatol*. 1995;23:71-78.
16. Hann LE, Getrajdman GI, Brown KT, et al. Hepatic lobar atrophy: association with ipsilateral portal vein obstruction. *AJR Am J Roentgenol*. 1996;167:1017-1021.
17. Matthieu D, Kracht M, Zafrani E, Dhumeaux D, Vasile N. Budd-Chiari syndrome. In: Ferrucci J, Matthieu D, eds. *Advances in Hepatobiliary Radiology*. St. Louis: CV Mosby Company; 1990:3-28.
18. Lemasters JJ, Ji S, Thurman RG. Centrilobular injury following hypoxia in isolated, perfused rat liver. *Science*. 1981;213:661-663.
19. Jungermann K, Kietzmann T. Oxygen: modulator of metabolic zonation and disease of the liver. *Hepatology*. 2000;31: 255-260.
20. Kim JS, He L, Lemasters JJ. Mitochondrial permeability transition: a common pathway to necrosis and apoptosis. *Biochem Biophys Res Commun*. 2003;304:463-470.
21. Gores GJ, Nieminen AL, Wray BE, et al. Intracellular pH during "chemical hypoxia" in cultured rat hepatocytes. Protection by intracellular acidosis against the onset of cell death. *J Clin Invest*. 1989;83:386-396.
22. Qian T, Nieminen AL, Herman B, et al. Mitochondrial permeability transition in pH-dependent reperfusion injury to rat hepatocytes. *Am J Physiol*. 1997;273:C1783-C1792.
23. Currin RT, Gores GJ, Thurman RG, et al. Protection by acidotic pH against anoxic cell killing in perfused rat liver: evidence for a pH paradox. *FASEB J*. 1991;5:207-210.
24. Kim JS, He L, Qian T, et al. Role of the mitochondrial permeability transition in apoptotic and necrotic death after ischemia/reperfusion injury to hepatocytes. *Curr Mol Med*. 2003;3:527-535.
25. Kim JS, Qian T, Lemasters JJ. Mitochondrial permeability transition in the switch from necrotic to apoptotic cell death in ischemic rat hepatocytes. *Gastroenterology*. 2003;124: 494-503.
26. Hunter DR, Haworth RA, Southard JH. Relationship between configuration, function, and permeability in calcium-treated mitochondria. *J Biol Chem*. 1976;251:5069-5077.
27. Bernardi P. Mitochondrial transport of cations: channels, exchangers, and permeability transition. *Physiol Rev*. 1999;79:1127-1155.
28. Kim JS, Jin Y, Lemasters JJ. Reactive oxygen species, but not Ca^{2+} overloading, trigger pH- and mitochondrial permeability transition-dependent death of adult rat myocytes after ischemia-reperfusion. *Am J Physiol Heart Circ Physiol*. 2006;290:H2024-H2034.
29. Kim JS, Ohshima S, Pediaditakis P, et al. Nitric oxide protects rat hepatocytes against reperfusion injury mediated by the mitochondrial permeability transition. *Hepatology*. 2004;39:1533-1543.
30. Kim RD, Kim JS, Watanabe G, Mohuczy D, Behrns KE. Liver regeneration and the atrophy-hypertrophy complex. *Semin Intervent Radiol*. 2008;25:92-103.
31. Herman B, Nieminen AL, Gores GJ, et al. Irreversible injury in anoxic hepatocytes precipitated by an abrupt increase in plasma membrane permeability. *FASEB J*. 1988;2:146-151.
32. Nieminen AL, Gores GJ, Wray BE, et al. Calcium dependence of bleb formation and cell death in hepatocytes. *Cell Calcium*. 1988;9:237-246.
33. Gao W, Bentley RC, Madden JF, et al. Apoptosis of sinusoidal endothelial cells is a critical mechanism of preservation injury in rat liver transplantation. *Hepatology*. 1998;27:1652-1660.
34. Natori S, Selzner M, Valentino KL, et al. Apoptosis of sinusoidal endothelial cells occurs during liver preservation injury by a caspase-dependent mechanism. *Transplantation*. 1999;68:89-96.
35. Richter C, Schweizer M, Cossarizza A, et al. Control of apoptosis by the cellular ATP level. *FEBS Lett*. 1996;378:107-110.
36. Leist M, Single B, Castoldi AF, et al. Intracellular adenosine triphosphate (ATP) concentration: a switch in the decision between apoptosis and necrosis. *J Exp Med*. 1997;185: 1481-1486.
37. Galluzzi L, Larochette N, Zamzami N, et al. Mitochondria as therapeutic targets for cancer chemotherapy. *Oncogene*. 2006;25:4812-4830.
38. Scaffidi C, Fulda S, Srinivasan A, et al. Two CD95 (APO-1/Fas) signaling pathways. *EMBO J*. 1998;17:1675-1687.
39. Hatano E, Bradham CA, Stark A, et al. The mitochondrial permeability transition augments Fas-induced apoptosis in mouse hepatocytes. *J Biol Chem*. 2000;275:11814-11823.

40. Wang X. The expanding role of mitochondria in apoptosis. *Genes Dev*. 2001;15:2922-2933.
41. Wei MC, Zong WX, Cheng EH, et al. Proapoptotic BAX and BAK: a requisite gateway to mitochondrial dysfunction and death. *Science*. 2001;292:727-730.
42. Zamzami N, Susin SA, Marchetti P, et al. Mitochondrial control of nuclear apoptosis. *J Exp Med*. 1996;183:1533-1544.
43. Gujral JS, Bucci TJ, Farhood A, et al. Mechanism of cell death during warm hepatic ischemia-reperfusion in rats: apoptosis or necrosis? *Hepatology*. 2001;33:397-405.
44. Kohli V, Madden JF, Bentley RC, et al. Calpain mediates ischemic injury of the liver through modulation of apoptosis and necrosis. *Gastroenterology*. 1999;116:168-178.
45. Michalopoulos GK, DeFrances MC. Liver regeneration. *Science*. 1997;276:60-66.
46. Barbason H, Bouzahzah B, Herens C, et al. Circadian synchronization of liver regeneration in adult rats: the role played by adrenal hormones. *Cell Tissue Kinet*. 1989;22:451-460.
47. Kim RD, Stein GS, Chari RS. Impact of cell swelling on proliferative signal transduction in the liver. *J Cell Biochem*. 2001;83:56-69.
48. Lambotte L, Li B, Leclercq I, et al. The compensatory hyperplasia (liver regeneration) following ligation of a portal branch is initiated before the atrophy of the deprived lobes. *J Hepatol*. 2000;32:940-945.
49. Hortelano S, Dewez B, Genaro AM, et al. Nitric oxide is released in regenerating liver after partial hepatectomy. *Hepatology*. 1995;21:776-786.
50. Rai RM, Lee FY, Rosen A, et al. Impaired liver regeneration in inducible nitric oxide synthase deficient mice. *Proc Natl Acad Sci USA*. 1998;95:13829-13834.
51. Garcia-Trevijano ER, Martinez-Chantar ML, Latasa MU, et al. NO sensitizes rat hepatocytes to proliferation by modifying S-adenosylmethionine levels. *Gastroenterology*. 2002;122: 1355-1363.
52. Uemura T, Miyazaki M, Hirai R, et al. Different expression of positive and negative regulators of hepatocyte growth in growing and shrinking hepatic lobes after portal vein branch ligation in rats. *Int J Mol Med*. 2000;5:173-179.
53. Kaido T, Yoshikawa A, Seto S, et al. Hepatocyte growth factor supply accelerates compensatory hypertrophy caused by portal branch ligation in normal and jaundiced rats. *J Surg Res*. 1999;85:115-119.
54. Kusaka K, Imamura H, Tomiya T, et al. Expression of transforming growth factor-alpha and -beta in hepatic lobes after hemihepatic portal vein embolization. *Dig Dis Sci*. 2006;51: 1404-1412.
55. Vejda S, Cranfield M, Peter B, et al. Expression and dimerization of the rat activin subunits betaC and betaE: evidence for the ormation of novel activin dimers. *J Mol Endocrinol*. 2002;28:137-148.
56. Takamura K, Tsuchida K, Miyake H, et al. Activin and activin receptor expression changes in liver regeneration in rat. *J Surg Res*. 2005;126:3-11.
57. Akerman P, Cote P, Yang SQ, et al. Antibodies to tumor necrosis factor-alpha inhibit liver regeneration after partial hepatectomy. *Am J Physiol*. 1992;263:G579-G585.
58. Yamada Y, Kirillova I, Peschon JJ, et al. Initiation of liver growth by tumor necrosis factor: deficient liver regeneration in mice lacking type I tumor necrosis factor receptor. *Proc Natl Acad Sci USA*. 1997;94:1441-1446.
59. Yokoyama S, Yokoyama Y, Kawai T, et al. Biphasic activation of liver regeneration-associated signals in an early stage after portal vein branch ligation. *Biochem Biophys Res Commun*. 2006;349:732-739.
60. Hayashi H, Nagaki M, Imose M, et al. Normal liver regeneration and liver cell apoptosis after partial hepatectomy in tumor necrosis factor-alpha-deficient mice. *Liver Int*. 2005; 25:162-170.
61. Starkel P, Horsmans Y, Sempoux C, et al. After portal branch ligation in rat, nuclear factor kappaB, interleukin-6, signal transducers and activators of transcription 3, c-fos, c-myc, and c-jun are similarly induced in the ligated and nonligated lobes. *Hepatology*. 1999;29:1463-1470.
62. Kobayashi S, Nagino M, Yokoyama Y, et al. Evaluation of hepatic interleukin-6 secretion following portal vein ligation using a minimal surgical stress model. *J Surg Res*. 2006;135: 27-33.
63. Wrana JL, Attisano L, Wieser R, et al. Mechanism of activation of the TGF-beta receptor. *Nature*. 1994;370:341-347.
64. Abdollah S, Ias-Silva M, Tsukazaki T. TbetaRI phosphorylation of Smad2 on Ser465 and Ser467 is required for Smad2-Smad4 complex formation and signaling. *J Biol Chem*. 1997;272:27678-27685.
65. Wu G, Chen YG, Ozdamar B, et al. Structural basis of Smad2 recognition by the Smad anchor for receptor activation. *Science*. 2000;287:92-97.
66. Hocevar BA, Smine A, Xu XX, et al. The adaptor molecule Disabled-2 links the transforming growth factor beta receptors to the Smad pathway. *EMBO J*. 2001;20:2789-2801.
67. Mishra L, Marshall B. Adaptor proteins and ubiquinators in TGF-beta signaling. *Cytokine Growth Factor Rev*. 2006;17: 75-87.
68. Dong C, Li Z, Alvarez R Jr, et al. Microtubule binding to Smads may regulate TGF beta activity. *Mol Cell*. 2000;5:27-34.
69. Macias-Silva M, Li W, Leu JI, et al. Up-regulated transcriptional repressors SnoN and Ski bind Smad proteins to antagonize transforming growth factor-beta signals during liver regeneration. *J Biol Chem*. 2002;277:28483-28490.
70. Stroschein SL, Wang W, Zhou S, et al. Negative feedback regulation of TGF-beta signaling by the SnoN oncoprotein. *Science*. 1999;286:771-774.
71. Albrecht JH, Meyer AH, Hu MY. Regulation of cyclin-dependent kinase inhibitor p21(WAF1/Cip1/Sdi1) gene expression in hepatic regeneration. *Hepatology*. 1997;25:557-563.
72. Farges O, Belghiti J, Kianmanesh R, et al. Portal vein embolization before right hepatectomy: prospective clinical trial. *Ann Surg*. 2003;237:208-217.
73. Lee KC, Kinoshita H, Hirohashi K, et al. Extension of surgical indications for hepatocellular carcinoma by portal vein embolization. *World J Surg*. 1993;17:109-115.
74. Azoulay D, Castaing D, Krissat J, et al. Percutaneous portal vein embolization increases the feasibility and safety of major liver resection for hepatocellular carcinoma in injured liver. *Ann Surg*. 2000;232:665-672.
75. Wakabayashi H, Ishimura K, Okano K, et al. Application of preoperative portal vein embolization before major hepatic resection in patients with normal or abnormal liver parenchyma. *Surgery*. 2002;131:26-33.
76. Imamura H, Shimada R, Kubota M, et al. Preoperative portal vein embolization: an audit of 84 patients. *Hepatology*. 1999;29:1099-1105.

77. Nagino M, Nimura Y, Kamiya J, et al. Changes in hepatic lobe volume in biliary tract cancer patients after right portal vein embolization. *Hepatology*. 1995;21:434-439.
78. Xing X, Burgermeister E, Geisler F, et al. Hematopoietically expressed homeobox is a target gene of farnesoid X receptor in chenodeoxycholic acid-induced liver hypertrophy. *Hepatology*. 2009;49(3):979-988.
79. Ezaki H, Yoshida Y, Saji Y, et al. Delayed liver regeneration after partial hepatectomy in adiponectin knockout mice. *Biochem Biophys Res Commun*. 2009;378:68-72.
80. Mizuno S, Nimura Y, Suzuki H, et al. Portal vein branch occlusion induces cell proliferation of cholestatic rat liver. *J Surg Res*. 1996;60:249-257.
81. Michalopoulos GK. Liver regeneration. *J Cell Physiol*. 2007;213(2):286-300.
82. Blasi F. Urokinase and urokinase receptor: a paracrine/autocrine system regulating cell migration and invasiveness. *Bioessays*. 1993;15:105-111.
83. Mars WM, Liu ML, Kitson RP, et al. Immediate early detection of urokinase receptor after partial hepatectomy and its implications for initiation of liver regeneration. *Hepatology*. 1995;21:1695-1701.
84. Liu ML, Mars WM, Zarnegar R, et al. Uptake and distribution of hepatocyte growth factor in normal and regenerating adult rat liver. *Am J Pathol*. 1994;144:129-140.
85. Shimizu M, Hara A, Okuno M, et al. Mechanism of retarded liver regeneration in plasminogen activator-deficient mice: impaired activation of hepatocyte growth factor after Fas-mediated massive hepatic apoptosis. *Hepatology*. 2001;33: 569-576.
86. Gordon GJ, Coleman WB, Grisham JW. Temporal analysis of hepatocyte differentiation by small hepatocyte-like progenitor cells during liver regeneration in retrorsine-exposed rats. *Am J Pathol*. 2000;157:771-786.
87. Ruddell RG, Knight B, Tirnitz-Parker JE, et al. Lymphotoxin-beta receptor signaling regulates hepatic stellate cell function and wound healing in a murine model of chronic liver injury. *Hepatology*. 2009;49:227-239.
88. Roskams TA, Libbrecht L, Desmet VJ. Progenitor cells in diseased human liver. *Semin Liver Dis*. 2003;23:385-396.
89. Wang X, Willenbring H, Akkari Y, et al. Cell fusion is the principal source of bone-marrow-derived hepatocytes. *Nature*. 2003;422:897-901.
90. Sugimoto H, Yang C, LeBleu VS, et al. BMP-7 functions as a novel hormone to facilitate liver regeneration. *FASEB J*. 2007;21:256-264.
91. Ando K, Miyazaki M, Shimizu H, et al. Beneficial effects of prostaglandin E(1) incorporated in lipid microspheres on liver injury and regeneration after 90% partial hepatectomy in rats. *Eur Surg Res*. 2000;32:155-161.
92. Gatzidou E, Kouraklis G, Theocharis S. Insights on augmenter of liver regeneration cloning and function. *World J Gastroenterol*. 2006;12:4951-4958.
93. Yuan H, Zhang H, Wu X, et al. Hepatocyte-specific deletion of Cdc42 results in delayed liver regeneration after partial hepatectomy in mice. *Hepatology*. 2009;49:240-249.
94. Jaeschke H. Molecular mechanisms of hepatic ischemia-reperfusion injury and preconditioning. *Am J Physiol Gastrointest Liver Physiol*. 2003;284:G15-G26.
95. Furst G, Schulte am EJ, Poll LW. Portal vein embolization and autologous CD133+ bone marrow stem cells for liver regeneration: initial experience. *Radiology*. 2007;243:171-179.
96. Dorrell C, Grompe M. Liver repair by intra- and extrahepatic progenitors. *Stem Cell Rev*. 2005;1:61-64.

Part II

Preoperative Assessment

7 Preoperative Imaging of Liver Cancers: Hepatocellular Carcinoma

Byung Ihn Choi and Jeong Min Lee

Abstract

Hepatocellular carcinoma (HCC) is a tumor of increasing incidence that usually arises in cirrhotic liver. Worldwide, HCC is the sixth most common cancer with 626,000 new cases in 2002, and is also the third most common cause of cancer death. Both surgical resection and transplantation are highly effective in the treatment of patients with localized HCC. Typically, these surgical modalities complement each other, as patients with preserved liver function are candidates for resection and those with poor underlying liver function would be directed toward liver transplantation. Liver resection for HCC requires rigorous patient selection, including evaluation of the stage of the tumor and of the functional reserve of the liver. Cross-sectional imaging modalities such as ultrasound (US), computed tomography (CT), and magnetic resonance imaging (MRI) play a crucial role in the diagnosis and tumor staging of HCC and thus enhance the safety and efficacy of hepatic resection. These modalities, along with biologic scanning techniques such as positron emission tomography (PET), are also invaluable for staging malignancies so as to improve patient selection and thereby optimize long-term surgical outcome.

Keywords

Imaging of liver cancers • Hepatocellular carcinoma • Liver cancer • MRI of liver • CT of liver • PET imaging of liver

Hepatocellular carcinoma (HCC) is a tumor of increasing incidence that usually arises in cirrhotic liver.[1] Worldwide, HCC is the sixth most common cancer with 626,000 new cases in 2002, and is also the third most common cause of cancer death.[2] Recent evidence would suggest that its incidence is on the rise in Western world.[3,4] The median survival in unresectable cases is less than 4 months and under a year for untreated patients with less advanced disease.[5-7] Both surgical resection and transplantation are highly effective in the treatment of patients with localized HCC. Typically, these surgical modalities complement each other, as patients with preserved liver function are candidates for resection and those with poor underlying liver function would be directed toward liver transplantation.[8] Liver resection for HCC requires rigorous patient selection, including evaluation of the stage of the tumor and of the functional reserve of the liver.[9] According to the

B.I. Choi (✉)
Department of Radiology, Seoul National University Hospital, 101 Daehangno, Jongno-gu, Seoul 110-744, South Korea
e-mail: bichoi@snu.ac.kr

D.C. Madoff et al. (eds.), *Venous Embolization of the Liver*,
DOI 10.1007/978-1-84882-122-4_7,

current TNM/UICC staging system for HCC,[10] most consider stage IIIB, IIIC, or IV disease to be incurable by resection.[10] Cross-sectional imaging modalities such as ultrasound (US), computed tomography (CT), and magnetic resonance imaging (MRI) play a crucial role in the diagnosis and tumor staging of HCC and thus enhance the safety and efficacy of hepatic resection. These modalities, along with biologic scanning techniques such as positron emission tomography (PET), are also invaluable for staging malignancies so as to improve patient selection and thereby optimize long-term surgical outcome.[8]

The diagnosis of HCC has significantly changed over the past decade from the use of invasive procedures such as angiography or biopsy to noninvasive imaging including contrast-enhanced ultrasound (US), multidetector row CT (MDCT), and magnetic resonance imaging (MRI).[11] The hallmark of HCC during CT scan or MRI is the presence of arterial enhancement followed by washout.[12] The most recent guideline issued by the American Association for the Study of Liver Diseases (AASLD) states that a noninvasive diagnosis of HCC can be made if a lesion greater than 2 cm shows typical vascular enhancement pattern on a single dynamic imaging study or if a lesion measuring 1–2 cm shows these features at two dynamic imaging studies.[13,14] The use of such criteria avoids the need to biopsy most lesions and thus removes the small (<2%) risk of tumor seeding down the needle tract. An atypical enhancement pattern on either dynamic study requires a formal biopsy of the nodule for the diagnosis. Unlike most other solid organ malignancies in which there is universal agreement on a single staging system, there are several staging systems that have been established for HCC. These include the modified TNM,[10] Barcelona Clinic Liver Cancer (BCLC),[15] Okuda et al.,[7] Cancer of the Liver Italian Program, and other classifications.[16] The lack of a consensus on an HCC staging system is attributed to several factors: (a) the heterogeneity in diagnostic criteria of HCC when histological confirmation is not available and (b) the outcome is influenced not only by the cancer burden but also by the underlying liver function and the patient's general physical status.[14] In Western countries, Barcelona Clinic Liver Cancer (BCLC) staging classification is most commonly used as the criteria of hepatectomy for patients with HCC, which is based mainly on portal hypertension. On the other hand, in eastern countries, the result of indocyanine green (ICG) retention test is employed. In recent years, reports have been made on cases in which patients who did not meet the BCLC criteria because of portal hypertension and tumor numbers but who met the eastern criteria underwent hepatectomy with good surgical results. Thus, criteria for hepatectomy are still debated.[17,18] Although there is no consensus as to which staging system is best in predicting the survivals of patients with HCC, many have adopted the BCLC group's proposal of five stages, providing a link to a treatment algorithm.[13]

The role of imaging in the diagnosis and staging of HCC is thus: (1) to offer sensitive and specific screening in patients at risk; (2) to definitively characterize lesions and diagnose HCC without the need for biopsy; (3) to evaluate tumor burden by determining the number and location of hepatic lesions, tumor size, the presence of major vascular invasion, nodal disease, and distant metastases; and (4) to radiologically contribute to the evaluation of the extent of chronic liver disease and portal hypertension.[14] Elucidation of the last two issues will enable the treating physician to determine resectability and suitability for transplantation, ablative therapies, embolization, or systemic antitumor agents. At a minimum, all candidates for hepatic resection should undergo either CT or MRI. Typically, patients with the firm diagnosis of HCC should undergo staging with a triphasic CT of the abdomen and a CT of the chest and pelvis. An MRI may alternatively be used to stage the abdominal cavity. Adjunctive studies such as bone scan or positron emission tomography (PET) imaging should be used more selectively.

7.1 Imaging Diagnosis of HCC

7.1.1 Ultrasound

Ultrasound (US) has a dual role in the diagnostic algorithm for HCC. In addition to being a primary screening modality in patients at risk, contrast-enhanced US offers the potential for definitive diagnosis.[14] HCC develops in approximately 4% of cirrhotic patients each year, so new focal lesions in cirrhotic livers with typical imaging characteristics have a high probability of being HCCs.[1,4,12] The typical US appearance of HCC is a heterogeneous nodule with peripheral sonolucency, lateral shadowing caused by a fibrotic pseudocapsule, and posterior acoustic enhancement[19] (Fig. 7.1). However, there is considerable variability in the appearance of HCC, and therefore, any nodule detected in the cirrhotic liver should be regarded with suspicion.[11] A systemic

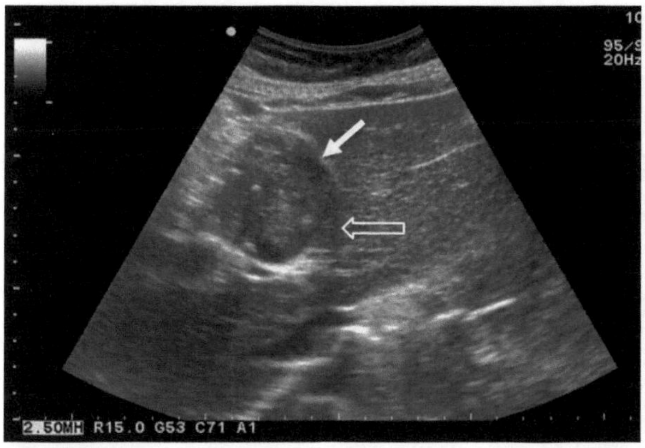

Fig. 7.1 Ultrasound examination demonstrates a round-shaped HCC with hypoechogenicity (*arrow*). It also shows subtle lateral shadows (*open arrow*)

review[20] evaluating the accuracy of US for deterring HCC demonstrated that the sensitivity was 60% and specificity was 97%. Contrast-enhanced US using microbubbles provides microflow imaging of nodules and demonstrates detailed vascular features of HCC[21]: strong intratumoral enhancement in the arterial phase (AP) followed by rapid washout in the portal venous phase (PVP) or delayed phases (DP). Recent studies of contrast-enhanced US[21-24] demonstrated that it provides sensitivities, specificities, and positive predictive values of greater than 90% in diagnosing HCC. Although in expert hands, US can determine the number and extent of lesions, the presence of hepatic portal vein tumor invasion or intrabiliary extension of tumor, and presence of portal hypertension, it is generally used as an initial assessment tool at most centers. For further characterization and staging of HCC detected with US, CT, or MRI is commonly used.

7.1.2 Computed Tomography

CT is the most commonly used imaging modality in diagnosing HCC due to its widespread availability and short examination time. A triphasic examination of the liver with AP, PVP, and DP scan can be regarded as standard today.[11] HCC typically presents as a hyperattenuated lesion in AP with following washout to iso- or mostly hypoattenuation in the PVP or DP (Fig. 7.2). The added value of DP scans for improving detection of HCC by showing washout has been demonstrated in the literature.[14] It is likely due to arterial neovascularization and is greater in HCC nodules than in the surrounding nonneoplastic hepatic parenchyma, and in delayed phases, there is early venous drainage.[25] Although other morphologic features of HCC such as the peripheral enhancing rim on DP images suggest-

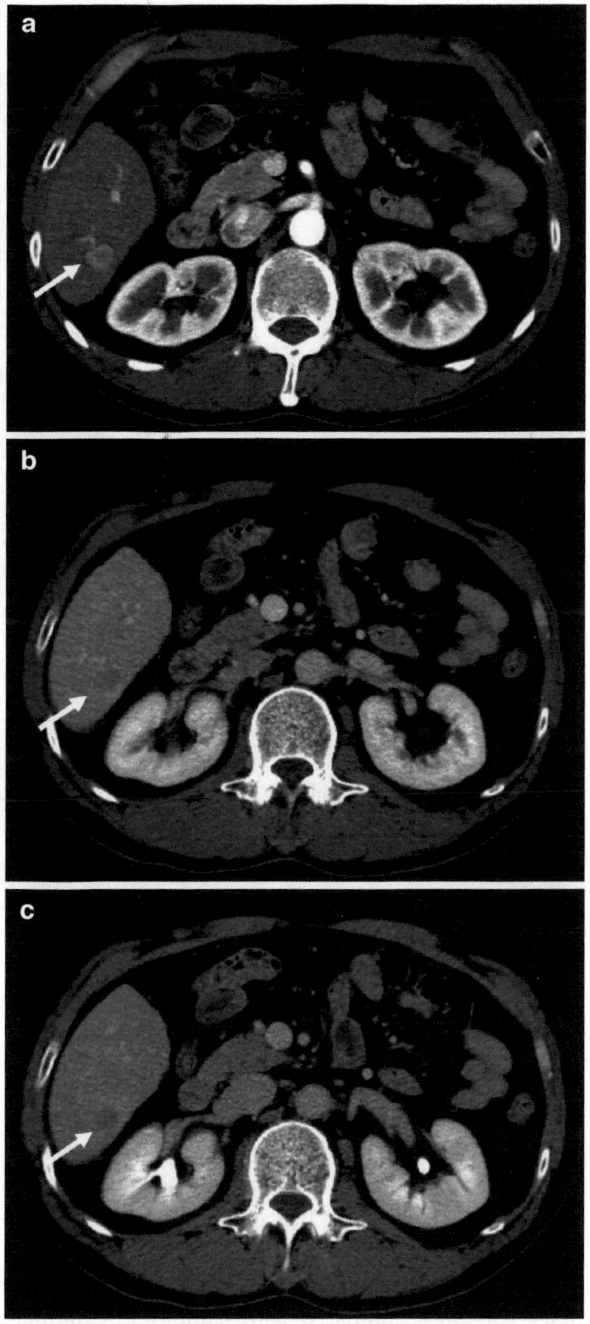

Fig. 7.2 Small classic hepatocellular carcinoma in hepatitis B virus-related liver cirrhosis. Transverse images obtained at (**a**) the arterial, (**b**) portal venous, and (**c**) delayed phase show a HCC in the right lobe of the liver (*arrow*) with arterial hyperenhancement and washout

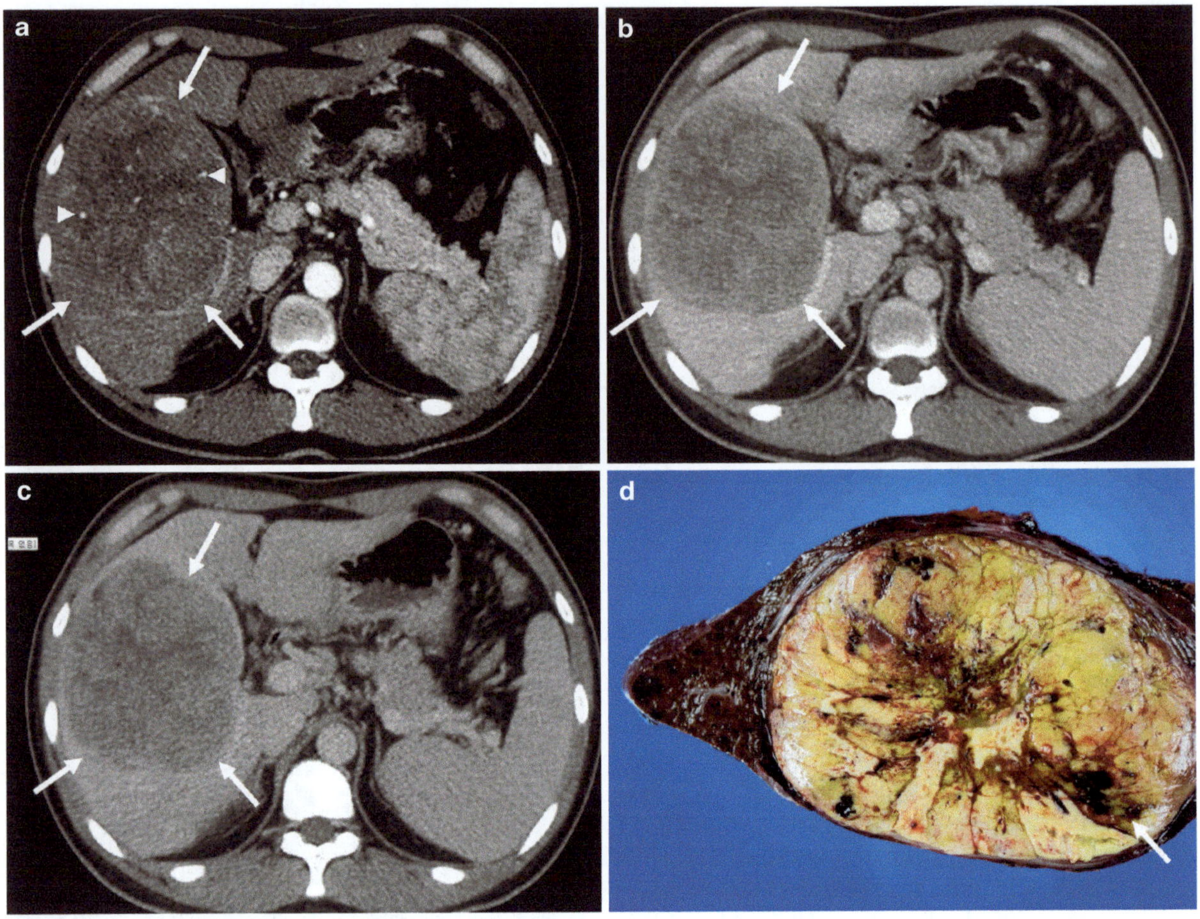

Fig. 7.3 Large hepatocellular carcinoma in hepatitis B virus-associated liver cirrhosis. Transverse dynamic CT during (**a**) the arterial, (**b**) portal venous, and (**c**) delayed phase shows a 9.2 cm hyperenhancing mass (*arrows*) with washout in the right lobe of the liver. Note the intratumoral vessels (*arrowheads*) at the arterial phase (**a**). (**d**) Cut section of the resected specimen shows a large tumor in yellow color with hemorrhagic foci (*arrow*)

ing fibrous capsule, internal mosaic architecture, invasion of portal vein branches may support the diagnosis of HCC, the depiction of typical enhancement pattern of HCC is crucial since this is the most reliable criteria to characterize HCC[26-28] (Fig. 7.3). A systemic review[7] estimated that sensitivity was 68% and specificity was 93% compared with pathologic examination. However, much of published data are reflective on previous-generation CT scanner. Using a modern MDCT scanner which allows rapid, extremely thin-sliced scanning, improved sensitivities and specificities were reported[29]: MDCT (65–79%) showed better sensitivity than spiral CT for detecting HCC (37–54%) when CT was correlated with whole-liver explants. However, despite substantial technological advances, CT remains relatively insensitive for the detection of subcentimeter HCC (33–45%).[29] In addition, MDCT provides detailed mapping and assessment of hepatic arteries, portal veins, and hepatic veins. In fact, data from thin-slice (1–2 mm) images captured by current MDCT scanners can be reconstructed to provide angiographic pictures and are able to replace direct angiograms. The anatomic and vascular pathologic details provided by the state-of-the-art MDCT scanners have become extraordinarily useful for surgical planning.[14] In some countries, especially in Japan, a CT variant known as angio-assisted CT (CT hepatic arteriography and CT portography), in which CT scanning is performed after the infusion of contrast into the superior mesenteric artery (CT portography) and

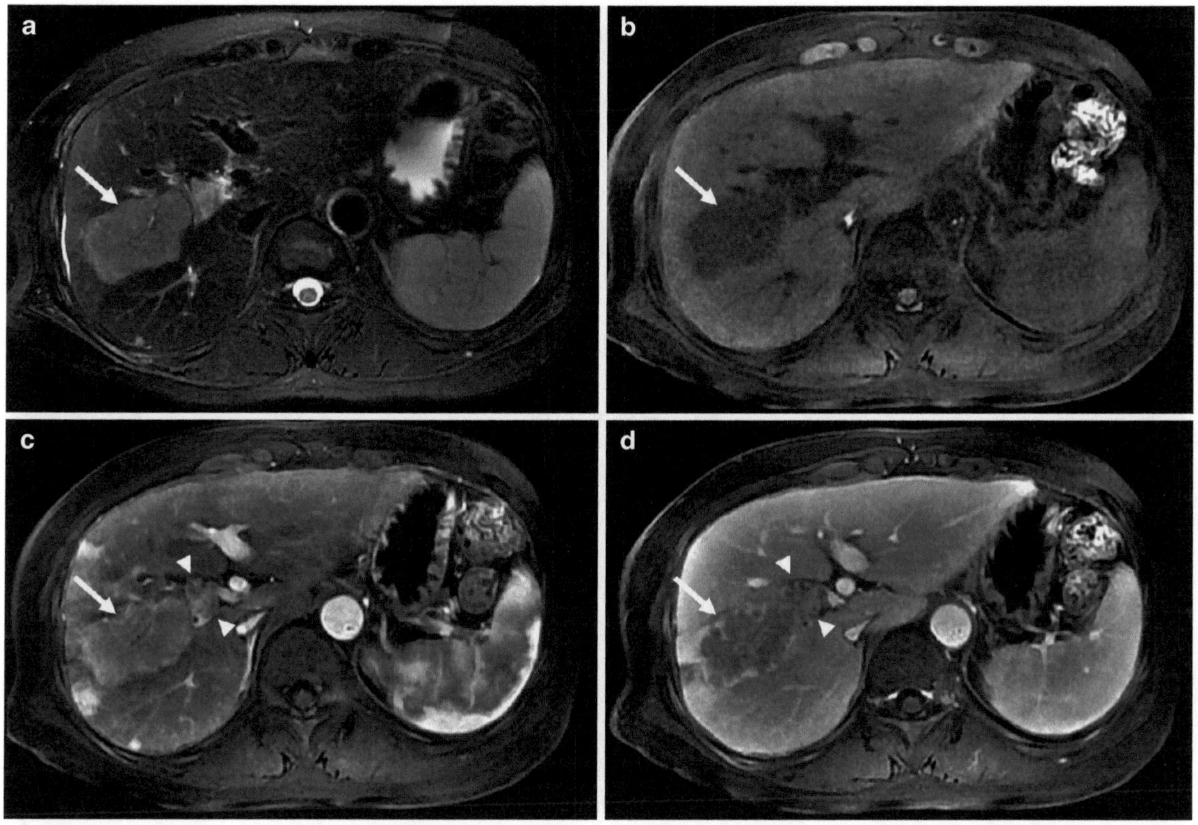

Fig. 7.4 Hepatocellular carcinoma with a tumor thrombus in the portal vein. (**a**) Transverse T2-weighted image shows a hyperintense lesion (*arrow*) in the right lobe of the liver. (**b**) On transverse T1-weighted image, the lesion (*arrow*) shows hypointensity. Transverse images obtained at (**c**) the arterial and (**d**) portal phase show a well enhancing HCC in the right lobe of the liver (*arrow*) with extension into the right portal vein (*arrowheads*)

then hepatic artery via catheters, is still widely used. In fact, angio-assisted CT scan has been regarded as being the most sensitive test available for identifying small hepatic tumors, but is an invasive procedure. Currently, with improvement in CT and MRI technologies, it has fallen out of favor and is not regarded as an essential test for the assessment of HCC in most practice settings except in Japan, mainly due to its invasiveness and high incidence of false positive diagnosis.[12]

7.1.3 Magnetic Resonance Imaging

MRI provides higher lesion to liver contrast than CT, which is a significant advantage over CT.[30] Thus, MRI provides better performance in distinguishing HCC from other hepatic lesions, including regenerative or dysplastic nodules in cirrhotic liver. The standard examination protocol for the evaluation of HCC includes T1-weighted images, T2-weighted images with fat saturation, and dynamic images using T1-weighted gradient echo sequences with fat saturation.[26] HCC shows a variety of MR imaging features on T1- and T2-weighted images.[27] On T1-weighted images, approximately 35% have high signal intensity, 25% have isointensity, and 40% have low signal intensity compared with the surrounding liver.[31] Homogeneous hyperintensity on T1 is more typical of dysplastic nodules but may be seen in small well-differentiated HCCs. Conversely, on T2-weighted sequences, HCCs are typically hyperintense, whereas dysplastic nodules are iso- to hypointense, although there is an overlap between the dysplastic nodule and the well-differentiated HCC[32] (Fig. 7.4). Furthermore, a focus of high signal intensity within a dysplastic

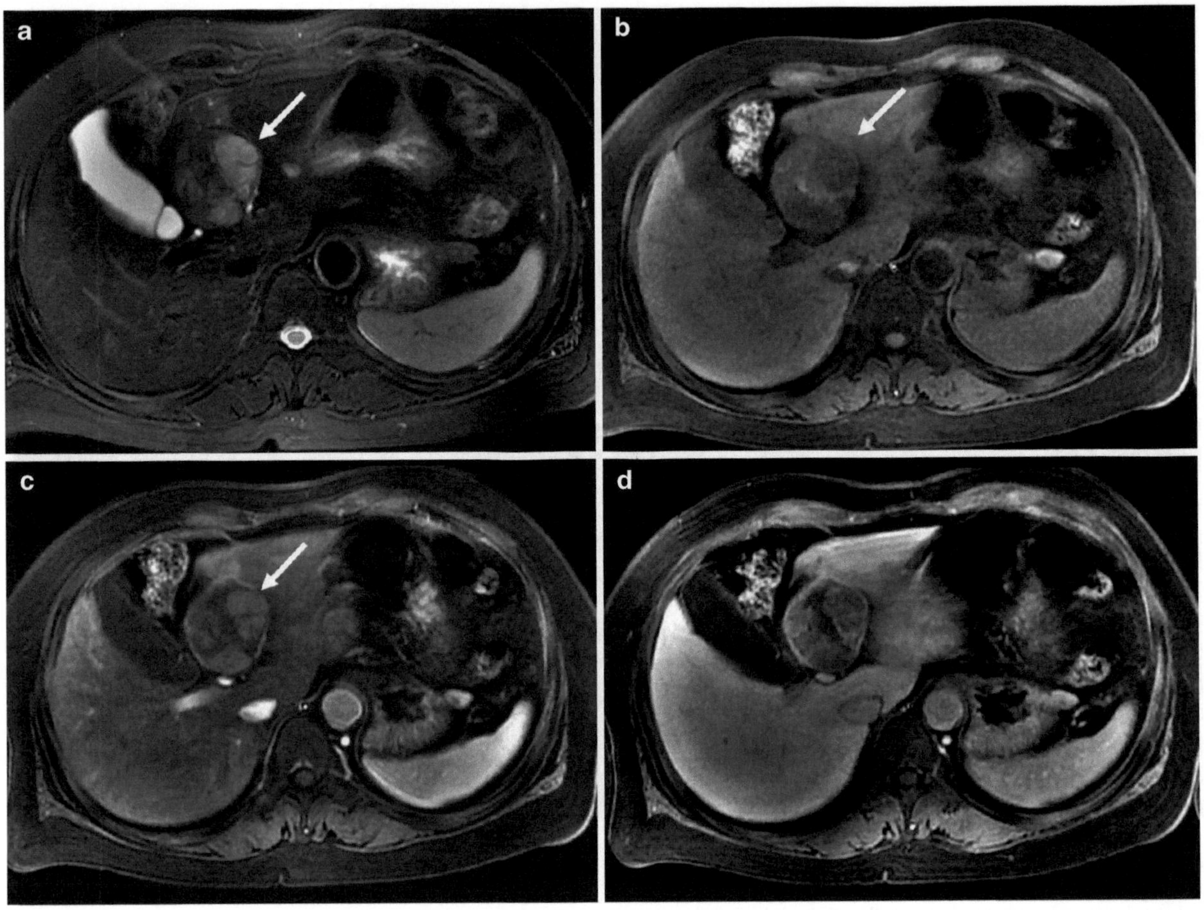

Fig. 7.5 Large hepatocellular carcinoma in hepatitis B virus-associated liver cirrhosis. (**a**) Transverse T2-weighted image shows a large hyperintense mass lesion (*arrow*) with internal mosaic architecture and a surrounding hypointense fibrous capsule in the left lobe of the liver. (**b**) On transverse T1-weighted image, the lesion (*arrow*) shows hypointensity. (**c**) Transverse arterial and (**d**) delayed phase show an internal mosaic architecture and the peripheral enhancing rim at the delayed phase (**c**) suggesting a pseudocapsule (*arrow*)

nodule suggests an area of development of HCC.[33] A large HCC lesion may present with additional characteristic MRI features such as a mosaic pattern, a tumor capsule, an extracapsular extension with satellite nodules, and vascular invasion (Fig. 7.5). Dynamic MRI with gadolinium enhancement well demonstrates the typical vascular feature of HCC, that is, arterial hyperenhancement and washout during PVP or DP (Figs. 7.4 and 7.5). The presence of arterial enhancement followed by washout has a sensitivity and specificity of 90% and 95%, respectively.[34] However, 71% of patients with HCC will have arterial enhancement and washout on more than one test, whereas the rest do not have these features and, therefore, will require liver biopsy for the diagnosis of HCC.[12,34]

A previous study of systematic review on the accuracies of US, spiral CT, and MRI in diagnosing HCC in patients with chronic liver disease revealed that the pooled estimates of the 14 US studies were 60% for sensitivity and 97% for specificity; for the 10 CT studies, the sensitivity was 68% and the specificity 93%; for the nine MRI studies, sensitivity was 81% and specificity 85%.[20] The operative characteristics of CT are comparable, whereas MRI is more sensitive. In fact, the performance of CT and MRI is affected by the size of the lesions.[29,35] Several studies that have compared the accuracy of CT and MRI for HCC diagnosis, using the explanted liver as the gold standard, show that MRI is slightly better in the diagnosis of HCC when compared with CT.[29,35,36] It was due to improved detection of small lesions 1–2 cm.[37] However, MRI remains relatively insensitive for the detection of small HCC nodules: in tumors larger than 2 cm, MRI is reported to have accuracy more than >90%; however, in tumors smaller than <1 cm, this level is reduced to 33–67%.[32,36,38] Therefore, the most important issue remains the identification of small tumors because curative treatments can be optimally applied to improve outcome.[39,40]

More recently, the development of rapid, high-quality MR techniques with new cell-specific contrast agents may induce further improvement of the detection and characterization of small nodules in the cirrhotic liver.[14] With MR angiography or MR cholangiography using faster three-dimensional sequences on a single breath-hold, a detailed analysis of vascular and of biliary involvement by tumor is now possible with great accuracy. Superparamagnetic iron oxide (SPIO) particles used alone[41] or in conjunction with gadolinium-based contrast agents[42,43] have been shown to be highly sensitive for the detection of HCC, particularly for small tumors. The reported sensitivity of double-contrast MR imaging (SPIO and gadolinium) for the detection of HCC measuring 1–2 cm is 92%.[42-44] More recently, two hepatobiliary agents with also extracellular properties, Gd-BOPTA and Gd-EOB-DTPA, were introduced. They can provide both dynamic imaging and hepatobiliary phase (Fig. 7.6). Recent studies with Gd-BOPTA or Gd-EOB-DPTA showed that the missing hepatobiliary uptake of the contrasts is an additional criterion for HCC[45] and demonstrated that MRI with those hepatobiliary agents was able to provide superior results to MDCT for the detection of small HCC[46,47] as well as for the differentiation of HCC from other benign arterial enhancing lesions.[48]

7.1.4 Positron Emission Tomography

Although 18F-fluorodeoxyglucose (FDG)-PET has proven to be a useful diagnostic and staging modality in a variety of oncologic conditions, the role of FDG-PET in the workup of patients with HCC is less clear, in that many tumors cannot be distinguished from the surrounding liver through assessment of glucose metabolism alone. Although the overall sensitivity of FDG-PET in detecting primary HCC is only 50–64%,[49,50] it may be

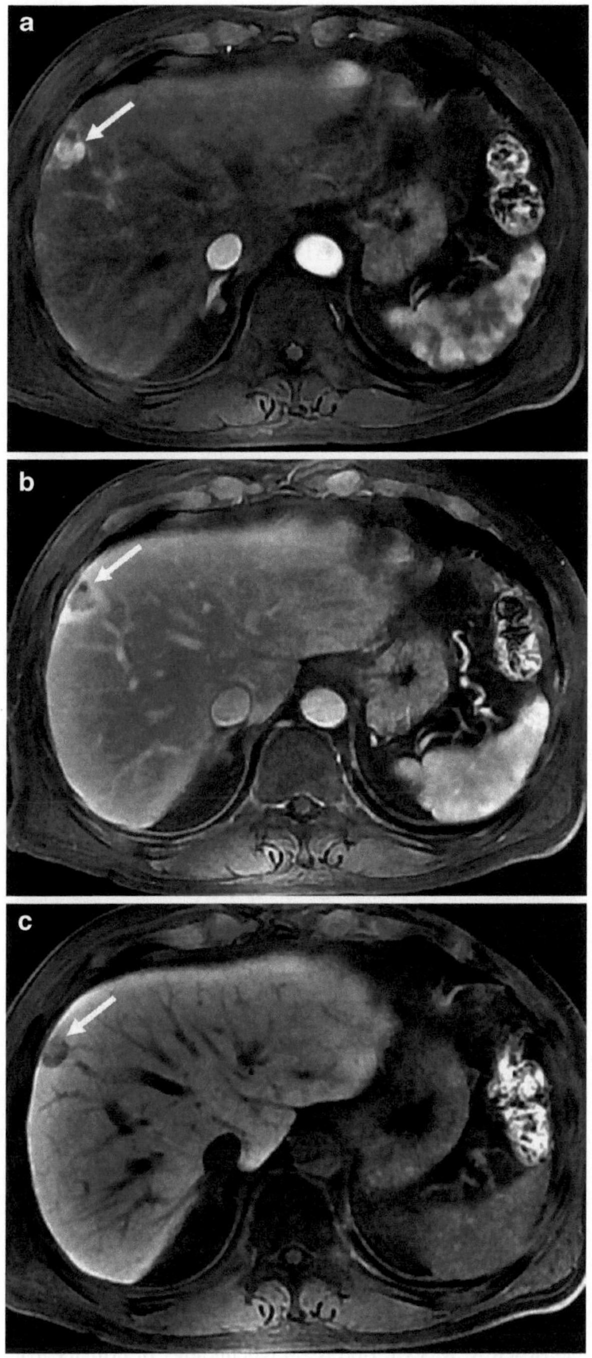

Fig. 7.6 Small hepatocellular carcinoma in the right hepatic lobe imaged with a new hepatobiliary MR contrast medium, Gd-EOB-DTPA. Transverse images obtained at (**a**) the arterial, (**b**) delayed, and (**c**) hepatobiliary phase show a HCC in segment VIII (*arrow*) with arterial hyperenhancement, washout, and decreased biliary uptake

useful for evaluating tumor differentiation and detecting metastatic disease as well as occult recurrence.[51-53] Another possible role for FDG-PET in HCC may be in the prediction of outcome and in the selection of optimal candidates for orthotopic liver transplantation. In a Korean study of 38 patients who underwent liver transplantation for HCC, the 2-year recurrence-free survival rate for FDG-PET-negative patients was 85% compared with 46% for FDG-PET-positive patients ($P = 0.0005$).[54] However, currently, there are insufficient data to recommend the routine use of PET imaging in primary HCC.[14]

7.1.5 Choice of Diagnostic and Staging Modalities

US, CT, and MRI are complementary in diagnosis, staging, and assessment of resectability for HCC. US should be the first tool in the evaluation of HCC, as it is noninvasive and free of ionizing radiation as well as risks of contrast allergy.[55] Typically, patients with liver lesions depicted on US should undergo staging with a contrast-enhanced multiphasic CT of the abdomen in order to better characterize the lesion and to assess the hepatic parenchyma and the effect of portal hypertension. If available, CT angiography should be used. An MRI may alternatively be used to stage the abdominal cavity and can be used to evaluate lesions with indeterminate findings on CT, especially with functional MR contrast agents or in patients with allergy to iodinated contrast. However, the choice between CT and MRI might depend on the available equipment and expertise in any given treatment center. Adjunctive studies such as bone scan or positron emission tomography imaging should be used more selectively.[14,55]

References

1. Bosch X, Ribes J, Borras J. Epidemiology of primary liver cancer. *Semin Liver Dis*. 1999;19:271-285.
2. Parkin DM, Bray F, Ferlay J, Pisani P. Global cancer statistics 2002. *CA Cancer J Clin*. 2005;55:74-108.
3. Taylor-Robinson SD, Foster GR, Arora S, Hargreaves S, Thomas HC. Increase in primary liver cancer in the U.K., 1979-1994. *Lancet*. 1997;350:1142-1143.
4. El-Serag HB, Mason AC. Rising incidence of hepatocellular carcinoma in the United States. *N Engl J Med*. 1999;340:745-750.
5. Llovet JM, Ricci S, Mazzaferro V, et al. Sorafenib in advanced hepatocellular carcinoma. *N Engl J Med*. 2008;359:378-390.
6. Nagasue N, Yukaya H, Hamada T, et al. The natural history of hepatocellular carcinoma. A study of 100 untreated cases. *Cancer*. 1984;54:1461-1465.
7. Okuda K, Ohtsuki T, Obata H, et al. Natural history of hepatocellular carcinoma and prognosis in relation to treatment. Study of 850 patients. *Cancer*. 1985;56:918-928.
8. Cha CH, Saif MW, Yamane BH, Weber SM. Hepatocellular carcinoma: current management. *Curr Probl Surg*. 2010; 47:10-67.
9. Bryant R, Laurent A, Tayar C, et al. Liver resection for hepatocellular carcinoma. *Surg Oncol Clin N Am*. 2008;17: 607-633.
10. Edge S, American Joint Committee on Cancer, American Cancer Society. *AJCC Cancer Staging Manual*. 7th ed. New York: Springer; 2009.
11. Choi BI, Lee JM. Advancement in HCC imaging: diagnosis, staging and treatment efficacy assessments: imaging diagnosis and staging of hepatocellular carcinoma. *J Hepatobiliary Pancreat Surg*. 2010;17(4):369-373. Epub 2009 Nov 19.
12. El-Serag HB, Marrero JA, Rudolph L, Reddy KR. Diagnosis and treatment of hepatocellular carcinoma. *Gastroenterology*. 2008;134:1752-1763.
13. Bruix J, Sherman M, Practice Guidelines Committee, American Association for the Study of Liver Diseases. Management of hepatocellular carcinoma. *Hepatology*. 2005; 42(42):1208-1236.
14. Miller G, Schwartz LH, D'Angelica M. The use of imaging in the diagnosis and staging of hepatobiliary malignancies. *Surg Oncol Clin N Am*. 2007;16:343-368.
15. Llovet JM, Bru C, Bruix J. Prognosis of hepatocellular carcinoma: the BCLC staging classification. *Semin Liver Dis*. 1999;19:329-338.
16. The Cancer of the Liver Italian Program (CLIP) Investigators. Prospective validation of the CLIP score: a new prognostic system for patients with cirrhosis and hepatocellular carcinoma. *Hepatology*. 2000;31:840-845.
17. Makuuchi M, Kosuge T, Takayama T, et al. Surgery for small liver cancers. *Semin Surg Oncol*. 1993;9(4):298-304.
18. Ishizawa T, Hasegawa K, Aoki T, et al. Neither multiple tumors nor portal hypertension are surgical contraindications for hepatocellular carcinoma. *Gastroenterology*. 2009; 44(7):733-741.
19. Choi BI. The current status of imaging diagnosis of hepatocellular carcinoma. *Liver Transplant*. 2004;10:S20-S25.
20. Colli A, Fraquelli M, Casazza G, et al. Accuracy of ultrasonography, spiral CT, magnetic resonance and alpha-fetoprotein in diagnosing hepatocellular carcinoma: a systematic review. *Am J Gastroenterol*. 2006;101:513-523.
21. Wilson SR, Burns PN. An algorithm for the diagnosis of focal liver masses using microbubble contrast-enhanced pulse-inversion sonography. *AJR*. 2006;186:1401-1412.
22. Hatanaka K, Kudo M, Minami Y, et al. Differential diagnosis of hepatic tumors: value of contrast-enhanced harmonic sonography using the newly developed contrast agent, Sonazoid. *Intervirology*. 2008;51(suppl 1):61-69.
23. Hatanaka K, Kudo M, Minami Y, Maekawa K. Sonazoid-enhanced ultrasonography for diagnosis of hepatic malignancies: comparison with contrast-enhanced CT. *Oncology*. 2008;75(suppl 1):42-47.
24. Korenaga K, Korenaga M, Furukawa M, Yamasaki T, Sakaida I. Usefulness of Sonazoid contrast-enhanced ultrasonography for

hepatocellular carcinoma: comparison with pathological diagnosis and superparamagnetic iron oxide magnetic resonance images. *J Gastroenterol.* 2009;44(7):733-741.
25. Lim JH, Kim EY, Lee WJ, et al. Regenerative nodules in liver cirrhosis: findings at CT during arterial portography and CT hepatic arteriography with histopathologic correlation. *Radiology.* 1999;210:451-458.
26. Zech CJ, Reiser MF, Herrmann KA. Imaging of hepatocellular carcinoma by computed tomography and magnetic resonance imaging: state of the art. *Dig Dis.* 2009;27:114-124.
27. Lencioni R, Cioni D, Pina CD, Crocetti L, Bartolozzi C. Hepatocellular carcinoma: imaging diagnosis. *Semin Liver Dis.* 2005;25:162-170.
28. Iannaccone R, Laghi A, Catalano C, et al. Hepatocellular carcinoma: role of unenhanced and delayed-phase multidetector row helical CT in patients with cirrhosis. *Radiology.* 2005;234:460-467.
29. Kim SH, Choi BI, Lee JY, et al. Diagnostic accuracy of multi-/single-detector row CT and contrast-enhanced MRI in the detection of hepatocellular carcinomas meeting the Milan criteria before liver transplantation. *Intervirology.* 2008;51(suppl 1):52-60.
30. Ariff B, Lloyd CR, Khan S, et al. Imaging of liver cancer. *World J Gastroenterol.* 2009;15:1289-1300.
31. Kamel IR, Bluemke DA. MR imaging of liver tumors. *Radiol Clin North Am.* 2003;41:51-65.
32. Ebara M, Ohto M, Watanabe Y, et al. Diagnosis of small hepatocellular carcinoma: correlation of MR imaging and tumor histologic studies. *Radiology.* 1986;159:371-377.
33. Mitchell DG, Rubin R, Siegelman ES, et al. Hepatocellular carcinoma within siderotic regenerative nodules: appearance as a nodule within a nodule on MR images. *Radiology.* 1991;178:101-103.
34. Marrero JA, Hussain HK, Nghiem HV, et al. Improving the prediction of heaptocellular carcinoma in cirrhotic patients with an arterial enhancing liver mass. *Liver Transpl.* 2005; 11:281-289.
35. Willatt JM, Hussain HK, Adusumilli S, Marrero JA. MR Imaging of hepatocellular carcinoma in the cirrhotic liver: challenges and controversies. *Radiology.* 2008;247:311-330.
36. Rode A, Bancel B, Douek P, et al. Small nodule detection in cirrhotic livers: evaluation with US, spiral CT, and MRI and correlation with pathologic examination of explanted liver. *J Comput Assist Tomogr.* 2001;25:327-336.
37. Kim YK, Kim CS, Chung GH, et al. Comparison of gadobenate dimeglumine-enhanced dynamic MRI and 16-MDCT for the detection of hepatocellular carcinoma. *AJR.* 2006;186: 149-157.
38. Krinsky GA, Lee VS, Theise ND, et al. Hepatocellular carcinoma and dysplastic nodules in patients with cirrhosis: prospective diagnosis with MR imaging and explanation correlation. *Radiology.* 2001;219:445-454.
39. Llovet JM, Burroughs A, Bruix J. Hepatocellular carcinoma. *Lancet.* 2003;362:1907-1917.
40. Arii S, Yamaoka Y, Futagawa S, et al. Results of surgical and nonsurgical treatment for small-sized hepatocellular carcinomas: a retrospective and nationwide survey in Japan. The Liver Cancer Study Group of Japan. *Hepatology.* 2000;32: 1224-1229.
41. Kim YK, Kwak HS, Kim CS, Chung GH, Han YM, Lee JM. Hepatocellular carcinoma in patients with chronic liver disease: comparison of SPIO-enhanced MR imaging and 16-detector row CT. *Radiology.* 2006;238:531-541.
42. Bhartia B, Ward J, Guthrie JA, Robinson PJ. Hepatocellular carcinoma in cirrhotic livers: double-contrast thin-section MR imaging with pathologic correlation of explanted tissue. *AJR Am J Roentgenol.* 2003;180:577-584.
43. Ward J, Guthrie JA, Scott DJ, et al. Hepatocellular carcinoma in the cirrhotic liver: double-contrast MR imaging for diagnosis. *Radiology.* 2000;216:154-162.
44. Yoo HJ, Lee JM, Lee MW, et al. Hepatocellular carcinoma in cirrhotic liver: double-contrast-enhanced, high-resolution 3.0T-MR imaging with pathologic correlation. *Invest Radiol.* 2008;43:538-546.
45. Kim JI, Lee JM, Choi JY, et al. The value of gadobenate dimeglumine-enhanced delayed-phase MR imaging for characterization of hepatocellular nodules in the cirrhotic liver. *Invest Radiol.* 2008;43:202-210.
46. Marin D, Di Martino M, Guerrisi A, et al. Hepatocellular carcinoma in patients with cirrhosis: qualitative comparison of gadobenate dimeglumine-enhanced MR imaging and multiphasic 64-section CT. *Radiology.* 2009;251:85-95.
47. Kim SH, Kim SH, Lee J, et al. Gadoxetic acid-enhanced MRI versus triple-phase MDCT for the preoperative detection of hepatocellular carcinoma. *AJR.* 2009;192:1675-1681.
48. Sun HY, Lee JM, Shin CI, et al. Gadoxetic acid-enhanced magnetic resonance imaging for differentiating small hepatocellular carcinomas (2 cm in diameter) from arterial enhancing pseudolesions: special emphasis on hepatobiliary phase imaging. *Invest Radiol.* 2010;45(2):96-103.
49. Wudel LJ Jr, Delbeke D, Morris D, et al. The role of [18F] fluorodeoxyglucose positron emission tomography imaging in the evaluation of hepatocellular carcinoma. *Am Surg.* 2003;69:117-124.
50. Trojan J, Schroeder O, Raedle J, et al. Fluorine-18 FDG positron emission tomography for imaging of hepatocellular carcinoma. *Am J Gastroenterol.* 1999;94:3314-3319.
51. Sugiyama M, Sakahara H, Torizuka T, et al. 18F-FDG PET in the detection of extrahepatic metastases from hepatocellular carcinoma. *J Gastroenterol.* 2004;39:961-968.
52. Nagaoka S, Itano S, Ishibashi M, et al. Value of fusing PET plus CT images in hepatocellular carcinoma and combined hepatocellular and cholangiocarcinoma patients with extrahepatic metastases: preliminary findings. *Liver Int.* 2006;26:781-788.
53. Chen YK, Hsieh DS, Liao CS, et al. Utility of FDG-PET for investigating unexplained serum AFP elevation in patients with suspected hepatocellular carcinoma recurrence. *Anticancer Res.* 2005;25:4719-4725.
54. Yang SH, Suh KS, Lee HW, et al. The role of (18)F-FDG-PET imaging for the selection of liver transplantation candidates among hepatocellular carcinoma patients. *Liver Transpl.* 2006;12:1655-1660.
55. Song T, Kit EW, Fong Y. Hepatocellular carcinoma: current surgical management. *Gastroenterology.* 2004;127:S248-S260.

Preoperative Imaging of Liver Cancers: Hilar Cholangiocarcinoma

8

Harmeet Kaur, Evelyne M. Loyer, and Chusilp Charnsangavej

Abstract

Patients with suspected hilar cholagiocarcinoma frequently present with obstructive jaundice. The conventional algorithm for imaging studies of those patients usually starts with an ultrasonography of the abdomen to exclude more common and benign conditions, such as choledocholithiasis, gallstones, cholecystitis, and Mirizzi syndrome.[2,29,30] An MR cholangiography and CT of the abdomen has been advocated and increasingly used in clinical practices to fully evaluate the causes of jaundice. Once the benign conditions are excluded, or in patients with a highly suspicious malignant cause of obstructive jaundice such as a hilar cholangiocarcinoma, pancreatic carcinoma, or gallbladder carcinoma, a more tailored examination will be needed to evaluate the cause, the extent, and the staging of the malignant disease. The primary signs of hilar cholangiocarcinoma on CT or MR imaging are the presence of soft tissue mass and the focal thickening of the ductal wall with periductal infiltration associated with constriction of the lumen, and the intraluminal nodule in the dilated duct.

Keywords

Hilar cholangiocarcinoma • Liver imaging • Imaging of liver • Imaging of hilar cholangiocarcinoma

Cholangiocarcinomas are uncommon tumors arising from the biliary epithelium. Its incidence is approximately 1 per 100,000/year in the United States with the peak occurring between age 70 and 74 years and at a median age of 69 years.[1-3] In most series, males and females have nearly an equal incidence, while people of Asian and Hispanic descent have an incidence almost twice of whites and African-Americans.[2,3]

There are certain conditions that are associated with an increased risk of cholangiocarcinoma, including primary sclerosing cholangitis, infection with food-borne trematodes such as *O. viverrini* and *C. sinensis*, typhoid carriers, and congenital malformations of the pancreatico-biliary tract. These malformations include choledochal cysts, Caroli's disease, and anomalous arrangements of the pancreatic and bile duct (AAPBD), which are associated with a 25% incidence of gallbladder cancer. The predisposing factors underlying these varied etiologies are an inflammation induced by an

C. Charnsangavej (✉)
Department of Diagnostic Radiology, The University of Texas M.D. Anderson Cancer Center, 1400 Pressler St, Unit 1473, Houston, TX 77030, USA
e-mail: ccharn@mdanderson.org

D.C. Madoff et al. (eds.), *Venous Embolization of the Liver*,
DOI 10.1007/978-1-84882-122-4_8, © Springer-Verlag London Limited 2011

infection, an autoimmune process, or a reflux of pancreatic juices into the bile ducts. Chronic inflammation and genetic alterations may induce dysplasia of the epithelium and may progress into a carcinoma in situ and subsequently into a carcinoma.

These tumors may arise from intrahepatic or extrahepatic bile ducts. According to the Japanese Society of Biliary Surgery, the point at which first order bile ducts (left and right hepatic ducts) become second order or segmental ducts is the separation between the intra- and extrahepatic bile ducts.[4] The clinical presentation, prognosis, and treatment of intrahepatic and extrahepatic cholangiocarcinoma are distinctly different – intrahepatic tumors frequently present as hepatic masses while extrahepatic tumors often cause biliary obstruction and jaundice. However, these presentations may overlap because intrahepatic tumors may extend into the hilum/hilar fissure and obstruct the bile duct and because extrahepatic tumors may form masses similar to intrahepatic tumors.[5]

Tumors of the extrahepatic bile duct are rare comprising 2% of all cancer in the United States. Perihilar or Klatskin tumors are the most common accounting for 40–67% of all cholangiocarcinomas. These tumors may involve the hepatic ducts, the confluence, and/or the common hepatic duct down to the level of the cystic duct.[2,3,6]

Surgical resection with negative margins (R0) offers the only possibility for prolonged survival in hilar cholangiocarcinoma. During the past two decades, the resection of extrahepatic cholangiocarcinoma has changed significantly from a local excision which was associated with a high recurrent rate to a more aggressive surgery that combines the resection of the bile duct and the resection of the anatomic liver.[2,7-10] In recent years, these techniques, in combination with portal vein grafting, have improved the proportion of R0 or margin-negative resections resulting in 5-year survival rates of up to 56% of surgical cases.[8,11-14] To avoid the morbidity of unnecessary surgery or limited resection that conveys no significant survival benefit, accurate preoperative staging is of the greatest importance. This is a challenge in hilar cholangiocarcinoma, given the infiltrative nature of the tumors which are commonly associated with perineural, perivascular, and lymphatic infiltration and the variable anatomy of the portal vein, hepatic artery, and bile duct which are closely situated in the hilar plate. Cross-sectional imaging, cholangiography, and MRCP are the mainstays of tumor staging for hilar cholangiocarcinoma.[15-22] Laparoscopic staging, while appropriate for the evaluation of peritoneal implants and small liver metastasis that may be missed on cross-sectional imaging, is inadequate for the assessment of the tumor spread along the bile ducts and of vascular involvement in the porta hepatis.[2,23]

The focus of this chapter is primarily extrahepatic cholangiocarcinoma. Extrahepatic cholangiocarcinomas have traditionally been classified as: (1) perihilar – that is, tumors involving the bifurcation and the portion of the hepatic duct above its junction with the cystic duct, (2) mid-duct tumors arising from the bile duct between the origin of the cystic duct and the upper border of the duodenum, and (3) distal tumors that are located in the intrapancreatic portion of the common bile duct.[5] However, the most recent AJCC classification (7th edition) has eliminated the uncommon mid-duct subgroup of cholangiocarcinomas, which is now grouped with either perihilar or distal tumors depending upon the type of surgery performed.[24]

8.1 Pathology

Adenocarcinoma accounts for more than 90% of tumors of the bile duct.[2,25-27] Few histologic variants such as papillary, mucinous, clear cells, and signet ring cells may be seen. Other epithelial tumors such as adenosquamous, squamous, small cell, and undifferentiated tumors are rare.

There are three morphologic patterns of the adenocarcinoma (cholangiocarcinoma) of the extrahepatic bile duct: (1) periductal infiltrating, also known as sclerosing, (2) mass forming, and (3) intraductal papillary tumors.[26,27] These gross morphologic patterns reflect how the tumors grow and spread and correlate well with the imaging characteristics on various cross-sectional imaging studies.[28]

8.2 Clinical and Pathologic Staging Classification of Hilar Cholangiocarcinoma

The staging classifications of extrahepatic cholangiocarcinoma are the Bismuth classification for hilar cholangiocarcinoma, which defines the longitudinal spread of the tumor, and the TNM classification, which defines the extent of the tumor based on the depth of invasion, nodal involvement, and the presence of distant metastasis.[2,3,24] Both systems are useful for surgical planning.

8.2.1 Bismuth–Corlette Classification

This classification describes the extent and patterns of biliary involvement around the confluence of hepatic ducts. It is commonly used to determine the extent of the anatomic resection of the hepatic segments for which their bile ducts are involved by the tumor in the hilar region. There are four types of Bismuth–Corlette staging classification. Type I tumors involve the biliary confluence, but do not touch the "roof" of the confluence. Type II lesions also involve the confluence but extend to abut the "roof." Type III lesions extend to involve the second order bile ducts with IIIa extending into the right hepatic duct and IIIb the left hepatic duct. Type IV tumors extend to involve the sectorial or second order ducts of both right and left hepatic ducts. This classification is mainly used to determine surgical approach and has not been widely applied for clinical prognosis.

8.2.2 TNM/AJCC Classification

The TNM staging classification defines the depth of tumor invasion locally, the presence of nodal metastases, and distant metastases (Table 8.1).[24] In the seventh edition, T-staging identifies those with T1–T3 as resectable tumors and distinguishes them from T4-lesions as unresectable tumors. N-staging characterizes nodal metastases to the N1 group for those with metastasis to regional nodes that are usually included in the routine surgical resection and to the N2 group for those with distant nodal metastases that are not routinely resected such as the celiac node, para-aortic nodes, and superior mesenteric nodes.

These T-, N-, and M-staging categories are then grouped together to form stage I to IV staging groups based on clinical or pathologic data so that they can be used as prognostic indicators.

The Japanese Society of Biliary Surgery has refined the definitions of nodal spread in greater detail than the AJCC classification, with the N1 and N2 depending upon the location of the primary tumor.[4] While the definition of regional or N1 nodes for perihilar tumors is the same as the AJCC classification (see above), in tumors of the distal pancreatic duct, nodes on the posterior surface of the pancreatic head qualify as N1 while a majority of nodes in the hepatoduodenal ligament are N2.

Table 8.1 TNM classification of extrahepatic cholangiocarcinoma

Primary tumor	
TX	Primary tumor cannot be assessed
T0	No evidence of primary tumor
Tis	Carcinoma in situ
T1	Tumor confined to the bile duct, with extension up to the muscle layer or fibrous tissue
T2a	Tumor invades beyond the wall of bile duct to surrounding adipose tissue
T2b	Tumor invades adjacent hepatic parenchyma
T3	Tumor invades unilateral branch of portal vein or hepatic artery
T4	Tumor invades main portal vein or its branches bilaterally; or the common hepatic artery; or second order biliary radicals bilaterally; or unilateral second order biliary radicals with contralateral portal vein or hepatic artery involvement
Regional lymph nodes	
NX	Regional lymph nodes cannot be assessed
N0	No regional lymph node metastasis
N1	Regional lymph node metastasis (including nodes along the cystic duct, common bile duct, hepatic artery, and portal vein)
N2	Metastasis to periaortic, pericaval, superior mesenteric artery, and /or celiac artery lymph nodes
Distant metastasis	
MX	Distant metastasis cannot be assessed
M0	No distant metastasis
M1	Distant metastasis

Anatomic stage			
Group	T	N	M
0	Tis	N0	M0
I	T1	N0	M0
II	T2a-b	N0	M0
IIIA	T3	N0	M0
IIIB	T1–3	N1	M0
IVA	T4	N0-1	M0
IVB	Any T	N2	M0
	Any T	Any N	M1

Used with the permission of the American Joint Committee on Cancer (AJCC), Chicago, Illinois. The original source for this material is the AJCC Cancer Staging Manual, 7th edn. (2010) published by Springer Science and Business Media LLC, www.springer.com

8.3 Imaging of Hilar Cholangiocarcinoma

Patients with suspected hilar cholagiocarcinoma frequently present with obstructive jaundice. The conventional algorithm for imaging studies of those patients usually starts with an ultrasonography of the abdomen to exclude more common and benign conditions such as choledocholithiasis, gallstones, cholecystitis, and Mirizzi syndrome.[2,29,30] An MR cholangiography and CT of the abdomen has been advocated and increasingly used in clinical practices to fully evaluate the causes of jaundice. Once the benign conditions are excluded, or in patients with a highly suspicious malignant cause of obstructive jaundice such as a hilar cholangiocarcinoma, pancreatic carcinoma, or gallbladder carcinoma, a more tailored examination will be needed to evaluate the cause, the extent, and the staging of the malignant disease.

The goals of imaging in such patients are: (1) to localize the precise location of the tumor, (2) to define the extent of longitudinal extension of the tumor in the right and left hepatic duct and the downward extension in the common hepatic duct, (3) to determine the radial extent of the tumor outside the wall of the duct, particularly the involvement of the adjacent portal vein and hepatic artery in the hilar plate and in the hepatoduodenal ligament, (4) to estimate or measure the volume of the affected and unaffected hepatic segments and lobes for surgical planning, (5) to identify potential site of nodal metastasis, and (6) to detect distant metastases.

Because the right and left hepatic duct and its confluence are tubular structures smaller than 5 mm with a wall thinner than 1 mm and are located in the hilar plate adjacent to the liver, the identification of the abnormalities in this region requires images with a higher spatial resolution and a higher tissue contrast resolution than conventional imaging techniques. The two most common noninvasive imaging studies that serve these purposes are the MR cholangiography and contrast-enhanced MR, and the multiphasic, contrast-enhanced, thin-section, multidetector helical CT of the abdomen.[15-22] An MR cholangiography uses a heavily T-2 weighted, breath-hold sequence to visualize intraductal bile, and dynamic, post-contrast, rapid data acquisition T-1 weighted images to provide excellent tissue contrast between the tumors and the surrounding normal structures.[19,20,22] On the other hand, CT imaging data can be acquired rapidly during the late arterial and portal venous phases after a rapid IV contrast administration on the 64-detector CT scanner at 2.5-mm section thickness. The scan data is then reconstructed to a 0.625-mm section thickness and used for image processing to display the images in coronal and sagittal plane as well as in 3-D volume rendering. This technique provides excellent images with the spatial resolution and enhancement characteristics of the tumor.

Transhepatic cholangiography and endoscopic retrograde cholangiopancreatography and endoscopic ultrasonography are more invasive techniques but can provide additional diagnostic and staging information and to relief jaundice. The studies can be used in conjunction with MR imaging and CT to guide treatment and intervention. Currently, there are no large prospective clinical trials to compare the efficacy of these imaging techniques for the preoperative assessment of patients with hilar cholangiocarcinoma. Most of the published reports are based on the experiences of single institutions, the imaging expertise that meets the need of hepatobiliary surgeons, and the preferences of clinical specialists.

8.3.1 CT and MR Imaging in the Diagnosis of Hilar Cholangiocarcinoma

The imaging diagnosis of hilar cholangiocarcinoma can be challenging because the tumor is often small as compared to the size of the liver and because it is located in the hilar plate containing the vital structures essential to the function of the liver. The density of the tumor can also be difficult to distinguish from the surrounding hepatic parenchyma. Moreover, its appearance may be similar to chronic inflammatory processes such as sclerosing cholangitis that causes benign ductal stricture. Despite those challenges, the imaging appearances correlate well with the three gross morphologic patterns described earlier, including the periductal infiltrative form (Fig. 8.1), the nodular or mass form (Fig. 8.2), and the intraductal papillary form. The nodular and periductal infiltrative forms account for about 95% of hilar cholangiocarcinoma, and about 5% is the intraductal papillary type.

The primary signs of hilar cholangiocarcinoma on CT or MR imaging are the presence of soft tissue mass and the focal thickening of the ductal wall with periductal infiltration associated with constriction of the lumen and an intraluminal nodule in the dilated duct. In practice, each segmental duct should be evaluated individually and followed downstream to where it becomes the right or left hepatic duct and to the point of obstruction. The density of the tumor may be variable depending on tumor vascularity and degree of

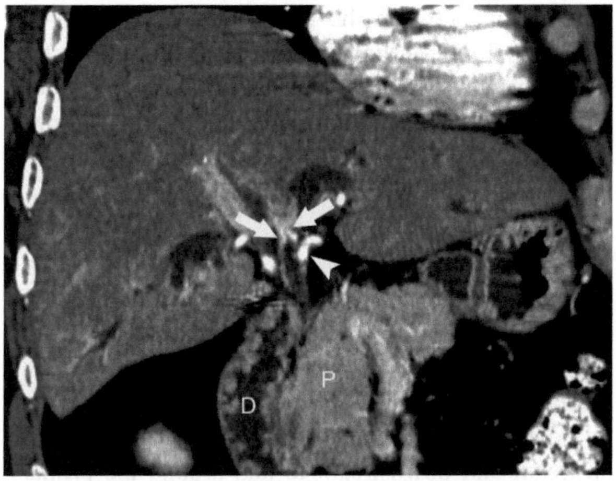

Fig. 8.1 Infiltrative form of hilar cholangiocarcinoma. CT image in coronal plane shows infiltrative tumor (*arrows*) constricting the common hepatic duct at the hilar region. Note the hepatic artery (*arrowhead*) coursing behind the duct below the tumor. *P* pancreas, *D* duodenum

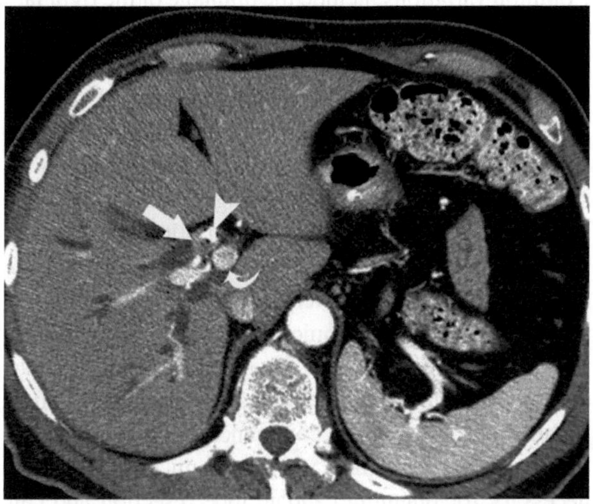

Fig. 8.2 Nodular form of hilar cholangiocarcinoma. Axial CT image shows a nodular tumor (*arrow*) obstructing the right hepatic duct. Note a stent (*arrowhead*) in the bile duct anterior to the right portal vein (*curve arrow*)

fibrosis within the tumor. They can be hyperdense, hypodense, or isodense relative to the wall of the normal duct and the adjacent hepatic parenchyma, but often have a higher density during the delayed phase. The secondary sign of lobar or segmental atrophy can complement the diagnosis and can be used to localize the primary site of the tumor because chronic ductal obstruction with or without portal vein involvement often results in parenchymal atrophy.

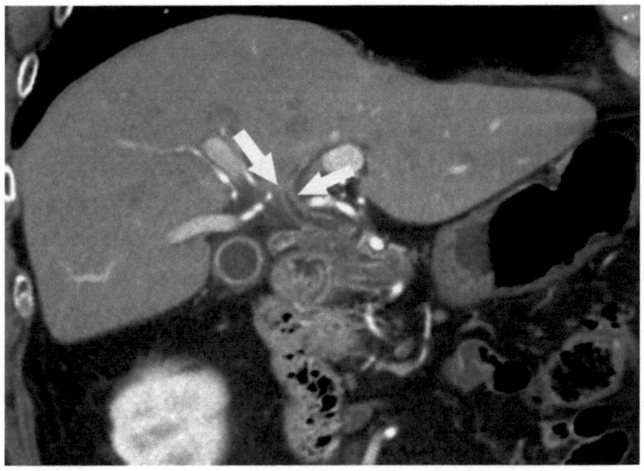

Fig. 8.3 Inflammatory stricture of the confluence of hepatic ducts from cholecystitis simulating hilar cholangiocarcinoma. CT image in coronal plane demonstrates infiltrative lesion (*arrows*) with narrowing of the confluence of the hepatic ducts due to inflammatory process from cholecystitis

Both CT and MR imaging have limitations in the diagnosis because the infiltrating form of hilar cholangiocarcinoma can present as the focal thickening of the duct and is indistinguishable from inflammatory strictures due to fibrosis or scar tissue[29-31] (Fig. 8.3). A definitive diagnosis, on rare occasion, can be difficult to obtain preoperatively. Consequently, a small number of these patients may undergo hepatic or bile duct resection despite the lack of preoperative pathologic diagnosis. In addition, the presence of biliary drainage catheters or stent could produce artifacts on CT or MR imaging precluding the characterization of the cause of biliary stricture.

8.3.2 Preoperative Imaging Staging of Hilar Cholangiocarcinoma

The growth patterns of the most common types of hilar cholangiocarcinoma are characterized by longitudinal submucosal infiltration beyond the gross tumor margin, radial growth into periductal tissue to involve the adjacent portal vein, hepatic artery, nerves, and lymphatics in the hilar plate and hepatoduodenal ligament, and the adjacent hepatic parenchyma.[2,25,26] They are also associated with inflammatory fibrotic tissues that are grossly indistinguishable from the tumor.

The basic principles of surgery for hilar cholangiocarcinoma to achieve a margin-negative resection are: (1) to resect the hepatic lobe and segment of which its main hepatic duct is the primary site of tumor or involved by the tumor, (2) to resect the contralateral duct away from the confluence but leave enough bile duct of the uninvolved segment or lobe for anastomosis with the small bowel (jejunum), and (3) to preserve its arterial and portal venous supply. The resection of hilar cholangiocarcinoma is usually performed at major centers with experienced hepatobiliary surgeons because of the complex anatomy of the vital structures in the hilar plate.

Because of the rarity of this tumor, the low resection rate and the complexity of surgery, and the potentially high morbidity, the goals of imaging must try to exclude those patients who are not likely surgical candidates and to identify those who are potentially resectable candidates. The unresectable patients can be defined by imaging studies as those who have distant metastases and those with locally advanced tumors. Distant metastases generally include hepatic metastases, pulmonary metastases, and peritoneal metastases. Metastatic nodes beyond the hepatoduodenal ligament such as the nodes at the celiac axis, the nodes in the mesentery along the superior mesenteric artery, and the periaortic nodes in the retroperitoneum are considered distant metastasis. However, they should be confirmed by tissue diagnosis.

Jarnagin and Blumgart et al. defined locally advanced disease that is considered unresectable[10] using the following criteria:

- Tumor extension to segmental duct or sectional duct bilaterally (Type 4 Bismuth–Corlette classification)
- Encasement or occlusion of the main portal vein proximal to its bifurcation
- Atrophy of one hepatic lobe with encasement or occlusion of the contralateral portal vein branch
- Atrophy of one hepatic lobe with contralateral tumor extension to segmental or sectional bile duct
- Unilateral tumor extension to sectional bile ducts with occlusion or encasement of the contralateral portal vein branch

These criteria have been accepted by many major surgical centers, but some have applied additional guidelines to include portal venous encasement shorter than 2 cm to allow venous resection as part of their resectable criteria.[8]

It is, therefore, important for preoperative imaging studies to provide the following information in the report, including: (1) the anatomy of the bile duct and the longitudinal extent of tumor involvement in the hilar plate and hepatoduodenal ligament, (2) the anatomy of the portal vein and segmental branches and the relationship between the tumor and the portal vein, (3) the anatomy of the hepatic artery and its branches, (4) the presence of enlarged nodes or abnormal nodes at the celiac axis, superior mesenteric artery, and periaortic nodes, and (5) the presence or absence of distant metastasis in the liver, lung, or peritoneal cavity.

8.3.3 Assessment of Anatomy of the Bile Duct and Ductal Involvement

The anatomy of the bile duct in the hilar plate and its confluence and the extent of tumor involvement upstream and downstream to and around the primary tumor are critical for planning surgery, particularly for the extent of the surgery and for the reconstruction of the anastomosis between the uninvolved duct and the jejunum. The right and left hepatic ducts joining to form the common hepatic duct are seen in 53–72% of cases. Common variations include the drainage of the right lateral duct into the left duct (6–22%), the right paramedian duct into the common hepatic duct (17%), the right lateral duct into the common hepatic duct (5%), and the right paramedian duct into the left duct (3–6%).[32,33] In spite of these numerous variations, the left hepatic duct and portal vein are consistently longer than the right and present in 97% of cases. Unusual variations such as two left ducts joining just above the confluence (Fig. 8.4) or low insertion of the segmental or sectional duct of the right liver into the common bile duct are important information. Moreover, the location where the caudate duct inserts into the right and left hepatic duct is often within 1 or 2 cm from the confluence, making it likely to be involved by the tumor.[34] This anatomic information is necessary for planning caudate lobe resection and can minimize complications such as bile leak and can lower the risk of local recurrent disease. Our practical approach to the analysis of ductal anatomy is by tracing each segmental duct individually in order to accurately describe the anatomy and the extent of ductal involvement.

The accuracies of CT and MRI to define the longitudinal extent of ductal involvement are similar and have been reported in the range of 85–95% when compared to surgical inspection.[15-17,19] However, detailed histological sections have shown that gross surgical morphology underestimated tumor infiltration in the submucosal layer of the duct by 1.7 cm toward the liver and by 7 mm toward the duodenum.[35] Therefore, the length of "normal-appearing" duct in the hilar plate and in the hepatoduodenal ligament would be useful for surgery.

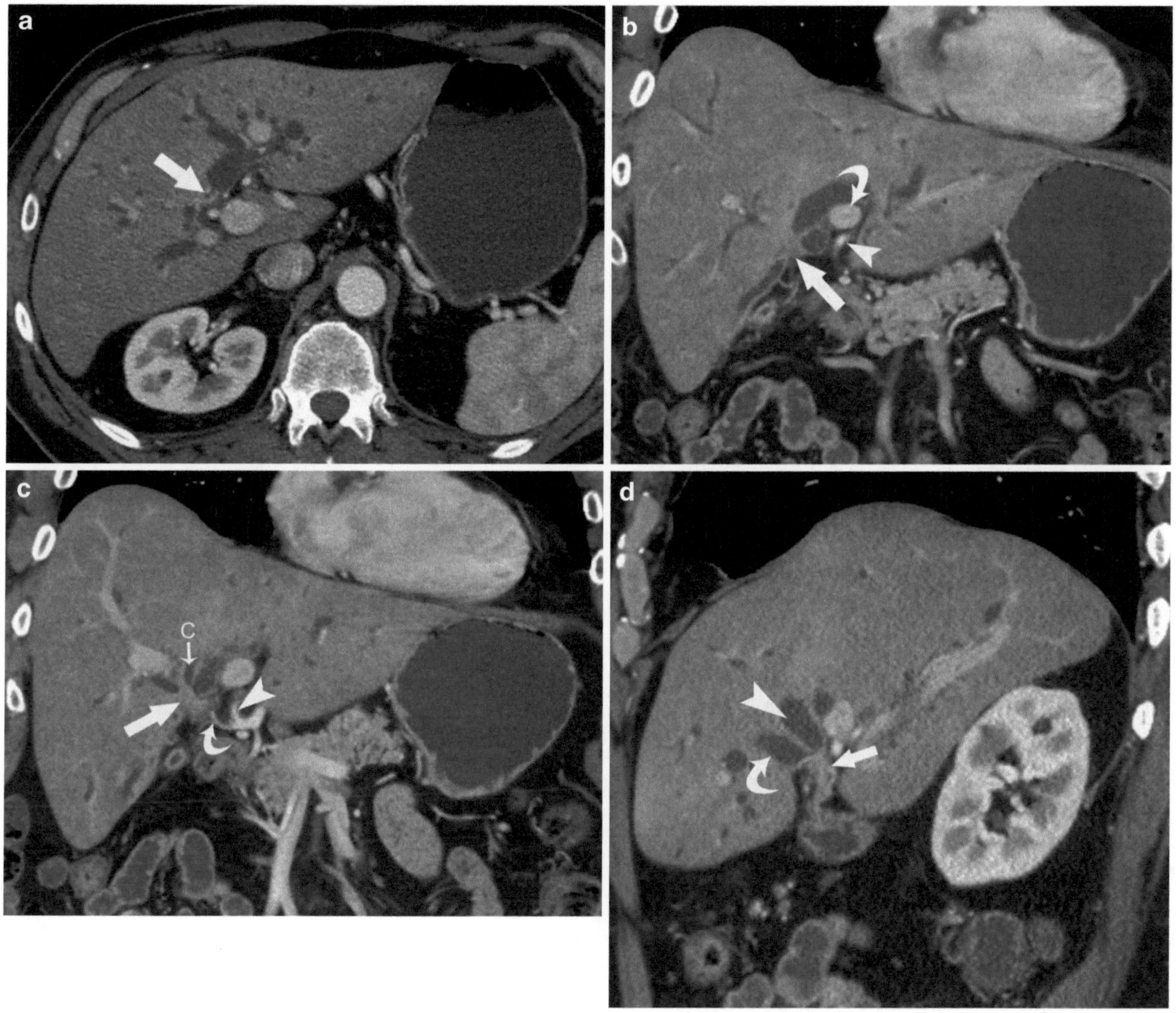

Fig. 8.4 Hilar cholangiocarcinoma with two left ducts just above the confluence. (**a**) A 2.5-mm axial CT image identifies a constricting lesion (*arrow*) of one of the two left hepatic ducts above the confluence due to hilar cholangiocarcinoma. (**b**) A 2-mm CT image on a coronal plane shows the stricture site (*arrow*) about 1 cm away from the left hepatic artery (*arrowhead*) and the left portal vein (*curve arrow*). (**c**) Another CT image on a coronal plane demonstrates the origin of the left hepatic artery (*arrowhead*) and the common hepatic artery away from the infiltrative tumor (*arrow*), but the hepatic artery supplying segment IV (*curve arrow*) is inseparable from the tumor. Note the caudate duct (**c**) joining the confluence and involved by the tumor. (**d**) CT image on a sagittal plane shows the two ducts draining segment II (*arrowhead*) and segments III and IV (*curve arrow*) just above the confluence that is involved by the infiltrative tumor (*arrow*)

8.3.4 Preoperative Imaging Assessment of Vascular Anatomy and Vascular Involvement in Hilar Cholangiocarcinoma

Multiphasic MDCT and dynamic contrast-enhanced MRI, as described earlier, provide excellent hepatic arterial and portal venous anatomy and can be displayed in multiple planes. The accuracies in identifying vascular anatomy and vascular involvement are similar. At our institution, we prefer to use multiphasic scanning with 64-detector helical scanners because of better spatial resolution, and the results in preoperative staging for local tumor vascular involvement were excellent and have been well accepted by our hepatobiliary surgeons[18,36]; the results have also been supported by others.[15,19,21]

The criteria of vascular involvement by tumors on CT and MR imaging are based on those observed in pancreatic ductal carcinoma, which include: (1) the abutment of the vessels, referring to a tumor inseparable from the vessels by less than 180°, (2) the encasement of the vessels, meaning a tumor encircling the vessel or in contact by more than 180°, and (3) the occlusion of the vessels.[37,38]

8.3.4.1 Portal Venous Anatomy and Its Involvement

Although the portal vein accompanies the bile duct in the portal triads in the hepatic lobules and in the hilar plate, the branching patterns of the main portal vein are not always similar or corresponding to the branching of the bile duct. The bifurcation of the portal vein into left and right branches occurs in 60–94% cases, with the right branch dividing into anterior and posterior sectorial branches supplying segments V/VIII and VI/VII, respectively. The variations of this pattern include the trifurcation of the main portal vein into left, right paramedian, and right lateral branches (8–10%), the right lateral branch from the main portal vein (5–10%) (Fig. 8.5), and the right paramedian branch from the left portal vein (3–4%).[33] However, the confluence of the right and left hepatic duct often lies anterior to the right portal vein, and the right portal vein always courses behind the right hepatic duct in the right hilar plate, whereas the left portal vein courses anteriorly medial to the left hepatic duct in the left hilar plate.

Because of this close relationship, the periductal growth of the tumor of the extrahepatic bile duct frequently involves the adjacent portal vein and can compromise surgical resectability. The anatomy of the branching patterns of the portal vein and the tumor involvement should be described in an imaging report with special attention on the anatomy of the contralateral portal vein, its adjacency to the tumor, and the presence or absence of tumor involvement (Figs. 8.6–8.8). However, it should be noted that the abutment of the contralateral portal vein shorter than 2 cm may be considered for resection with the venous construction in the center with such expertise. Moreover, in isolated cases, anatomic variations of the portal vein could significantly change surgical approach.

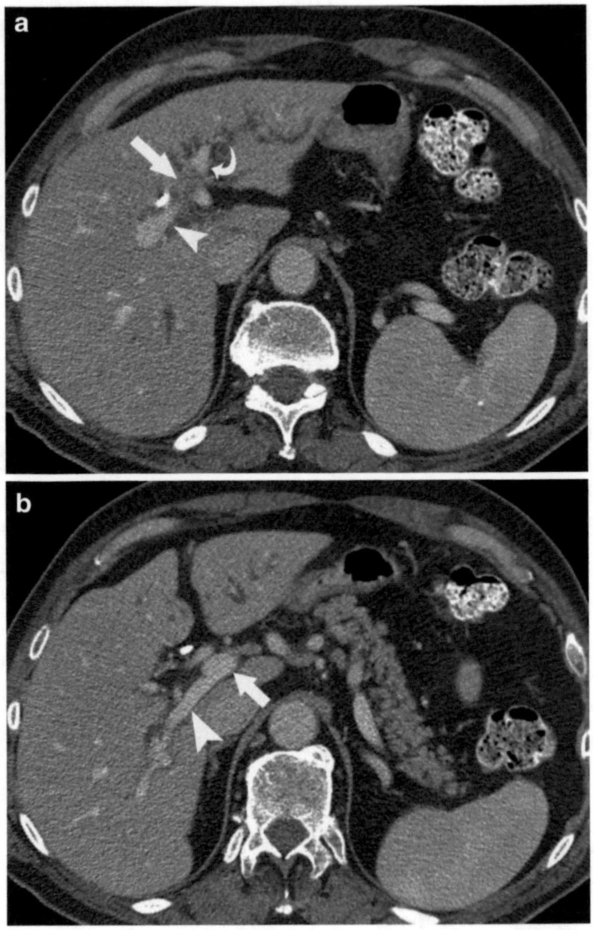

Fig. 8.5 Variation of lateral sectorial branch of the right portal vein arising from the main portal vein. (**a**) Axial CT image demonstrates an infiltrative tumor (*arrow*) involving the left hepatic duct and left portal vein (*curve arrow*). The paramedian sectorial branch of the right portal vein (*arrowhead*) is also encased. (**b**) Axial CT image at a lower level shows the lateral sectorial branch of the right liver (*arrowhead*) originated from the main portal vein (*arrow*) and was not involved by the tumor. This anatomic variation allowed a margin-negative left liver resection and the paramedian sectoral liver resection leaving the lateral sector of the right liver intact

8.3.4.2 Hepatic Arterial Anatomy and Its Involvement

The variations of hepatic arterial anatomy are well recognized, and Michel's classification has been the standard of reference in imaging and surgical literature.[33,39] This information should be included in imaging reports. The branching patterns of the segmental and lobar artery and its adjacency to the tumor can be demonstrated on CT. Most commonly, the right hepatic artery courses between the right hepatic duct and the right portal vein or anterior to the duct in the hilar plate, while the left hepatic artery is medial to the left hepatic duct.

Once tumor growth penetrates into the periductal tissues, it often infiltrates along the hepatic nerve and hepatic artery in the hilar plate and can grow along the

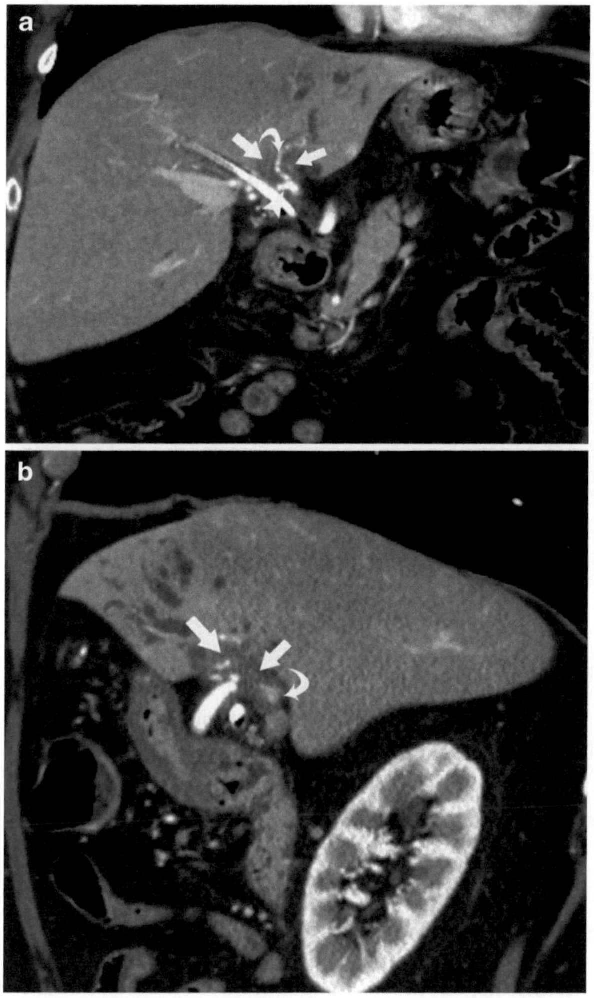

Fig. 8.6 Locally advanced, unresectable hilar cholangiocarcinoma involving the left hepatic artery, right hepatic artery, occlusion of the left portal vein, and encasement of the right portal vein. (**a**) CT image on a coronal plane shows infiltrative tumor (*arrows*) in the left hilar plate encasing the left hepatic artery (*curve arrow*) and the origin of the right hepatic artery (*arrowhead*). Note a stent on the bile duct of segment VIII. (**b**) CT image on a sagittal plane identifies the infiltrative tumor (*arrows*) involving the right portal vein (*curve arrow*)

hepatic artery toward the celiac axis or the superior mesenteric artery. The detailed anatomic information of the hepatic artery of the involved hepatic lobe and segment may not be as important as that of the uninvolved segment or lobe, and the extent of the tumor along the hepatic artery. This is because the artery and portal vein of the involved lobe or segment will be removed as part of anatomic resection. The branching patterns and the course of the hepatic artery of the uninvolved liver and its adjacency to the tumor are

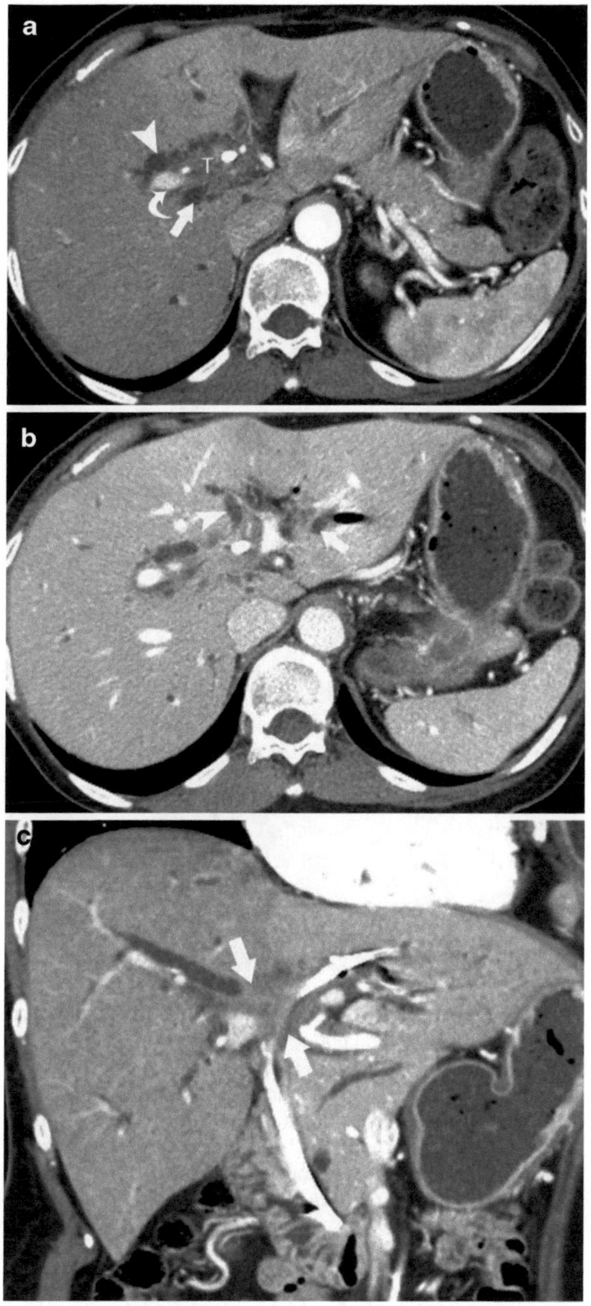

Fig. 8.7 Locally advanced, unresectable hilar cholangiocarcinoma, a type IV Bismuth–Corlette classification. (**a**) Axial CT image demonstrates diffuse infiltrative tumor (*T*) in the right hilar plate obstructing segment VIII bile duct (*arrowhead*) and segment VI and VII bile duct (*arrow*). The right portal vein (*curve arrow*) is also encased. (**b**) Axial CT image at a lower level shows the tumor in the left hilar plate obstructing segment IV bile duct (*arrowhead*) and segment II duct (*arrow*). (**c**) Coronal CT image shows extensive tumor (*arrows*) in both hilar plate involving the portal veins and hepatic arteries

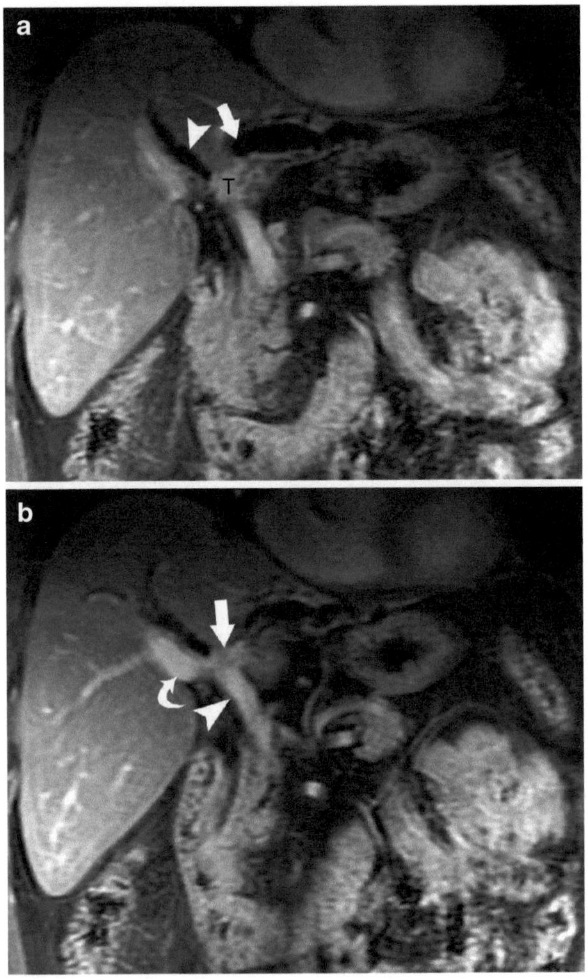

Fig. 8.8 Locally advanced, unresectable hilar cholangiocarcinoma due to contralateral portal vein involvement. (**a**) Post contrast, T1-weighted coronal MR image shows an enhancing, hilar cholangiocarcinoma (*T*) predominantly in the left hilar plate obstructing the left hepatic duct (*arrow*) and segment VIII duct (*arrowhead*). (**b**) Post contrast, T1-weighted coronal MR image posterior to image A demonstrates the tumor (*arrow*) encasing the main portal vein (*arrowhead*) and the origin of the right portal vein (*curve arrow*)

more important and should be identified for surgical planning in order to achieve a negative resection margin (see Fig. 8.4).

8.3.4.3 Preoperative Imaging Assessment of Nodal Metastasis in Hilar Cholangiocarcinoma

Lymphatic metastases are common in hilar cholangiocarcinoma and are correlated with poor survival. Nodal metastases are found in about 30–50% of patients undergoing surgical resection. Nodal metastases commonly occur along the lymphatic drainage pathways of the bile duct. The TNM/AJCC classification identifies the nodes in the hepatic hilum and the nodes along the portal vein and hepatic artery in the hepatoduodenal ligament as N1 nodal station. They are routinely removed at surgery for curative intent. Metastases to the nodes at the celiac axis, superior mesenteric artery, periaortic and pericaval region are considered N2 nodal station. They are associated with poorer outcome and are not considered resectable for curative intent. The Japanese classification adds the N3 nodal group and identifies the nodes along the common hepatic artery and posterior pancreaticoduodenal region as N2 nodal station and the nodes at the celiac axis, superior mesenteric artery, periaortic and pericaval region as N3 nodal station.[4] One of the studies focusing on lymph node metastasis in hilar cholangiocarcinoma showed that nodal metastases are most commonly found at the hilar region. Metastases to periaortic nodes occurred in about 10% and were usually associated with advanced disease and metastatic nodes far away from the primary tumor such as the nodes at the common hepatic artery and superior mesenteric artery.[40]

CT and MR imaging can identify lymph nodes in the hepatoduodenal ligament, at the celiac axis, at the mesentery, and in the retroperitoneum, but they lack specificity to determine if they are metastatic nodes. Nodal size alone cannot distinguish reactive nodes from metastatic nodes. Criteria such as central necrosis with ill-defined margins are more specific for metastasis, but those changes are not common and lack sensitivity. The suggested imaging criteria for nodal involvement including short axis measurements of greater than 10 mm, nodal enhancement, or central necrosis had an accuracy rate of 84%.[15]

Because of the lack of specificity in the diagnosis of metastatic nodes and the routine lymphadenectomy of nodes in the hepatoduodenal ligament at surgery with curative intent, our approach to image analysis regarding nodal metastasis focuses on using those criteria to identify the abnormal nodes that are away from the primary tumor and those that would not be included in the field of surgical resection. We then use those images to guide aspiration biopsy before planning definitive surgery.

8.3.4.4 Preoperative Imaging for Volume Analysis

Lobar atrophy is a secondary sign for hilar cholangiocarcinoma. The measurement of the volume of the normal liver that will be preserved for future liver remnant is essential for preoperative portal vein embolization and for planning extended liver resection.[41,42] The issues are described elsewhere in this book.

References

1. Carriega MT, Henson DE. Liver, gallbladder, extrahepatic bile ducts and pancreas. *Cancer*. 1995;75:171-190.
2. Ito F, Cho CS, Rikkers LF, Weber SM. Hilar cholangiocarcinoma: current management. *Ann Surg*. 2009;250:210-218.
3. Blechacz B, Gores GJ. Cholangiocarcinoma: advances in pathogenesis, diagnosis and treatment. *Hepatology*. 2008;48: 308-321.
4. Japanese Society of Biliary Surgery. *General Rules for Surgical and Pathological Studies on Cancer of the Biliary Tract*. Tokyo: Kanehara; 1986.
5. Nakeeb A, Pitt HA, Sohn T, et al. Cholangiocarcinoma: a spectrum of intrahepatic, perihilar, and distal tumors. *Ann Surg*. 1996;224:463-475.
6. Klatskin G. Adenocarcinoma of the hepatic duct at its bifurcation within the porta hepatis. An unusual tumor with distinctive clinical and pathological features. *Am J Med*. 1965;38:241-256.
7. Kosogue T, Yamamoto J, Shimada K, et al. Improved surgical results for hilar cholangiocarcinoma with procedures including major hepatic resection. *Ann Surg*. 1999;230:663-671.
8. Neuhaus P, Jonas S, Bechstein WO, et al. Extended resection for hilar cholangiocarcinoma. *Ann Surg*. 1999;230:808-818.
9. Launois B, Reding R, Lebeau G, et al. Surgery for hilar cholangiocarcinoma: French experience in a collective survey of 552 extrahepatic bile duct cancer. *J Hepatobiliary Pancreat Surg*. 2000;7:128-134.
10. Jarnagin WR, Fong Y, DeMatteo RP, et al. Staging, resectability, and outcome in 225 patients with hilar cholangiocarcinoma. *Ann Surg*. 2001;234:507-517.
11. Seyema Y, Kubota K, Sano K, et al. Long-term outcome of extended hemihepatectomy for hilar bile duct cancer with no mortality and high survival rate. *Ann Surg*. 2003;238: 73-83.
12. Ebata T, Nagino M, Kamiya J, et al. Hepatectomy with portal vein resection for hilar cholangiocarcinoma: audit of 52 consecutive cases. *Ann Surg*. 2003;238:720-727.
13. Hemming AW, Reed AI, Fujita S, et al. Surgical management of hilar cholangiocarcinoma. *Ann Surg*. 2005;241:693-699.
14. Hemming AW, Kim RD, Mekeel KL, et al. Portal vein resection for hilar cholangiocarcinoma. *Am Surg*. 2006;72:599-604.
15. Lee HY, Kim SH, Lee JM, et al. Preoperative assessment of resectability of hilar cholangiocarcinoma: combined CT and cholangiography with revised criteria. *Radiology*. 2006; 239:113-121.
16. Chen HW, Pan AZ, Zhen ZY, et al. Preoperative evaluation of resectability of Klatskin tumor with 16-MDCT angiography and cholangiography. *AJR*. 2006;186:1580-1586.
17. Kim HJ, Lee JM, Kim SH, et al. Evaluation of the longitudinal tumor extent of bile duct cancer: value of adding gadolinium-enhanced dynamic imaging to unenhanced imaged and magnetic resonance cholangiography. *J Comput Assist Tomogr*. 2007;31:469-474.
18. Aloia TA, Charnsangavej C, Faria S, et al. High-resolution computed tomography accurately predicts resectability in hilar cholangiocarcinoma. *Am J Surg*. 2007;193:702-706.
19. Choi J-Y, Kim M-J, Lee JM, et al. Hilar cholangiocarcinoma: role of preoperative imaging with sonography, MDCT, MRI, and direct cholangiography. *AJR*. 2008;191:1448-1457.
20. Park HS, Lee JM, Choi J-Y, et al. Preoperative evaluation of bile duct cancer: MRI combined with MR cholangiopancreatography. *AJR*. 2008;190:396-405.
21. Vilgrain V. Staging cholangiocarcinoma by imaging studies. *HPB (Oxford)*. 2008;10:106-109.
22. Masselli G, Manfredi R, Vecchioli A, Gualdi G. MR imaging and MR cholangiopancreatography in the preoperative evaluation of hilar cholangiocarcinoma: correlation with surgical and pathologic findings. *Eur Radiol*. 2008;18: 2213-2221.
23. Weber SM, DeMatteo RP, Fong Y, et al. Staging laparoscopy in patients with extrahepatic biliary carcinoma. Analysis of 100 patients. *Ann Surg*. 2002;235:392-399.
24. Edge SB, Byrd DR, Compton CC, et al., eds. Perihilar bile duct and distal bile duct. In: *Cancer Staging Manual*. 7th ed. New York: Springer; 2010:219–233.
25. Weinbren K, Mutum SS. Pathological aspects of cholangiocarcinoma. *J Pathol*. 1983;139:217-238.
26. Hayashi S, Miyazaki M, Kondo Y, et al. Invasive growth patterns of hepatic hilar ductal carcinoma. A histologic analysis of 18 surgical cases. *Cancer*. 1994;73:2922-2929.
27. Jarnagin WR, Bowne W, Klimstra DS, et al. Papillary phenotype confers improved survival after resection of hilar cholangiocarcinoma. *Ann Surg*. 2005;241:703-712.
28. Lim JH. Cholangiocarcinoma: morphologic classification according to growth pattern and imaging findings. *AJR*. 2003;181:819-827.
29. Verbeek PC, van Leeuwen DJ, de Wit LT, et al. Benign fibrosing disease at the hepatic confluence mimicking Klatskin tumors. *Surgery*. 1992;112:866-871.
30. Wetter LA, Ring EJ, Pellegrini CA, et al. Differential diagnosis of sclerosing cholangiocarcinomas of the common hepatic duct (Klatskin tumors). *Am J Surg*. 1991;161:57-62.
31. Kim JY, Lee JM, Han JK, et al. Contrast-enhanced MRI combined with MR cholangiopancreatography for the evaluation of patients with biliary strictures: differentiation of malignant from benign bile duct strictures. *J Magn Reson Imaging*. 2007;26:304-312.
32. Healy JE, Scroy PC. Anatomy of the biliary ducts within the human liver: analysis of the prevailing pattern of branching and the major variations of the biliary ducts. *Arch Surg*. 1953;66:599-616.
33. Charnsangavej C. Anatomy of the liver, bile duct and pancreas. In: Gazelle GC, Saini S, Mueller PR, eds. *Hepatobiliary and Pancreatic Radiology, Imaging and Intervention*. New York: Thieme Medical Publishers, Inc.; 1998:1-23.
34. Abdalla EK, Vauthey JN, Couinaud C. The caudate lobe of the liver: implications of embryology and anatomy for surgery. *Surg Oncol Clin N Am*. 2002;11:835-848.
35. Sakamoto E, Nimura Y, Hayakawa N, et al. The pattern of infiltration at the proximal border of hilar bile duct carcinoma: a histologic analysis of 62 resected cases. *Ann Surg*. 1998;227:405-411.
36. Parikh A, Abdala E, Vauthey JN. Operative considerations in the resection of hilar cholangiocarcinoma. *HPB (Oxford)*. 2005;7:254-258.

37. Loyer EM, David CL, DuBrow RA, Evans DB, Charnsangavej C. Vascular involvement in pancreatic adenocarcinoma: reassessment by thin-section CT. *Abdom Imaging*. 1996;21:202-206.
38. Katz MHG, Pisters PWT, Evans DB, et al. Borderline resectable pancreatic cancer: the importance of this emerging stage of disease. *J Am Coll Surg*. 2008;206:833-848.
39. Michels NA. Observations on the blood supply of the liver (200 dissections). In: *Blood Supply and Anatomy of the Upper Abdominal Organs*. Philadelphia: Lippincott JB; 1995:139-165.
40. Kitagawa Y, Nagino M, Kayima J, et al. Lymph node metastasis from hilar cholangiocarcinoma: audit of 110 patients who underwent regional and paraaortic node dissection. *Ann Surg*. 2001;233:385-392.
41. Vauthey JN, Chaoui A, Do KA, et al. Standardized measurement of the future liver remnant prior to extended liver resection; methodology and clinical associations. *Surgery*. 2000;127:512-519.
42. Hemming AW, Reed AI, Howard RJ, et al. Preoperative portal vein embolization for extended hepatectomy. *Ann Surg*. 2003;237:686-691.

Preoperative Imaging of Liver Cancers: Metastases

9

Richard K.G. Do and Bachir Taouli

Abstract

Imaging plays a pivotal role in patients with suspected liver metastases not only for diagnosis but also for staging and for presurgical evaluation. Several modalities are available; these include ultrasound, CT, MRI, and PET or PET/CT. Ultrasound is operator-dependent and has *generally* low sensitivity for detection, especially for small lesions. CT is the most frequently used technique as it is quick, widely available, and accurate; however, it is limited by radiation exposure and has limited characterization of subcentimeter hepatic lesions. MRI is accurate and free of radiation exposure; however, it is limited by cost and availability. PET and PET/CT have a role mostly for detection of extrahepatic disease. The role and results of these modalities will be discussed in this review.

Keywords

Liver metastases • Imaging of liver cancer • MDCT of liver cancer • MRI of liver cancer • Staging of liver cancer

Liver metastases are the most frequently encountered malignant liver lesions, commonly arising from colon, breast, lung, pancreas, melanoma, and sarcoma. A large proportion (up to 70%) of patients with primary colorectal carcinoma (CRC) will develop synchronous or metachronous hepatic metastases.[1,2]

B. Taouli (✉)
Department of Radiology, Mount Sinai Medical Center, New York, NY, USA
e-mail: bachir.taouli@mountsinai.org

9.1 Diagnosis: Impact and Considerations

Accurate diagnosis of liver metastases is increasingly critical as surgical resection has been shown to improve patient survival, especially in patients with CRC.[3] From an economic perspective, improving our sensitivity in the detection of liver metastases can also spare patients unnecessary surgery.[4] The goals of preoperative imaging were recently outlined in an expert consensus statement in the selection of patients for resection of hepatic colorectal metastases.[5] Briefly,

D.C. Madoff et al. (eds.), *Venous Embolization of the Liver*,
DOI 10.1007/978-1-84882-122-4_9, © Springer-Verlag London Limited 2011

these were to (1) define the number and extent of hepatic metastases and their segmental and lobar distribution and (2) identify any extrahepatic disease. These imaging goals can be broadly applied to other liver metastases, not only for surgical planning, but also for regional therapies such as chemoembolization, radiofrequency ablation, hepatic artery infusion pumps, etc., which may be performed alone or in combination with surgical resection.

Once liver metastases are identified, they should be characterized with respect to size and location. The segmental location and adjacent vessel should be identified, with attention to vascular anatomy variants.[6] Proximity to feeding vessels and draining veins should be identified as these may impact chemoembolization and radiofrequency ablation, respectively. Resectability based on preoperative imaging depends on the number of metastases and the presence of bilobar involvement, and it may be underestimated depending on the imaging technique.[7] As will be discussed below, intraoperative ultrasound at the time of surgery may alter the surgical plan.

9.1.1 Hypervascular Versus Hypovascular Liver Metastases

The literature on the imaging of liver metastases is skewed toward CRC, given evidence for improved survival following surgical resection of colorectal liver metastases. Insights from studies on CRC are potentially applicable to other malignancies. However, an important distinction should be made between hypovascular metastases (which include the majority of colorectal metastases) and hypervascular metastases.

The liver has a dual blood supply provided by the portal venous and hepatic arterial systems. Metastases are termed hyper- or hypovascular depending on their enhancement relative to background liver parenchyma after contrast injection. Primary hypervascular tumors that typically lead to hypervascular liver metastases include thyroid carcinomas, neuroendocrine tumors including carcinoid tumors, and renal cell carcinomas.[8] Metastases from breast, colon, and pancreatic carcinomas may also be hypervascular. Hypovascular metastases typically enhance less avidly than the surrounding liver parenchyma, but may exhibit perilesional enhancement.[9]

9.2 Available Imaging Modalities and Results for Detection of Liver Metastases

9.2.1 Ultrasound

Transabdominal ultrasound (US) plays a limited role in the diagnosis of liver metastases, given its limited sensitivity of approximately 50–75%.[10] The addition of intravenous contrast improves the sensitivity of transabdominal US by about 20%, approaching that of MDCT (multidetector CT).[10-12]

Recent studies using perflubutane ultrasound microbubbles (Sonazoid, Amersham Health) showed promising results for the detection and characterization of focal liver lesions.[13] Contrast-enhanced US with perflubutane microbubbles has two phases of contrast enhancement: a vascular and a Kupffer phase (perflubutane microbubbles are taken up by Kupffer cells in the reticuloendothelial system of the liver, and these images are typically performed 10 min after contrast injection). Recent studies have revealed perflubutane-enhanced ultrasound to have a higher sensitivity in detecting liver lesions when compared to contrast-enhanced CT, especially for small tumors.[14,15] Note that this agent is not FDA-approved in the United States.

However, the best practical reference standard for detection of liver metastases is intraoperative ultrasound (IOUS) combined with surgical exploration, which are often performed at the time of hepatic surgery.[16,17] IOUS often alters the surgical plan, demonstrating unresectability or altering a surgical approach.[18]

In a comparison between IOUS and helical CT on 250 patients undergoing surgical resection, IOUS detected additional tumors in 27% of patients.[19] In a later study, improvements in cross-sectional imaging did not alter the beneficial role of IOUS, which altered surgical management in 20% of cases in two different time periods to account for improvements in CT scanning.[20] However, advances in MDCT and MRI may ultimately reduce the utility of IOUS.[21,22]

Similar to transabdominal ultrasound, a limitation of IOUS is its operator dependence. CRC liver metastases can have a variable appearance on IOUS from hyperechoic to isoechoic and hypoechoic.[23] More recently, the utility of contrast-enhanced IOUS (CE-IOUS) has been advocated in a study of 60 patients with colorectal cancer.[24] CE-IOUS had greater sensitivity compared to CT/MRI and IOUS (96.1% vs. 76.7% and 81.5%).

9.2.2 Multidetector CT (MDCT)

MDCT is now routinely used for the detection of liver metastases.[25] State-of-the-art MDCT offers high temporal and spatial resolution and is widely available and relatively inexpensive. Bolus-tracking technique is required for the optimization of arterial and portal venous phase imaging. The arterial phase of enhancement is typically obtained at 20–30 s after the injection of contrast, while the portal venous phase is obtained at approximately 60 s. The exact timing depends on the rate and volume of contrast injection and the scanning technique. Hypovascular metastases are most evident during portal venous phase imaging,[26] while hypervascular metastases are typically more conspicuous on arterial phase imaging.[27,28] Hypovascular metastases are hypodense compared to normal liver parenchyma, but they may demonstrate rim enhancement that subsequently washes out on later phases.[21] Arterial phase imaging using a high-contrast injection rate is also useful for surgical or regional therapy planning, for delineation of vascular anatomy.

Liver metastases have a variable appearance on unenhanced CT, with the majority being hypodense. Calcifications may occur when the primary malignancy is a mucinous adenocarcinoma (Fig. 9.1); cystic liver metastases may occur in the setting of a cystic malignant tumor such as ovarian carcinoma. A drawback for unenhanced CT occurs in the imaging of patients with fatty livers, where typically hypodense lesions may blend imperceptibly with the low-attenuation fatty liver.

A limitation of CT is the patient exposure to ionizing radiation and the potential for reactions to iodinated contrast, discussed below. Another limitation of CT is in the limited characterization of subcentimeter lesions, too small to accurately characterize as metastatic or benign, even in patients with known primary malignancies.[29,30]

9.2.3 PET and PET/CT

State-of-the-art FDG-PET imaging is performed with concurrent CT, and it provides a metabolic map of

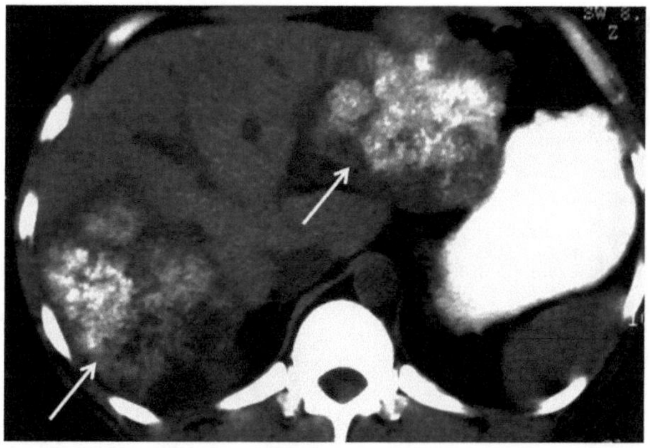

Fig. 9.1 Axial pre-contrast CT image shows two large calcified liver metastases from mucinous colon carcinoma (*arrows*)

glucose uptake throughout the whole body with the goal of detecting metabolically active tumor cells (Fig. 9.2). PET is routinely used in the evaluation of patients with malignancies, demonstrating high sensitivity and specificity for the detection of liver metastases, with the advantage of the detection of extrahepatic metastases that have profound implications in patient management.[31] PET has been shown to be superior to CT for the detection of extrahepatic metastases.[32,33]

The use of intravenous contrast in the CT portion of a PET/CT exam has been shown to improve the detection of colorectal liver metastases.[34] The authors of a retrospective study which included 39 patients advocated for the routine use of intravenous contrast in PET/CT in lieu of the usual low-dose unenhanced CT. Dual time point PET/CT, with a second PET acquisition at approximately 100 min, also appears to increase the detection of liver metastases.[35] This is due to the decrease in background FDG uptake in the liver at a later time, relative to FDG-avid metastases.

9.2.4 MRI

Liver metastases have a variable appearance on MRI, depending on the primary malignancy and their vascularity.[8] Compared to CT, MRI has the potential advantage of increased lesion conspicuity given the number of different imaging sequences employed. With noncontrast imaging, T1 weighted (T1W), T2 weighted (T2W), and diffusion weighted imaging (DWI) are used to detect and characterize liver lesions. Most liver

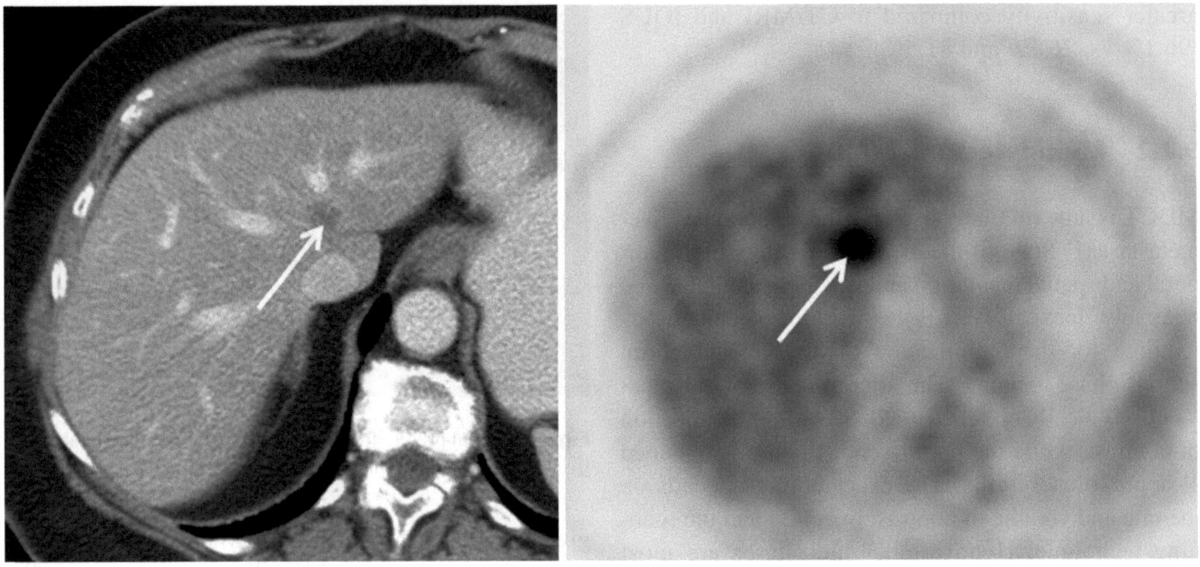

Fig. 9.2 Axial post-contrast CT (*left*) and PET (*right*) images in a patient with metastatic colon cancer. There is a left hepatic lobe lesion (*arrow*) with increased FDG uptake

metastases are hypointense on T1W and hyperintense on T2W images. DWI increases liver lesion conspicuity compared to T2W sequences.[36,37]

A number of different intravenous contrast agents can also be used to further detect and characterize liver lesions.[38] Extracellular gadolinium chelates such as gadopentetate dimeglumine (Gd-DTPA, Magnevist, Bayer Healthcare Pharmaceuticals) are used routinely in abdominal MRI. With these, liver lesion conspicuity depends on dynamic imaging protocols and the hyper- or hypovascular nature of the metastasis (Figs. 9.3 and 9.4). Peripheral rim enhancement is a common pattern; heterogeneous enhancement is seen more often in larger lesions (>3 cm), and homogeneous enhancement is seen more often in small hypervascular lesions.[8] Perilesional enhancement in the form of circular or wedge-shaped enhancement may also be seen, typically for hypovascular colorectal metastases, which can lead to overestimation in tumor size.[9]

Hepatobiliary agents such as gadobenate dimeglumine (Gd-BOPTA, MultiHance, Bracco Diagnostics, Princeton, NJ) or gadoxetate disodium (Gd-EOB-DTPA, Eovist, Bayer Healthcare Pharmaceuticals) potentially improve the characterization of small liver lesions as they are incorporated in normal liver, but excluded from metastatic lesions.[39,40] The use of contrast agents containing superparamagnetic iron oxide (SPIO) particles including ferumoxides and a newer agent, ferucarbotran (Resovist, Schering, Germany – approved for use in Europe and Japan),[41] is based on the differential uptake of contrast in normal liver parenchyma that contain Kupffer cells, compared to liver metastases that lack them. Uptake of SPIO agents causes T2W shortening, decreasing normal liver signal intensity on T2W images. In two recent studies, SPIO MRI using ferucarbotran was better than CT at detecting liver metastases.[42,43] For small liver lesions that are indeterminate on CT or PET/CT, MRI may serve as a problem-solving tool when the resectability of liver metastases is questioned.[44]

9.2.5 Comparisons Between Imaging Modalities

Each imaging modality has specific advantages and disadvantages (Table 9.1) related to cost, speed of acquisition, lack or presence of ionizing radiation, and risk of contrast reaction. The choice between CT and MRI for individual patients will depend on a number of factors, including the patient's renal function and a history of anaphylactoid or allergic reaction to contrast.[45] There is a risk of contrast-induced nephropathy following iodinated CT contrast administration in patients with impaired renal function.[46] In patients with severe renal failure, MRI contrast agents containing gadolinium chelates should be avoided given the risk of nephrogenic systemic fibrosis.[47,48] An abdominal MRI also

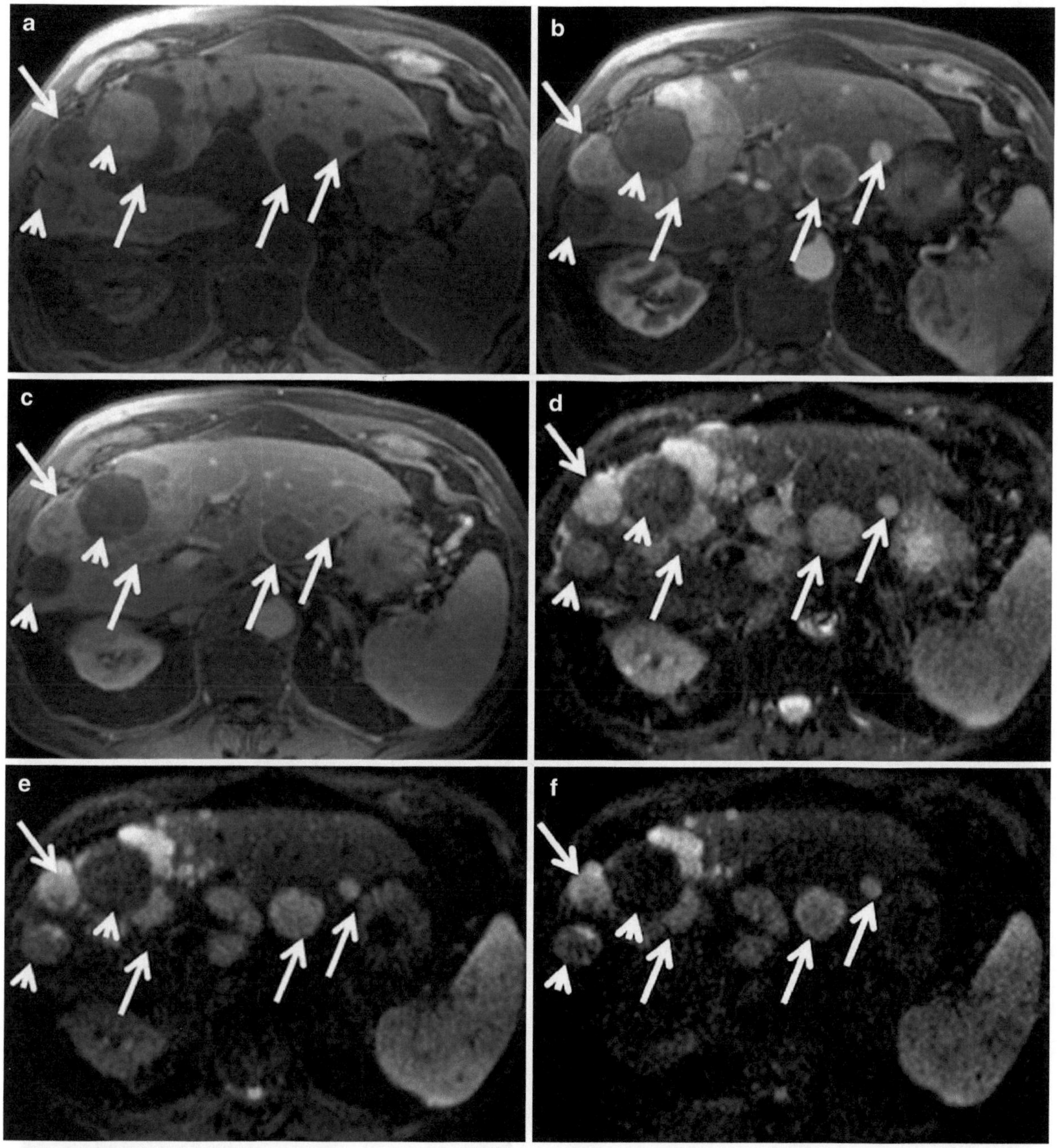

Fig. 9.3 MR images in a patient with liver metastases from carcinoid tumor treated with prior chemoembolization. Axial T1-weighted images obtained prior (**a**), and after contrast administration at the arterial (**b**) and portal venous phases (**c**). Axial fat suppressed single shot echoplanar diffusion images for $b=0$ (**d**), 500 (**e**), and 1,000 (**f**) s/mm^2. There are innumerable liver metastases which demonstrate early arterial enhancement with washout at the portal venous phase (*arrows*) and restricted diffusion (hyperintense at b500 and 1,000 s/mm^2). There are two necrotic lesions (secondary to prior chemoembolization) that show no evidence for enhancement or restricted diffusion (*arrowheads*)

requires a patient who is able to consistently breath hold, as image degradation by respiratory motion can easily render postcontrast images non-diagnostic. The sensitivity and specificity of individual modalities vary depending on the primary malignancy and, perhaps more importantly, on institution-specific expertise.

In a meta-analysis comparing CT, PET/CT, and MRI in the diagnosis of colorectal liver metastases,[49]

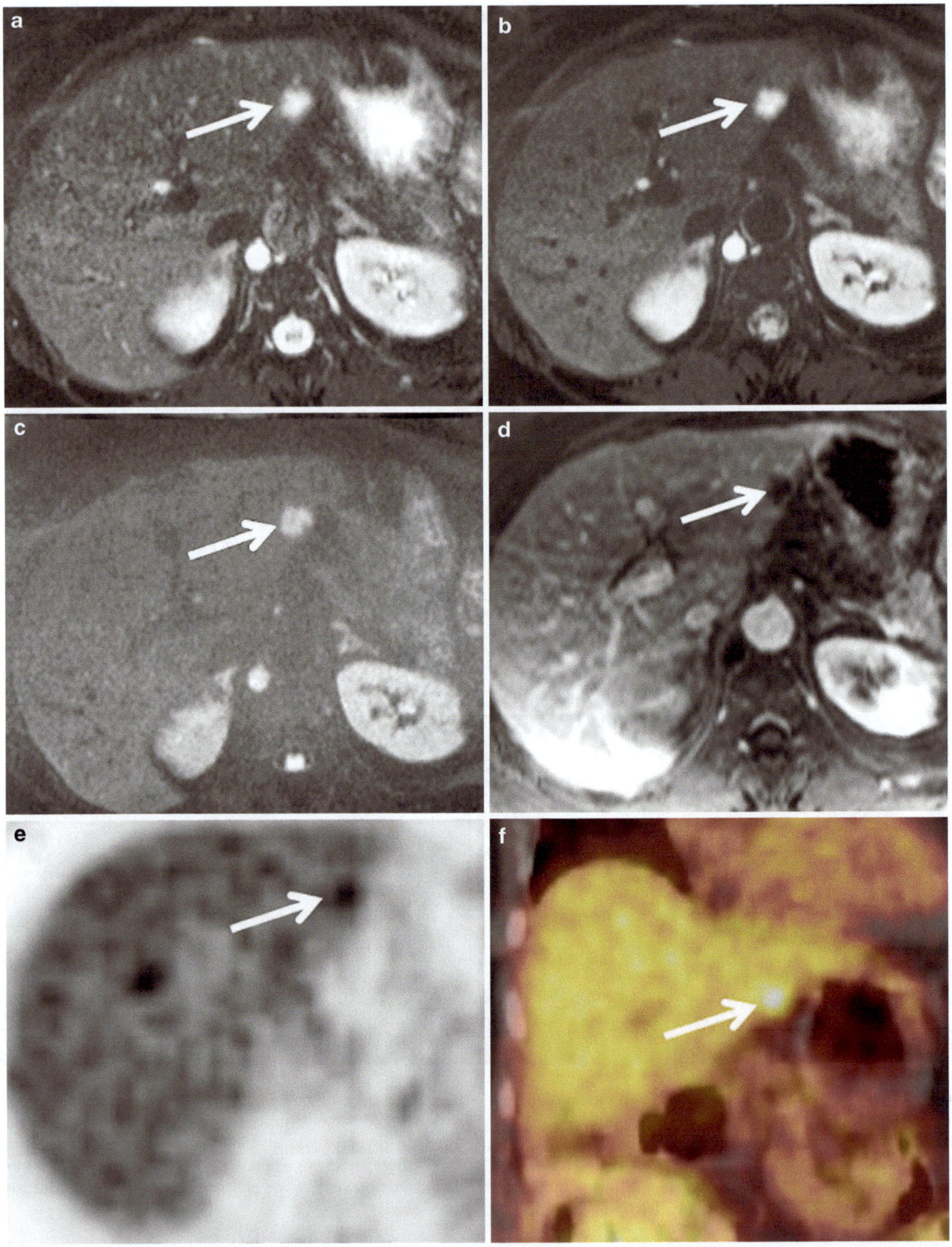

Fig. 9.4 MRI and PET in a patient with liver metastasis from colorectal cancer. Axial fat suppressed single shot echoplanar diffusion images for $b=0$ (**a**), 500 (**b**) and 1,000 (**c**) s/mm^2. Axial T1-weighted images after contrast administration at the portal venous phase (**d**). Axial FDG PET (**e**) and fused PET/CT coronal image (**f**). There is a lateral left hepatic lobe hypovascular metastasis, which demonstrates restricted diffusion (hyperintense on b500 and 1000 s/mm^2) and avid FDG uptake on PET (*arrow*)

Table 9.1 Overview of imaging modalities used for detection of colorectal liver metastases

Modality	Advantages	Disadvantages	Sensitivity (%)
MDCT	Speed	Ionizing radiation	60–80
	Availability and cost	Contrast reactions	
		Low accuracy for subcentimeter lesions	
MRI	No ionizing radiation	Risk of NSF	84–99
	Liver specific contrast	Respiratory motion artifact	
PET/CT	Detection of extrahepatic disease	Low resolution	85–97
		Ionizing radiation	

Sensitivity on a per lesion basis for each imaging modality were pooled from recent studies using MDCT (multidetector CT), PET/CT with CECT (contrast-enhanced CT), and MRI using a variety of contrast agents.[22,32,37,39,42,45,52] A single study[42] used for the calculation of sensitivities included 2 patients (out of 58) with a malignancy other than colorectal cancer

61 articles published between 1990 and 2003 were reviewed; the authors concluded that PET/CT had a significantly higher sensitivity on a per-patient basis, but not on a per-lesion basis. However, significant advances in technique have occurred since 2003. In a more recent retrospective study examining 33 patients with colorectal cancer with a total of 110 liver lesions, MRI was found to have higher accuracy than CE-PET/CT and NE-PET/CT based on ROC analysis (0.97 vs. 0.86 and 0.74).[50] In this study, the MRI study included T2W TSE, T1W in and out of phase, and pre- and postcontrast images using gadolinium chelates. Similarly, in a study of 24 patients with colorectal liver metastases, MRI (using SPIO with a spin echo echoplanar imaging sequence) demonstrated superior sensitivity to PET/CT, especially for small lesions.[51]

The sensitivity and specificity reported for different imaging modalities depend on a number of factors. These include the number of patients and their tumor burden (high tumor burden patients will have many subcentimeter lesions, lowering overall sensitivity), the reference standard used (preferably histological examination of resected specimens), the prevalence of incidental benign lesions (which will affect the specificity), and the contrast agent used for MRI (SPIO, hepatobiliary agents, extracellular Gd chelates).

Overall, PET/CT was shown to be superior to CE-CT for the detection of liver metastases on a per-patient basis, in a study of 131 patients, 75 of which had CRC.[33] A substantial limitation of MDCT and PET remains in the characterization of small subcentimeter lesions. In a study of 127 patients with 363 liver metastases from CRC, both multiphasic CT and PET missed the majority of lesions <1.0 cm and missed over 20% of lesions between 1.0 and 2.0 cm.[52] The use of dual time point PET/CT may improve the sensitivity of PET to small liver metastases.[35]

9.3 Conclusion

In preoperative imaging of oncologic patients, the detection of liver and extrahepatic metastases is initially best accomplished by PET/CT. Contrast-enhanced MDCT, with its widespread availability and relatively low cost, remains the workhouse for the detection of liver metastases and the evaluation of hepatic vasculature, which potentially influences therapeutic options. MRI is superior to both PET/CT and contrast-enhanced MDCT in the characterization of small liver lesions, but its disadvantages include limited availability and the requirement of a cooperative patient. The choice of MRI versus CT may ultimately depend on institution-specific expertise or patient-specific considerations such as impaired renal function and allergic history.

Several advances in liver imaging will improve our diagnostic accuracy. These include contrast-enhanced ultrasonography, quantitative perfusion imaging using MDCT and MRI, and the routine use of intravenous contrast in the CT portion of PET/CT. If surgical resection is considered, intraoperative ultrasound currently remains useful as it may alter surgical approach or patient resectability status in spite of state-of-the-art preoperative imaging.

References

1. Baker ME, Pelley R. Hepatic metastases: basic principles and implications for radiologists. *Radiology*. 1995;197(2): 329-337.
2. Martinez L, Puig I, et al. Colorectal liver metastases: radiological diagnosis and staging. *Eur J Surg Oncol*. 2007;33(suppl 2): S5-S16.
3. Adams RB, Haller DG, et al. Improving resectability of hepatic colorectal metastases: expert consensus statement by Abdalla et al. *Ann Surg Oncol*. 2006;13(10):1281-1283.

4. Annemans L, Lencioni R, et al. Health economic evaluation of ferucarbotran-enhanced MRI in the diagnosis of liver metastases in colorectal cancer patients. *Int J Colorectal Dis*. 2008;23(1):77-83.
5. Charnsangavej C, Clary B, et al. Selection of patients for resection of hepatic colorectal metastases: expert consensus statement. *Ann Surg Oncol*. 2006;13(10):1261-1268.
6. Catalano OA, Singh AH, et al. Vascular and biliary variants in the liver: implications for liver surgery. *Radiographics*. 2008;28(2):359-378.
7. Jarnagin WR, Fong Y, et al. Liver resection for metastatic colorectal cancer: assessing the risk of occult irresectable disease. *J Am Coll Surg*. 1999;188(1):33-42.
8. Danet IM, Semelka RC, et al. Spectrum of MRI appearances of untreated metastases of the liver. *AJR Am J Roentgenol*. 2003;181(3):809-817.
9. Semelka RC, Hussain SM, et al. Perilesional enhancement of hepatic metastases: correlation between MR imaging and histopathologic findings—initial observations. *Radiology*. 2000;215(1):89-94.
10. Konopke R, Kersting S, et al. Contrast-enhanced ultrasonography to detect liver metastases: a prospective trial to compare transcutaneous unenhanced and contrast-enhanced ultrasonography in patients undergoing laparotomy. *Int J Colorectal Dis*. 2007;22(2):201-207.
11. Dietrich CF, Kratzer W, et al. Assessment of metastatic liver disease in patients with primary extrahepatic tumors by contrast-enhanced sonography versus CT and MRI. *World J Gastroenterol*. 2006;12(11):1699-1705.
12. Larsen LP, Rosenkilde M, et al. The value of contrast enhanced ultrasonography in detection of liver metastases from colorectal cancer: a prospective double-blinded study. *Eur J Radiol*. 2007;62(2):302-307.
13. Sugimoto K, Shiraishi J, et al. Improved detection of hepatic metastases with contrast-enhanced low mechanical-index pulse inversion ultrasonography during the liver-specific phase of sonazoid: observer performance study with JAFROC analysis. *Acad Radiol*. 2009;16(7):798-809.
14. Hatanaka K, Kudo M, et al. Sonazoid-enhanced ultrasonography for diagnosis of hepatic malignancies: comparison with contrast-enhanced CT. *Oncology*. 2008;75(suppl 1): 42-47.
15. Moriyasu F, Itoh K. Efficacy of perflubutane microbubble-enhanced ultrasound in the characterization and detection of focal liver lesions: phase 3 multicenter clinical trial. *AJR Am J Roentgenol*. 2009;193(1):86-95.
16. Cervone A, Sardi A, et al. Intraoperative ultrasound (IOUS) is essential in the management of metastatic colorectal liver lesions. *Am Surg*. 2000;66(7):611-615.
17. Foroutani A, Garland AM, et al. Laparoscopic ultrasound vs triphasic computed tomography for detecting liver tumors. *Arch Surg*. 2000;135(8):933-938.
18. Kruskal JB, Kane RA. Intraoperative US of the liver: techniques and clinical applications. *Radiographics*. 2006;26(4): 1067-1084.
19. Scaife CL, Ng CS, et al. Accuracy of preoperative imaging of hepatic tumors with helical computed tomography. *Ann Surg Oncol*. 2006;13(4):542-546.
20. Ellsmere J, Kane R, et al. Intraoperative ultrasonography during planned liver resections: Why are we still performing it? *Surg Endosc*. 2007;21(8):1280-1283.
21. Sahani DV, Kalva SP, et al. Intraoperative US in patients undergoing surgery for liver neoplasms: comparison with MR imaging. *Radiology*. 2004;232(3):810-814.
22. Tamandl D, Herberger B, et al. Adequate preoperative staging rarely leads to a change of intraoperative strategy in patients undergoing surgery for colorectal cancer liver metastases. *Surgery*. 2008;143(5):648-657.
23. Choti MA, Kaloma F, et al. Patient variability in intraoperative ultrasonographic characteristics of colorectal liver metastases. *Arch Surg*. 2008;143(1):29-34; discussion 35.
24. Ong KO, Leen E. Radiological staging of colorectal liver metastases. *Surg Oncol*. 2007;16(1):7-14.
25. Kamel IR, Fishman EK. Recent advances in CT imaging of liver metastases. *Cancer J*. 2004;10(2):104-120.
26. Soyer P, Poccard M, et al. Detection of hypovascular hepatic metastases at triple-phase helical CT: sensitivity of phases and comparison with surgical and histopathologic findings. *Radiology*. 2004;231(2):413-420.
27. Bonaldi VM, Bret PM, et al. Helical CT of the liver: value of an early hepatic arterial phase. *Radiology*. 1995;197(2):357-363.
28. Francis IR, Cohan RH, et al. Multidetector CT of the liver and hepatic neoplasms: effect of multiphasic imaging on tumor conspicuity and vascular enhancement. *AJR Am J Roentgenol*. 2003;180(5):1217-1224.
29. Schwartz LH, Gandras EJ, et al. Prevalence and importance of small hepatic lesions found at CT in patients with cancer. *Radiology*. 1999;210(1):71-74.
30. Khalil HI, Patterson SA, et al. Hepatic lesions deemed too small to characterize at CT: prevalence and importance in women with breast cancer. *Radiology*. 2005;235(3):872-878.
31. Erturk SM, Ichikawa T, et al. PET imaging for evaluation of metastatic colorectal cancer of the liver. *Eur J Radiol*. 2006;58(2):229-235.
32. Truant S, Huglo D, et al. Prospective evaluation of the impact of [18F] fluoro-2-deoxy-D-glucose positron emission tomography of resectable colorectal liver metastases. *Br J Surg*. 2005;92(3):362-369.
33. Chua SC, Groves AM, et al. The impact of 18F-FDG PET/CT in patients with liver metastases. *Eur J Nucl Med Mol Imaging*. 2007;34(12):1906-1914.
34. Badiee S, Franc BL, et al. Role of IV iodinated contrast material in 18F-FDG PET/CT of liver metastases. *AJR Am J Roentgenol*. 2008;191(5):1436-1439.
35. Dirisamer A, Halpern BS, et al. Dual-time-point FDG-PET/CT for the detection of hepatic metastases. *Mol Imaging Biol*. 2008;10(6):335-340.
36. Bruegel M, Gaa J, et al. Diagnosis of hepatic metastasis: comparison of respiration-triggered diffusion-weighted echo-planar MRI and five t2-weighted turbo spin-echo sequences. *AJR Am J Roentgenol*. 2008;191(5):1421-1429.
37. Parikh T, Drew SJ, et al. Focal liver lesion detection and characterization with diffusion-weighted MR imaging: comparison with standard breath-hold T2-weighted imaging. *Radiology*. 2008;246(3):812-822.
38. Gandhi SN, Brown MA, et al. MR contrast agents for liver imaging: what, when, how. *Radiographics*. 2006;26(6):1621-1636.
39. Kim YK, Lee JM, et al. Detection of liver metastases: gadobenate dimeglumine-enhanced three-dimensional dynamic phases and one-hour delayed phase MR imaging versus superparamagnetic iron oxide-enhanced MR imaging. *Eur Radiol*. 2005;15(2):220-228.

40. Hammerstingl R, Huppertz A, et al. Diagnostic efficacy of gadoxetic acid (Primovist)-enhanced MRI and spiral CT for a therapeutic strategy: comparison with intraoperative and histopathologic findings in focal liver lesions. *Eur Radiol.* 2008;18(3):457-467.
41. Reimer P, Balzer T. Ferucarbotran (Resovist): a new clinically approved RES-specific contrast agent for contrast-enhanced MRI of the liver: properties, clinical development, and applications. *Eur Radiol.* 2003;13(6):1266-1276.
42. Ward J, Robinson PJ, et al. Liver metastases in candidates for hepatic resection: comparison of helical CT and gadolinium- and SPIO-enhanced MR imaging. *Radiology.* 2005; 237(1):170-180.
43. Kim HJ, Kim KW, et al. Comparison of mangafodipir trisodium- and ferucarbotran-enhanced MRI for detection and characterization of hepatic metastases in colorectal cancer patients. *AJR Am J Roentgenol.* 2006;186(4):1059-1066.
44. Mueller GC, Hussain HK, et al. Effectiveness of MR imaging in characterizing small hepatic lesions: routine versus expert interpretation. *AJR Am J Roentgenol.* 2003;180(3): 673-680.
45. Weinreb JC. Which study when? Is gadolinium-enhanced MR imaging safer than iodine-enhanced CT? *Radiology.* 2008;249(1):3-8.
46. Gleeson TG, Bulugahapitiya S. Contrast-induced nephropathy. *AJR Am J Roentgenol.* 2004;183(6):1673-1689.
47. Kanal E, Barkovich AJ, et al. ACR guidance document for safe MR practices: 2007. *AJR Am J Roentgenol.* 2007;188(6): 1447-1474.
48. Thomsen HS, Marckmann P, et al. Update on nephrogenic systemic fibrosis. *Magn Reson Imaging Clin N Am.* 2008;16(4): 551-560.
49. Bipat S, van Leeuwen MS, et al. Colorectal liver metastases: CT, MR imaging, and PET for diagnosis–meta-analysis. *Radiology.* 2005;237(1):123-131.
50. Cantwell CP, Setty BN, et al. Liver lesion detection and characterization in patients with colorectal cancer: a comparison of low radiation dose non-enhanced PET/CT, contrast-enhanced PET/CT, and liver MRI. *J Comput Assist Tomogr.* 2008;32(5):738-744.
51. Coenegrachts K, De Geeter F, et al. Comparison of MRI (including SS SE-EPI and SPIO-enhanced MRI) and FDG-PET/CT for the detection of colorectal liver metastases. *Eur Radiol.* 2008;16:16.
52. Wiering B, Ruers TJ, et al. Comparison of multiphase CT, FDG-PET and intra-operative ultrasound in patients with colorectal liver metastases selected for surgery. *Ann Surg Oncol.* 2007;14(2):818-826.

CT Volumetry: The Japanese Methodology

10

Keiichi Kubota

Abstract

Since the balance between the extent of liver resection and liver function is closely associated with postoperative morbidity and mortality, volumetric information is indispensable when deciding on the most appropriate liver resection procedure for hepatic tumors and any indications for portal embolization (PE), and when performing living-donor liver transplantation (LDLT). The extent of liver resection is usually evaluated by computed tomography (CT) volumetry using two-dimensional (2D) or three-dimensional (3D) CT images, both of which can calculate liver volume precisely. Furthermore, volumetry with 3D CT yields the total liver volume and automatically calculates the volumes of the territories of individual vessels (both portal vein branches and hepatic venous branches) from their diameters and lengths. Based on this volumetric data and liver function, the feasibility of a planned liver resection procedure can be decided. Any indications for PE in extended hemi-hepatectomy can also be evaluated. The volume of Couinaud's segment can also be estimated by volumetry using 3D CT. Because ensuring the donor's safety is of prime importance in LDLT, CT volumetry is routinely employed to assess the necessary graft size and determine whether an adequately sized graft can be procured. Furthermore, 3D CT volumetry can estimate the volume of congestion in the hepatic venous branch of the graft, which gives important information on which to base decisions regarding the reconstruction of the branch. Thus, CT volumetry is indispensable in hepatic surgery.

Keywords

Computed tomography • CT volumetry • Japanese methodology of CT volumetry • Liver resection • 3D CT

K. Kubota
Department of Gastroenterological Surgery,
Dokkyo Medical University, 880 Kitakobayashi, Mibu,
Shimotsuga-gun, Tochigi 321-0293, Japan
e-mail: kubotak@dokkyomed.ac.jp

D.C. Madoff et al. (eds.), *Venous Embolization of the Liver*,
DOI 10.1007/978-1-84882-122-4_10, © Springer-Verlag London Limited 2011

In spite of advances in therapeutic modalities in the field of abdominal diseases, liver resection is still the mainstay of treatment for hepatobiliary malignancies. Many kinds of hepatobiliary diseases require liver resection. The background status of the liver parenchyma differs with each type, and can be roughly classified as normal, icteric, or cirrhotic. These different characteristics of the liver parenchyma may lead to different degrees of regenerative power or functional reserve. Clinically, the treatment option is selected according to the tumor condition and liver function. The tumor condition includes the size, number, location, and invasiveness of the tumor(s). These factors are associated with the extent of liver parenchymal resection required to extirpate the tumor; however, the safe maximum extent of liver resection is restricted by each patient's individual liver function. In patients with normal liver function, about 70% of the liver parenchyma can be resected,[1] while in patients with liver cirrhosis, the extent of liver resection is limited. When there is curative intent, extensive liver resection is often required; however, this may lead to postoperative liver failure due to an inadequate liver remnant, and consequently has a major impact on morbidity and mortality after liver resection. It is therefore important to develop accurate diagnostic tools for evaluating liver function and measuring the future liver remnant (FLR) so that the risk of liver resection-related morbidity and mortality can be predicted.

Various laboratory data and imaging techniques have been used to complement the Child-Pugh score in order to predict liver failure after hepatectomy and to assess the functional hepatic reserve.[2] The aminopyrine breath test and galactosyl elimination capacity yield important information on liver function but are not accurate enough to determine whether hepatectomy is indicated in impaired livers.[3] The indocyanine green (ICG) retention test is the most widely used clearance test. In most cases, the most appropriate liver resection procedure can be determined using Makuuchi's criteria, which include the absence or presence of ascites, the serum total bilirubin level, and the indocyanine green retention rate at 15 min (ICG15).[4] However, these criteria remain imperfect because they depend on both the hepatic blood flow and the functional capacity of the liver. Nuclear imaging of the asialoglycoprotein receptors with radio-labeled synthetic asialoglycoproteins provides volumetric information as well as a functional assessment of the liver.[5] In a population that included patients with parenchymal disease and hilar cholangiocarcinoma, preoperative measurement of 99 mTc-mebrofenin uptake in the FLR by functional hepatobiliary scintigraphy proved more valuable than measurement of the actual volume of the FLR when assessing the risk of post-hepatectomy liver failure.[6] Since liver function is complex, a test that can successfully assess the quantitative functional hepatic reserve still needs to be established.

Volumetric information is mainly obtained by computed tomography (CT) volumetry. CT volumetry is now employed in many clinical fields, including the treatment of tumors of the lung, breast, stomach, oral cavity, and esophagus,[7-12] and of intracranial hemorrhage.[13] CT volumetry was first described by Heymsfield in 1979.[14] In the field of hepatobiliary surgery, CT volumetry is used for estimating the FLR and the necessary size of the liver graft in living-donor liver transplantation (LDLT) and in deciding whether there are indications for portal embolization (PE). Without the information gained from CT volumetry, the safety of liver resection and LDLT cannot be guaranteed. In this chapter, the status of CT volumetry in the field of liver surgery is described.

10.1 Methods of CT Volumetry

Volumetric information is essential when deciding on the most appropriate liver resection procedure for hepatic tumors and for any indications for PE, and when performing LDLT. The maximum extent of liver resection is determined according to liver function. In Japan, CT scanning with enhancement to measure liver volume and the ICG retention test to evaluate liver function are routinely performed before each hepatectomy.[15] The balance between the extent of liver resection and liver function is closely associated with postoperative morbidity and mortality. The extent of liver resection is usually evaluated by CT volumetry of the relevant liver segments. This detailed information contributes to a final decision regarding the most appropriate surgical procedure. CT volumetry can now be done using both two-dimensional (2D) CT and three-dimensional (3D) CT.

10.1.1 Volumetry with Two-Dimensional CT

Preoperative helical CT images are made using representations of 2- to 5-mm-thick slices of the liver on a

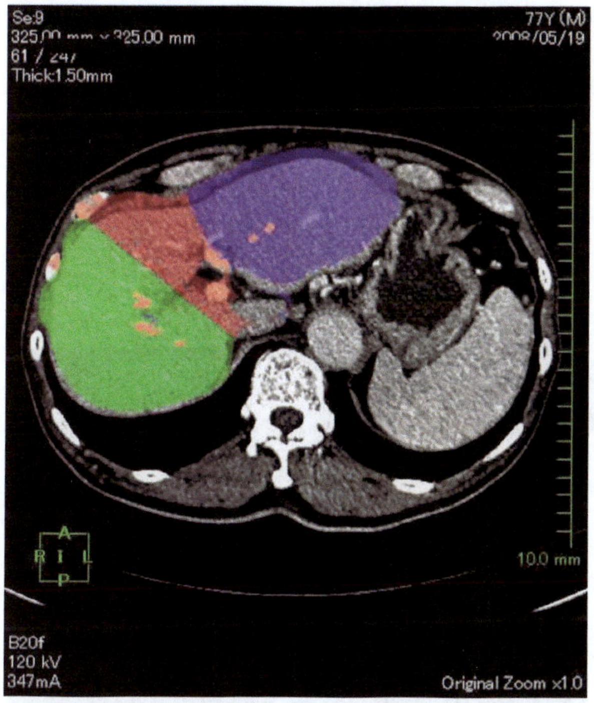

Fig. 10.1 Autocalculation of the enclosed area using two-dimensional computed tomography (2D CT) images. The *green*, *red*, and *violet* zones represent the right hepatic lobe, segment 4, and the left lateral lobe, respectively. The respective areas are calculated automatically. These areas and the slice thickness are used to calculate the volume of the slice

CT machine, including the segments between the dome of the diaphragm and the most caudal part of the liver. Enhancement is achieved using an intravenous bolus of contrast medium. This method allows for clear visualization of the intrahepatic portal veins and the hepatic veins. The liver volume (mL) is calculated by the method of Heymsfield with minor modifications.[14] The CT slices are scanned using a scanner (Epson GT-9500, Long Beach, CA) with a mouse ball device and image-handling software (PhotoShop 5.0, Adobe, San Jose, CA). The entire perimeter of the liver and the segment of each slice are outlined, and the enclosed area is automatically calculated using image-analysis software (NIH image 1.61) (Fig. 10.1).[16] The right and middle hepatic veins, falciform ligament, umbilical portion of the left portal vein, gallbladder, and inferior vena cava are used to determine the borderlines of each segment. Using these CT slices, the whole liver, tumor, non-tumor resected parenchymal area, and non-tumor preserved area can be traced, and their areas calculated as described above. The volume of each liver slice is then calculated using the following equation:

$$V = S \times A$$

V, the volume of one liver slice

S, the interval between the serial slices (cm)

A, the enclosed area (cm^2)

The same procedure is repeated for all the slices. The resection ratio (RR) is then calculated using the following formula:

$$\mathrm{VW} = \mathrm{VW}_1 + \mathrm{VW}_2 + \cdots + \mathrm{VW}_n$$

$$\mathrm{VT} = \mathrm{VT}_1 + \mathrm{VT}_2 + \cdots + \mathrm{VT}_n$$

$$\mathrm{VRP} = \mathrm{VRP}_1 + \mathrm{VRP}_2 + \cdots + \mathrm{VRP}_n$$

$$\mathrm{VPP} = \mathrm{VPP}_1 + \mathrm{VPP}_2 + \cdots + \mathrm{VPP}_n$$

$$\mathrm{RR} = \mathrm{VRP} / (\mathrm{VW} - \mathrm{VT}) \times 100(\%)$$

VW, volume of the whole liver, including the tumor (mL)

VT, tumor volume (mL)

VRP, volume of the non-tumor resected parenchyma (mL)

VPP, volume of the non-tumor preserved parenchyma (mL)

VW − VT = VRP + VPP (mL)

n, number of slices

The RR is the ratio of the non-tumor parenchymal volume of the resected liver to that of the whole liver.

This 2D CT volumetry technique yields a sufficiently accurate volume. However, it should be borne in mind that volumetric CT is subject to an absolute error, which tends to increase as the extent of liver resection increases (mean, 64.9 mL (13.8%).[17]

10.1.2 Volumetry with Three-Dimensional CT

In hepatic surgery, 3D visualization makes it possible to understand the stereoscopic relationship between a hepatic tumor and the hepatic vessels, including the portal veins and hepatic veins. In particular, 3D visualization is useful for hepatic venous reconstruction in the recipient, as well as for donor surgery, in LDLT using a right lobe graft.[18,19]

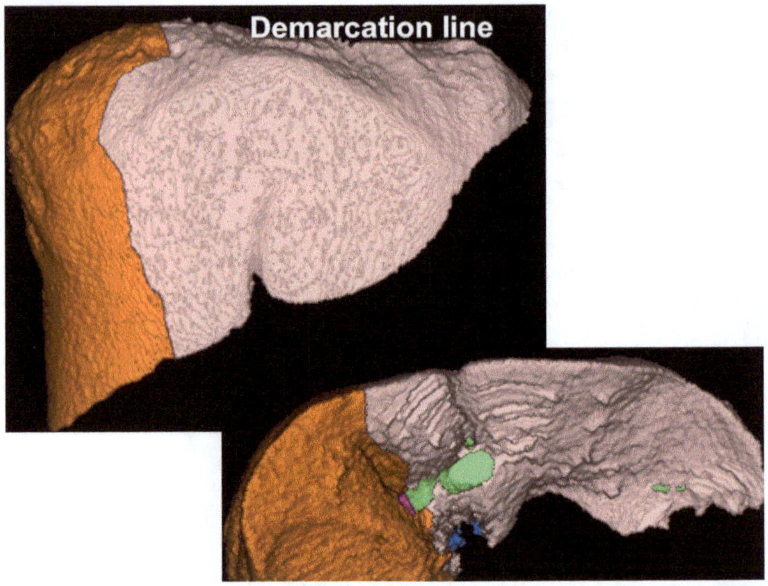

Fig. 10.2 Reconstructive imaging of the liver based on the territories of the portal branches (Region Growing Software, Hitachi, Tokyo, Japan). Using a region-growing method, images of the right and left liver have been reconstructed according to the ramifications of the portal branches. The border line can be clearly seen (Courtesy of Prof. Kokudo, Tokyo University)

The entire 3D image is visualized and reconstructed from a 0.2–3 mm slice of helical CT data. By selecting images of all abdominal structures except the liver (achieved by changing the contrast of the CT number), a rough 3D image of the liver can be reconstructed by subtracting these images from the entire image. The three-directional 2D images are rechecked and used to provide detailed 3D images. The color of the images and the contrast level of the CT number between the vessels and hepatic parenchyma are altered. Then, a picture of the vessels in and around the liver is constructed. Once the correct image of the liver has been selected, the volume of the liver can be calculated using a region-growing technique.

Region-growing is one of the simplest region-based segmentation methods. It can be classified as a pixel-based image segmentation technique because it involves the selection of initial seed points. Region-growing software enables one to calculate the total liver volume and the volumes of the territories of individual vessels (both the portal vein branches and hepatic venous branches) from their diameters and lengths.[20] The volume of the right lobe is calculated automatically from the right portal vein territories and the drainage volume of each hepatic venous branch (Figs. 10.2–10.4). This type of volumetry can also contribute to decisions regarding whether small hepatic branches should be reconstructed. It has been reported that 3D CT can reveal the anatomy of the hepatic vein bifurcation and the shape of the graft.[19] The error ratio is 12.8 ± 2.3% in 3D CT compared with 19.4 ± 2.5% in 2D CT. Thus, 3D CT volumetry appears to be more exact than the conventional 2D CT volumetry, but volumetry by 3D CT still produces an error ratio of approximately 13%. It should be taken into consideration that 3D CT volumetry based on venous phase CT is associated with considerable overestimation, while

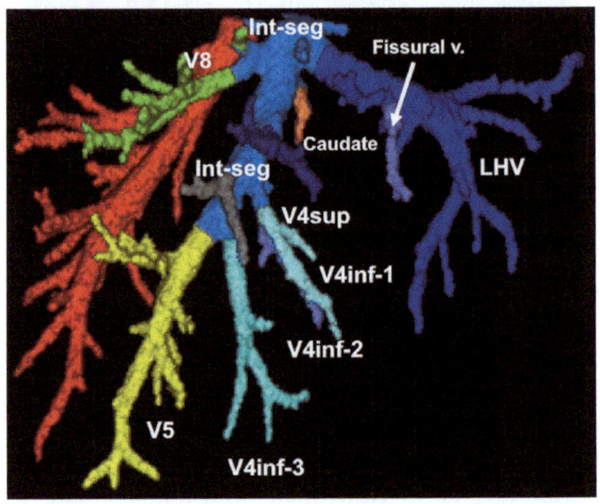

Fig. 10.3 Reconstructive imaging of the hepatic vein branches (Region Growing Software, Hitachi, Tokyo, Japan.). Three-dimensional images of the main hepatic venous branches have been reconstructed with color identification (Courtesy of Prof. Kokudo, Tokyo University, Japan)

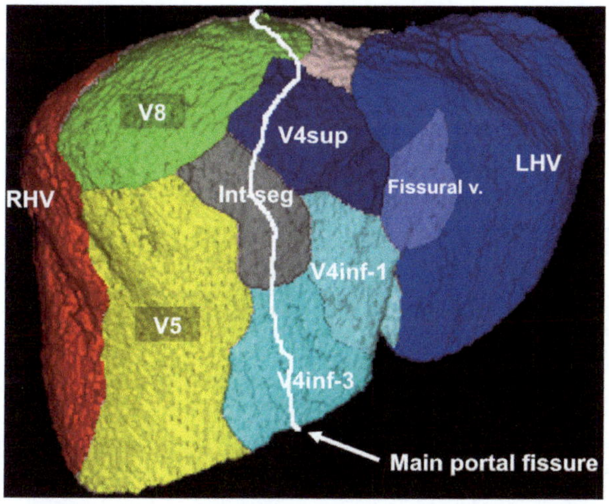

Fig. 10.4 Liver areas drained by the respective hepatic vein branches (Region Growing Software, Hitachi, Tokyo, Japan). The respective areas drained by the main hepatic venous branches shown in Fig. 10.3 are illustrated. The main portal fissure is identified by the ramification of the portal branches (Courtesy of Prof. Kokudo, Tokyo University, Japan)

3D CT volumetry based on the native CT phase accurately matches the intraoperative findings.[21]

Furthermore, 3D imaging can be used to simulate a planned hepatic resection. Three-dimensional graft images are advantageous because they allow both 3D visualization and three separate 2D perspectives, which are useful as reliability checks, and make a smooth cutting line possible in operative simulations. The error ratio may be attributed to a mismatch between the cutting line in the simulation and that in the actual hepatectomy. Although it has been reported that there were no significant differences between volumetry using a region-growing technique and conventional volumetry,[22] 3D CT volumetry is easier to perform than 2D CT volumetry and can be performed automatically.

10.2 CT Volumetry in Hepatobiliary Diseases

10.2.1 Hepatic Resection

10.2.1.1 Liver Function and Liver Resection Procedures

Makuuchi's criteria are one of the most widely accepted sets of criteria for selecting the most appropriate hepatic resection procedure according to liver function (Fig. 10.5).[4] Untreatable ascites is a contraindication for hepatic resection. Patients must have a serum total bilirubin level of less than 2 mg/dL to be accepted for hepatic resection. When the serum total bilirubin level is normal (less than 1 mg/dL), the hepatic procedure is selected according to the ICG15. In principle, a right hepatic lobectomy is indicated in patients with an ICG15 smaller than 10%. However, if an extensive liver resection is needed, resulting in a small remnant liver, there is an increased risk of postoperative mortality.[23] Therefore, even if the liver function is normal, estimation of the FLR after major hepatectomy is mandatory in order to justify the procedure and decide whether there are any indications for PE. Furthermore, although right hepatic lobectomy is not usually indicated in patients with slightly impaired liver function (i.e., an ICG15 of 10–20%), the procedure can be performed in such patients after PE, provided that the RR is 40–60%. Thus, CT volumetry is indispensable when planning hepatic surgery.

10.2.1.2 CT Volumetry for Hemi-hepatectomy and Segmentectomy

Major hepatectomy, including right hemi-hepatectomy, is always associated with some degree of postoperative liver failure. Only volumetric data can predict whether a patient should undergo right hemi-hepatectomy with or without PE. The resection range of the liver is determined from CT, and the volume of the FLR is calculated using CT volumetry.[24] Despite progress in surgical procedures and perioperative care, the possibility or extent of liver resection is still limited in many cases by liver dysfunction. It has been reported that the critical FLR values for safe hepatectomies should be 26.5% in patients with normal liver function and 31% in patients in whom impaired liver function is suspected preoperatively.[25] The postoperative liver function level and survival rate are related to the percentage of FLR and the grade of liver cirrhosis as determined by CT. Combining these two parameters forms an important prediction line for the estimation of hepatic functional reserve and likelihood of survival.[26] Furthermore, ICG values decrease significantly after surgery, depending on the reduction in liver volume, and the estimated ICG value based on the residual liver volume may be useful in predicting postoperative morbidity.[27] Based on our experience, an RR of up to 60% is possible in patients with normal liver function, while in patients with impaired liver function (i.e., an ICG15 of 10–20%) an RR of up

Fig. 10.5 Makuuchi's criteria

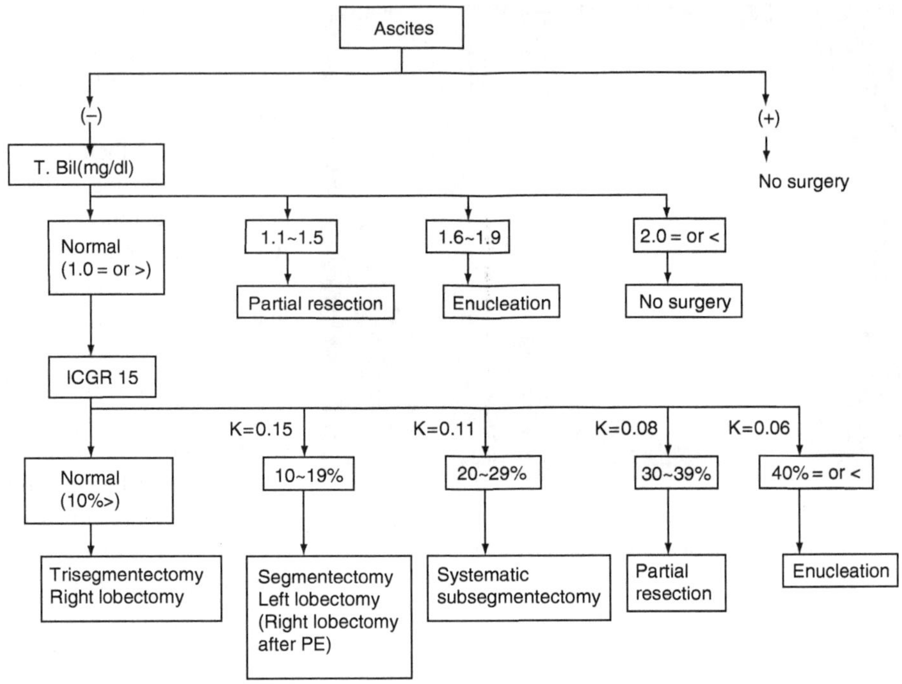

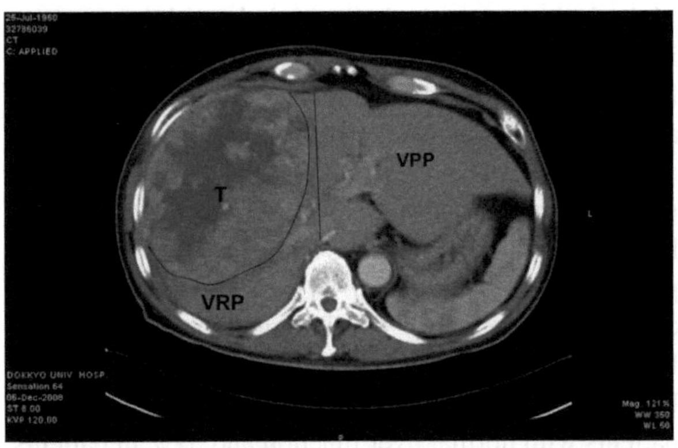

Fig. 10.6 Case 1: CT findings in a massive hepatocellular carcinoma (HCC). A 20-cm HCC occupied the right liver of a 58-year-old male patient. CT volumetry using 2D images estimated that the volume of the non-tumor resected liver parenchyma after right hemi-hepatectomy would be 23%. The patient successfully underwent right hemi-hepatectomy without portal embolization. *VRP* volume of non-tumor resected liver parenchyma (mL), *VPP* volume of non-tumor preserved liver (mL)

to 40% is possible. In order to decide whether hepatectomy with a large RR is possible, information on liver function and volumetric data are indispensable.

Case 1: A 58-year-old male patient was admitted to our department with a massive hepatic tumor. He was positive for hepatitis B virus antibody and hepatitis C virus antibody. CT showed a large hepatocellular carcinoma (HCC) with a maximum diameter of 20 cm. Volumetry using 2D CT images demonstrated that the non-tumor liver parenchymal volumes of the right and left hepatic lobes were 153 and 751 mL, respectively, with an RR of 17% (Fig. 10.6). ICG15 was 11%. He underwent right hemi-hepatectomy without PE. The postoperative course was uneventful.

10.2.1.3 Portal Embolization

Recently, PE has become widely accepted as a preoperative management technique for increasing the safety of subsequent extensive liver resection. Depending on the FLR, PE can be employed to reduce the size of the liver region to be resected and induce hypertrophy of the contra-lateral liver.[28] PE allows more patients with previously unresectable liver tumors to benefit from resection.[29] Thus, PE not only reduces the risk of postoperative liver failure but also increases the chances of a curative resection.[30,31] In fact, it has been reported that in icteric patients with hilar cholangiocarcinoma, there was no postoperative mortality after extended hemi-hepatectomy when PE was employed.[32] In order to select the most appropriate surgical procedure, including the need for PE, the extent of liver resection (in terms of the RR) should be estimated precisely.

The normal liver is reported to tolerate removal of up to 70% of its volume,[1] but the extent to which the liver parenchyma can be resected in patients with chronic liver diseases or jaundice has yet to be elucidated.

Several criteria for assessing the indications for PE have been proposed. Kubota et al. reported that PE is indicated when liver function is normal (i.e., the ICG15 is less than 10%) and the resection volume of the non-cancerous liver parenchyma is greater than 60% or when there is mild liver dysfunction (i.e., the ICG15 is 10–20%), and the resection volume of the non-cancerous liver parenchyma is 40–60%.[17] In principle, right hemi-hepatectomy and PE are contraindicated in patients with an ICG15 value of more than 20% or with an RR of more than 60% and an ICG15 of 10–20%. However, Abdalla et al. reported that preoperative PE is acceptable in patients with an RR of 75% or more if the liver is normal and in those with a RR of 60% or more if the liver is diseased.[33] Ferrero et al. also reported that patients with an FLR of less than 25% could undergo PE.[25] Thus, the indications for PE based on volumetric data for normal or impaired livers have not yet been standardized worldwide.

Two to four weeks after PE, CT volumetry is repeated to evaluate the regeneration of the FLR. It has been reported that PE increases the FLR by an average of 9%, thereby allowing resection in 50% of patients.[34] Confirmation of the regeneration of the contra-lateral lobe is also important. Only then can the feasibility and timing of an extended resection be finally decided.

Case 2: A 68-year-old male patient was referred to our department for treatment of hilar cholangiocarcinoma. After reduction of the serum total bilirubin to less than 5 mg/dL, he underwent right PE. After 2 weeks, CT showed an increase in the volume of the left hepatic lobe from 501 mL (33%) to 621 mL (45%) (Fig. 10.7a, b). On the 43 rd postoperative day after PE, he underwent extended right hemi-hepatectomy. The postoperative course was uneventful.

10.2.1.4 CT Volumetry for Partial Hepatectomy

In patients with an ICG15 value of 20–30%, Couinaud's segmentectomy is possible, while in patients with an ICG15 value greater than 30%, non-anatomical resection or partial resection is possible. These procedures are safer if the volume of the non-tumor resected parenchyma can be estimated. However, with 2D CT volumetry, it is difficult to calculate the volume

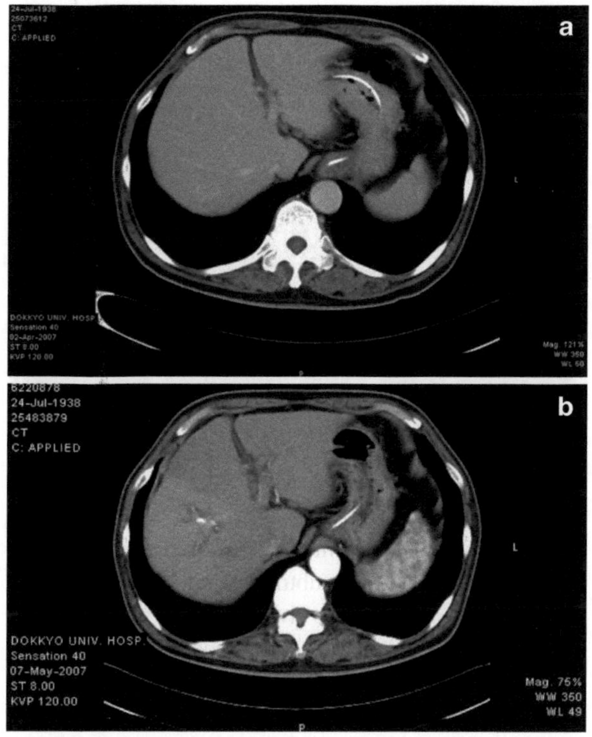

Fig. 10.7 Case 2: CT findings in the liver of a patient with hilar cholangiocarcinoma. (**a**) Before portal embolization, the volumes of the right and left livers were estimated to be 1,021 mL (67%) and 501 mL (33%), respectively, by volumetry using 2D images. (**b**) After portal embolization, the left liver regenerated to an estimated volume of 621 mL (45%). Arterial flow was predominant in the right liver and consequently the demarcation line between the right and left livers clearly shows a dent due to atrophy

correctly. Accurate assessment of the resection volume and the vascular anatomy is mandatory in preoperative planning to maximize the chances of a safe hepatectomy when cancer is being treated with curative intent. Hepatectomy simulations using 3D CT images and a region-growing technique can accurately predict the segmental liver volume at the level of Couinaud's segments and the resection margin. This virtual method can, thus, make a strong contribution to the preoperative planning of curative resection in HCC patients whose hepatic function is compromised.[35] This type of volumetry will also help to establish new criteria for the indications for hepatectomy in patients with impaired liver function.

Furthermore, the use of 3D images has made it possible to simulate hepatic procedures. A hepatectomy simulation consists of the following steps[1]: transmission of CT images to the 3D simulation system[2]; 3D

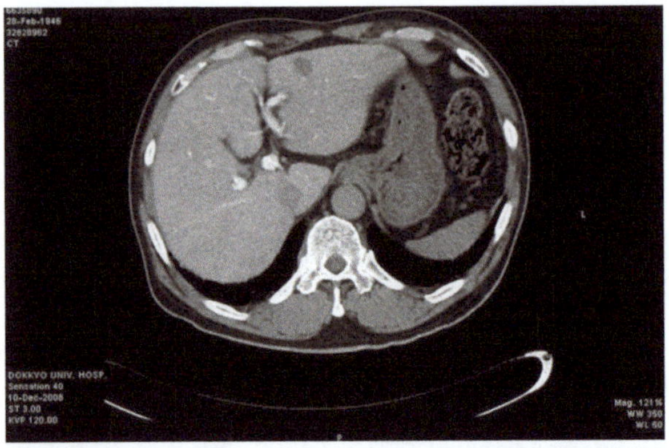

Fig. 10.8 Case 3: CT findings during arterial portography. A 1.7-cm HCC was demonstrated as a perfusion defect in segment 3 by CT during arterial portography

reconstruction of the tumor, portal vein, hepatic vein, and liver parenchyma[3]; subtraction of the intrahepatic vascular volume from the liver parenchymal volume[4]; editing of the intrahepatic vessel images to separate the portal system from the hepatic venous system[5]; calculation of the vascular perfusion area using an algorithm based on the directions and diameters of the hepatic vessels; and [6] calculation of multiple resection patterns and visualization of the results.[35] This type of simulation will increase the safety of hepatic resection.

Case 3: A 62-year-old male patient was referred to our department with a 1.7 cm hepatic tumor. CT findings indicated an HCC (Fig. 10.8). 3D CT images were made using 0.6 mm-thick slices. Volumetry was performed using a region-growing technique (Virtual Place Advance Plus Version 2.03, AZE, Tokyo, Japan). The volumes of the whole liver and segment 3 were calculated to be 1719.4 and 321.9 mL, respectively (Fig. 10.9 a, b, c). By volumetry using 2D

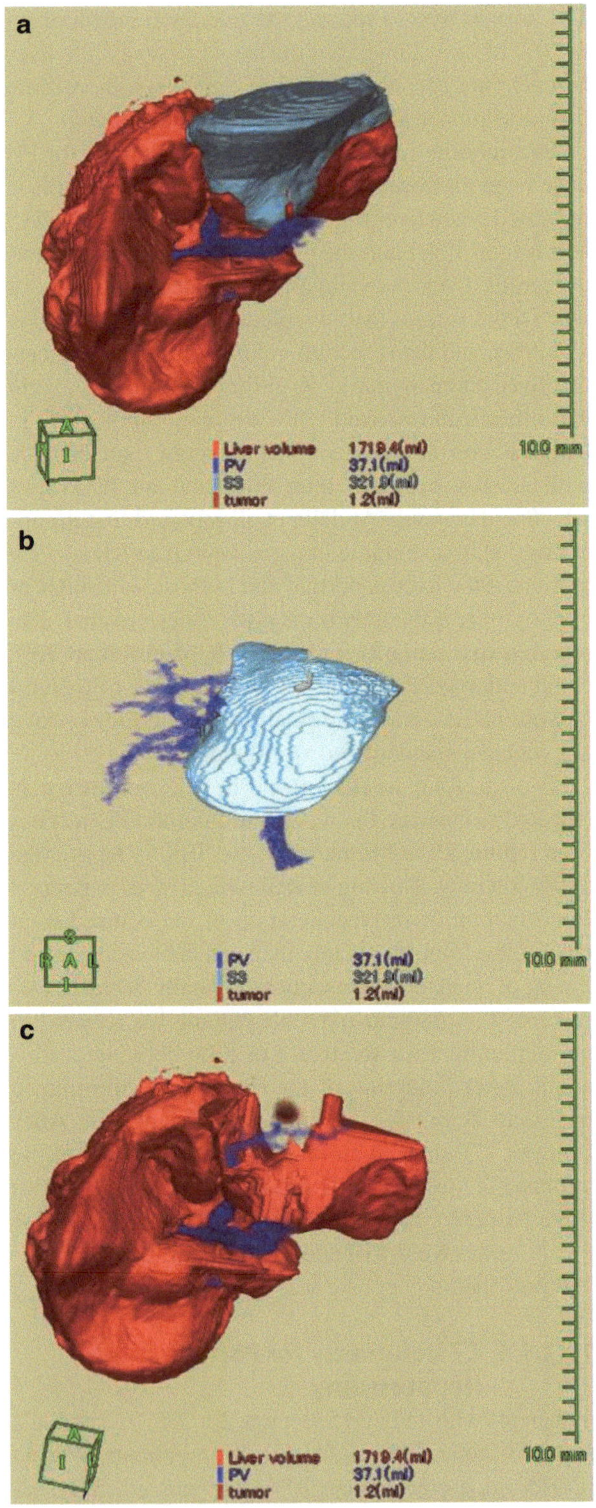

Fig. 10.9 Case 3: Findings on 3D imaging (Virtual Place Advance Plus Version 2.03, AZE, Tokyo, Japan). (**a**) Using 0.6-mm slice-thickness CT images, the liver has been reconstructed by a region-growing method based on the portal branches. The predicted resection area of segment 3 is shown as a *blue* region. Its volume was calculated automatically to be 321.9 mL. (**b**) Segment 3 can be depicted in isolation and checked from any angle using the portal branches as a reference. (**c**) Simulated surgery. The cut surface after resection of segment 3 is clearly demonstrated. The estimated volume of segment 3 correlated well with the actual weight of the resected specimen

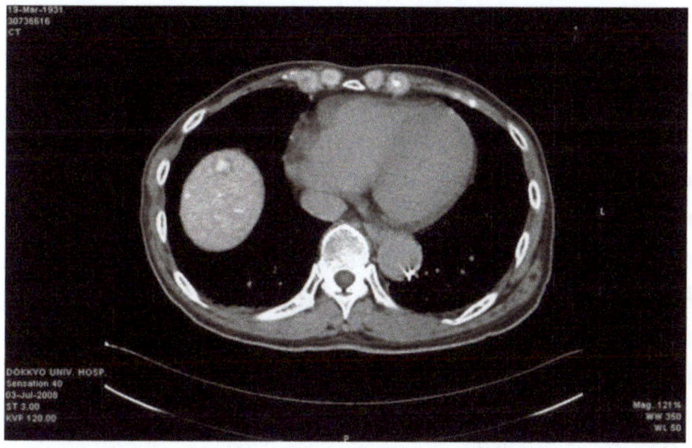

Fig. 10.10 Case 4: HCC in segment 3. CT visualized a small HCC with a diameter of 1.7 cm in the ventral part of segment 8

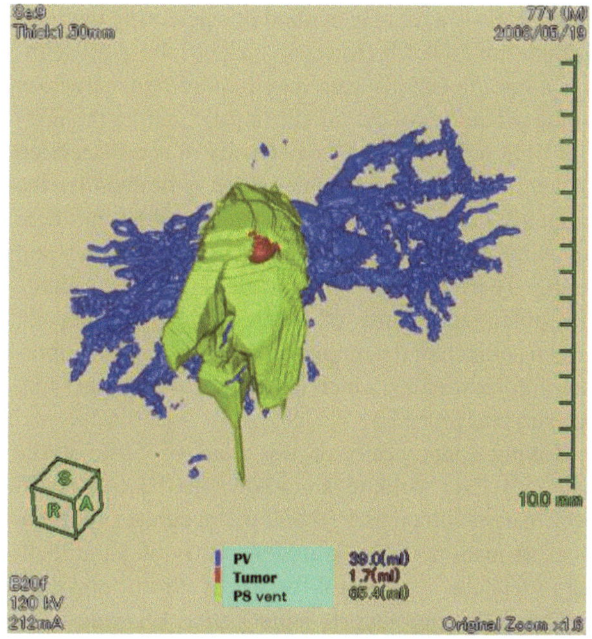

Fig. 10.11 Case 4: 3D images of the ventral part of segment 8 (Virtual Place Advance Plus Version 2.03, AZE, Tokyo, Japan). Using 3-mm slices, 3D images were reconstructed. The ventral part of segment 8 and the tumor can be seen. The estimated volume correlated well with the actual weight of the resected specimen. Note: 3D images reconstructed from 3-mm slice CT images do not have such good resolution as those reconstructed from thinner slices

images, the volume of the whole liver was estimated to be 1,730 mL. The patient was scheduled to undergo resection of segment 3. The weight of the resected specimen was 292 g. His postoperative course was uneventful.

Case 4: A 77-year-old male patient was found to have an HCC with a diameter of 1.7 cm (Fig. 10.10). 3D CT images were made using 3 mm-thick slices. The volume of the ventral part of segment 8 was estimated to be 65.4 mL (Fig. 10.11). He underwent resection of the ventral part of segment 8. The weight of the resected specimen was 71 g.

10.2.2 Living-Donor Liver Transplantation

Because ensuring the donor's safety is of prime importance in LDLT, CT volumetry is routinely employed to assess the necessary graft size[36] and determine whether an adequately sized graft can be procured. In the recipient, the ratio of the graft volume to the standard liver volume[37] should be greater than 30%, and in the donor, more than 40% of the whole liver should be preserved after harvesting. Liu and colleagues advocate other criteria, namely that when preoperative CT volumetry indicates that the volume of the remnant liver will be more than 35%, and the ratio of the right lobe graft to the recipient's standard liver volume will exceed 40%, adult-to-adult LDLT using a right lobe graft without the middle hepatic vein is likely to be a very safe procedure for both the donor and the recipient. When this is not the case, dual-graft liver transplantation should be considered.[38] Because impaired liver function after resection and transplantation is caused by an insufficient liver volume, reliable volumetric assessment of the hepatic segments of potential living donors is crucial for successful liver transplantation. It has been reported that the relationship between the volume of the liver calculated by CT and its actual weight is linear in both the recipient and the donor, and that a partial liver graft (reduced to about 30% of the recipient's expected liver weight) can result in successful LDLT.[39] Both 2D and 3D CT are suitable for calculating the graft volume, although there is a difference in their absolute error rates. For harvesting a left-lobe graft, either type of CT volumetry is acceptable. In fact, it has been reported that manual 2D CT volumetric calculation is a reliable method of calculating the liver volume for LDLT.[40] However, a right-lobe graft without a middle hepatic vein may require reconstruction of the tributaries of the middle hepatic vein or the inferior right hepatic vein. The necessity of reconstruction is determined by the volume which is drained by the branch.[41] Even if the tributaries are under 5 mm, there are potential risks such as the congestion volume being high.[20] Therefore, 3D CT volumetry is used to evaluate the potential volume of congestion in the hepatic venous branch of the remnant liver, which gives important information on which to base decisions regarding the surgical procedure.[42]

Living-donor grafts of less than 40–50% of the standard liver volume are known to be associated with worse outcomes.[43] Therefore, accurate preoperative estimation of the graft volume is of paramount importance to avoid small-for-size syndrome and graft failure following adult-to-adult LDLT. CT volumetry is the current gold standard for preoperative estimation of the graft volume. Overestimation of right graft volume has been frequently observed with CT volumetry, possibly due to scanning a perfused liver filled with blood, leading to expansion and volume increase, or to the level of hydration of the patient, variations in parenchymal densities, or even to the performance of the radiologist. The calculated liver volume, which is obtained from the percentage of the right lobe multiplied by the standard liver volume, has been reported to show a better correlation with the actual graft volume than the volume estimated from volumetry.[44] It has also been reported that automated CT volumetry of the liver using a region-growing technique yields acceptable measurements when compared with data obtained from the resected liver and is quicker than the manual method.[45] Furthermore, Itamoto stated that in order to ensure the donor's safety, precise evaluations of liver remnant volume by CT volumetry and of biliary variation at the hilum by CT cholangiography are mandatory when performing right hepatectomy in a donor because they prevent not only serious complications such as hepatic insufficiency but also biliary tract complications.[46]

After LDLT, it is important to evaluate graft regeneration. CT volumetry has been reported to be useful for following up the regeneration of grafted livers, as determined by an increase in volume, after LDLT.[47,48] Thus, CT volumetry is indispensable when performing LDLT.

10.2.3 Other Uses of CT Volumetry

CT volumetry can be used not only to evaluate regeneration of the remnant liver and graft[47-49] but also to monitor tumor size and evaluate the response of a tumor to chemotherapy.[50-52] Beal reported that periprocedural chemotherapy reduced but did not prevent hypertrophy caused by PE, and a trend towards tumor regression was observed.[34] Furthermore, CT volumetry has been used to demonstrate that oncogenesis is promoted by PE, with tumor doubling time reduced from 92 to 76 days.[50] Thus, precise evaluation of tumor size is possible using CT volumetry.

This technique is also employed in other clinical fields. Hashiba et al. reported that CT volumetry is useful for the follow-up of small or irregularly shaped gastric submucosal tumors and for making decisions regarding surgical interventions.[51]

References

1. Stone HH, Long WD, Smith RB III, Haynes CD. Physiological considerations in major hepatic resection. *Am J Surg*. 1969;117:78-84.
2. Schneider PD. Preoperative assessment of liver function. *Surg Clin North Am*. 2004;84:355-373.
3. Redaelli CA, Wagner M, Krahenbuhl L, et al. Liver surgery in the era of tissue-preserving resections: early and late outcome in patients with primary and secondary hepatic tumors. *World J Surg*. 2002;26:1126-1132.
4. Miyagawa S, Makuuchi M, Kawasaki S, et al. Criteria for safe hepatic resection. *Am J Surg*. 1995;169:589-594.
5. Yanaga K. Current status of hepatic resection for hepatocellular carcinoma. *J Gastroenterol*. 2004;39:919-926.
6. Dinant S, de Graaf W, Verwer BJ, et al. Risk assessment of posthepatectomy liver failure using hepatobiliary scintigraphy and CT volumetry. *J Nucl Med*. 2007;48:685-692.
7. Wiemker R, Rogalla P, Blaffert T, et al. Aspects of computed-aided detection (CAD) and volumetry of pulmonary nodules using multislice CT. *Br J Radiol*. 2005;78:S46-S56.
8. Das M, Ley-Zaporoshan J, Gietema HA, et al. Accuracy of automated volumetry of pulmonary nodules across different multislice CT scanners. *Eur Radiol*. 2007;17:1979-1984.
9. Marten K, Engelke C. Computed-aided detection and automated CT volumetry of pulmonary nodules. *Eur Radiol*. 2007;17:888-901.
10. Beer AJ, Wieder HA, Lordick F, et al. Adenocarcinoma of esophagogastric junction: multi-detector row CT to evaluate early response to neoadjuvant chemotherapy. *Radiology*. 2006;239:472-480.
11. Rohde S, Kovacs AF, Berkefeld J, Turowski B. Reliability of CT-based tumor volumetry after intraarterial chemotherapy in patients with small carcinoma of the oral cavity and the oropharynx. *Neuroradiology*. 2006;48:415-421.

12. Yamamoto S, Fukuda T, Hamada S, et al. Technical application of three-dimensional visualization and measurement for breast cancer using multidetector-row CT scanner. *Nippon Hoshasen Gijutsu Gakkai Zasshi*. 2002;58:1666-1675.
13. Strik HM, Borchert H, Fels C, et al. Three-dimensional reconstruction and volumetry of intracranial haemorrhage and its mass effect. *Neuroradiology*. 2005;47:417-424.
14. Heymsfield SB, Fulenwider T, Nordlinger B, et al. Accurate measurement of liver, kidney and spleen volume and mass by computerized axial tomography. *Ann Intern Med*. 1979; 90:185-187.
15. Togo S, Nagano Y, Masui H, et al. Two-stage hepatectomy for multiple bilobar liver metastases from colorectal cancer. *Hepatogastroenterology*. 2005;52:913-919.
16. Masumoto J, Sato Y, Hori M, et al. A new similarity measure for nongrid volume registration using known joint distribution of target tissue: application to dynamic CT data of the liver. *Med Image Anal*. 2003;7:553-564.
17. Kubota K, Makuuchi M, Kusaka K, et al. Measurement of liver volume and hepatic functional reserve as a guide to decision-making in resectional surgery for hepatic tumors. *Hepatology*. 1997;26:1176-1181.
18. Hiroshige S, Nishizaki T, Soejima Y, et al. Beneficial effects of 3-dimensional visualization on hepatic vein reconstruction using right lobe graft. *Transplantation*. 2001;72:1993-1996.
19. Hiroshige S, Shimada M, Harada N, et al. Accurate preoperative estimation of liver-graft volumetry using three-dimensional computed tomography. *Transplantation*. 2003;75:1561-1564.
20. Yonemura Y, Taketomi A, Soejima Y, et al. Validity of preoperative volumetric analysis of congestion volume in living donor liver transplantation using three-dimensional computed tomography. *Liver Transpl*. 2005;11:1556-1562.
21. Radtke A, Sotiropoulos GC, Nadalin S, et al. Preoperative volume prediction in adult living donor liver transplantation: how much can we rely on it? Essen experience based on virtual three-dimensional computed tomography-volume assessment. *Am J Transplant*. 2007;7:672-679.
22. Frericks BB, Caldarone FC, Nashan B, et al. 3D CT modeling of hepatic vessel architecture and volume calculation in living donated liver transplantation. *Eur Radiol*. 2004;14:326-333.
23. Schindl MJ, Redhead DN, Fearon KC, et al. The value of residual liver volume as a predictor of hepatic dysfunction and infection after major liver resection. *Gut*. 2005;54:289-296.
24. Katsuramaki T, Fujimori K, Furuhata T, et al. Preoperative estimation of risk in hepatectomy using technetium-99 m-galactosyl human serum albumin receptor amount by nonlinear 3-compartment model. *Hepatogastroenterology*. 2003;50:174-177.
25. Ferrero A, Vigano L, Polastri R, et al. Postoperative liver dysfunction and future remnant liver: where is the limit? *World J Surg*. 2007;31:1643-1651.
26. Tu R, Xia LP, Wu L. Assessment of hepatic functional reserve by cirrhosis grading and liver volume measurement using CT. *World J Gastroenterol*. 2007;13:3956-3961.
27. Okochi O, Kaneko T, Sugimoto H, et al. ICG pulse spectrophotometry for perioperative liver function in hepatectomy. *J Surg Res*. 2002;103:109-113.
28. Makuuchi M, Thai BL, Takayasu K, et al. Preoperative portal embolization to increase safety of major hepatectomy for hilar bile duct carcinoma: a preliminary report. *Surgery*. 1990;107:521-527.
29. Azoulay D, Castaing D, Smail A, et al. Resection of nonresectable liver metastases from colorectal cancer after percutaneous portal vein embolization. *Ann Surg*. 2000;231: 480-486.
30. Sirichindakul B, Nonthasoot B, Thienpaitoon P, et al. Preoperative portal vein embolization in hepatobiliary tract malignancy: an experience at King Chulalongkorn Memorial Hospital. *J Med Assoc Thai*. 2005;88:1115-1119.
31. Hiramatsu K, Sano T, Nagino M, Nimura Y. Repeat hepatectomy for colonic liver metastasis presenting intrabiliary growth – application of percutaneous transhepatic portal vein embolization for impaired liver. *Hepatogastroenterology*. 2007;54:1554-1556.
32. Seyama Y, Kubota K, Sano K, et al. Long-term outcome of extended hemihepatectomy for hilar bile duct cancer with no mortality and high survival rate. *Ann Surg*. 2003;238: 73-83.
33. Abdalla EK, Hicks ME, Vauthey JN. Portal vein embolization: rationale, technique and future prospects. *Br J Surg*. 2001;88:165-175.
34. Beal IK, Anthony S, Papadopoulou A, et al. Portal vein embolization prior to hepatic resection for colorectal liver metastases and the effects of periprocedure chemotherapy. *Br J Radiol*. 2006;79:473-478.
35. Yamanaka J, Saito S, Fujimoto J. Impact of preoperative planning using virtual segmental volumetry on liver resection for hepatocellular carcinoma. *World J Surg*. 2007;31: 1249-1255.
36. Fan ST, Lo CM, Liu CL. Experience of donor right lobe hepatectomy in adult-to-adult live donor liver transplantation: clinical analysis of 89 cases. *Hepatobiliary Pancreat Dis Int*. 2002;1:166-171.
37. Urata K, Kawasaki S, Matsunami H, et al. Calculation of child and adult standard liver volume for liver transplantation. *Hepatology*. 1995;21:1317-1321.
38. Liu B, Yan LN, Wang WT, et al. Clinical study on safety of adult-to-adult living donor liver transplantation in both donors and recipients. *World J Gastroenterol*. 2007;13: 955-959.
39. Higashiyama H, Yamaguchi T, Mori K, et al. Graft size assessment by preoperative computed tomography in living related partial liver transplantation. *Br J Surg*. 1993;80: 489-492.
40. Emiroglu R, Coskun M, Yilmaz U, et al. Safety of multidetector computed tomography in calculating liver volume for living-donor liver transplantation. *Transplant Proc*. 2006;38: 3576-3578.
41. Ishifuro M, Horiguchi J, Nakashige A, et al. Use of multidetector row CT with volume renderings in right lobe living liver transplantation. *Eur Radiol*. 2002;12:2477-2483.
42. Kishi Y, Sugawara Y, Akamatsu N, et al. Sharing the middle hepatic vein between donor and recipient: left liver graft procurement preserving a large segment VIII branch in donor. *Liver Transpl*. 2004;10:1208-1212.
43. Lo CM, Fan ST, Liu CL, et al. Applicability of living donor liver transplantation to high-urgency patients. *Transplantation*. 1999;67:73-77.
44. Khalaf H, Shoukri M, Al-Kadhi Y, et al. Accurate method for preoperative estimation of the right graft volume in

adult-to-adult living donor liver transplantation. *Transplant Proc*. 2007;39:1491-1495.

45. Nakayama Y, Katsuragawa S, Ikeda R, et al. Automated hepatic volumetry for living related liver transplantation at multisection CT. *Radiology*. 2006;240:743-748.
46. Itamoto T, Emoto K, Mitsuta H, et al. Safety of donor right hepatectomy for adult-to-adult living donor liver transplantation. *Transpl Int*. 2006;19:177-183.
47. Maetani Y, Itoh K, Egawa H, et al. Factors influencing liver regeneration following living-donor liver transplantation of the right hepatic lobe. *Transplantation*. 2003;75:97-102.
48. Tutar NU, Kirbas I, Ozturk A, et al. Computed tomography volumetric follow-up of graft volume in living related liver recipients. *Transplant Proc*. 2007;39:1175-1177.
49. Morimoto T, Honda G, Kawai Y, et al. Right hepatic lobectomy for hepatocellular carcinoma which developed in primary biliary cirrhosis: report of a case. *Surg Today*. 1999;29:646-650.
50. Kokudo N, Tada K, Seki M, et al. Proliferative activity of intrahepatic colorectal metastases after preoperative hemihepatic portal vein embolization. *Hepatology*. 2001;34:267-272.
51. Hashiba T, Oda K, Koda K, et al. A gastrointestinal stromal tumor in the stomach: usefulness of computed tomographic volumetry. *Gastric Cancer*. 2004;7:260-265.
52. Lee SM, Kim SH, Lee JM, et al. Usefulness of CT volumetry for primary gastric lesions in predicting pathologic response to neoadjuvant chemotherapy in advanced gastric cancer. *Abdom Imaging*. 2009;34(4):430-440.

Morphometric Imaging Techniques and the Functional Liver Remnant

11

Mathew M. Augustine, Ihab R. Kamel, and Timothy M. Pawlik

Abstract

Surgical resection is the treatment of choice for select patients with primary and secondary hepatic malignancies. The goal of hepatic surgery is complete resection with preservation of sufficient liver parenchyma. Inadequate hepatic reserve can result in the development of hepatic dysfunction and failure. One parameter used to assess the adequacy of liver reserve is to measure the future liver remnant (FLR) volume. Accurate measurement of FLR is important not only as a surrogate marker for liver function, but also assists in the selection of patients for preoperative portal vein embolization (PVE). The preferred modality to provide accurate and reproducible measurements of FLR is computer tomography (CT) volumetry. CT volumetry measurements can be performed utilizing either manual or automated techniques. The measured FLR is standardized to the patient's total liver volume (TLV), which is derived from the body surface area (BSA). Various equations have been derived that relate TLV to BSA. CT volumetry provides hepatic surgeons and radiologists an informed approach toward the surgical management of patients with complex liver disease.

Keywords

Computer tomography (CT) volumetry • Functional liver remnant • Future liver remnant volume • Morphometric imaging techniques and the functional liver remnant • MRI of the liver

Abbreviations

BH	Body Height
BSA	Body Surface Area
BW	Body Weight
CRM	Colorectal Metastasis
CT	Computed Tomography
CTAP	CT Angioportograms
FLR	Future Liver Remnant
FLV	Functional Liver Volume
HCC	Hepatocellular Carcinoma
ICG	Indocyanine Green Clearance
INR	International Normalized Ratio
LV	Liver Volume
MRI	Magnetic Resonance Imaging
PVE	Portal Vein Embolization
RLV	Remnant Liver Volume
sFLR	Standardized Future Liver Remnant

T.M. Pawlik (✉)
Division of Surgical Oncology, Department of Surgery, Johns Hopkins Hospital, Baltimore, MD, USA
e-mail: tpawlik1@jhmi.edu

D.C. Madoff et al. (eds.), *Venous Embolization of the Liver*,
DOI 10.1007/978-1-84882-122-4_11,

TLV	Total Liver Volume
^{99m}Tc-GSA	Technetium-99 m Galactosyl Serum Albumin

11.1 Introduction

When appropriate, surgical resection remains the best therapeutic option in patients with both primary and secondary hepatic malignancies. In fact, over the past decade, the criteria for resectability of hepatocellular cancer (HCC), colorectal metastasis (CRM), as well as other secondary metastatic diseases such as neuroendocrine have expanded.[1] Specifically, some clinicians have begun to advocate a more "aggressive" surgical approach to the management of patients with hepatic malignancies.[2-8] The reason for this shift toward expanding the criteria of resectability for liver malignancies, and in turn, the adoption of more "aggressive" surgical approaches, is multifactorial. One factor that is often cited is the decreased mortality rates and increased safety associated with major hepatic resection.[9-11] Traditionally, hepatic resection was associated with large-volume blood loss, varying degrees of liver failure, and significant morbidity. As such, the perioperative mortality associated with hepatic resection before the 1990s was reported to be as high as 10–20%.[12-14] However, over the past decades, with better patient selection, operative techniques, and improved anesthesia and critical care, the reported mortality associated with hepatic resection has decreased to well less than 5%.[11,15]

Extended hepatic resections are sometimes necessary to allow for a curative resection in patients with multiple or large tumors. In fact, in a significant proportion of patients, extended hepatectomy may be the only means available to achieve complete resection and provide a chance for cure. While extended hepatectomy can be performed with a near-zero operative mortality rate in some high-volume centers,[9] there can be risk associated with this operation. Specifically, one risk associated with extended hepatic resection is postoperative liver insufficiency. When too much liver parenchyma is resected, the risk of liver insufficiency increases due to the small postoperative liver remnant volume. Postoperative liver insufficiency can be manifested by coagulopathy, increased risk of complications, nonobstructive cholestasis, and jaundice. Postoperative liver insufficiency and failure can lead to prolonged recovery, prolonged time in the intensive care unit, long hospital stays, and increased risk of death. The ascertainment of preoperative liver volumes has been shown to help reduce the incidence of complications due to insufficient residual liver volume.

The future liver remnant (FLR) defines the expected volume of functional liver that will remain following hepatic resection. Determining the FLR is important for two main reasons. First, defining the FLR ensures that an adequate minimal functional volume of liver will be left following resection to avoid liver insufficiency. In general, in patients with normal underlying hepatic parenchyma, 20–30% of the total liver volume appears to be the minimum safe volume that can be left following extended resection.[16] Stone et al.[17] estimated that the removal of approximately 70% of total liver volume could be well tolerated by patients with normal livers. A recent study corroborated this finding, noting that the cutoff of 30% was safe for donation of a right lobe graft for adult-to-adult liver transplantation.[18] In patients with parenchymal disease, 40–50% should be left following resection, depending on the degree of underlying liver injury. The second role of defining the FLR is that patients who do not meet the criteria for minimal FLR volume can be considered for preoperative portal vein embolization (PVE). PVE is a safe and effective modality to increase the FLR.[16,19] As such, defining the FLR plays an essential role in determining which patients can safely undergo a major liver resection. The relative contributions of the hepatic segments to total liver volume may vary significantly between patients. In fact, Abdalla et al.[20] noted that there was clinically significant interpatient variation in hepatic volumes, with right liver volumes ranging from 49% to 82% and left liver volumes ranging from 17% to 49%. Therefore, one cannot assume the volume of the FLR. Rather, in patients being considered for a major hepatic resection, the FLR must be routinely and empirically measured. In general, computed tomography (CT) has become the preferred method to obtain accurate, reproducible images for preoperatively assessing the FLR volume.

11.2 Measuring the Future Liver Remnant

The basic principles of morphometric measurements were first published in 1847[21] and introduced formally into the practice of medicine by Weibel[22] and Hennig[23] in the 1950s and 1960s. Organ volume measurements are based on these morphometric principles, and the application of morphometric volume assessment has been described utilizing ultrasonography,[24] CT,[25-27] and magnetic resonance imaging (MRI).[28]

11.2.1 Ultrasonography and Magnetic Resonance Imaging

Prior to the widespread adoption of more sophisticated cross-sectional imaging, a morphometric method to calculate liver volumes utilizing ultrasonography had been described.[24] After obtaining ultrasound images of the liver, the sonographic tomograms were analyzed using the point-integrating method.[24] Specifically, the liver contour would be delineated on square paper as a morphometric screen. All points of the square paper within the liver contour would be taken into account, and the points of each scan would be summarized and multiplied by the interscan distance, the square of the interpoint distance, and a correction factor. Although very cumbersome, measurement of liver volume utilizing this technique has been shown to correlate with CT examination.[24] This technique, however, has been abandoned in favor of much more reproducible and less labor-intense techniques. One such technique is the use of MRI. MRI has been shown to allow for accurate volumetric assessment of solid organs in animals,[29] phantoms,[30] as well as in humans.[28,31] While MRI may allow for volumetric analysis of the liver, its widespread acceptance has been limited. Rather, CT has been the most widely accepted method to determine liver volumetry.

11.2.2 Computed Tomography

In 1979, Heymsfield et al.[32] first validated the technique of CT volumetry by showing an agreement between the liver volume as assessed by CT and the actual ex vivo volume of the liver. In a subsequent study by the same group,[25] hand tracings of the liver were performed, and the volume was calculated by multiplying the area within the tracings by two since each CT cut was taken at 2-cm intervals (summation of areas). While the CT volumetric determinations in this study were never compared to actual liver volumes, as was the case in the previous study from this group, the authors indicated that the calculated volumes were representative of volumes estimated by other methods. These early reports established the utility of CT as a simple, accurate, and reproducible modality for liver volume determination.

More recently, sophisticated algorithms have been established for the use of CT volumetry. Using 3-D reconstructions from CT portography, Soyer et al.[33] reported on 25 patients with hepatic metastasis from colorectal cancer. In this study, total liver volume, resected liver volume, and estimated postoperative liver volume were assessed. The authors found a strong correlation between the preoperative resection volume as assessed by CT and the actual volume of the resected specimen as determined by water displacement. The tumor volume was not subtracted from the resected liver volume, which did result in an underestimation of the relative postoperative FLR. As a result, two patients were identified as having an estimated FLR less than 35% and underwent preoperative PVE prior to resection. In retrospect, the underestimation of the FLR due to the failure to subtract the tumor volume may have led to potentially unnecessary PVE procedures in these patients. Nevertheless, results from this study proved that CT volumetry could accurately estimate liver volume and provided a framework upon which to stratify patients who might have borderline liver function by anatomy, facilitating referral for PVE.

Wigmore et al.[34] similarly reported on the use of 3-D models constructed from CT angioportograms (CTAP) to assess liver volume in patients with metastatic disease and nondysfunctional livers. In this study, the authors reconstructed images of the liver from 7-mm cut sections and computed the total liver volume, tumor volume, and FLR. A close correlation was identified between the preoperative 3-D CT volumetrics and the actual resected specimen weight (e.g., 1 g of liver was equivalent to a volume of 1 mL). The authors also noted a correlation between the volume of the FLR and the body weight. In a separate study utilizing multidetector, multiphasic CT to image the livers of 52 potential donors for liver transplantation, Kamel et al.[35] calculated right and left lobar volumes. Hand tracings of liver volumes were performed independently by two fellowship-trained radiologists using axial portal venous images. The tracings excluded major vascular and liver-related structures including the inferior vena cava, extrahepatic veins, as well as other nonhepatic structures that could falsely add to the estimated liver volumes. From these tracings, an automated "paintbrush" method was used to create a 3-D reconstruction of the liver from which the volumes were automatically computed. A virtual right hepatectomy was subsequently performed using an avascular plane to the right of the middle hepatic vein. The volume of the right hemi-liver was then calculated. Doing this, the authors established a significant correlation between the calculated right lobar volume and the explanted graft weight. In a subsequent study from the same group,[35] a multidetector, multiphasic CT was used to determine not only hepatic volume, but also levels of fatty infiltration and variants of hepatic vasculature in potential liver donors. In this study, the authors were able to exclude 37.5% of potential liver donors through volumetric and parenchymal assessment, which identified small liver remnants and severe fatty liver infiltration in a subset of patients.

Studies have shown that assessment of hepatic volumes with CT not only correlates with explanted liver volumes, but also with clinical outcomes. Shirabe et al.[36] reported on 80 patients with hepatitis B- or C-associated HCC who underwent major hepatic resection. Liver volumes were calculated based on CT images obtained at 1-cm intervals, and the FLR was expressed as milliliter/body surface area. Seven out of 80 patients developed liver insufficiency. Importantly, the authors noted that only patients with a preoperative FLR of less than 250 mL/m^2 developed liver insufficiency. In contrast, there was no association between the risk of liver failure and the volume of liver that was resected. The authors therefore concluded that a volume of 250 mL/m^2 should be adopted as a cutoff for selecting patients with an adequate hepatic reserve for liver resection.

In a separate study, Shoup et al.[37] assessed the impact of remnant liver volume on the risk for liver dysfunction. CT-based volumetric analysis was used to calculate total liver volume, tumor volume, as well as FLR. A significant correlation between FLR and the risk of hepatic dysfunction was identified. Specifically, 90% of those patients with an FLR less than 25% developed some element of liver insufficiency as part of their postoperative course. In fact, patients with an FLR less than 25% were more likely to develop postoperative complications and had a longer hospital length of stay. Despite the increased risk of developing liver dysfunction, no patient in this study succumbed to fulminant liver failure. Based on these findings, the authors concluded that patients with less than 25% FLR determined by preoperative CT volumetrics should be considered for PVE prior to hepatic resection. Schindl et al.[38] corroborated these findings in a study of 104 patients who underwent CT volumetry prior to hepatic resection. In the study by Schindl et al.,[38] the percent residual liver volume (%RLV) was strongly correlated with the risk of hepatic dysfunction in the postoperative period. Using receiver operating characteristic (ROC) curve analysis, the authors determined that the appropriate cutoff for the % RLV to avoid an increased risk of liver insufficiency was 26.6%. In aggregate, these data, as well as those published by others,[16] strongly suggest that CT volumetry of the liver is an integral part of the preoperative workup of patients being considered for a major extended hepatic resection. In patients with normal underlying hepatic parenchyma, an FLR threshold of 20–25% is necessary to avoid an increased risk of postoperative liver insufficiency.

11.2.2.1 CT Volumetry Techniques

The accuracy of CT-based volumetric techniques depends on the quality of the imaging data, as well as the segmentation algorithm used.[26,30] The advent of multidetector, thin-slice CT has allowed for the acquisition of high-speed, high-resolution helical imaging of the entire liver volume during a single breath-hold, thereby minimizing volume averaging and artifactual volume estimation. Segmentation algorithms are fundamental to the processing of image-based CT volumetric techniques. Ideal CT image-based volumetric measurements should yield accurate and reproducible calculations of liver volumes. After obtaining the CT-based images, volumetry can be performed either by measuring the liver volumes manually or with automated techniques.

The manual method of CT liver volumetry involves the radiologist to manually trace the contours of all liver sections using an electronic cursor (Fig. 11.1). The total liver, tumors, and FLR are delineated on the images using hepatic and portal vein anatomy as landmarks for segmental division. Utilizing the appropriate integrated software, the number of pixels included within the hand-traced contours on each section can be calculated, and the cross-sectional area of the liver on a section-by-section basis is provided. Following this, coronal plane images are obtained after a computer interpolation of the hand-traced images to ensure adequate coverage of the liver outline (Fig. 11.2). The circumscribed areas are then multiplied by the CT section thickness, yielding an approximate volume for

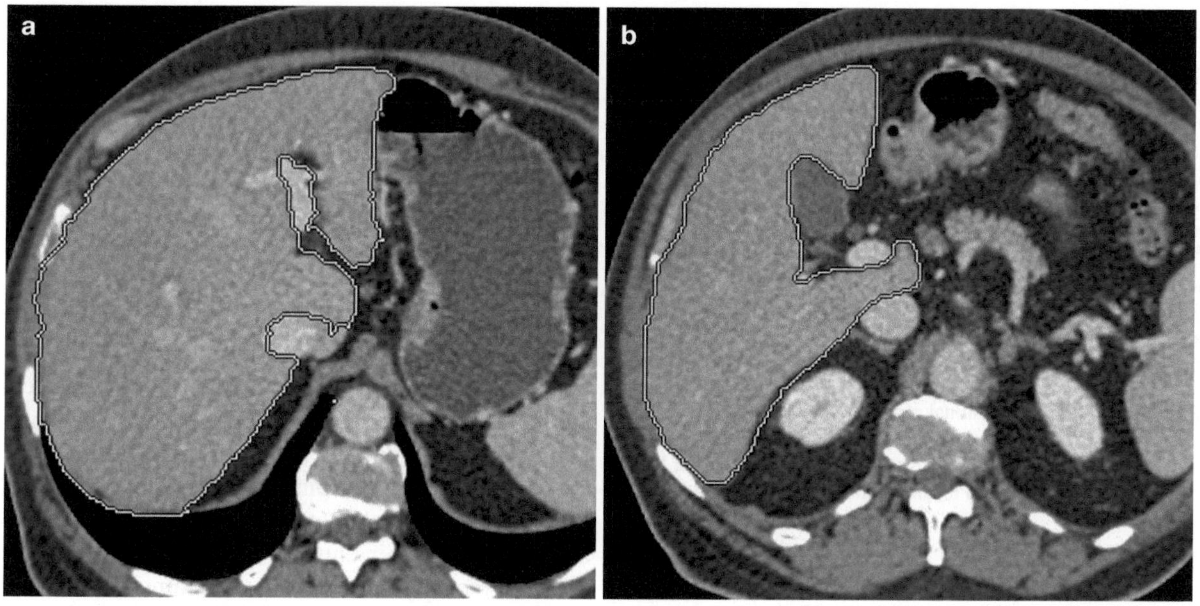

Fig. 11.1 Hand tracing of the liver outline using axial CT images. Hand tracing enables the radiologist to provide a more accurate estimate of liver volume by excluding nearby structures such as the gallbladder, vasculature, and major fissures such as the fissure for the ligamentum teres. In this image (**a**), the radiologist has carefully isolated the liver from the inferior vena cava, left portal vein, and right kidney. This axial CT image (**b**) depicts a more inferior cut and demonstrates how the hand tracing has excluded the gallbladder, portal vein, and IVC from the liver

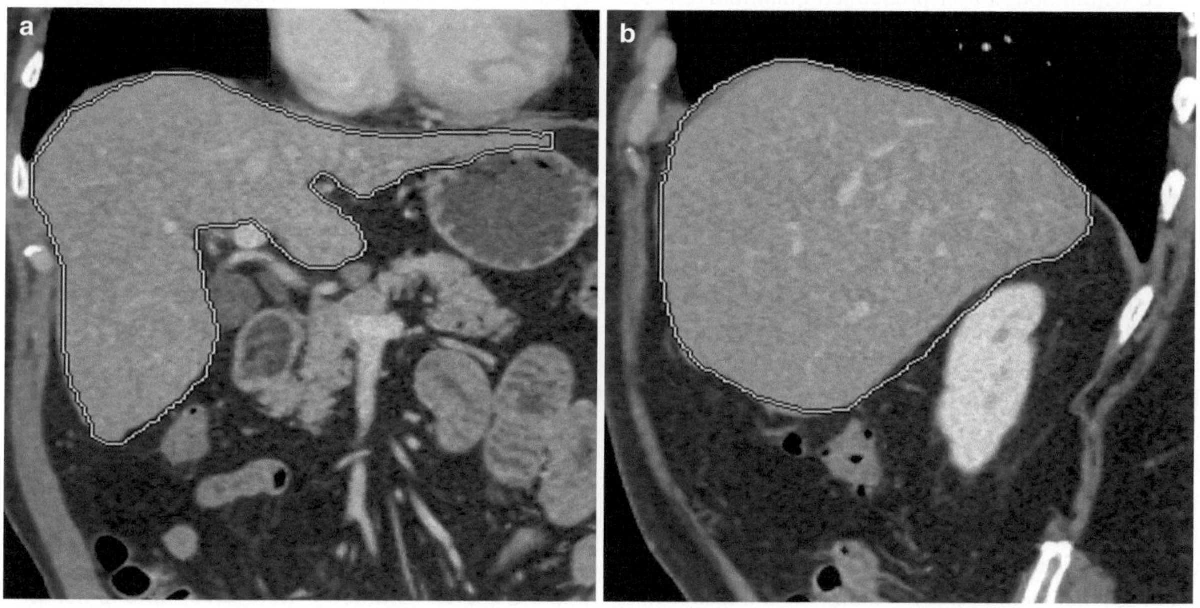

Fig. 11.2 Hand tracing of the liver outline utilizing CT images reconstructed in the coronal plane. In this image (**a**), the radiologist has isolated the liver from the stomach, gallbladder, and porta hepatis vessels. Volumetrics in the coronal plane verify the accuracy of measurements performed in the axial plane. This image (**b**) depicts hand tracing of the liver outline from a sagittal CT image

each liver section. The volumes of each section that are manually outlined can then be summed to give the total liver volume. The tumor volume is then subtracted from the total hepatic volume (Fig. 11.3).

Because the manual method of liver volumetry requires considerable user involvement in the segmentation of the liver on each section, the process can be time-consuming.[39] As such, there has been interest in

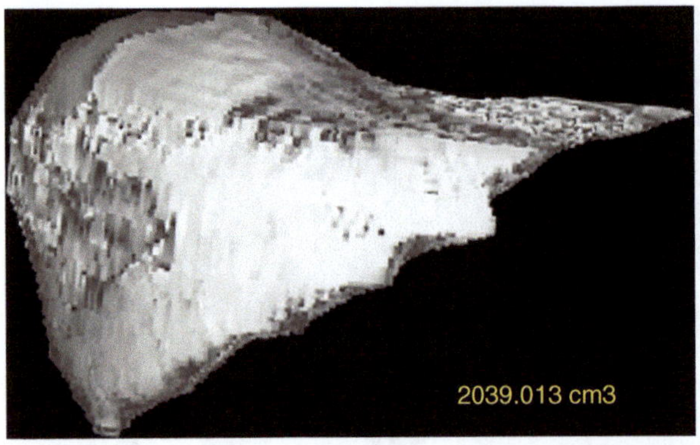

Fig. 11.3 Three-dimensional model of the total liver in frontal projection with the calculated volume displayed. These models are generated using commercially available software after hand tracing the liver outline in the axial plane

automating the process of CT-based liver volumetry.[39,40] Farraher et al.[28] reported on liver volumetry utilizing a semiautomated dual-space clustering segmentation technique with MRI-based images. The algorithm operates by interrogating each voxel in the image data set to determine whether the voxel is contained within both a user-predefined quantitative MRI space subvolume and a predefined anatomic space volume. Linear regression analysis was used to assess agreement regarding the volumes calculated by using semiautomated versus manual tracing techniques. The authors noted strong agreement between the regression parameters for the liver volumes obtained using the two techniques ($r=0.98$), with the mean volume difference between the two techniques being only 1.2%.[28] In a separate study, Nakayama et al.[39] compared multisection CT-based image hepatic volumetry using a manual versus automated technique for living-related liver transplantation. Manual volumetry was performed using a standard hand-tracing technique, while the automated volumetry algorithm had no human input throughout image processing. The computerized automated method of liver volumetry initially estimated the mean CT number of the liver by means of an analysis of CT numbers in a 3-D volume of interest with a 32×32-pixel in-section matrix and an automatically determined height. The location of the in-section 32×32-pixel region was determined empirically at a location where the liver was likely to be included. The initial candidate regions of the liver on each slice were selected using an estimated CT value of the liver. The liver was then separated from other adjacent organs by analyzing edge information inside the initially estimated liver. The 3-D region with the maximum volume was selected by the use of a 3-D connected-component labeling technique with final refinement of the liver using a restricted region growing technique. The liver volume was then automatically calculated by the summation of the products of the section thickness and the area of the segmented liver in each section. The authors noted a good correlation between the measured and estimated hepatic volumes obtained with the manual versus the automated method ($r=0.80$). In addition, the automated method required significantly less time than the manual technique (4.4 min versus 32.8 min). The authors concluded that the automated method reduced the time required for volumetry of the liver and provided acceptable measurements.

More recently, there has been an attempt to bring CT volumetry of the liver to the surgeon's desktop to reduce costs and to increase the accessibility of the technique.[40,41] Lu et al.[41] reported on the use of transformed digitized CT-based images analyzed using PhotoShop. While the authors reported that this approach was reliable, the use of PhotoShop to calculate liver volumes cannot be standardized, is laborious, and is dependent on surgeons who may be unfamiliar with volumetry techniques. An alternative "plug and play" method that has been proposed is the use of a freely downloadable image analysis software package developed at the National Institute of Health.[42] The accuracy of the software package, known as ImageJ, was assessed in a small study by Dello et al.[40] In this study, the authors assessed the liver volumes with CT-based images utilizing ImageJ and compared them to the specimen weights and calculated volumes obtained during pathology examination of the explant. Dello et al.[40] noted that there was good correlation between the volumes calculated with ImageJ and the actual measured weights of the resection specimens ($r^2=0.98$). The authors noted that such desktop-based programming may make CT liver volumetry more accessible to hepatobiliary surgeons.

Accurate segmentation and measurement of liver volumes from CT-based imaging is critical to ensure high-quality volumetry (Figs. 11.4–11.6). The determination of volumes based on CT imaging can be obtained either by manual hand tracing, semiautomated, or automated techniques. At most centers, manual hand tracing remains

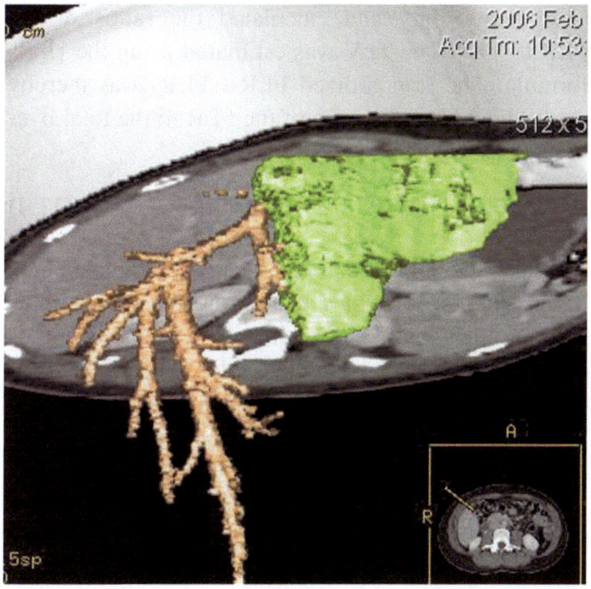

Fig. 11.4 Three-dimensional imaging of the right and middle hepatic veins coursing through the liver parenchyma, as seen from a superior view. This image displays the hepatic venous anatomy and provides "virtual guidance" for the surgeon in performing a right hepatectomy. The remnant left lobe (*green*) is outlined. Reconstructions of the left lobe provide remnant volume measurements which inform the surgeon preoperatively of the need for portal vein embolization

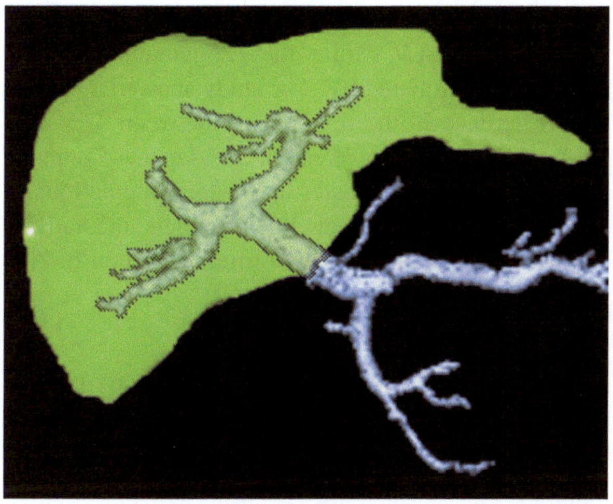

Fig. 11.5 Cross-sectional image of the liver (*green*) is displayed with superimposed portal vein anatomy. From an inferior projection, tributaries of the portal vein (splenic vein and superior mesenteric vein) are seen converging from the right. The main portal vein is seen branching within the outline of the liver into anterior, posterior, and left branches. In addition to providing volumetric data, these images inform the surgeon of potential vascular variants and guide hepatectomy by illustrating planes for resection

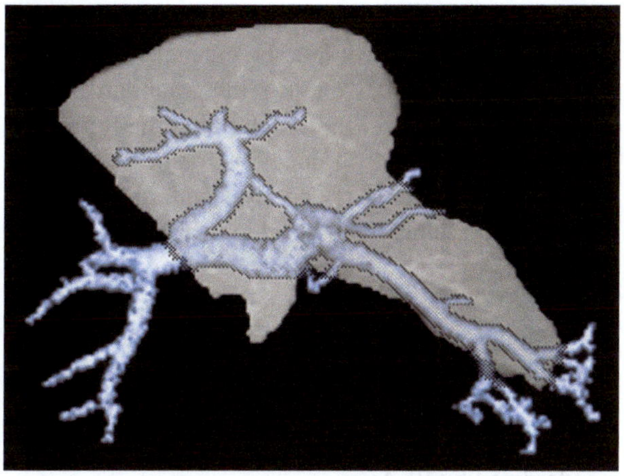

Fig. 11.6 This image illustrates how radiologic images can be used for preoperative planning of right hepatic lobectomy. The left lobe of the liver is outlined and isolated. Inferior projection of the main portal vein, splenic and superior mesenteric vein tributaries, and branches of the portal vein are superimposed on a cross section of the left liver lobe. By determining a virtual resection plane based on anatomic and vascular structures, the remnant liver volume can be calculated from the summation of the areas of the outlined left liver

the prevalent technique of choice, with subsequent calculations determined from computer-calculated estimates of the circumscribed areas. Manual methods of liver volumetry should be performed by skilled, experienced radiologists in cooperation with hepatobiliary surgeons. Fully automated techniques to determine liver volumes, although promising, have not been widely adopted and still have limited applicability.

11.3 Formulas Utilized to Calculate the Future Liver Remnant

Images obtained from CT are used to calculate the volume based on a number of models that use various published equations for liver size.[43-45] Early efforts aimed at estimating liver volume indicated a linear but disproportional (non-zero intercept) relationship to body size.[45,46] In patients with underlying chronic liver disease, this linear relationship, however, does not appear to hold.[47] Moreover, there is empiric evidence that variations in liver size for a given body size may differ based on other covariates such as age, gender, and ethnicity.[48-50] In addition, there has been debate as to whether the volume of the remnant liver should be normalized to body weight (BW) or body surface area

(BSA).[51] For live-donor liver transplantation, the CT-measured graft volume is equated with graft weight.[32,44] The graft weight is then standardized to the recipient body weight to determine the minimum graft requirement.[52,53] In contrast, for hepatic resection, the FLR volume is usually standardized to the total liver volume (TLV), which is based on the patient BSA.[45]

Using CT-based images of 96 Japanese children and adults without underlying liver abnormalities, Urata et al.[44] noted a direct proportional relationship between BSA and liver volume. The authors defined the following formula for estimating the liver volume standardized by BSA:

$$\text{LV (mL)} = 706.2 \times \text{BSA (m}^2) + 2.4 \qquad (11.1)$$

The formula espoused by Urata et al.[44] was widely adopted to estimate standardized liver volumes to determine the minimally acceptable donor liver size for living-donor liver transplantation. Subsequently, other groups,[45,49,54,55] however, have questioned the generalizablity of this equation. Heinemann et al.[49] applied the Urata equation to a population of over 1,000 German individuals in whom liver volume was measured at autopsy. Heinemann et al.[49] noted that the Urata formula underestimated the Caucasian liver volume by approximately 323 mL. As such, Heinemann proposed a modified formula for Caucasian adults:

$$\text{LV (mL)} = 1072.8 \times \text{BSA (m}^2) - 345.7 \qquad (11.2)$$

Application of the Urata and Heinemann equations to the adult data of Yoshizumi et al.[55] was associated with underestimation and overestimation, respectively, of liver volume. Yu et al.[56] subsequently performed a study assessing the correlation between BSA and liver volume in a Korean population. Unlike the Urata and Heinemann findings, Yu et al.[56] noted a non-linear relationship between liver volume and BSA in the Korean population. As such, the authors proposed a further modified equation specifically for use in the Korean population:

$$\text{LV (mL)} = 21.585 \times \text{BW (kg)}^{0.732} \times \text{BH (cm)}^{0.225} \qquad (11.3)$$

where BW and BH refer to body weight and height, respectively.

In a small study by Vauthey et al.,[57] the authors obtained CT volumetric measurements of the FLR (segments 2 and 3 ± 1) prior to extended right trisegmentectomy and calculated the ratios of the FLR to TLV. The TLV was estimated using the Urata formula. The standardized FLR (sFLR) was thereby determined from the ratio of the FLR to the total liver volume as follows:

$$\text{sFLR} = \text{FLR}/706.2 \times \text{BSA (m}^2) + 2.4 \qquad (11.4)$$

The authors noted that this relatively simple method of measurement provided an accurate assessment of the liver remnant before resection. In addition, Vauthey et al.[57] noted a strong association between small sFLR and postoperative peak alkaline phosphatase, prothrombin time, bilirubin levels, as well as increased length of stay. Abdalla et al.[16] subsequently showed that the preoperative estimation of sFLR utilizing this formula was effective in selecting patients for PVE prior to extended right hepatectomy. By identifying the sFLR prior to surgery, Abdalla et al.[16] showed that patients with an anticipated small FLR could be referred for PVE. Following PVE, there was an average increase in FLR of 8%. Of note, patients with a percent FLR less than 20% had more complications as a group.

More recently, Vauthey et al.[45] examined a multicenter cohort of patients containing North American/North European patients. In this study, Vauthey et al.[45] utilized CT-based images to calculate LV. Vauthey and colleagues found that the Urata equation actually underestimated LV, while the Heinemann equation slightly overestimated LV. The study showed a noticeable difference in the relationship between TLV and BSA when comparing Western and Japanese populations. The TLV was greater in Western populations at any BSA value. Using new linear models, the authors empirically developed a new formula based on BSA:

$$\text{TLV} = -794.41 + 1267.28 \times \text{BSA} \qquad (11.5)$$

Utilizing this modified formula, Ribero et al.[58] reported on a series of patients in whom the sFLR was assessed in conjunction with the degree of hypertrophy of the sFLR following PVE. The authors found that estimation of the sFLR utilizing the modified formula strongly correlated with outcome. Specifically, an estimated sFLR of less than 20% or less than a 5% degree of hypertrophy based on this formula was associated with increased complications. In a separate study, Vauthey et al.[9] noted that an sFLR less than 20% based on this formula was again associated with an increased risk of hyperbilirubinemia (greater than

10 mg/dL), elevated INR, and hepatic insufficiency. As such, the authors concluded that estimated liver volumes utilizing CT-images should be standardized to BSA to ensure accuracy. In a separate series, Yigitler et al.[59] reported on the impact of a small liver remnant on outcome following major liver resections using a different equation. In this study, the authors calculated the ratio of the remnant liver volume (RLV) to functional liver volume (FLV) utilizing a formula derived by Lin et al.[60]:

$$\text{FLV (mL)} = [13 \times \text{height (cm)}] + [12 \times \text{weight (kg)}] - 1{,}530 \qquad (11.6)$$

The authors noted that liver volume determined by CT volumetry utilizing this formula was accurate.

In an attempt to assess the accuracy of the diversity of equations available for the estimation of liver volume, Johnson et al.[43]performed a meta-analysis that integrated all published data. The authors recommended the equation espoused by Vauthey et al.[45] as the best model to predict liver volume. Specifically, the authors noted that the incorporation of BSA was associated with the most parsimonious and the least biased model. In a separate study, Chun et al.[51] compared FLR volumes standardized to BW versus BSA to assess their utility in predicting postoperative hepatic dysfunction after hepatic resection. The authors noted that regression analysis revealed that the FLR/TLV and FLR/BW ratios were highly correlated (Pearson correlation coefficient, 0.98). The area under the ROC curve was 0.85 for FLR/TLV and 0.84 for FLR/BW. Based on the strong correlation between the FLR measurements standardized to BW and BSA and their similar ability to predict postoperative hepatic dysfunction, both methods were deemed to be appropriate for assessing liver volume.

11.4 Special Considerations: The Liver with Underlying Parenchymal Disease

In patients with underlying parenchymal disease such as cirrhosis or steatosis, preoperative functional, as well as anatomical volumetric data may be beneficial to help stratify patients with regard to their anticipated functional FLR. In most Western centers, for patients with underlying parenchymal disease, most centers still utilize CT volumetry alone and simply increase the percent FLR deemed acceptable. For example, while an FLR of 20–30% may be acceptable for patients with normal hepatic parenchyma, an FLR of 40–50% is needed for those patients with cirrhosis. In Asia, indocyanine green clearance (ICG) is utilized more frequently to identify patients with potential inadequate functional reserve. More recently, several investigators have suggested combining functional tests such as ICG[61] or technetium-99 m galactosyl serum albumin (^{99m}Tc-GSA) scintigraphy[62] with anatomical CT volumetry measurements.

Nanashima et al.[62] examined the relationship between morphological hepatic volume versus functional volume by ^{99m}Tc-GSA. Asialoglycoprotein receptors on hepatocytes reflect functional liver cells.[63] As such, utilizing ^{99m}Tc-GSA scintigraphy, the functional and anatomic hepatic volume in the liver can be measured. In the study by Nanashima et al.,[62] there were no significant differences, however, in the volume measurements utilizing CT versus ^{99m}Tc-GSA scintigraphy. Even in patients with cirrhosis, the correlation between CT and ^{99m}Tc-GSA scintigraphy was high, questioning the added benefit of this latter technique. The authors did note that following PVE, the mean values of liver volumes of the right hemi-liver – but not the left hemi-liver – as assessed by CT versus ^{99m}Tc-GSA scintigraphy were significantly different. The authors concluded that the volumetric measurement by ^{99m}Tc-GSA scintigraphy may be useful in conjunction with CT volumetry in detecting changes in the functional volume of the liver following PVE.

In the East, the use of ICG is routinely assessed in patients with underlying hepatic parenchymal disease who are being considered for surgery.[61,64] PVE has been advocated for FLR volumes of ≤40% when the ICG R15 is ≤10% and for FLR volumes of ≤50% when the ICG R15 is 10–20%.[61] In the study by Kubota et al.,[64] the authors demonstrate how the integration of volumetric data from CT volumetry in conjunction with functional data from ICG can increase the ability to stratify patients with underlying liver disease/cirrhosis with regard to their need for PVE.

11.5 Conclusion

CT volumetry is as an essential tool in the modern day approach to patients with complex hepatic disease. High-quality CT images can now be routinely obtained with relative ease with the currently available technology and widely available scanners. The actual measurement of the liver volume based on these images can be performed either manually or with automated techniques. However, the active participation of experienced radiologists and hepatobiliary surgeons is necessary to ensure accurate measurements. The liver volume and FLR can be calculated with these measurements using various published formulas. However, based on the current data, the formula espoused by Vauthey et al.[45] appears to be associated with the least bias and therefore is the most widely applicable. In patients with advanced liver malignancies requiring major hepatic resection, CT volumetry should inform both the operative approach and the identification of patients for preoperative PVE.

References

1. Pawlik TM, Schulick RD, Choti MA. Expanding criteria for resectability of colorectal liver metastases. *Oncologist*. 2008;13(1):51-64.
2. Adam R, Lucidi V, Bismuth H. Hepatic colorectal metastases: methods of improving resectability. *Surg Clin North Am*. 2004;84(2):659-671.
3. Elias D, Baton O, Sideris L, et al. Hepatectomy plus intraoperative radiofrequency ablation and chemotherapy to treat technically unresectable multiple colorectal liver metastases. *J Surg Oncol*. 2005;90(1):36-42.
4. Elias D, Manganas D, Benizri E, et al. Trans-metastasis hepatectomy: results of a 21-case study. *Eur J Surg Oncol*. 2006;32(2):213-217.
5. Hemming AW, Reed AI, Howard RJ, et al. Preoperative portal vein embolization for extended hepatectomy. *Ann Surg*. 2003;237(5):686-691. discussion 691-693.
6. Pawlik TM, Choti MA. Surgical therapy for colorectal metastases to the liver. *J Gastrointest Surg*. 2007;11(8):1057-1077.
7. Ng KK, Vauthey JN, Pawlik TM, et al. Is hepatic resection for large or multinodular hepatocellular carcinoma justified? Results from a multi-institutional database. *Ann Surg Oncol*. 2005;12(5):364-373.
8. Takizawa D, Kakizaki S, Sohara N, et al. Hepatocellular carcinoma with portal vein tumor thrombosis: clinical characteristics, prognosis, and patient survival analysis. *Dig Dis Sci*. 2007;52(11):3290-3295.
9. Vauthey JN, Pawlik TM, Abdalla EK, et al. Is extended hepatectomy for hepatobiliary malignancy justified? *Ann Surg*. 2004;239(5):722-730. discussion 730-732.
10. Virani S, Michaelson JS, Hutter MM, et al. Morbidity and mortality after liver resection: results of the patient safety in surgery study. *J Am Coll Surg*. 2007;204(6):1284-1292.
11. Zhou L, Rui JA, Wang SB, et al. Outcomes and prognostic factors of cirrhotic patients with hepatocellular carcinoma after radical major hepatectomy. *World J Surg*. 2007;31(9):1782-1787.
12. Fan ST, Lai EC, Lo CM, et al. Hospital mortality of major hepatectomy for hepatocellular carcinoma associated with cirrhosis. *Arch Surg*. 1995;130(2):198-203.
13. Nagasue N, Yukaya H. Liver resection for hepatocellular carcinoma: results from 150 consecutive patients. *Cancer Chemother Pharmacol*. 1989;23(suppl):S78-S82.
14. Thompson HH, Tompkins RK, Longmire WP Jr. Major hepatic resection. A 25-year experience. *Ann Surg*. 1983; 197(4):375-388.
15. Jarnagin WR, Gonen M, Fong Y, et al. Improvement in perioperative outcome after hepatic resection: analysis of 1,803 consecutive cases over the past decade. *Ann Surg*. 2002; 236(4):397-406. discussion 406-407.
16. Abdalla EK, Barnett CC, Doherty D, et al. Extended hepatectomy in patients with hepatobiliary malignancies with and without preoperative portal vein embolization. *Arch Surg*. 2002;137(6):675-680. discussion 680-681.
17. Stone HH, Long WD, Smith RB III, Haynes CD. Physiologic considerations in major hepatic resections. *Am J Surg*. 1969;117(1):78-84.
18. Fan ST, Lo CM, Liu CL, et al. Safety of donors in live donor liver transplantation using right lobe grafts. *Arch Surg*. 2000;135(3):336-340.
19. Farges O, Belghiti J, Kianmanesh R, et al. Portal vein embolization before right hepatectomy: prospective clinical trial. *Ann Surg*. 2003;237(2):208-217.
20. Abdalla EK, Denys A, Chevalier P, et al. Total and segmental liver volume variations: implications for liver surgery. *Surgery*. 2004;135(4):404-410.
21. Delesse MA. Procede mechanique pour determiner la composition des roches. *C R Acad Sci*. 1847;25:544-545.
22. Weibel ER. Principles and methods for the morphometric study of the lung and other organs. *Lab Invest*. 1963;12:131-155.
23. Hennig A. Kritische btrachtungen zur volumenund Oberflachenmessung in der mikroskopie. *Zeiss Werkz*. 1958;30:76-86.
24. Fritschy P, Robotti G, Schneekloth G, Vock P. Measurement of liver volume by ultrasound and computed tomography. *J Clin Ultrasound*. 1983;11(6):299-303.
25. Henderson JM, Heymsfield SB, Horowitz J, Kutner MH. Measurement of liver and spleen volume by computed tomography. Assessment of reproducibility and changes found following a selective distal splenorenal shunt. *Radiology*. 1981;141(2):525-527.
26. Kamel IR, Kruskal JB, Pomfret EA, et al. Impact of multidetector CT on donor selection and surgical planning before living adult right lobe liver transplantation. *AJR Am J Roentgenol*. 2001;176(1):193-200.
27. Leelaudomlipi S, Sugawara Y, Kaneko J, et al. Volumetric analysis of liver segments in 155 living donors. *Liver Transpl*. 2002;8(7):612-614.
28. Farraher SW, Jara H, Chang KJ, et al. Liver and spleen volumetry with quantitative MR imaging and dual-space clustering segmentation. *Radiology*. 2005;237(1):322-328.
29. Caldwell SH, de Lange EE, Gaffey MJ, et al. Accuracy and significance of pretransplant liver volume measured by magnetic resonance imaging. *Liver Transpl Surg*. 1996;2(6): 438-442.
30. Luft AR, Skalej M, Welte D, et al. Reliability and exactness of MRI-based volumetry: a phantom study. *J Magn Reson Imaging*. 1996;6(4):700-704.
31. Zacharia TT. Assessment of future remnant liver regeneration after portal vein embolization using three-dimensional CT and MR volumetric analyses. *Australas Radiol*. 2006; 50(6):543-548.
32. Heymsfield SB, Fulenwider T, Nordlinger B, et al. Accurate measurement of liver, kidney, and spleen volume and mass by computerized axial tomography. *Ann Intern Med*. 1979; 90(2):185-187.

33. Soyer P, Roche A, Elias D, Levesque M. Hepatic metastases from colorectal cancer: influence of hepatic volumetric analysis on surgical decision making. *Radiology*. 1992;184(3):695-697.
34. Wigmore SJ, Redhead DN, Yan XJ, et al. Virtual hepatic resection using three-dimensional reconstruction of helical computed tomography angioportograms. *Ann Surg*. 2001; 233(2):221-226.
35. Kamel IR, Kruskal JB, Warmbrand G, et al. Accuracy of volumetric measurements after virtual right hepatectomy in potential donors undergoing living adult liver transplantation. *AJR Am J Roentgenol*. 2001;176(2):483-487.
36. Shirabe K, Shimada M, Gion T, et al. Postoperative liver failure after major hepatic resection for hepatocellular carcinoma in the modern era with special reference to remnant liver volume. *J Am Coll Surg*. 1999;188(3):304-309.
37. Shoup M, Gonen M, D'Angelica M, et al. Volumetric analysis predicts hepatic dysfunction in patients undergoing major liver resection. *J Gastrointest Surg*. 2003;7(3):325-330.
38. Schindl MJ, Redhead DN, Fearon KC, et al. The value of residual liver volume as a predictor of hepatic dysfunction and infection after major liver resection. *Gut*. 2005;54(2):289-296.
39. Nakayama Y, Li Q, Katsuragawa S, et al. Automated hepatic volumetry for living related liver transplantation at multisection CT. *Radiology*. 2006;240(3):743-748.
40. Dello SA, van Dam RM, Slangen JJ, et al. Liver volumetry plug and play: do it yourself with ImageJ. *World J Surg*. 2007;31(11):2215-2221.
41. Lu Y, Wu Z, Liu C, Wang HH. Hepatic volumetry with PhotoShop in personal computer. *Hepatobiliary Pancreat Dis Int*. 2004;3(1):82-85.
42. Rasband W. ImageJ. U.S. National Institutes of Health, Bethesda, 1997–2005.
43. Johnson TN, Tucker GT, Tanner MS, Rostami-Hodjegan A. Changes in liver volume from birth to adulthood: a meta-analysis. *Liver Transpl*. 2005;11(12):1481-1493.
44. Urata K, Kawasaki S, Matsunami H, et al. Calculation of child and adult standard liver volume for liver transplantation. *Hepatology*. 1995;21(5):1317-1321.
45. Vauthey JN, Abdalla EK, Doherty DA, et al. Body surface area and body weight predict total liver volume in Western adults. *Liver Transpl*. 2002;8(3):233-240.
46. DeLand FH, North WA. Relationship between liver size and body size. *Radiology*. 1968;91(6):1195-1198.
47. Zoli M, Magalotti D, Grimaldi M, et al. Physical examination of the liver: is it still worth it? *Am J Gastroenterol*. 1995;90(9):1428-1432.
48. Chandramohan A, Eapen A, Govil S, et al. Determining standard liver volume: assessment of existing formulae in Indian population. *Indian J Gastroenterol*. 2007;26(1):22-25.
49. Heinemann A, Wischhusen F, Puschel K, Rogiers X. Standard liver volume in the Caucasian population. *Liver Transpl Surg*. 1999;5(5):366-368.
50. Urata K, Hashikura Y, Ikegami T, et al. Standard liver volume in adults. *Transplant Proc*. 2000;32(7):2093-2094.
51. Chun YS, Ribero D, Abdalla EK, et al. Comparison of two methods of future liver remnant volume measurement. *J Gastrointest Surg*. 2008;12(1):123-128.
52. Kiuchi T, Kasahara M, Uryuhara K, et al. Impact of graft size mismatching on graft prognosis in liver transplantation from living donors. *Transplantation*. 1999;67(2): 321-327.
53. Lo CM, Fan ST, Liu CL, et al. Minimum graft size for successful living donor liver transplantation. *Transplantation*. 1999;68(8):1112-1116.
54. Ogiu N, Nakamura Y, Ijiri I, et al. A statistical analysis of the internal organ weights of normal Japanese people. *Health Phys*. 1997;72(3):368-383.
55. Yoshizumi T, Gondolesi GE, Bodian CA, et al. A simple new formula to assess liver weight. *Transplant Proc*. 2003; 35(4):1415-1420.
56. Yu HC, You H, Lee H, et al. Estimation of standard liver volume for liver transplantation in the Korean population. *Liver Transpl*. 2004;10(6):779-783.
57. Vauthey JN, Chaoui A, Do KA, et al. Standardized measurement of the future liver remnant prior to extended liver resection: methodology and clinical associations. *Surgery*. 2000;127(5):512-519.
58. Ribero D, Abdalla EK, Madoff DC, et al. Portal vein embolization before major hepatectomy and its effects on regeneration, resectability and outcome. *Br J Surg*. 2007;94(11): 1386-1394.
59. Yigitler C, Farges O, Kianmanesh R, et al. The small remnant liver after major liver resection: how common and how relevant? *Liver Transpl*. 2003;9(9):S18-S25.
60. Lin XZ, Sun YN, Liu YH, et al. Liver volume in patients withorwithoutchronicliverdiseases.*Hepatogastroenterology*. 1998;45(22):1069-1074.
61. Ribero D, Curley SA, Imamura H, et al. Selection for resection of hepatocellular carcinoma and surgical strategy: indications for resection, evaluation of liver function, portal vein embolization, and resection. *Ann Surg Oncol*. 2008;15(4): 986-992.
62. Nanashima A, Yamaguchi H, Shibasaki S, et al. Relationship between CT volumetry and functional liver volume using technetium-99 m galactosyl serum albumin scintigraphy in patients undergoing preoperative portal vein embolization before major hepatectomy: a preliminary study. *Dig Dis Sci*. 2006;51(7):1190-1195.
63. Ashwell G, Harford J. Carbohydrate-specific receptors of the liver. *Annu Rev Biochem*. 1982;51:531-554.
64. Kubota K, Makuuchi M, Kusaka K, et al. Measurement of liver volume and hepatic functional reserve as a guide to decision-making in resectional surgery for hepatic tumors. *Hepatology*. 1997;26(5):1176-1181.

Preoperative Assessment with Functional Studies of the Liver

12

Thomas M. van Gulik, Wilmar de Graaf, and Roelof J. Bennink

Abstract

Whereas imaging studies such as CT or MRI allow volumetric assessment of the liver segments, only indirect information is provided concerning the quality of the liver parenchyma and its actual functional capacity. Assessment of liver function is therefore crucial in the preoperative work-up of patients who require extensive liver resection and in whom PVE is considered. As the regenerative capacity of the liver is related to the quality of liver parenchyma, the success of PVE largely depends on parameters of liver function. This chapter deals with several tests for the measurement of liver function. Passive liver function tests include biochemical parameters and clinical grading systems such as the Child-Pugh and MELD scores. Dynamic quantitative tests of liver function can be based on clearance capacity tests such as the ICG clearance test, galactose elimination capacity, and lidocaine clearance test. Although widely used, discrepancies have been reported of the ICG clearance test in relation with clinical outcome. Nuclear imaging studies have the advantage of providing simultaneous morphologic (visual) and physiologic (quantitative functional) information of the liver. In addition, regional (segmental) differences in liver function can be determined. The use of SPECT-CT cameras enables measurements of volume and function of the future remnant liver. ^{99m}Tc-galactosl serum albumin (GSA) scintigraphy and ^{99m}Tc-mebrofenin hepatobiliary scintigraphy potentially identify patients at risk for post-resectional liver failure who might benefit from PVE. Bioenergetic tests are based on the energy state of the liver and the availability of ATP. The caffeine clearance test, aminopyrine breath test and MEGX test measure the microsomal or cytosolic capacity of the liver. As there is not one test that can measure all the components of liver function, liver functional reserve remains to be estimated from a combination of clinical parameters and quantitative liver function tests.

Keywords

Child-Pugh score • Functional studies in the liver • GSA scintigraphy • ICG clearance test • Liver function tests

T.M. van Gulik (✉)
Department of Surgery, Academic Medical Center, University of Amsterdam, Meibergdreef 9, Amsterdam NL-1105AZ, The Netherlands
e-mail: t.m.vangulik@amc.uva.nl

D.C. Madoff et al. (eds.), *Venous Embolization of the Liver*,
DOI 10.1007/978-1-84882-122-4_12, © Springer-Verlag London Limited 2011

Liver failure is the major cause of mortality and morbidity after partial liver resection.[1] Post-resectional liver function largely depends on the quantity and quality of the remnant liver and the ability of the parenchyma to regenerate. Preoperative assessment of risk factors for insufficient function of the future remnant liver is therefore mandatory in the selection of candidates for safe partial liver resection. The quantity of the remnant liver is determined by the extent of resection. CT volumetry is useful to assess the volume of the remnant liver relative to total liver volume as has been dealt with above (see Chap. 11). Imaging studies such as CT or MRI, however, only provide indirect information on the quality of the liver parenchyma and its actual functional capacity.

The quality of liver parenchyma is first of all determined by any underlying liver disease such as cirrhosis, cholestasis, or steatosis. Steatosis is becoming more and more a problem in the Western world because of its increasing incidence.[2,3] Also, as a result of neoadjuvant chemotherapy, the liver may have sustained considerable injury characterized as steatohepatitis or veno-occlusive disease.[4] Under these circumstances, postoperative liver function may be overestimated when based only on volumetric analysis.

Postoperative recovery, especially after resection of critical liver cell mass, relies on the regenerative capacity of the liver remnant. The potential of the liver remnant to regenerate also depends on the quality of the parenchyma and is hampered by concomitant cirrhosis, cholestasis, or steatosis, conditions in which ATP production is impaired.[5] In the context of preoperative portal vein embolization, the regenerative capacity of the liver is essential, and failure of the non-embolized liver lobe to hypertrophy is considered a sign of poor liver function.[6,7]

Assessment of liver function is therefore crucial in the preoperative work-up of patients who require extensive liver resection. This chapter will focus on several dynamic quantitative tests for the measurement of liver function and their application in patients undergoing portal vein embolization.

12.1 How Is Liver Function Defined?

The liver is responsible for a spectrum of functions including the uptake, metabolism, conjugation, and excretion of various endogenous and foreign substances, as well as the syntheses of vital plasma proteins.[8] The liver also provides an immunologic function and the reticuloendothelial capacity of the liver plays a role in phagocytosis and clearance of microorgansims and endotoxins from the portal blood.[9] The excretion of bile is an important end point of liver function and the production of bile immediately ceases when perfusion of the liver is arrested. The complexity of liver function is best reflected by our inability to restore full liver function in liver failure as liver assist devices and bioartificial livers have not proven to fully substitute all the components of liver function.[10,11] In recent years, several prognostic tools have been employed for the assessment of liver function. These can be grossly divided into passive liver tests, dynamic quantitative liver function tests, and bioenergetic tests.

12.2 Passive Liver Function Tests

Passive liver function tests include biochemical parameters and clinical grading systems. The term "liver function tests" to indicate a set of conventional plasma parameters is confusing because they do not represent functional components of the liver except for clotting factors which are synthesized by the liver. The aminotransaminase enzymes, aspartate transferase (AST) and alanine transferase (ALT) are markers of liver damage and correlate with the extent of hepatocellular necrosis. Although a persisting release of these enzymes will ultimately result in the loss of liver functional capacity, they are not parameters of function per se. Albumin and clotting factors however, are exclusively synthesized by the liver and their plasma concentrations are therefore used as indirect indicators of liver function. Plasma bilirubin concentration provides indirect information on the uptake, conjugation and excretion function of the liver. Plasma bilirubin levels are, however, also influenced by extrahepatic factors such as increased production of bilirubin or bile duct obstruction.

One of the crucial metabolic functions of the liver is the synthesis of urea from ammonia and amino acids. Insufficient liver function leads to diminished urea synthesis and consequently, hyperammonemia and encephalopathy. Increased plasma ammonia levels therefore indicate severely compromised liver function, and most patients with hyperammonemia are not candidates for major liver resection. In the setting of postresectional

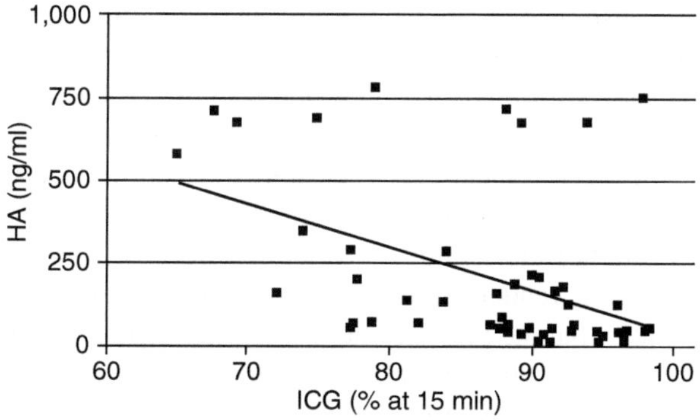

Fig. 12.1 Significant correlation between ICG-C 15 and plasma hyarulonic acid (*HA*) values ($N=50$, $r=-0.52$)

Table 12.1 Quantitative tests of liver function

Clearance tests	Indocyanin green clearance test (ICG)
	Galactose elimination test
	Lidocaine elimination test (MEGX test)
Nuclear imaging studies	^{99m}Tc-galactosyl serum albumin (GSA) scintigraphy
	^{99m}Tc-mebrofenin hepatobiliary scintigraphy
Cytochrome P450 activity test	Caffeine elimination test
	Aminopyrine breath test
Bioenergetic tests	Assessment of ketone bodies
	31-Phosphorus (^{31}P) magnetic resonance spectroscopy

liver function, progressive increase in plasma ammonia is an ominous sign of remnant liver failure.

Hyaluronic acid (HA), a more recent biochemical parameter, is a glycosaminoglycan which is produced by connective tissue cells and synovial cells and is exclusively taken up from the blood and metabolized by the sinusoidal endothelial cells of the liver. Hyaluronic acid concentration in the blood may therefore be considered a functional test of the liver sinusoidal endothelial cell and as such, of the whole liver. In a series of patients with primary and secondary liver tumors, we found a significant positive correlation of HA and almost every conventional liver parameter. A significant correlation was demonstrated between plasma concentrations of hyaluronic acid and the ICG retention test in which ICG retention of 15% corresponded with a hyaluronic acid level of 233 ng/mL (normal plasma values of hyaluronic acid: 0–75 ng/mL). [Unpublished results] (Fig. 12.1) A similar correlation of plasma hyaluronic acid and ICG-15 has been reported by Nanashima et al.[12]

Clinical grading systems combine several biochemical parameters together with clinical symptoms of insufficient liver function. The Child-Pugh (CP) score is a widely used clinical scoring system which includes total bilirubin plasma level, albumin plasma level, and prothrombin time together with the presence or absence of encephalopathy and ascites. The CP scoring system is particularly useful in selecting patients with HCC and cirrhosis for resection or transplantation as most class Child B and class Child C patients are candidates for transplantation, leaving the class Child A patients for resection. In patients with liver metastases who usually have normal liver parenchyma and who are all classified as class Child A, the question then arises how to predict those patients at risk of post-resectional liver failure.[13] In these patients, the Child-Pugh score has been shown to be quite variable and may be unreliable for predicting the outcome of liver resections, especially in patients with non-cirrhotic livers.[14]

The MELD score was originally developed to predict short-term survival in patients undergoing transcutaneous intrahepatic portosystemic shunt procedures (TIPS), and has been adopted to stratify patients with end-stage liver disease awaiting transplantation. MELD scores, however, did not predict morbidity or mortality after elective liver resection.[15]

12.3 Dynamic Quantitative Liver Function Tests

Biochemical liver function tests and clinical grading systems only provide indirect information about liver function. Therefore, especially in patients with non-cirrhotic livers, there is a need for objective tests to evaluate liver function in addition to clinical judgment. To this end, several dynamic quantitative tests of liver function have been devised. (Table 12.1) Some of these tests such as the ICG clearance test, lidocaine clearance test, and galactose elimination capacity are influenced by perfusion of the hepatocyte mass and are therefore bloodflow dependent.[13] A bloodflow independent test is the aminopyrine breath test, discussed below. The various function tests are also based on different metabolic pathways, which makes it difficult to compare the value of each test in the context of risk assessment for liver resection. Several of these tests are discussed in more detail below.

12.4 Indocyanin Green (ICG) Clearance Test

The indocyanine green (ICG) clearance test was initially devised for the measurement of blood flow, and later found clinical application in the assessment of liver function. It is now the most widely used quantitative liver function test. ICG is a tricarbocyanine dye that binds to albumin and distributes uniformly in the blood within 2–3 min after intravenous injection. ICG is exclusively removed by the liver and excreted into the bile without intrahepatic conjugation.[16] Following administration, the blood level falls exponentially for about 20 min, by which time approximately 97% of the dye is excreted. ICG clearance is determined by serum sampling or pulse dye densitometry using an optical sensor placed on the finger.[17,18]

The disappearance of ICG from the blood reflects the liver's capacity to transport organic anions and metabolize drugs providing indirect measurement of global liver function. The uptake of ICG by the hepatocytes is mediated by members of the bile canalicular organic anion transporting polypeptides (OATPs).[19] Excretion of ICG into the bile is governed by the ATP-dependent export pump multidrug-resistance associated protein 2 (MRP 2). ICG is excreted without undergoing biotransformation during transit through the hepatocyte.[20]

The results of ICG tests are expressed by several parameters including the plasma disappearance rate (ICG-PDR), ICG elimination rate constant (ICG-k), and the ICG-R15, which describes the percent of clearance or conversely, the retention of ICG in 15 min. Several cut-off values for safe resection have been mentioned in literature.[5] An ICG clearance rate of more than 86% was found to correlate with sufficient liver functional reserve, which equals a retention rate of less than 14%.[21] It has been reported that the ICG-R15 value is a better indicator of liver function in comparison with Child-Pugh classification in patients who underwent cardiac surgery. In these patients a high ICG-R15 correlated with a high rate of mortality.[22]

The ICG clearance test was found to be the best discriminating preoperative test for evaluating the hepatic functional reserve in patients with HCC.[23] However, there are some drawbacks that may lead to discrepancies in relation with histological findings and clinical outcomes. Discrepancies have been reported between ICG-15 clearance rates and histological liver findings, and also clinical outcomes.[24,25] Mortality has been noted in patients with normal ICG-15, and survival in patients with predicted poor outcome on the basis of preoperative ICG-15.[21] One of the confounding factors in the measurement of ICG clearance is its flow dependency. Variations in hepatic bloodflow such as caused by intrahepatic shunting will influence the ICG clearance rate, rendering the test less predictive. Another point is that the ICG clearance test reflects global liver function but does not take into account regional variations which may occur within the liver obscuring a possible functional disadvantage of the segments to be preserved.

Cholestasis affects ICG clearance since the excretion of ICG into bile is impeded. Also, hyperbilirubinemia by itself confounds the uptake of ICG because there is a competition between bilirubin and ICG for the same cellular transporter systems. Assessment using the ICG clearance test therefore requires complete biliary drainage in patients with concomitant obstruction of (part of) the biliary tree. Alternatively, when percutaneous transhepatic biliary drainage has been performed, ICG excretion can be measured directly in the drained bile. The rate of excretion into the drained bile was found to be more representative of hepatic ATP stores than plasma ICG-15.[26,27]

12.4.1 The ICG Clearance Test After PVE

A decreased clearance rate of ICG is one of the factors for considering preoperative PVE in patients requiring major liver resection in order to augment function of the remnant liver. However, since abnormal ICG clearance rates are usually found in compromised livers, an impaired regenerative response should be taken into account.[6] As mentioned above, failure of the non-embolized liver segments to hypertrophy is considered a significant sign of deficient functional reserve of the liver increasing the risk of liver failure associated with liver resection. As postresectional regeneration also depends on the same mechanisms; insufficient volume increase of the future remnant liver after PVE is a strong predictor of postoperative liver failure.[7,28]

Interestingly, Wakabyashi et al.[29] who tested ICG-15 after PVE in patients with HCC showed a decrease of the ICG clearance rate in 2 weeks time after PVE. This finding is compatible with changed bloodflow in the non-embolized liver lobe after occlusion of the portal venous branches in the embolized liver lobe, emphasizing the dependency of the ICG-15 test on hepatic blood flow. ICG values returned to base line levels after 6–8 weeks after PVE, suggesting equilibration of portal and hepatic arterial blood flow by that time. As the time interval between PVE and resection tends to be chosen in the range of 3–4 weeks to prevent further tumor progression after PVE, the use of the ICG-15 test in the assessment of liver function following PVE is doubtful.[28,30] Conceivably, as ICG clearance measures the global liver function, an increase in function of the non-embolized lobe is accompanied by a decreased function of the embolized, atrophied lobe resulting in no net effect on total liver function. The ICG clearance test is therefore not able to measure the increase in future remnant liver function after PVE.

12.5 ^{99m}Tc-Galactosyl Serum Albumin Scintigraphy

The asialoglycoprotein (ASGP) receptor is only present in mammalian hepatocytes and is specific for asialoglycoproteins. The ASGP receptor consists of two subunits (human hepatic lectins 1 and 2) and is expressed on the hepatocyte sinusoidal surface adjoining the extracellular space of Disse.[31] Asialoglycoproteins bind to ASGP receptors and are subsequently taken up by receptor mediated endocytosis. A significant decrease in ASGP receptors is seen in patients with chronic liver diseases together with accumulation of asialoglycoproteins in the blood plasma.[32] At first, technetium-99 m (^{99m}Tc), labeled galactosyl-neoglyoalbumin (^{99m}Tc-GNA), was developed as a synthetic asialoglyoprotein to visualize and quantify its hepatic binding to the ASGP receptor.[33] For clinical analyses, ^{99m}Tc-GSA was developed in Japan as a synthetic asialoglycoprotein.[34] The liver is the only uptake site for ^{99m}Tc-GSA and it is therefore an ideal agent for receptor-targeted, functional liver scintigraphy. The parameters obtained from planar ^{99m}Tc-GSA scintigraphy proved valuable parameters for the assessment of liver function in cirrhotic patients, and demonstrated a correlation with conventional liver function tests, including antithrombin III, total and direct bilirubin, prothrombin time, ICG clearance, Child-Pugh classification, and histology (hepatic activity index (HAI) score).[25,35] A discrepancy between the ICG clearance test and ^{99m}Tc-GSA scintigraphy has been described in 9–20% of the patients in whom the histological severity of disease was better reflected by ^{99m}Tc-GSA scintigraphy.[36,37] Since bilirubin does not bind to the ASGP receptor, ^{99m}Tc-GSA scintigraphy is also effective in assessing hepatic function in patients with hyperbilirubinemia.[38]

12.5.1 Kinetics and Quantitative Measurement of Liver Function by ^{99m}Tc-GSA Scintigraphy

Several imaging modalities have been developed including planar dynamic scintigraphy, static SPECT and dynamic SPECT. In dynamic ^{99m}Tc-GSA scintigraphy, images are obtained after an intravenous bolus of ^{99m}Tc-GSA using a gamma camera positioned over the heart and liver region. The blood clearance and hepatic uptake are obtained by generating regions of interest (ROIs) from heart and liver, respectively. For the actual kinetics of the ^{99m}Tc-GSA receptor binding, several complex kinetic models have been developed. Although many different parameters can be calculated from different kinetic models, these are highly complex and therefore not widely used in the context of liver surgery. The hepatic uptake ratio of ^{99m}Tc-GSA (LHL15) and the blood clearance ratio (HH15) are the most commonly used parameters in planar dynamic ^{99m}Tc-GSA scintigraphy (Fig. 12.2). The HH15 is calculated by dividing the radioactivity of the heart ROI at 15 min after ^{99m}Tc-GSA injection by that of 3 min after injection. LHL15 is calculated by dividing the radioactivity of the liver ROI by the radioactivity of the liver plus heart ROIs at 15 min after injection.[34,36,39] The modified receptor index (MRI) is determined by dividing the LHL15 by the HH15.[36]

Static ^{99m}Tc-GSA Single Photon Emission Computed Tomography (SPECT) and dynamic SPECT have been introduced to improve the assessment of segmental liver function and to measure functional liver volume.[40,41] The outline extraction method is a simple technique to calculate the functional liver volume using a specific cut-off value to automatically outline the liver.[40] It, however, does not take into account the regional functional differences within the included volume.

In addition to static SPECT, dynamic SPECT has been applied. Dynamic SPECT measures the uptake dynamics of ^{99m}Tc-GSA in a 3-dimentional way but requires a fast rotating, multidetector gamma camera, which is not available in every institution.

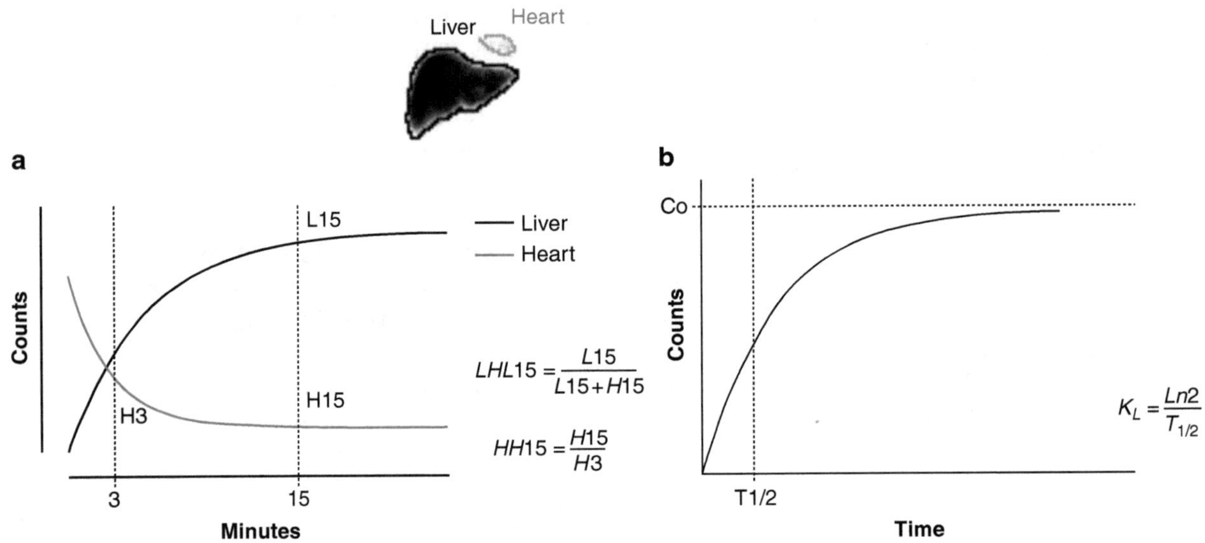

Fig. 12.2 Planar ^{99m}Tc-GSA scintigraphy. The hepatic uptake ratio (*LHL15*) and blood disappearance ratio (*HH15*) is calculated from the ^{99m}Tc-GSA time–activity curves from the heart (*gray*) and the liver (*black*) (*panel* **a**). Blood disappearance constant (K_L) is calculated from the liver uptake curve, with the use of the disappearance halftime ($T_{1/2}$) (*panel* **b**).

12.5.2 Preoperative Assessment of Liver Function Using of ^{99m}Tc-GSA Liver Scintigraphy

Multiple studies have described the use of preoperative planar dynamic ^{99m}Tc-GSA scintigraphy for predicting postoperative complications.[37,42-44] Preoperative hepatic uptake ratio of ^{99m}Tc-GSA (LHL15) proved a reliable indicator for predicting postoperative complications in patients with hepatocellular carcinoma (HCC) and chronic liver disease, showing significantly lower values in patients with major postoperative complications.[25,43] Specific cut-off values for LHL15 (i.e., 0.90 and 0.875) have been described to select patients with a high risk for complications. Cut-off values were however, mostly not based on accurate risk analysis but rather set arbitrarily. Postoperative liver failure was also observed in patients with a relatively normal liver function (LHL15 > 0.875). This can be explained by the fact that LHL15 only measures the preoperative total liver function and not the function of the FRL.

For a more accurate assessment of FRL function, static ^{99m}Tc-GSA SPECT was introduced to estimate total and segmental liver functional volume.[41,45] Preoperative functional volume measured by ^{99m}Tc-GSA SPECT proved more suitable for predicting remnant liver function than CT volumetry in a study group with predominantly cirrhotic patients.[40,41] In cirrhotic patients, advanced fibrosis is accompanied by a reduction of functional hepatocytes. While functional volume measured by ^{99m}Tc-GSA SPECT reflects the functional hepatocyte mass,[45] CT volumetry cannot distinguish between functional and non-functional liver tissue. In addition, tumor compression on surrounding liver tissue, bile ducts[40], and/or blood vessels[46] can impact regional liver function, while liver volume is maintained over a longer time period. Although the outline extraction method is regularly used to calculate functional hepatic volume,[40,41,46-48] it is based on the assumption that liver function is uniformly distributed in the tissue included within the cut-off value. Especially in tumor bearing and compromised livers, function is not distributed homogeneously. Therefore, total functional liver volume does not necessarily correlate with the intrinsic liver function measured by dynamic planar GSA scintigraphy.[39,45] Alternatively, dynamic SPECT can be used to measure FRL function and it has been demonstrated in studies with small numbers of patients that this technique can be used to predict postoperative complications.[45,49]

12.5.3 Increase of Liver Function After PVE

Multiple studies evaluated the increase of the FRL function after PVE using ^{99m}Tc-GSA scintigraphy.[47,50-53]

In three studies, the increase of FRL function after PVE, measured by the dynamic ^{99m}Tc-GSA SPECT, was compared with morphologic hypertrophy of the FRL, measured by CT volumetry, in cirrhotic and non-cirrhotic patients.[47,52,53] The uptake of ^{99m}Tc-GSA showed a rapid increase during the first week following PVE but little in the second week. The increase in ^{99m}Tc-GSA uptake in the FRL was more extensive than the increase in FRL volume. Therefore, it was concluded that ^{99m}Tc-GSA scintigraphy was useful in evaluating the functional increase of the FRL after PVE, which could not be evaluated with CT volumetry. Patients with a small liver volume and a low ^{99m}Tc-GSA uptake in the non-embolized lobe had an increased risk of developing postoperative liver failure.

12.6 ^{99m}Tc-Mebrofenin Hepatobiliary Scintigraphy

^{99m}Tc-mebrofenin is an iminodiacetic acid (IDA) analogue which is transported to the liver predominantly bound to albumin.[23,54] Dissociation between albumin and IDA agents occurs in the hepatic space of Disse, after which it is taken up by the hepatocytes. The hepatic uptake of IDA analogues is suggested to be similar to the uptake of organic anions such as bilirubin and ICG[54] involving organic anion transporter polypeptide transporters (OATP). Similar to ICG, IDA agents are excreted into the bile canaliculi, without undergoing biotransformation during their transport through the hepatocyte, and are therefore ideal tracers for the biliary tract.[20] The suggested bile canalicular transporters include multidrug resistance proteins-2, and -3.[55] Although ^{99m}Tc-mebrofenin is not metabolized, the uptake and intracellular transit is similar to various endogenous and exogenous substances including bilirubin, hormones, drugs and several toxins, and therefore reflects an important function of the liver.

^{99m}Tc-labeled IDA analogues were first used for the diagnosis of multiple biliary diseases.[54,56,57] More recently, the application of ^{99m}Tc-labeled IDA agents have been proposed for the assessment of liver function.[58] Liver uptake of IDA agents can be affected by high plasma levels of bilirubin as mentioned previously in connection with the measurement of ICG clearance. Of all IDA analogues, ^{99m}Tc-mebrofenin shows the highest hepatic uptake, minimal urinary excretion and resists strongly the displacement by high plasma bilirubin concentration.[59,60] Therefore, ^{99m}Tc-mebrofenin is considered the most suitable agent for hepatic and biliary diagnostic procedures. ^{99m}Tc-mebrofenin uptake can be hindered by hypoalbuminemia, as albumin is the main plasma carrier of mebrofenin.[59] Conversely, hypoalbuminemia and hyperbilirubinemia in liver disease can be a sign of impaired liver function and therefore decreased uptake of ^{99m}Tc-mebrofenin in patients with hypoalbuminemia can still reflect liver function under these circumstances.

12.6.1 The Kinetics and Quantitative Measurement of Liver Function Using ^{99m}Tc-Mebrofenin Hepatobiliary Scintigraphy

Measurement of hepatic uptake function by the clearance rate of the IDA analogue Iodida was first described by Ekman et al.[61] The hepatic uptake of mebrofenin is calculated similar to Iodida. After intravenous injection of ^{99m}Tc-mebrofenin, a dynamic scintigraphy is obtained with the use of a gamma camera. The hepatic uptake of ^{99m}Tc mebrofenin is determined by drawing a ROI around the liver, the heart (serving as blood pool) and the total field of view (Fig. 12.3a). Three different time–activity curves are generated based on these ROIs (Fig. 12.3b). With these three parameters, the hepatic ^{99m}Tc-mebrofenin uptake rate (%/min) can be calculated. Radioactivity values acquired between 150 and 350 s post injection are used to ensure that the calculations are made during a phase of homogenous distribution of the agent in the blood pool, before biliary excretion takes place.[62,63] Furthermore, ROIs can be drawn around parts of the liver to calculate regional differences in the ^{99m}Tc-mebrofenin uptake rate. The regional uptake of ^{99m}Tc-mebrofenin can be assessed with small intra- and interobserver variation.[62,64] Other quantitative parameters such as the hepatic extraction fraction of mebrofenin can also be used.

Owing to technical advances, new rotating gamma cameras have been developed which enable fast 3-dimensional single photon emission computed tomography (SPECT). With ^{99m}Tc-mebrofenin SPECT, it is possible to assess liver function in a three-dimensional manner and it enables the measurement of liver functional volume. Modern SPECT cameras can be combined with a CT scan which allows the measurement of segmental liver function using the CT scan as reference

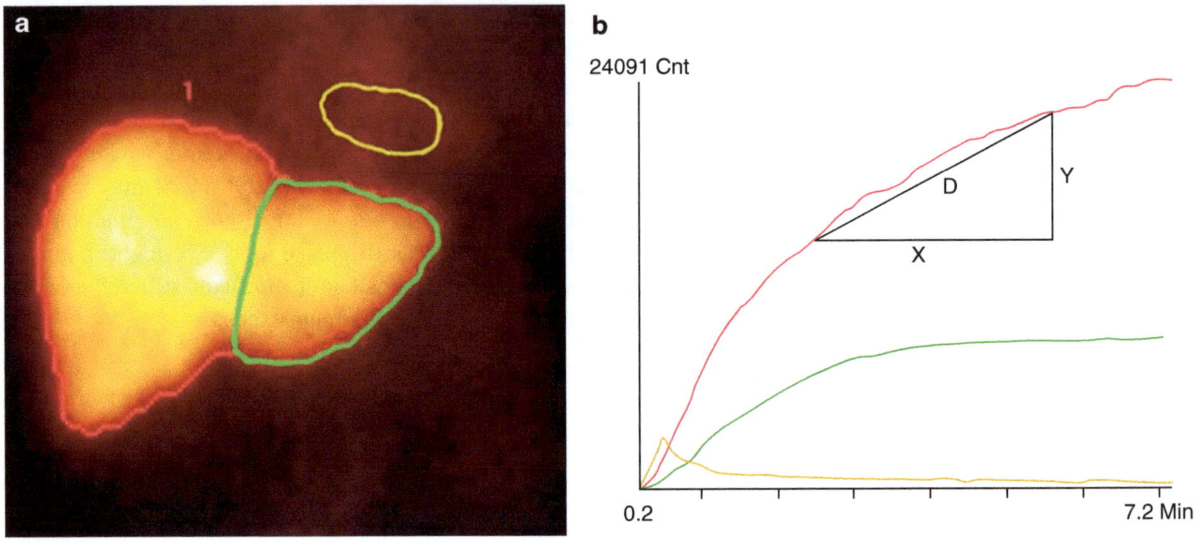

Fig. 12.3 Dynamic image of planar ^{99m}Tc-mebrofenin hepatobiliary scintigraphy (HBS). (**a**) This panel shows an example of summed HBS images from 150 to 300 s after intravenous injection of ^{99m}Tc-mebrofenin. A region of interest (ROI) is drawn around the entire liver (*red line*). A second ROI is drawn around the mediastinum (*blood pool*) (*yellow line*). A third ROI is drawn around the future remnant liver (*green line*), indicating segments two and three after extended right hemihepatectomy. (**b**) This panel shows a blood pool corrected liver-uptake time–activity curve. The liver uptake of mebrofenin is calculated as an increase of blood pool corrected ^{99m}Tc-mebrofenin uptake (*y-axis*) per minute over a time period of 200 s.

for accurate delineation of liver segments. The timing of the SPECT is a challenge when a dynamic tracer such as ^{99m}Tc-mebrofenin is used which is first taken up by the liver and subsequently excreted in the bile. The SPECT acquisition is therefore centered around the peak of the hepatic time–activity curve, since the amount of radioactivity within the liver is relatively stable during this phase. In patients with fast hepatic uptake, biliary excretion is already visible during the SPECT phase. Accumulation of radioactivity in the small bile ducts results in voxels with relatively large counts, disturbing calculation of total and regional liver function and volume. Therefore, the activity within the extrahepatic bile ducts must be masked-out. The outline extraction method is subsequently used to automatically outline the liver and calculate total functional liver volume. The FRL can be outlined manually on a low-dose CT linked to the SPECT images. The delineated FRL on contrast enhanced CT scans can be used as a constant reference. Regional distribution of liver function can be measured by dividing the counts within the FRL by the total counts within the entire liver. For calculation of the FRL function, this count ratio is multiplied by total liver ^{99m}Tc-mebrofenin uptake as measured by the dynamic hepatobiliary scintigraphy (Fig. 12.4).

12.6.2 Preoperative Assessment of Liver Function Using of ^{99m}Tc-Mebrofenin Hepatobiliairy Scintigraphy

To examine correlation of the ICG clearance test with the uptake of ^{99m}Tc-mebrofenin, both tests were sequentially performed in patients planned to undergo partial liver resection for primary or metastatic liver tumors. The ICG-C15 value and the ^{99m}Tc-mebrofenin clearance rate in blood in 15 min showed a significant, positive correlation (Fig. 12.5). A significant, positive correlation was obtained between the ^{99m}Tc-mebrofenin clearance rate at 15 min and ^{99m}Tc-mebrofenin uptake by scintigraphy. Also, the ICG-C15 value and the ^{99m}Tc-mebrofenin uptake rate, as evaluated by scintigraphy, showed a significant, positive correlation (Fig. 12.6). In addition, ^{99m}Tc-mebrofenin scintigraphy provided information on segmental functional liver tissue which is of additional use when planning liver resection.[63]

^{99m}Tc-mebrofenin scintigraphy was used to determine function of the future remnant liver preoperatively. A strong positive correlation ($r = 0.95$) was found between future remnant liver function determined preoperatively and the actually measured value 24 h after resection. Also, 3 months after the resection, there was

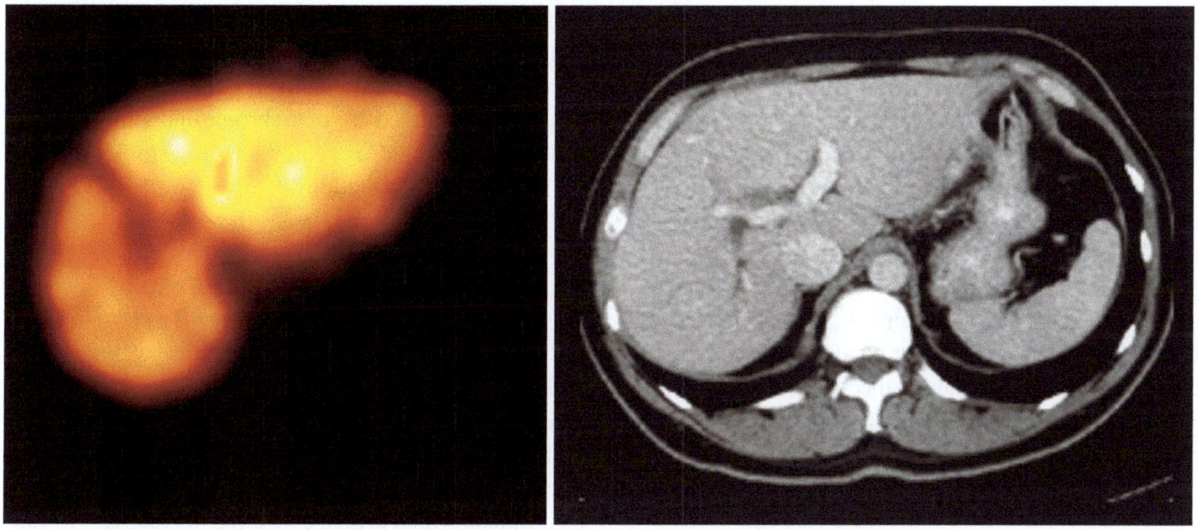

Fig. 12.4 Regional differences in liver function as shown by ^{99m}Tc-mebrofenin SPECT in a patient with colon carcinoma metastases compressing the right bile ducts at the liver hilus. Percentage of counts relative to total liver counts is higher in the FRL (left liver segments) and exceeds volume percentage of the FRL

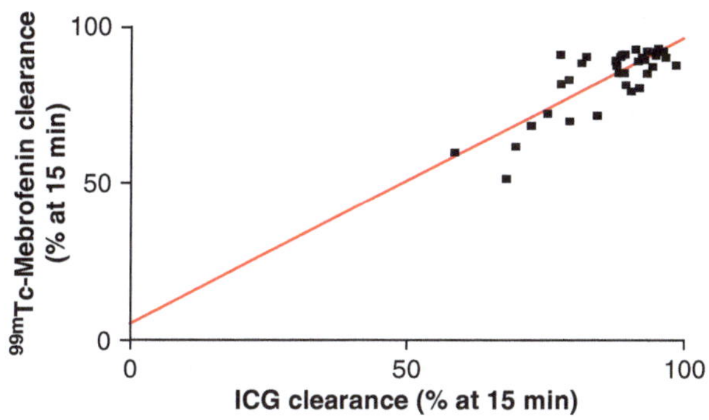

Fig. 12.5 Correlation between clearance at 15 min of ICG and ^{99m}Tc-mebrofenin (%/15 min; $r=0.81$, $P<0.0001$, $N=36$) (From Erdogan et al.[63], with permission)

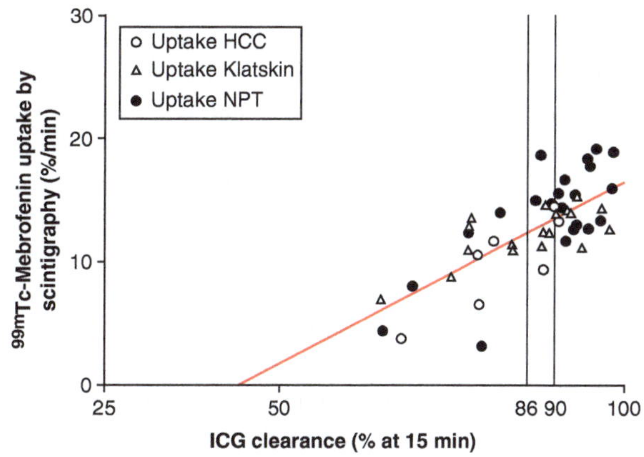

Fig. 12.6 Correlation between blood ICG clearance at 15 min and ^{99m}Tc-Mebrofenin uptake as measured by scintigraphy ($y=0{,}2925x-12{,}745$; $r=0.73$, $P<0.0001$, $N=54$) (From Erdogan et al.[63], with permission)

a strong positive correlation ($r=0.81$) between liver function assessed by ^{99m}Tc-mebrofenin scintigraphy and the ICG clearance test. However, only a weak association ($r=0.61$) was found between functional liver regeneration and liver volume increase after 3 months, which may account for some of the discrepancies between volumetric regeneration of the liver remnant and clinical outcome after liver resection.[62]

In a series including patients with parenchymal disease and hilar cholangiocarcinoma the accuracy of preoperative ^{99m}Tc-mebrofenin scintigraphy was compared with CT volumetric measurement of the future remnant liver, in predicting outcome of liver resections. Preoperative measurement of FRL ^{99m}Tc-mebrofenin uptake proved more valuable than FRL volume in post-resectional risk assessment of liver failure and liver failure related mortality.[64]

12.6.3 Increase of Liver Function After PVE

Although to date there are no published studies regarding the application of ^{99m}Tc-mebrofenin scintigraphy after PVE, it could potentially be used to evaluate the functional increase of the FRL. In addition, because of the ability to select patients with a high risk of postoperative liver failure,[64] ^{99m}Tc-mebrofenin scintigraphy could be used for the selection of candidates for PVE.

Postoperative regeneration of the remnant liver is usually evaluated by CT volumetry. As mentioned above, only a weak association between functional recovery measured with ^{99m}Tc-mebrofenin scintigraphy and ICG on the one hand, and volumetric regeneration measured by CT volumetry on the other hand, was observed. This discrepancy suggests that the mechanisms of functional recovery may be independent of those controlling volumetric regeneration.[64]

12.7 Other Tests of Liver Function

12.7.1 Bioenergetic Tests

The key determinant of liver functional status and reserve is the energy state of the organ. The availability of adenosine triphosphate (ATP) is therefore crucial for the maintenance of integrity and function of the liver cells. When the ATP generating ability of the liver cells falls short as in chronic parenchymal diseases, the energy state of the liver decreases resulting in compensatory suppression of energy consuming processes such as active anionic transport and protein and nucleic acid synthesis. The latter is important for liver cell proliferation as the key feature of liver regeneration. Assessment of the energy state of the liver, therefore, provides direct evidence of the liver functional reserve.[8] This can be estimated by measurement of ketone bodies reflecting the redox state in liver mitochondria[65] or by 31-phosphorus (^{31}P) magnetic resonance spectroscopy. The naturally abundant ^{31}P isotope is central to biologic energy transformation.[66,67]

12.7.2 Aminopyrine Breath Test

The aminopyrine breath test measures microsomal cytosolic capacity of the liver by way of cytochrome P450 dependent pathways. Aminopyrine with radioactive isotope (^{14}C) labeled methyl groups undergoes N-demethylation in liver microsomes to form aminoantipyrine and formaldehyde. The latter is converted to labeled carbon dioxide which is exhaled. Analysis of the breath allows quantitative assessment of liver function.[68] Decreased results have been associated with chronic liver disease and liver fibrosis.[69] The results may be confounded by cytochrome-inducing (phenytoin) or inhibiting drugs (omeprazole), smoking, ethanol and biliary obstruction.[3,68]

12.7.3 Galactose Elimination Test and Caffeine Clearance Test

Both the galactose elimination test and caffeine clearance test determine microsomal capacity of the liver. Caffeine is metabolized by the cytochrome P450 system. Galactose is phosphorylated in the liver to galactose-1-phosphate which is then converted to glucose. The rate of elimination which depends on the phophorylating activity of galactokinase has shown prognostic significance in chronic liver disease.[69,70] The galactose elimination capacity has been reported to decrease with age in patients with normal liver, suggesting a decline of liver functional reserve in older patients.[71] Carbon-13-caffeine is also a metabolic liver function test which has served as a prognostic indicator in patients with cirrhosis.[72]

12.7.4 MEGX Test

Lidocaine is metabolized in the liver by the cytochrome P450 pathway with the formation of monoethylglycinexylidide (MEGX) which can be measured in the blood using an immunofluorescence assay. The clearance of lidocaine is reduced in chronic liver disease with consequently, decreased generation of MEGX. Decreased MEGX levels have been correlated with increased complication rates after liver resection[73] and have been used to determine the risk of liver failure in patients with HCC undergoing transcatheter arterial chemoembolization (TACE).[74] The MEGX test has been widely used in the setting of liver transplantation, both for the evaluation of liver function in potential donors and for the prediction of survival after transplantation.[75,76]

12.8 Discussion

Accurate measurement of liver function before liver resection is crucial in the assessment of hepatic functional reserve and resectability, especially in patients who require major resection and patients with underlying parenchymal disease. Several quantitative tests have been employed for the assessment of liver functional reserve, each technique reflecting a separate component of the spectrum of liver function. Because of the complexity of liver function, one single test cannot represent overall liver function and reliably determine the safe limits of resection in any given patient undergoing major liver resection.[3]

Several clinical and quantitative liver function tests have been described in literature. The Child-Pugh classification, based on clinical symptoms of insufficient liver function (ascites/encephalopathy) and laboratory analysis of parameters of liver function (albumin, bilirubin and PT) can be used to identify high risk patients, i.e., class Child B and class Child C patients. The challenge is, however, to select in class Child A patients those who are good risk and poor risk patients.[13] In these patients, the need for reliable quantitative liver function tests is crucial.

Specific liver function tests such as the ICG clearance rate can complement the clinical Child-Pugh classification.[77] The ICG clearance rate has been reported not to unequivocally correlate with morbidity and mortality after partial liver resection. The reported studies however, vary in respect with the extent of liver resections performed and the type of patients included (i.e., patients with hepatocellular carcinoma and cirrhosis, vs. patients with normal liver parenchyma). Another drawback of the ICG clearance test is that only global liver function is measured whereas one would be particularly interested in the functional capacity of the part of the liver to be preserved during liver resection.

Nuclear imaging studies have been introduced for the quantitative testing of liver function. Potential advantages of these techniques are the possibility to provide simultaneous morphologic (visual) and physiologic (functional) information of the liver, especially when SPECT-CT cameras are used. Functional capacity may vary within the liver and with nuclear imaging studies, regional differences in hepatic function are detected. SPECT allows measurement of volume and function of specifically, the future remnant liver. In addition, when using radiopharmaceutical agents that are excreted into the bile, two dynamic phases can be examined, i.e., hepatic uptake of the agent and secretion into the biliary system.

^{99m}Tc-GSA is a receptor-targeted ligand that specifically binds to asialoglycoprotein receptors on the hepatocyte cell membrane. A good correlation was found between ^{99m}Tc-GSA, ICG clearance, and conventional liver function parameters.[78] There is a problem of availability of the radiopharmaceutical, since as yet, it is not certified in Europe and the USA and its use is mainly limited to Japan. Both preoperative ^{99m}Tc-GSA and ^{99m}Tc-mebrofenin scintigraphy have been shown to be accurate methods for preoperative assessment of liver function and prediction of postoperative complications.[37,63,64] Both examinations are especially suitable for evaluation of liver function in patients with parenchymal liver disease. Unlike ^{99m}Tc-GSA, ^{99m}Tc-mebrofenin is excreted into the bile, and therefore can be used to visualize the biliary system which may be helpful to diagnose biliary complications after liver resection.

Both ^{99m}Tc-GSA and ^{99m}Tc-mebrofenin scintigraphy have the potential to preoperatively select patients with a high risk of developing postoperative liver insufficiency and who might therefore, benefit from PVE. After PVE, hypertrophy of the non-embolized liver segments is commonly monitored by CT volumetry, showing only morphological increase of the future remnant liver. Little is, however, known about the increase of FRL function after PVE while only few methods are available to measure FRL function. Although the indocyanine green clearance test and the galactose elimination capacity (GEC) are able to measure liver function, these tests only quantify overall liver function, and are therefore not suitable to assess post-PVE increase in FRL function. Nuclear imaging studies however, provide information on augmented function of the future remnant liver. A discrepancy between volumetric hypertrophy and functional increase has been described in several studies indicating that functional gain of the future remnant liver is more rapid and of greater magnitude than the volumetric increase.[47,52] Since after PVE, the functional advantage of the remnant liver exceeds the volume increase of residual liver mass, the recommended waiting time following PVE may therefore be shorter than suggested by volumetric studies.

Many quantitative liver function tests such as the aminopyrine breath test, caffeine clearance test and MEGX test are based on measuring microsomal or cytosolic capacity of the liver. The major disadvantage of these tests is the fact that they only measure global liver function and not specifically the function of the future remnant liver. Another limitation is that all these tests are affected by numerous factors including cytochrome-inducing or -inhibiting drugs, smoking, fever and chronic disease.[68]

There is not one test that can accurately predict operative risk in patients considered for major liver resection. We still rely on the combination of clinical parameters and quantitative liver function tests to estimate liver functional reserve and to decide whether we can perform a safe resection in any patient presented to us. Clearly, scoring methods need to be developed in which clinical parameters, CT volumetric criteria and the results of dynamic quantitative liver function tests guide our decision making in patients requiring major liver resection.[79] Objective functional criteria are necessary to define patients at increased risk and select patients who are candidates for preoperative PVE.

References

1. Van den Broek MA, Olde Damink SW, Dejong CH, et al. Liver failure after partial hepatic resection: definition, pathophysiology, risk factors and treatment. *Liver Int*. 2008;28(6):767-780.
2. Vetelainen RL, van Vliet AK, Gouma DJ, van Gulik TM. Steatosis as a risk factor in liver surgery. *Ann Surg*. 2007;245(1): 20-30.
3. Mullin EJ, Metcalfe MS, Maddern GJ. How much liver resection is too much? *Am J Surg*. 2005;190(1):87-89.
4. Abdalla EK, Vauthey JN. Chemotherapy prior to hepatic resection for colorectal liver metastases: helpful until harmful? *Dig Surg*. 2008;25(6):421-429.
5. Morris-Stiff G, Gomez D, Prasad R. Quantitative assessment of hepatic function and its relevance to the liver surgeon. *J Gastrointest Surg*. 2009;13:374-385.
6. Nagasue N, Yukaya H, Ogawa Y, Kohno H, Nakamura T. Human liver regeneration after major hepatic resection. A study of normal liver and livers with chronic hepatitis and cirrhosis. *Ann Surg*. 1987;206(1):30-39.
7. Ribero D, Abdalla EK, Madoff DC, Donadon M, Loyer EM, Vauthey JN. Portal vein embolization before major hepatectomy and its effects on regeneration, resectability and outcome. *Br J Surg*. 2007;94:1386-1394.
8. Mann DV. Assessment of liver function. In: Lau J, ed. *Hepatocellular Carcinoma*. Republic of Singapore: World Scientific Publishing Co. Pte Ltd; 2008:51-83.
9. Schindl MJ, Millar AM, Redhead DN, et al. The adaptive response of the reticuloendothelial system to major liver resection in humans. *Ann Surg*. 2006;243(4):507-514.
10. Van de Kerkhove MP, Hoekstra R, Chamuleau RAFM, Van Gulik TM. Clinical application of bioartificial liver support systems. *Ann Surg*. 2004;240:216-230.
11. Demetriou AA, Brown RS Jr, Busuttil RW, et al. Prospective, randomized, multicenter, controlled trial of a bioartificial liver in treating acute liver failure. *Ann Surg*. 2004;239(5): 660-667, discussion 667-670.
12. Nanashima A, Yamaguchi H, Shibasaki S, et al. Measurement of serum hyaluronic acid level during the perioperative period of liver resection for evaluation of functional liver reserve. *J Gastroenterol Hepatol*. 2001;16(10):1158-1163.
13. Schneider PD. Preoperative assessment of liver function. *Surg Clin North Am*. 2004;84:355-373.
14. Nagashima I, Takada T, Okinaga K, et al. A scoring system for the assessment of the risk of mortality after partial hepatectomy in patients with chronic liver dysfunction. *J Hepatobiliary Pancreat Surg*. 2005;12:44-48.
15. Schroeder RA, Marroquin CE, Bute BP, Khuri S, Henderson WG, Kuo PC. Predictive indices of morbidity and mortality after liver resection. *Ann Surg*. 2006;243:373-379.
16. Paumgartner G. The handling of indocyanine green by the liver. *Schweiz Med Wochenschr*. 1975;105:1-30.
17. Okuchi O, Kaneko T, Sugimoto H, Inoue S, Takeda S, Nakao A. ICG pulse spectrophotometry for perioperative liver function in hepatectomy. *J Surg Res*. 2002;103(1):109-113.
18. Akita H, Sasaki Y, Yamada T, et al. Real-time intraoperative assessment of residual liver functional reserve using pulse dye densitrometry. *World J Surg*. 2008;32(12):2668-2674.
19. Cui Y, Konig J, Leier I, Buchholz U, Keppler D. Hepatic uptake of bilirubin and its conjugates by the human organic anion transporter SLC21A6. *J Biol Chem*. 2001;276:9626-9630.
20. Trauner M, Meier PJ, Boyer JL. Molecular pathogenesis of cholestasis. *N Engl J Med*. 1998;339:1217-1227.
21. Fan ST, Lai ECS, Lo CM, Ng IOL, Wong J. Hospital mortality of major hepatectomy for hepatocellular carcinoma associated with cirrhosis. *Arch Surg*. 1995;130:198-203.
22. Watanabe Y, Kumon K. Assessment by pulse dye-densitometry indocyanine green (ICG) clearance test of hepatic function of patients before cardiac surgery: its value as a predictor of serious postoperative liver dysfunction. *J Cardiothorac Vasc Anesth*. 1999;13:299-303.
23. Lau H, Man K, Fan ST, et al. Evaluation of preoperative hepatic function in patients with hepatocellular carcinoma undergoing hepatectomy. *Br J Surg*. 1997;84:1255-1259.
24. Lam CM, Fan ST, Lo CM, Wong J. Major hepatectomy for hepatocellular carcinoma in patients with an unsatisfactory indocyanine green clearance test. *Br J Surg*. 1999;86: 1012-1017.
25. Kwon AH, Ha-Kawa SK, Uetsuji S, Inoue T, Matsui Y, Kamiyama Y. Preoperative determination of the surgical procedure for hepatectomy using technetium-99 m-galactosyl human serum albumin (99mTc-GSA) liver scintigraphy. *Hepatology*. 1997;25:426-429.
26. Uesaka N, Nimura Y, Nagino M. Changes in hepatic lobar function after right portal vein embolization: an appraisal by biliary indocyanine green excretion. *Ann Surg*. 1996;223: 77-83.
27. Chijiiwa K, Watanabe M, Nakano K, Noshiro H, Tanaka M. Biliary indocyanine green excretion as a predictor of hepatic adenosine triphosphate levels in patients with obstructive jaundice. *Am J Surg*. 2000;179:161-166.
28. Van Gulik TM, Van den Esschert JW, De Graaf W, et al. Controversies in the use of portal vein embolization (PVE). *Dig Surg*. 2008;25(6):436-444.
29. Wakabayashi H, Okada S, Maeba T, Maeta H. Effect of preoperative portal vein embolization on major hepatectomy for advanced-stage hepatocellular carcinomas in injured livers: a preliminary report. *Surg Today*. 1997;27: 403-410.
30. De Graaf W, van den Esschert JW, van Lienden KP, van Gulik TM. Induction of tumor growth after preoperative

portal vein embolization; is it a real problem? *Ann Surg Oncol*. 2009;16:423-430.
31. Akaki S, Mitsumori A, Kanazawa S, et al. Technetium-99 m-DTPA-galactosyl human serum albumin liver scintigraphy evaluation of regional CT/MRI attenuation/signal intensity differences. *J Nucl Med*. 1998;39:529-532.
32. Sawamura T, Kawasato S, Shiozaki Y, et al. Decrease of a hepatic binding protein specific for asialoglycoproteins with accumulation of serum asialoglycoproteins in galactosamine-treated rats. *Gastroenterology*. 1981;81:527-533.
33. Vera DR, Krohn KA, Stadalnik RC, et al. Tc-99 m-galactosyl-neoglycoalbumin: in vivo characterization of receptor-mediated binding to hepatocytes. *Radiology*. 1984;151:191-196.
34. Kokudo N, Vera DR, Makuuchi M. Clinical application of TcGSA. *Nucl Med Biol*. 2003;30:845-849.
35. Sasaki N, Shiomi S, Iwata Y, et al. Clinical usefulness of scintigraphy with 99mTc-galactosyl-human serum albumin for prognosis of cirrhosis of the liver. *J Nucl Med*. 1999;40:1652-1656.
36. Kwon AH, Ha-Kawa SK, Uetsuji S, et al. Use of technetium 99 m diethylenetriamine-pentaacetic acid-galactosyl-human serum albumin liver scintigraphy in the evaluation of preoperative and postoperative hepatic functional reserve for hepatectomy. *Surgery*. 1995;117:429-434.
37. Nanashima A, Yamaguchi H, Shibasaki S, et al. Relationship between indocyanine green test and technetium-99 m galactosyl serum albumin scintigraphy in patients scheduled for hepatectomy: clinical evaluation and patient outcome. *Hepatol Res*. 2004;28:184-190.
38. Mimura T, Hamazaki K, Sakai H, et al. Evaluation of hepatic functional reserve in rats with obstructive jaundice by asyaloglycoprotein receptor. *Hepatogastroenterology*. 2001;48:777-782.
39. Tanaka A, Shinohara H, Hatano E, et al. Perioperative changes in hepatic function as assessed by asialoglycoprotein receptor indices by technetium 99 m galactosyl human serum albumin. *Hepatogastroenterology*. 1999;46:369-375.
40. Mitsumori A, Nagaya I, Kimoto S, et al. Preoperative evaluation of hepatic functional reserve following hepatectomy by technetium-99 m galactosyl human serum albumin liver scintigraphy and computed tomography. *Eur J Nucl Med*. 1998;25:1377-1382.
41. Kwon AH, Matsui Y, Ha-Kawa SK, et al. Functional hepatic volume measured by technetium-99 m-galactosyl-human serum albumin liver scintigraphy: comparison between hepatocyte volume and liver volume by computed tomography. *Am J Gastroenterol*. 2001;96:541-546.
42. Kim YK, Nakano H, Yamaguchi M, et al. Prediction of postoperative decompensated liver function by technetium-99 m galactosyl-human serum albumin liver scintigraphy in patients with hepatocellular carcinoma complicating chronic liver disease. *Br J Surg*. 1997;84:793-796.
43. Takeuchi S, Nakano H, Kim YK, et al. Predicting survival and post-operative complications with Tc-GSA liver scintigraphy in hepatocellular carcinoma. *Hepatogastroenterology*. 1999;46:1855-1861.
44. Kokudo N, Vera DR, Tada K, et al. Predictors of successful hepatic resection: prognostic usefulness of hepatic asialoglycoprotein receptor analysis. *World J Surg*. 2002;26:1342-1347.
45. Satoh K, Yamamoto Y, Nishiyama Y, et al. 99mTc-GSA liver dynamic SPECT for the preoperative assessment of hepatectomy. *Ann Nucl Med*. 2003;17:61-67.
46. Akaki S, Okumura Y, Sasai N, et al. Hepatectomy simulation discrepancy between radionuclide receptor imaging and CT volumetry: influence of decreased unilateral portal venous flow. *Ann Nucl Med*. 2003;17:23-29.
47. Hirai I, Kimura W, Fuse A, et al. Evaluation of preoperative portal embolization for safe hepatectomy, with special reference to assessment of nonembolized lobe function with 99mTc-GSA SPECT scintigraphy. *Surgery*. 2003;133:495-506.
48. Kwon AH, Matsui Y, Kaibori M, et al. Functional hepatic regeneration following hepatectomy using galactosyl-human serum albumin liver scintigraphy. *Transplant Proc*. 2004;36:2257-2260.
49. Hwang EH, Taki J, Shuke N, et al. Preoperative assessment of residual hepatic functional reserve using ^{99m}Tc-DTPA-Galacttosyl-human serum albumin dynamic SPECT. *J Nucl Med*. 1999;40(10):1644-1651.
50. Sugai Y, Komatani A, Hosoya T, et al. Response to percutaneous transhepatic portal embolization: new proposed parameters by 99mTc-GSA SPECT and their usefulness in prognostic estimation after hepatectomy. *J Nucl Med*. 2000;41:421-425.
51. Kubo S, Shiomi S, Tanaka H, et al. Evaluation of the effect of portal vein embolization on liver function by (99 m)tc-galactosyl human serum albumin scintigraphy. *J Surg Res*. 2002;107:113-118.
52. Nishiyama Y, Yamamoto Y, Hino I, et al. 99mTc galactosyl human serum albumin liver dynamic SPET for pre-operative assessment of hepatectomy in relation to percutaneous transhepatic portal embolization. *Nucl Med Commun*. 2003;24:809-817.
53. Nanashima A, Yamaguchi H, Shibasaki S, et al. Relationship between CT volumetry and functional liver volume using technetium-99 m galactosyl serum albumin scintigraphy in patients undergoing preoperative portal vein embolization before major hepatectomy: a preliminary study. *Dig Dis Sci*. 2006;51:1190-1195.
54. Krishnamurthy S, Krishnamurthy GT. Technetium-99 m-iminodiacetic acid organic anions: review of biokinetics and clinical application in hepatology. *Hepatology*. 1989;9:139-153.
55. Hendrikse NH, Kuipers F, Meijer C, et al. In vivo imaging of hepatobiliary transport function mediated by multidrug resistance associated protein and P-glycoprotein. *Cancer Chemother Pharmacol*. 2004;54:131-138.
56. Krishnamurthy S, Krishnamurthy GT, Lieberman D, et al. Scintigraphic criteria for the diagnosis of obstructive hepatobiliary diseases with Tc-99 m IDA. *Clin Nucl Med*. 1988;13:704-709.
57. Krishnamurthy GT, Lieberman DA, Brar HS. Detection, localization and quantitation of degree of common bile duct obstruction by scintigraphy. *J Nucl Med*. 1985;26:726-735.
58. Heyman S. Hepatobiliary scintigraphy as a liver function test. *J Nucl Med*. 1994;35:436-437.
59. Krishnamurthy GT, Krishnamurthy S. *Nuclear Hepatology: A Textbook of Hepatobiliary Diseases*. Berlin/Heidelberg/New York: Springer; 2000.
60. Lan JA, Chervu LR, Johansen KL, et al. Uptake of technetium 99 m hepatobiliary imaging agents by cultured rat hepatocytes. *Gastroenterology*. 1988;95:1625-1631.
61. Ekman M, Fjalling M, Holmberg S, et al. IODIDA clearance rate: a method for measuring hepatocyte uptake function. *Transplant Proc*. 1992;24:387-388.

62. Bennink RJ, Dinant S, Erdogan D, et al. Preoperative assessment of postoperative remnant liver function using hepatobiliary scintigraphy. *J Nucl Med*. 2004;45:965-971.
63. Erdogan D, Heijnen BHM, Bennink RJ, et al. Preoperative assessment of liver function: a comparison of 99mTc-Mebrofenin scintigraphy with indocyanine green clearance test. *Liver Int*. 2004;24:117-123.
64. Dinant S, de Graaf W, Verwer BJ, et al. Risk assessment of posthepatectomy liver failure using hepatobiliary scintigraphy and CT volumetry. *J Nucl Med*. 2007;48(5): 685-692.
65. Mori K, Ozawa K, Yamamoto Y, et al. Response of hepatic mitochondrial redox state to oral glucose load. Redox tolerance test as a new predictor of surgical risk in hepatectomy. *Ann Surg*. 1990;211(4):438-446.
66. Mann DV, Lam WW, Hjelm NM, et al. Metabolic control patterns in acute phase and regenerating human liver determined in vivo by 31-phosphorus magnetic resonance spectroscopy. *Ann Surg*. 2002;235(3):408-416.
67. Mann DV, Lam WW, Hjelm NM, et al. Human liver regeneration: hepatic energy economy is less efficient when the organ is diseased. *Hepatology*. 2001;34(3):557-565.
68. Armuzzi A, Candelli M, Zocco MA, et al. Review article: breath testing for human liver function assessment. *Aliment Pharmacol Ther*. 2002;16(12):1977-1996.
69. Herold C, Heinz R, Niedobitek G, Schneider T, Hahn EG, Schuppan D. Quantitative testing of liver function in relation to fibrosis in patients with chronic hepatitis B and C. *Liver*. 2001;21(4):260-265.
70. Redaelli CA, Dufour JF, Wagner M, et al. Preoperative galactose elimination capacity predicts complications and survival after hepatic resection. *Ann Surg*. 2002;235(1):77-85.
71. Marchesini G, Bua V, Brunori A, et al. Galactose elimination capacity and liver volume in aging man. *Hepatology*. 1988; 8(5):1079-1083.
72. Jover R, Carnicer F, Sanchez-Paya J, et al. Salivary caffeine clearance predicts survival in patients with liver cirrhosis. *Am J Gastroenterol*. 1997;92:1905-1908.
73. Ercolani G, Grazi GL, Callivà R, et al. The lidocaine (MEGX) test as an index of hepatic function: its clinical usefulness in liver surgery. *Surgery*. 2000;127(4):464-471.
74. Huang YS, Chiang J, Wu J, Chang F, Lee S. Risk of hepatic failure after transcatheter arterial chemoembolization for hepatocellular carcinoma: predictive value of the monoethylglycinexylidide test. *Am J Gastroenterol*. 2002;97:1223-1227.
75. Oellerich M, Armstrong VW. The MEGX test: a tool for the real-time assessment of hepatic function. *Ther Drug Monit*. 2001;23:81-92.
76. Oellerich M, Burdelski M, Ringe B, et al. Functional state of the donor liver and early outcome of transplantation. *Transplant Proc*. 1991;23:1575-1578.
77. Nonami T, Nakao A, Kurokawa T, et al. Blood loss and ICG clearance as best prognostic markers of post-hepatectomy liver failure. *Hepatogastroenterology*. 1999;46:1669-1672.
78. Onodera Y, Takahashi K, Togashi T, Sugai Y, Tamaki N, Miyasaka K. Clinical assessment of hepatic functional reserve using 99mTc DTPA galactosyl human serum albumin SPECT to prognosticate chronic hepatic diseases–validation of the use of SPECT and a new indicator. *Ann Nucl Med*. 2003;17:181-188.
79. Torzilli G, Makuuchi M, Inoue K, et al. No-mortality liver resection for hepatocellular carcinoma in cirrhotic and noncirrhotic patients: is there a way? A prospective analysis of our approach. *Arch Surg*. 1999;134(9):984-992.

Part III

Embolization Techniques

13 Indications and Contraindications for Portal Vein Embolization

David C. Madoff and Jean-Nicolas Vauthey

Abstract

Multiple factors are considered when determining whether or not a particular patient will benefit from portal vein embolization (PVE). First, an evaluation for underlying liver disease must be made to ascertain the necessary future liver remnant (sFLR) volume following resection – those patients with an otherwise healthy liver will not require as large an FLR mass as those with cirrhosis. Next, the patient's body size must be taken into account. Then, the planned surgical intervention must be considered (i.e., the size and complexity of the surgical resection as well as the possibility of any other nonhepatic surgery to be performed concomitantly). These three factors are considered in the setting of the patient's age and comorbidities (e.g., diabetes mellitus) that may affect hypertrophy and ultimately, the perioperative outcome. Thus, after all of these factors have been evaluated and the patient remains a surgical candidate, appropriate liver CT volumetry is performed so that the standardized FLR volume expressed as a percentage of the estimated total liver volume (TLV) can be used to determine the need for PVE. In addition, contraindications with regards to the use of PVE are also discussed.

Keywords

Chemotherapy before portal vein embolization • Future liver remnant volume • Indications and contraindications for portal vein embolization • Portal vein embolization

Multiple factors are considered when determining whether or not a particular patient will benefit from portal vein embolization (PVE).[1] First, an evaluation for underlying liver disease must be made to ascertain the necessary future liver remnant (sFLR) volume following resection – those patients with an otherwise healthy liver will not require as large an FLR mass as those with cirrhosis. Next, the patient's body size must be taken into account. Larger patients will inevitably require larger FLRs than smaller patients under otherwise similar circumstances. Then, the planned surgical intervention must be considered (i.e., the size and complexity of the surgical resection as well as the possibility of any other nonhepatic surgery to be performed concomitantly). These three factors are considered in

D.C. Madoff (✉)
Division of Interventional Radiology, Department of Radiology, New York-Presbyterian Hospital/Weill Cornell Medical Center, 525 E 68th Street, P-518, New York, NY 10065, USA
e-mail: dcm9006@med.cornell.edu

D.C. Madoff et al. (eds.), *Venous Embolization of the Liver*,
DOI 10.1007/978-1-84882-122-4_13,

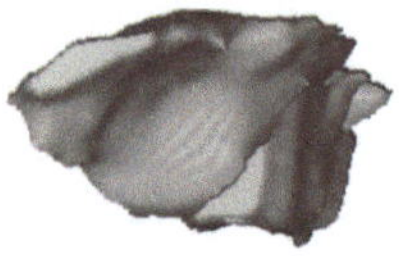

Segments I + II + III = 233 cm^3

$$\frac{\text{Measured FLR volume}}{\text{TLV (calculated*)}} = \frac{233}{1{,}853} = 13\% \text{ of TLV}$$

PVE indicated

*TLV = −794 + 1,267 x BSA

Fig. 13.1 An example of standardized future liver remnant (sFLR) calculation using the formula based on body surface area to estimate total liver volume. *FLR* future liver remnant, *TLV* total liver volume, *BSA* body surface area

the setting of the patient's age and comorbidities (e.g., diabetes mellitus) that may affect hypertrophy and ultimately, the perioperative outcome. Thus, after all of these factors have been evaluated and the patient remains a surgical candidate, appropriate liver CT volumetry is performed so that the standardized FLR volume expressed as a percentage of the estimated total liver volume (TLV) can be used to determine the need for PVE (Fig. 13.1).

As mentioned previously, a "healthy" liver has a greater regenerative capability than a cirrhotic liver, tolerates injury better, and functions more efficiently. Patients with normal liver can survive resection of up to 90% of the liver, but in cirrhotic patients, survival after resection beyond 60% of the functional parenchyma is unlikely.[2] Therefore, chronic liver disease often limits the amount of liver parenchyma that can be resected due to diminished functional reserve. Further, complications of the poorly functioning remnant liver and fatal postoperative liver failure occur with greater frequency in patients with cirrhosis, and the relatively poor synthetic function of such diseased liver can lead to fluid retention, ascites, and wound breakdown more often than with normal liver.

With regards to liver volume specifically, there is a limit to how small a liver can remain after resection. If too little liver remains after resection, immediate postresection hepatic failure leads to multisystem organ failure and death. If a marginal volume of liver remains, cirrhotic or not, the lack of reserve often leads to a cascade of complications, prolonged hospital and intensive-care unit stays, and slow recovery or slowly progressive liver failure over weeks to months with eventual death.[3-5] Therefore, the usefulness of PVE with regards to patients with normal liver, those who have steatosis or have undergone high-dose chemotherapy, and those with advanced fibrosis or cirrhosis will be reviewed. In addition, contraindications with regards to the use of PVE will also be discussed.

13.1 Normal Liver

In patients with normal liver, the indications for PVE have evolved with the greater accuracy of liver CT volumetric measurements and the use of standardized liver volumes. Although extensive resections are now achieved with a very low risk of death from liver failure, small-for-patient-size normal liver remnants are still associated with an increased number of complications and slower postoperative recovery.[3] An sFLR of more than 20% is associated with a fourfold reduction in complications, compared with an sFLR of 20% or less.[2] This finding was corroborated in a retrospective series that revealed that residual liver volume, not resected volume, more accurately predicts postoperative course.[6]

Despite the studies that demonstrate the 20%-sFLR cut off for safe resection and the potential utilization of PVE in this patient population,[2,7] there remains considerable debate regarding how small a liver remnant can remain in situ without developing unacceptable perioperative complications. Many physicians still use 30% as a cutoff for safe resection,[8] and therefore, many patients that may be considered resectable at one institution may be considered unresectable at another. Recently, a study from M. D. Anderson Cancer Center assessed the development of hepatic insufficiency and death from liver failure after 301 consecutive extended right hepatectomies based on CT volumetric data and the utilization of PVE (Fig. 13.2).[9] The authors again found that there was a statistically significant difference in the outcomes in patients that had less than 20% sFLR when compared to those that had more than 20% sFLR. However, they also found that there was no difference in patients that had more than 20% sFLR as compared to those who had more than 30% sFLR. Therefore, patients who have a normal underlying liver – requiring an extended right hepatectomy for cure but have more than the necessary 20% sFLR – do not benefit greatly from the addition of PVE. The authors, however, recommend using these data as a guideline as each patient must be assessed individually for the need for resection whether or not PVE is to be performed.

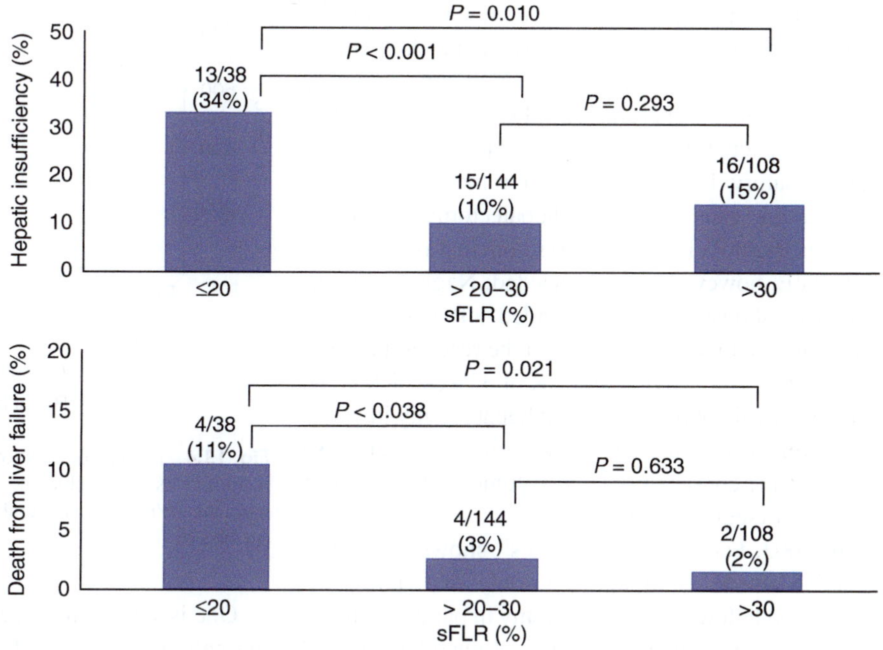

Fig. 13.2 Incidence of hepatic insufficiency and death from liver failure based on standardized future liver remnant (sFLR) in 301 patients who underwent extended right hepatectomy (From Kishi et al.[9], with permission)

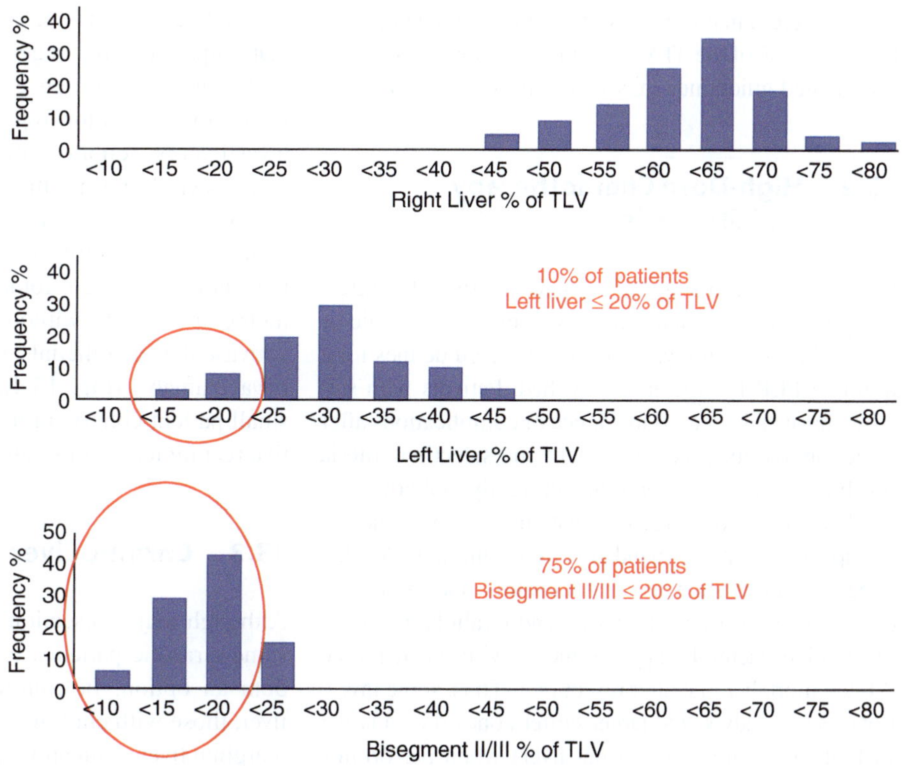

Fig. 13.3 Anatomical variation in the intrahepatic volumes. *TLV* total liver volume (From Abdalla et al.[10], with permission)

Also critical to the discussion of performing PVE in the setting of normal liver is the recognition that there is considerable intrahepatic segmental variability (Fig. 13.3). Therefore, the volumes of liver must be systematically evaluated for each patient so as to avoid overutilization of PVE. Liver CT volumetric analysis revealed that the lateral left liver (segments 2 and 3) contributes less than 20% of the TLV in more than

75% of patients, in the absence of compensatory hypertrophy. In contrast, the left liver (segments 2, 3, and 4) contributes less than 20% of the TLV in approximately 10% of patients.[10] Therefore, an sFLR of less than 20% can be expected in most patients who do not develop compensatory hypertrophy from tumor growth and require an extended right hepatectomy. In these patients, right PVE extended to segment 4 is indicated. Left PVE, however, is rarely needed; Nagino and colleagues[11] showed that an extended left hepatectomy with caudate lobectomy results in the resection of only 67% of the liver, leaving an FLR of 33%, which is the same residual volume after right hepatectomy in a normal liver. Volumetric analysis of normal livers also confirms the consistently large volume of the posterior right liver (segments 6 and 7).[12]

In 2003, Farges and colleagues[13] showed in a prospective albeit nonrandomized study that right PVE performed before right hepatectomy in patients with an otherwise normal liver showed no clinical benefit, and they concluded that in this setting, PVE may be unnecessary (except in the small subset of patients whose left liver is <20% of the TLV). Failure to follow these well-established guidelines may result in overuse of PVE.

13.2 High-Dose Chemotherapy and Steatosis

Retrospective data suggest an increased risk of surgical complications in patients after preoperative systemic or regional chemotherapy,[14] but no definite guidelines for a minimal FLR have been established. Patients with steatosis have an increased incidence of complications after resection, but the potential benefit and selection criteria for PVE in these patients are currently unknown.[15,16] Furthermore, knowledge of a patient's specific chemotherapeutic regimen is mandatory as patients may develop hepatic injuries such as steatohepatitis and sinusoidal dilatation from irinotecan-based and oxaliplatin fluoropyrimidine chemotherapy regimens, with an increased 90-day mortality rate after resection.[17] Thus, some investigators have advocated larger buffer zones (i.e., a larger FLR than required for normal liver) when performing extended resection in selected patients who have received prolonged (>4 months) preoperative chemotherapy. Although such patients have been less well studied than patients with normal liver, PVE may be indicated when the FLR is ≤30% of the TLV.[18,19]

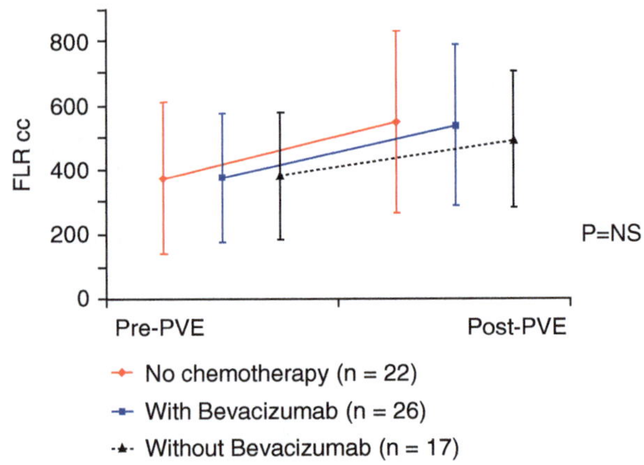

Fig. 13.4 The use of chemotherapy prior to portal vein embolization does not preclude hepatic regeneration. *FLR* future liver remnant, *PVE* portal vein embolization (From Zorzi et al.[24], with permission)

One issue that has been raised is whether maintaining patients on chemotherapy will have an impact on hepatic hypertrophy, especially in the setting of colorectal liver metastases. Some investigators do suggest that impaired liver regeneration occurs after portal occlusion in the presence of chemotherapy but with a trend toward tumor regression.[20,21] However, other investigators reported that systemic chemotherapy administered during the period between PVE and resection does not affect FLR hypertrophy or outcome.[22,23] In addition, no differences in regeneration rates after PVE were found in patients receiving chemotherapy with or without prior administration of the antivascular endothelial growth factor agents such as bevacizumab[24] (Fig. 13.4). Unfortunately, due to the small patient cohorts in the various studies, no definitive recommendations can be made.

13.3 Chronic Liver Disease

Although major resection can be performed safely in some cirrhotic patients, extended hepatectomy is seldom an option. In contrast to patients with normal liver, those with chronic liver disease or cirrhosis with marginal liver remnant volumes are at a greater risk for both postoperative complications and death from liver failure.[4] However, in carefully selected patients with cirrhosis with preserved liver function (Child's Class A and ICGR15 <10%), major hepatectomy can be performed safely, and PVE is indicated when the sFLR is

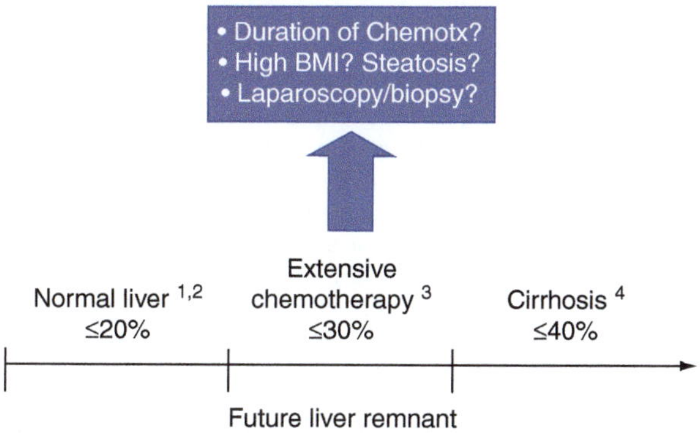

Fig. 13.5 Indications for preoperative portal vein embolization. *Chemotx* chemotherapy, *BMI* body mass index

less than 40%[25] (Fig. 13.5). This guideline is supported by the finding that when liver volume is standardized to BSA, sFLR volume predicts death from liver failure after hepatectomy in chronic liver disease.[4]

These studies were validated by the only prospective study that assessed the use of PVE prior to right hepatectomy.[13] This study showed that patients with chronic liver disease who underwent PVE before right hepatectomy had fewer complications and shorter intensive care unit and hospital stays than those with chronic liver disease who did not have PVE before right hepatectomy. This guideline has been expanded to include patients in whom the liver is compromised by prolonged biliary obstruction who need extended hepatectomy.[5,26-28]

Highly selected patients with advanced liver disease might be able to undergo safe resection. Specifically, in patients with cirrhosis with a moderately abnormal ICGR15 (10–20%) but with preserved liver function, sequential chemoembolization and PVE have been advocated.[29] Recent studies have shown that this strategy leads to increased atrophy of the embolized liver and greater hypertrophy of the FLR than PVE alone.[30]

At M. D. Anderson Cancer Center, portal pressures are routinely measured before and after PVE because of the lack of reliability of assessment of hepatic fibrosis by core needle biopsy.[31] Patients with overt portal hypertension (splenomegaly, low platelets, imaging evidence of varices) are not candidates for major hepatectomy and therefore are not candidates for PVE. Mild portal hypertension, however, is not a contraindication to PVE followed by hepatectomy provided liver function test results are otherwise normal (Child-Pugh A). However, because "liver disease" is a continuum, the specific indications for PVE in patients with chronic liver disease remain to be precisely defined and will require an individualized approach. However, it is anticipated that refined criteria will be developed with the accumulation of additional experience with the standardized measurement of FLR.

13.4 Contraindications

There are only two absolute contraindications to PVE: established portal hypertension and extensive tumor thrombus of the ipsilateral portal vein (as portal flow is already diverted and may preclude safe catheter manipulation and optimal delivery of embolic material).[1,32] For patients with established portal hypertension, major hepatectomy is usually not feasible and PVE therefore should not be performed. However, mild portal hypertension and advanced fibrosis are not absolute contraindications but relative ones, as long as the patient has otherwise normal liver function tests. Despite reports that suggest limited hypertrophy in patients with cirrhosis and advanced fibrosis, investigators have shown significant hypertrophy after PVE in this setting.[33] Patients with portal hypertension may have considerable hepatofugal flow such that distal embolization of the material used for PVE will not occur and may, in fact, result in nontarget embolization.[1] In addition, PVE in the setting of portal hypertension has resulted in the development of bleeding esophageal varices.[34]

Relative contraindications to PVE include tumor extension to the FLR (PVE may still be performed if part of aggressive therapy involving multistage hepatectomy or thermal ablation of the lesions within the FLR), biliary dilatation in the FLR (if the biliary tree is obstructed, drainage prior to PVE is recommended), mild portal hypertension, uncorrectable coagulopathy, and renal insufficiency. Rarely, the presence of a large tumor may preclude safe transhepatic ipsilateral access, and the contralateral approach is used.

References

1. Madoff DC, Abdalla EK, Vauthey JN. Portal vein embolization in preparation for major hepatic resection: evolution of a new standard of care. *J Vasc Interv Radiol*. 2005;16: 779-790.
2. Abdalla EK, Barnett CC, Doherty D, Curley SA, Vauthey JN. Extended hepatectomy in patients with hepatobiliary malignancies with and without preoperative portal vein embolization. *Arch Surg*. 2002;137:675-680.

3. Tsao JI, Loftus JP, Nagorney DM, Adson MA, Ilstrup DM. Trends in morbidity and mortality of hepatic resection for malignancy: matched comparative analysis. *Ann Surg*. 1994; 220:199-205.
4. Shirabe K, Shimada M, Gion T, et al. Postoperative liver failure after major hepatic resection for hepatocellular carcinoma in the modern era with special reference to remnant liver volume. *J Am Coll Surg*. 1999;188:304-309.
5. Vauthey JN, Chaoui A, Do KA, et al. Standardized measurement of the future liver remnant prior to extended liver resection: methodology and clinical associations. *Surgery*. 2000;127:512-519.
6. Shoup M, Gonen M, D'Angelica M, et al. Volumetric analysis predicts hepatic dysfunction in patients undergoing major liver resection. *J Gastrointest Surg*. 2003;7:325-330.
7. Vauthey JN, Pawlik TM, Abdalla EK, et al. Is extended hepatectomy for hepatobiliary malignancy justified? *Ann Surg*. 2004;239:722-730.
8. Clavien PA, Petrowsky H, DeOliveira ML, Graf R. Strategies for safer liver surgery and partial liver transplantation. *N Engl J Med*. 2007;356:1545-1559.
9. Kishi Y, Abdalla EK, Chun YS, et al. Three hundred and one consecutive extended right hepatectomies: evaluation of outcome based on systematic liver volumetry. *Ann Surg*. 2009;250:540-548.
10. Abdalla EK, Denys A, Chevalier P, Nemr RA, Vauthey JN. Total and segmental liver volume variations: implications for liver surgery. *Surgery*. 2004;135:404-410.
11. Nagino M, Nimura Y, Kamiya J, et al. Right or left trisegment portal vein embolization before hepatic trisegmentectomy for hilar bile duct carcinoma. *Surgery*. 1995;117:677-681.
12. Leelaudomlipi S, Sugawara Y, Kaneko J, Matsui Y, Ohkubo T, Makuuchi M. Volumetric analysis of liver segments in 155 living donors. *Liver Transpl*. 2002;8:612-614.
13. Farges O, Belghiti J, Kianmanesh R, et al. Portal vein embolization before right hepatectomy: prospective clinical trial. *Ann Surg*. 2003;237:208-217.
14. Elias D, Lasser P, Spielmann M, et al. Surgical and chemotherapeutic treatment of hepatic metastases from carcinoma of the breast. *Surg Gynecol Obstet*. 1991;172:461-464.
15. Kooby DA, Fong Y, Suriawinata A, et al. Impact of steatosis on perioperative outcome following hepatic resection. *J Gastrointest Surg*. 2003;7:1034-1044.
16. McCormack L, Petrowsky H, Jochum W, et al. Hepatic steatosis is a risk factor for postoperative complications after major hepatectomy: a matched case-control study. *Ann Surg*. 2007;245:923-930.
17. Vauthey JN, Pawlik TM, Ribero D, et al. Chemotherapy regimen predicts steatohepatitis and an increase in 90-day mortality after surgery for hepatic colorectal metastases. *J Clin Oncol*. 2006;24:2065-2072.
18. Azoulay D, Castaing D, Krissat J, et al. Percutaneous portal vein embolization increases the feasibility and safety of major liver resection for hepatocellular carcinoma in injured liver. *Ann Surg*. 2000;232:665-672.
19. Adam R, Delvart V, Pascal G, et al. Rescue surgery for unresectable colorectal liver metastases downstaged by chemotherapy: a model to predict long-term survival. *Ann Surg*. 2004;240:644-657.
20. Beal IK, Anthony S, Papadopoulou A, et al. Portal vein embolisation prior to hepatic resection for colorectal liver metastases and the effects of periprocedure chemotherapy. *Br J Radiol*. 2006;79:473-478.
21. Sturesson C, Kuessen I, Tranberg KG. Prolonged chemotherapy impairs liver regeneration after portal vein occlusion – an audit of 26 patients. *Eur J Surg Oncol*. 2010;36:358-364.
22. Goere D, Farges O, Leporrier J, Sauvanet A, Vilgrain V, Belghiti J. Chemotherapy does not impair hypertrophy of the left liver after right portal vein obstruction. *J Gastrointest Surg*. 2006;10:365-370.
23. Covey AM, Brown KT, Jarnagin WR, et al. Combined portal vein embolization and neoadjuvant chemotherapy as a treatment strategy for resectable hepatic colorectal metastases. *Ann Surg*. 2008;247:451-455.
24. Zorzi D, Chun YS, Madoff DC, et al. Chemotherapy with bevacizumab does not affect liver regeneration after portal vein embolization in the treatment of colorectal liver metastases. *Ann Surg Oncol*. 2008;15:2765-2772.
25. Kubota K, Makuuchi M, Kusaka K, et al. Measurement of liver volume and hepatic functional reserve as a guide to decision-making in resectional surgery for hepatic tumors. *Hepatology*. 1997;26:1176-1181.
26. Abdalla EK, Hicks ME, Vauthey JN. Portal vein embolization: rationale, technique and future prospects. *Br J Surg*. 2001;88:165-175.
27. Makuuchi M, Thai BL, Takayasu K, et al. Preoperative portal vein embolization to increase safety of major hepatectomy for hilar bile duct carcinoma: a preliminary report. *Surgery*. 1990;107:521-527.
28. Nagino M, Nimura Y, Kamiya J, et al. Changes in hepatic lobe volume in biliary tract cancer patients after right portal vein embolization. *Hepatology*. 1995;21:434-439.
29. Aoki T, Imamura H, Hasegawa K, et al. Sequential preoperative arterial and portal venous embolizations in patients with hepatocellular carcinoma. *Arch Surg*. 2004;139:766-774.
30. Ogata S, Belghiti J, Farges O, Varma D, Sibert A, Vilgrain V. Sequential arterial and portal vein embolizations before right hepatectomy in patients with cirrhosis and hepatocellular carcinoma. *Br J Surg*. 2006;93:1091-1098.
31. Bedossa P, Dargere D, Paradis V. Sampling variability of liver fibrosis in chronic hepatitis C. *Hepatology*. 2003;38: 1449-1457.
32. Madoff DC, Hicks ME, Vauthey JN, et al. Transhepatic portal vein embolization: anatomy, indications, and technical considerations. *Radiographics*. 2002;22:1063-1076.
33. Denys A, Lacombe C, Schneider F, et al. Portal vein embolization with *N*-butyl cyanoacrylate before partial hepatectomy in patients with hepatocellular carcinoma and underlying cirrhosis or advanced fibrosis. *J Vasc Interv Radiol*. 2005; 16:1667-1674.
34. Ribero D, Abdalla EK, Madoff DC, Donadon M, Loyer EM, Vauthey JN. Portal vein embolization before major hepatectomy and its effects on regeneration, resectability and outcome. *Br J Surg*. 2007;94:1386-1394.

Embolic Materials Used for Portal Vein Embolization

14

Raymond H. Thornton, Anne M. Covey, and David C. Madoff

Abstract

The gamut of embolic materials has been used for portal venous embolization. Local preferences appear to dictate the choice of embolic material, as there are no clear data supporting a superior choice among absolute ethanol, cyanoacrylate, fibrin glue, and small particle embolization with or without coils – the techniques accounting for the majority of recent PVE series. Among these, differing technical demands include the need for specialized catheters for the delivery of ethanol and fibrin glue. The contralateral approach, which carries risk for injury to the future liver remnant, is most commonly used when ethanol or cyanoacrylate is used. Standard angiographic catheters inserted from an ipsilateral approach can be used to deliver small particles with or without coils, making this potentially the simplest technique. The results of embolization using any of these methods are fairly consistent and therefore the strategy best adapted to the skills of local operators should be employed.

Keywords

Embolic agents for portal venous embolization • Fibrin glue for portal vein embolization • *N*-Butyl cyanoacrylate • Portal venous embolization

Although numerous embolic agents have been used for portal venous embolization (PVE), no randomized, prospective comparison has been performed to systematically evaluate the effectiveness of different agents for the induction of liver hypertrophy after embolization. Impressions regarding the performance profile of the various options, therefore, must be derived from the comparison of retrospective series consisting of relatively small numbers of patients from institutions where one technique has evolved as the preferred method and where differing methods of liver volumetry have been practiced. With this state of evidence, it is convenient that the results of PVE appear similar across the range of commonly used embolic agents. As we consider each embolic agent in turn, it is useful to bear in mind the attributes of an ideal PVE agent set forth by Madoff et al.[1]: an agent that causes permanent portal venous embolization without recanalization, is well tolerated by the patient, and is easy to use.

A.M. Covey (✉)
Department of Diagnostic Radiology, Memorial Sloan-Kettering Cancer Center, 1275 York Avenue, New York, NY 10021, USA
e-mail: coveya@mskcc.org

D.C. Madoff et al. (eds.), *Venous Embolization of the Liver*,
DOI 10.1007/978-1-84882-122-4_14, © Springer-Verlag London Limited 2011

14.1 *N*-Butyl Cyanoacrylate

N-Butyl cyanoacrylate (NBCA, n-BCA), also known as butyl cyanoacrylate or enbucrilate, is the butyl ester of 2-cyano-2-propenoic acid ($C_8H_{11}NO_2$). A medical glue most often used for skin closure and marketed under a variety of trade names, the product Histoacryl™ or Histoacryl Blue™ (Braun, Melsungen, Germany) is commonly encountered in descriptions of its use for portal venous embolization (PVE), although it is not FDA-approved for this use. A clear, colorless liquid with a sharp and irritating odor, it is water insoluble and polymerizes within seconds in contact with weak bases, such as blood.[2] NBCA is a component of the Trufill™ Liquid Embolic System (Cordis Neurovascular, Miami Lakes, FL), which is FDA-approved for the presurgical devascularization of cerebral arteriovenous malformations.[3] Its off-label utility in a variety of extracranial applications includes descriptions of successful bronchial artery embolization[4], varicocele treatment,[5] embolization of gastrointestinal bleeding,[6] and PVE.[7-12] The durability of PVE by NBCA was described by Matsuoka, who demonstrated portal occlusion more than 4 weeks post-procedure using the glue, compared to shorter-lived portal venous occlusions produced by either thrombin (1 week) or fibrin adhesive mixtures (2 weeks).[7]

14.2 Technique

A mixture of NBCA and ethiodized oil is usually delivered through an end-hole angiographic catheter into the portal veins targeted for occlusion. Ethiodized oil both confers radiopacity and functions as a polymerizing retardant for the glue. The dilution ratio of NBCA with lipiodol, therefore, can be adapted according to portal flow dynamics and operator preference. One author describes using an NBCA/lipiodol ratio of 1:2 for the initial portion of the embolization when flow is rapid and distal embolization is desired. For reduced portal flow rates, including the final stages of embolization when the closure of the proximal portal venous trunks is the objective, a more rapidly polymerizing 1:1 dilution is used to assist in avoiding nontarget embolization.[8] Typical portal embolizations require 1–3 mL of NBCA.[9] While some operators prefer a contralateral approach through the future liver remnant (FLR) in order to minimize the chance of gluing the catheter into the liver, others use an ipsilateral approach with reverse-curve catheters.

Cyanoacrylate rapidly polymerizes on contact with blood, and strategies to prevent nontarget embolization are important. To minimize the risk of nontarget embolization with NBCA, the selective embolization of second- or third-order portal branches rather than main trunks is one such safeguard.[8] Additionally, Di Stefano et al. recommend that the catheter tip should be maintained in the targeted portal venous branches following embolization until the catheter has been abundantly flushed and/or a guidewire has been inserted through it.[10] This is meant to protect against the unintended shedding of NBCA fragments attached to the catheter shaft or lumen following embolization. Similarly, the placement of an introducer sheath into the veins targeted for embolization may protect against the nontarget shedding of NBCA fragments from the embolization catheter. In cases where segment IV branches are intended for embolization in addition to the right portal vein, special care must be taken to avoid the delivery or dislodgement of embolic material into the segment II and III portal branches, since this could cause total portal obstruction. In such instances, particle embolization of the segment IV branches – performed prior to right side NBCA embolization – may be the most prudent strategy.

14.3 Results

In 1996, DeBaere compared the results of PVE among 31 patients, of whom 24 received NBCA, 3 received thrombin with gelatin sponge, and 4 received coils only. Increase in the size of the FLR was $90\% \pm 52\%$ when NBCA was used, compared with only $53\% \pm 6\%$ and $44\% \pm 30\%$ with thrombin/gelatin sponge and coils, respectively.[9] Pathologic analysis of 19 of the livers embolized with NBCA revealed intense peribiliary fibrosis. In 2000, Azoulay demonstrated that PVE using NBCA was effective for the induction of hypertrophy of the FLR in patients with underlying chronic liver disease, increasing the number of patients eligible for resection of three or more segments by 47%.[11] There were no major complications in this group of 29 patients, but one patient with hemochromatosis and cirrhosis had inadequate liver regeneration for resection. Using NBCA as their embolic agent, Farges et al. showed that the hypertrophy induced by PVE significantly decreased the rate of post-hepatectomy complications in patients with chronic liver disease.[12] In this study, there were no major complications of PVE but two patients with chronic liver disease had insufficient regeneration to permit resection. In 2005, Denys et al. reported on 40 patients with HCC and underlying cirrhosis/fibrosis who underwent NBCA right PVE with a 41% increase in the volume of the left lobe. Among these patients, there were two cases of non-target embolization (one of which could ultimately be resected) and two cases of inadequate regeneration (one diabetic and another s/p prior hepatic arterial chemoembolization).

In 2005, Di Stefano et al. published the largest review to date of NBCA PVE complications.[10] Reviewing 188 patients over 10 years, the robust clinical performance of the technique was confirmed with FLR increases of 62% in noncirrhotics and of 41% in cirrhotic patients. Only three patients had an inadequate liver regeneration response to the NBCA PVE. Twenty-four complications were recognized, but only half were deemed clinically relevant. Three of the twelve clinically relevant complications (25%) involved nontarget embolization of NBCA – in one case, leading to total portal thrombosis; and in two others, to NBCA fragment migration into left-sided FLR portal veins. Other clinically relevant complications included a case of hemoperitoneum, rupture of a liver metastasis into the gallbladder, and six cases of transient liver failure. Notably, 10 of the 12 complications deemed to be clinically irrelevant imaging findings involved nontarget migration of NBCA fragments.

In 2009, Bent et al. reported results in 16 patients who underwent right PVE with histoacryl glue following the placement of a nitinol plug in the right portal vein. Using this novel method, the mean procedure time was about 30 min, and the mean absolute increase in FLR volume was 68.9% ± 12%. No instances of nontarget embolization were identified.[13]

14.4 Summary

Advantages of NBCA as an embolic agent for PVE include durability of portal venous occlusion, ability to achieve both proximal and distal occlusion with a single agent, and rates of liver regeneration believed to be as good or better than other embolic agents. The major disadvantage is the technical learning curve associated with its use, including titration of proportion of NBCA to ethiodized oil, contralateral approach through the future liver remnant (or care not to glue the catheter in place from an ipsilateral approach), and special precautions for avoidance of nontarget embolization by embolic material injected through or shed from the delivery catheter.

14.5 Fibrin Glue

Fibrin glue is created when separate solutions of fibrinogen and thrombin are mixed. The combination causes a fibrin clot to form in 10–60 s, depending upon the concentration of thrombin used.[14] The mechanism of action recapitulates the final steps of the normal coagulation cascade.

14.5.1 Technique

The addition of iodized oil to the fibrinogen–thrombin mixture is necessary to confer radiopacity. The administration of fibrin glue requires a specialized balloon catheter with separate lumens for balloon inflation and for delivery of both fibrinogen and thrombin. Nagino and colleagues were successful in using 5.5-Fr triple-lumen balloon catheters with end holes both distal and proximal to the balloon for ipsilateral fibrin glue PVE.[15] Gibo et al. subsequently described the modification of a commercially available four-lumen catheter for ipsilateral fibrin glue PVE.[16] The authors preferred the four-lumen catheter over the triple-lumen catheter since a guidewire or pressure-monitoring lumen was continuously available for use during the procedure.

14.5.2 Results

Nagino et al. reported a 55% increase in FLR following ipsilateral fibrin glue PVE of segments 4–8 and a 27% increase in FLR following ipsilateral fibrin glue PVE of segments 5–8.[15] Two patients had minimal nontarget embolization of the contralateral portal vein, and two others had recanalization of the embolized portal vein, requiring repeat embolization. The durability of fibrin glue embolization was previously characterized by Matsuoka who showed less than 75% portal occlusion at 2 weeks and less than 25% portal occlusion at 4 weeks.[7] The importance of the duration of portal vein occlusion necessary to achieve maximal contralateral hypertrophy has not been rigorously evaluated. Gibo et al. reported a 131% increase in the future liver remnant without nontarget embolization or other procedural complication.[16]

14.5.3 Summary

The portal infusion of an opacified mixture of fibrinogen and thrombin (fibrin glue) requires specialized multilumen balloon catheters and can be accomplished by an ipsilateral approach. While results do suggest similar hypertrophy of the FLR compared to other embolic agents, portal recanalization appears to occur within 4 weeks when this technique is used. Nevertheless, it is the preferred agent in most Asian series.[17]

14.6 Absolute Ethanol

Ethanol is a colorless, odorless straight-chain alcohol with molecular formula C_2H_5OH. Absolute ethanol, also known as anhydrous alcohol, is the purified form of ethanol containing less than 1% water. A low viscosity liquid, it is a strong sclerosant, rapidly denaturing, and coagulating protein. This property has found use in several medical applications, including injection into bleeding esophageal and gastric varices, treatment of peripheral arteriovenous malformations, intravascular treatment of renal cell carcinomas, and direct injection into hepatomas.[18-22] The vascular endothelium is destroyed by absolute ethanol, and local tissue effects including inflammation, fibrosis, and necrosis are pronounced.

14.6.1 Technique

Absolute ethanol is typically delivered through a balloon catheter placed from a contralateral approach.

14.6.2 Results

In 1995, Yamakado et al. published work comparing portal embolization using steel coils or absolute ethanol in a canine model.[23] The findings of portography, arteriography, and histology were compared between groups. In the five dogs treated by coil embolization of the portal vein, portography revealed occlusion of the target vessel at all time points up to 4 weeks. In four of the five dogs, however, non-embolized portal venous branches developed constriction or obstruction, believed due to propagation of thrombus from the coils. Arteriography showed intense arterial staining of the embolized liver segments, indicative of compensatory increase in arterial flow to these areas. Histopathologically, there was no difference in appearance of embolized and non-embolized segments. No liver parenchymal damage was detected in the coil-embolized segments. Twelve other dogs underwent portal embolization with escalating doses of ethanol ranging from 0.2 to 0.8 cm^3/kg body weight. In these animals, portal occlusion was similarly durable throughout the study period for doses greater than 0.2 cm^3/kg, but none had findings of nontarget portal vein occlusion. Angiography in the ethanol group also did not show hyper-arterialization of the embolized segments. Except at the lowest, ineffective dose of ethanol (0.2 cm^3/kg), liver parenchymal damage was noted in all embolized segments. The degree of liver parenchymal damage was proportional to ethanol dose, as was the degree of adherence of greater omentum to the surface of the embolized liver segment. Histopathologically, the portal endothelium was destroyed, and hepatocytes around the portal triad were degenerated and necrotic.

In 1996, Osgasawara et al. described a study of portal venous embolization using absolute ethanol in rats.[24] Two groups of rats underwent portal venous embolization using either low-dose (0.5 mL/kg body weight) or high-dose (1.2 mL/kg body weight) absolute ethanol injection into the target portal vein. A third group had surgical resection of the same lobes which were embolized in the other groups. The investigators found that "complete obstruction of portal venous branches and massive necrosis were the main histopathologic observations after portal vein embolization with all doses of ethanol." Although the rats treated with higher dose ethanol had faster initial regeneration of the non-embolized liver, by the end of the observation period, there was no difference between the low-dose and high-dose groups in the volume changes of non-embolized liver. Final results of hypertrophy from both ethanol doses nearly equaled the hypertrophy induced by resection. Mortality, on the other hand, was significantly higher for those rats treated with higher dose ethanol. The work illustrated the efficacy of portal embolization using ethanol and highlighted the dose-dependent "strong contact destructivity" of the agent.

Shimamura et al. reported on seven patients who underwent ethanol PVE via the contralateral approach. Twenty-milliliter absolute ethanol was found to be effective in producing complete portal occlusion and a 27% increase in FLR volume.[25] Ogasawara et al. reported near doubling of left liver volumes within 4 weeks after ethanol PVE in HCC patients with chronic liver dysfunction.[24]

In 2003, Ji et al. reported their clinical experience of ethanol PVE in 47 patients with HCC using a novel technique.[26] A 21-gauge needle was placed percutaneously under ultrasound guidance into the targeted right portal vein. Under sonographic observation, 0.4-mL/kg ethanol mixed with iodized oil was administered through the needle into the vein. No major complications were encountered. The mean left liver volume increased from 352 to 509 cm^3 within 3 weeks, permitting 52% of patients to have resection.

14.6.3 Summary

Absolute ethanol is effective in producing durable portal venous occlusion, and the rates of FLR hypertrophy following its use are among the highest reported. The need for occlusion balloon catheters to prevent reflux into nontarget veins increases the complexity of its use. While responsible for its efficacy as an embolic agent, the cytotoxic nature of ethanol causes hepatocyte necrosis, characterized by transaminase and bilirubin elevation. Because some patients who undergo PVE in anticipation of major hepatectomy do not undergo resection because of failure to regenerate or extent of disease, agents that cause irreversible parenchymal damage should be used with caution. Other potential systemic effects of intravascular alcohol administration include intoxication, abdominal pain, and thrombocytopenia.[27]

14.7 Particle Embolization

A variety of particulate agents have been used to perform portal venous embolization, including Gelfoam, polyvinyl alcohol, and tris-acryl microspheres. The armamentarium of embolic particulates is constantly expanding. The mechanical obstruction produced by injected particulates is augmented by clot formation to produce thrombosis of target vessels.

14.7.1 Gelfoam®

A sterile compressed sponge prepared from purified porcine skin gelatin, Gelfoam® is a water-insoluble temporary hemostatic device.[27] Capable of absorbing more than 45 times its weight of whole blood,[28] its hemostatic mechanism of action is mechanical,[29] forming a matrix that supports and facilitates blood clot formation.[30] The sponge form can be modified for intravascular injection by trimming the foam into injectable pledgets or by production of a slurry created by forcefully exchanging a solution of contrast material and small Gelfoam® pieces between two syringes through a three-way stopcock. Alternatively, a powderized form is available, prepared by the milling of gelatin sponge.[27] Gelfoam® is a temporary embolic agent, and its absorption is dependent upon the amount used, the site of use, and the degree of saturation with blood.[20]

14.7.2 Polyvinyl Alcohol

PVA is a nontoxic, synthetic polymer with chemical formula $(C_2H_4O)_x$. In addition to its well-known medical use as an embolic agent, PVA is widely used in a variety of applications, including as a paint thickener, as an essential component of Elmer's glue, as a lubricant in eye drop and contact solutions, and as a moisture-retentive agent in confections. Available in a variety of sizes, the aggregation of PVA particles in blood vessels leads to clot formation and thrombosis. Used alone, PVA embolization durability is typically reported to be measured in weeks rather than months.

14.7.3 Tris-acryl Microspheres

Microspheres are biocompatible, nonresorbable tris-acryl gelatin spherical embolic agents available in calibrated sizes. Prior to use as a vascular embolic agent, microspheres were used as a base material in chromatography columns and as a microcarrier for cell culture.[31] Inert and compressible by up to 33%, the hydrophilic surface and spherical shape prevent the clumping/aggregation commonly encountered with nonspherical agents such as PVA. The agent was cleared by the FDA in 2000 for use as an embolic agent in hypervascular tumors and arteriovenous malformations.

14.7.4 Technique

Particulate agents are administered into target portal vein branches through end-hole catheters. Ipsilateral approach utilizing reverse-curve catheters permits the procedure to be performed through the lobe destined for resection, minimizing risk of injury to the future liver remnant. The particulate embolic agent is diluted in contrast material and injected through the reverse-curve catheter or through a co-axially placed, selectively positioned microcatheter. The endpoint is the cessation of flow into the target branches. Some augment particle embolization with placement of coils into secondary portal branches.

14.7.5 Results

In 1999, Duncan et al. reported animal data demonstrating induction of hepatocyte replication following portal venous embolizaton using PVA and coils.[32] Eight pigs underwent embolization of the median and left portal vein using 350–750 μm PVA. Three- to ten-millimeter embolization coils were deposited in the proximal portal vein branches at the conclusion of particle embolization. No recanalization of occluded portal veins was found in animals sacrificed up to 35 days after embolization. Histologic findings in the embolized lobe included hepatocyte and lobular atrophy without widespread coagulative necrosis, PVA particles occluding portal vein branches with only mild surrounding inflammatory changes, occasional regenerative nodules, and rare apoptotic hepatocytes. In the non-embolized lobe, histologic findings included findings of hepatocyte replication with little change in lobule size, suggesting that the mechanism of post-embolization hypertrophy involves the addition of new hepatic lobules rather than an increase in the size of preexisting lobules.

In 2003, Madoff reported safety and efficacy of preoperative PVE using PVA and coils in patients with liver metastases.[1] Twenty-one patients underwent right PVE, and five underwent right plus segment 4 PVE using 300–1,000 μm PVA for the occlusion of third-order and smaller portal branches and microcoils for the occlusion of second-order branches. After embolization, the mean FLR/TELV ratio increase was 7.7%. Two complications occurred after PVE. One patient in the group developed main and left PV thrombosis after PVE, successfully treated by tPA infusion. Another developed a subcapsular hematoma, evacuated at time of successful resection. Sixteen of twenty-six (62%) patients were ultimately resected. Of the ten patients not resected, only two had inadequate hypertrophy for safe operation, and one of these was diabetic.

In 2005, Covey and colleagues described safety and efficacy of preoperative PVE using PVA particles in 58 patients with liver metastases.[33] Forty-seven underwent right PVE, three underwent right plus segment four PVE, and eight underwent left PVE using 100–300 μm PVA. Mean FLR/TELV increases were 9%, 10%, and 3%, respectively. Fever without bacteremia was noted in 36% after embolization. Mean hospital stay was 1.6 days, and there were no major complications of embolization. Of the group, 38 patients (65.5%) ultimately underwent planned resection, and there were no instances of sustained postoperative liver failure.

The same year, Madoff updated his earlier series, reporting 44 patients who underwent preoperative right plus segment 4 PVE with either PVA (355–1,000 μm) or tris-acryl microspheres (100–700 μm) and coils.[34] As in the earlier report, the smallest particles were used to achieve distal portal embolization; larger particles were used to achieve embolization to the level of third-order branches, and microcoils were then used to occlude second-order branches. Comparing the 23 patients embolized with nonspherical PVA and the 21 embolized with microspheres, embolization with the spherical agent was associated with significant improvements in volumetric outcomes and resection rates. This was believed the result of more distal embolization made possible by the smaller spheres, limiting the development of collateral blood supply to the embolized segments. Seventy-one percent of patients ultimately underwent extended right hepatectomy, 86% after receiving microspheres, and 57% after receiving PVA as embolic agent. No instances of postembolization syndrome or liver insufficiency occurred.

14.7.6 Summary

Particle embolization of the portal vein, with or without coil embolization of second-order branches, can be performed from the ipsilateral approach using standard angiographic catheters. Hypertrophy results appear equivalent to the alternate embolic agents.

14.8 Novel Techniques

Fürst et al. reported a small series comparing seven patients who underwent PVE using particles and coils (segments I and IV) or particles and cyanoacrylate (segments V–VIII) with six patients who had PVE in addition to intraportal infusion of CD133+ bone marrow stem cells into the FLR.[35] Those patients receiving stem cells had significantly greater gain in FRLV (77.3% vs. 39.1%, $p=0.039$) and a trend toward shorter time to surgery (27 vs. 45 days, $p=0.057$). In addition, the search for an ideal embolic material continues. For example, a new liquid embolic material (Embol-78), formed from the product of partial hydrolysis of PVA dissolved in absolute ethanol and water-soluble contrast material, was shown to be safe and effective for preoperative PVE.[36]

14.9 Conclusion

The gamut of embolic materials has been used for portal venous embolization. Local preferences appear to dictate the choice of embolic material, as there are no clear data supporting a superior choice among absolute ethanol, cyanoacrylate, fibrin glue, and small particle embolization with or without coils – the techniques accounting for the majority of recent PVE series. Among these, differing technical demands include the need for specialized catheters for the delivery of ethanol and fibrin glue. The contralateral approach, which carries risk for injury to the future liver remnant, is most commonly utilized when ethanol or cyanoacrylate is used. Standard angiographic catheters inserted from an ipsilateral approach can be used to deliver small particles with or without coils, making this potentially the simplest technique. The results of embolization using any of these methods are fairly consistent and therefore the strategy best adapted to the skills of local operators should be employed.

References

1. Madoff DC, Hicks ME, Abdalla EK, Morris JS, Vauthey JN. Portal vein embolization with polyvinyl alcohol particles and coils in preparation for major liver resection for hepatobiliary malignancy: safety and effectiveness—study in 26 patients. *Radiology*. 2003;227(1):251-260.
2. http://www.osha.gov/dts/chemicalsampling/data/CH_223320.html. Accessed 17 Jan 2009.
3. http://www.fda.gov/cdrh/pdf/p990040.html. Accessed 17 Jan 2009.
4. Baltacioglu F, Cimsit NC, Bostanci K, Yuksel M, Kodalli N. Transarterial microcatheter glue embolization of the bronchial artery for life-threatening hemoptysis: technical and clinical results. *Eur J Radiol*. 2008;73(2):380-384.
5. Sze DY, Kao JS, Frisoli JK, McCallum SW, Kennedy WA 2nd, Razavi MK. Persistent and recurrent post-surgical varicoceles: venographic anatomy and treatment with N-butyl cyanoacrylate embolization. *J Vasc Interv Radiol*. 2008;19(4): 539-545.
6. Jae HJ, Chung JW, Jung AY, Lee W, Park JH. Transcatheter arterial embolization of nonvariceal upper gastrointestinal bleeding with N-butyl cyanoacrylate. *Korean J Radiol*. 2007;8(1):48-56.
7. Matsuoka T. Experimental studies of intrahepatic portal vein embolization and embolic materials. *Nippon Igaku Hoshasen Gakkai Zasshi*. 1989;49(5):593-606.
8. Denys A, Lacombe C, Schneider F, et al. Portal vein embolization with *N*-butyl cyanoacrylate before partial hepatectomy in patients with hepatocellular carcinoma and underlying cirrhosis or advanced fibrosis. *J Vasc Interv Radiol*. 2005;16:1667-1674.
9. de Baere T, Roche A, Elias D, Lasser P, Lagrange C, Bousson V. Preoperative portal vein embolization for extension of hepatectomy indications. *Hepatology*. 1996;24(6):1386-1391.
10. Di Stefano DR, de Baere T, Denys A, et al. Preoperative percutaneous portal vein embolization: evaluation of adverse events in 188 patients. *Radiology*. 2005;234(2):625-630.
11. Azoulay D, Castaing D, Krissat J, et al. Percutaneous portal vein embolization increases the feasibility and safety of major liver resection for hepatocellular carcinoma in injured liver. *Ann Surg*. 2000;232(5):665-672.
12. Farges O, Belghiti J, Kianmanesh R, et al. Portal vein embolization before right hepatectomy: prospective clinical trial. *Ann Surg*. 2003;237(2):208-217.
13. Bent CL, Low D, Matson MB, Renfrew I, Fotheringham T. Portal vein embolization using a nitinol plug (Amplatzer vascular plug) in combination with histoacryl glue and iodinized oil: adequate hypertrophy with a reduced risk of nontarget embolization. *Cardiovasc Intervent Radiol*. 2009; 32(3):471-477.
14. Thompson DF, Letassy NA, Thompson GD. Fibrin glue: a review of its preparation, efficacy, and adverse effects as a topical hemostat. *Drug Intell Clin Pharm*. 1988;22(12): 946-952.
15. Nagino M, Nimura Y, Kamiya J, Kondo S, Kanai M. Selective percutaneous transhepatic embolization of the portal vein in preparation for extensive liver resection: the ipsilateral approach. *Radiology*. 1996;200(2):559-563.
16. Gibo M, Unten S, Yogi A, et al. Percutaneous ipsilateral portal vein embolization using a modified four-lumen balloon catheter with fibrin glue: initial clinical experience. *Radiat Med*. 2007;25(4):164-172.
17. Denys A, Madoff DC, Doenz F, et al. Indications for and limitations of portal vein embolization before major hepatic resection for hepatobiliary malignancy. *Surg Oncol Clin N Am*. 2002;11(4):955-968.

18. Danila M, Sporea I, Sirli R, Popescu A. Percutaneous ethanol injection therapy in the treatment of hepatocarcinoma—results obtained from a series of 88 cases. *J Gastrointestin Liver Dis*. 2009;18(3):317-322.
19. Ferrari AP, de Paulo GA, de Macedo CM, Araujo I, Della Libera E Jr. Efficacy of absolute alcohol injection compared with band ligation in the eradication of esophageal varices. *Arq Gastroenterol*. 2005;42(2):72-76.
20. Ginat DT, Saad WE, Turba UC. Transcatheter renal artery embolization: clinical applications and techniques. *Tech Vasc Interv Radiol*. 2009;12(4):224-239.
21. Gloviczki P, Duncan A, Kalra M, et al. Vascular malformations: an update. *Perspect Vasc Surg Endovasc Ther*. 2009;21(2):133-148.
22. Jutabha R, Jensen DM, See J, Machicado G, Hirabayashi K. Randomized, controlled study of various agents for endoscopic injection sclerotherapy of bleeding canine gastric varices. *Gastrointest Endosc*. 1995;41(3):206-211.
23. Yamakado K, Takeda K, Nishide Y, et al. Portal vein embolization with steel coils and absolute ethanol: a comparative experimental study with canine liver. *Hepatology*. 1995; 22(6):1812-1818.
24. Ogasawara K, Uchino J, Une Y, Fujioka Y. Selective portal vein embolization with absolute ethanol induces hepatic hypertrophy and makes more extensive hepatectomy possible. *Hepatology*. 1996;23(2):338-345.
25. Shimamura T, Nakajima Y, Une Y, et al. Efficacy and safety of preoperative percutaneous transhepatic portal embolization with absolute ethanol: a clinical study. *Surgery*. 1997;121(2): 135-141.
26. Ji W, Li JS, Li LT, et al. Role of preoperative selective portal vein embolization in two-step curative hepatectomy for hepatocellular carcinoma. *World J Gastroenterol*. 2003;9(8):1702-1706.
27. http://www.pfizer.com/files/products/uspi_gelfoam_sponge.pdf. Accessed 20 Mar 2009.
28. Council on Pharmacy and Chemistry. Absorbable gelatin sponge—new and nonofficial remedies. *JAMA*. 1947; 135:921.
29. Goodman LS, Gilman AG, Gilman A. Surface-acting drugs. In: *The Pharmacologic Basis of Therapeutics*. 6th ed. New York: Macmillan; 1980:955.
30. Guralnick W, Berg L. GELFOAM in oral surgery. *Oral Surg Oral Med Oral Pathol*. 1948;1:629-632.
31. Spies JB, Benenati JF, Worthington-Kirsch RL, Pelage JP. Initial experience with use of tris-acryl gelatin microspheres for uterine artery embolization for leiomyomata. *J Vasc Interv Radiol*. 2001;12(9):1059-1063.
32. Duncan JR, Hicks ME, Cai SR, Brunt EM, Ponder KP. Embolization of portal vein branches induces hepatocyte replication in swine: a potential step in hepatic gene therapy. *Radiology*. 1999;210(2):467-477.
33. Covey AM, Tuorto S, Brody LA, et al. Safety and efficacy of preoperative portal vein embolization with polyvinyl alcohol in 58 patients with liver metastases. *AJR Am J Roentgenol*. 2005;185(6):1620-1626.
34. Madoff DC, Abdalla EK, Gupta S, et al. Transhepatic ipsilateral right portal vein embolization extended to segment IV: improving hypertrophy and resection outcomes with spherical particles and coils. *J Vasc Interv Radiol*. 2005;16 (2 Pt 1):215-225.
35. Furst G, Poll LW, et al. Portal vein embolization and autologous CD133+ bone marrow stem cells for liver regeneration: initial experience. *Radiology*. 2007;243(1):171-179.
36. Ko GY, Sung KB, Yoon HK, Kim JH, Weon YC, Song HY. Preoperative portal vein embolization with a new liquid embolic agent. *Radiology*. 2003;227(2):407-413.

15 Transileocolic Portal Vein Embolization

Yoji Kishi, Yasuji Seyama, and Masatoshi Makuuchi

Abstract

Transileocolic portal vein embolization (TIPE) is invasive compared to percutaneous transhepatic portal vein embolization (PTPE) because the procedure requires general anesthesia. There are, however, several advantages: First, it enables the examination of extrahepatic diseases; second, catheter manipulation is easier compared to ipsilateral PTPE because the catheter should not be passed through ramifications with a narrow angle (e.g., from the segment 5 portal vein branch to the segment 6 portal vein branch); third, it provides the opportunity to perform completion portography after embolization. Furthermore, PTPE is not appropriate in cases with multiple or large hepatic tumors considering the risk of puncturing tumors that result in rupture of the tumor and cancer cell seeding. Selection of each approach may principally be based on each operator's preference, but must be decided according to each patient's condition.

Keywords

Transileocolic portal vein embolization • Percutaneous transhepatic portal vein embolization • Portal vein embolization

Transileocolic portal vein embolization (TIPE) was originally reported by Makuuchi et al.[1] The procedure requires general anesthesia because catheters are inserted through the ileocolic vein branch. With the increase in the popularity of portal vein embolization (PVE), most institutions now favor the percutaneous approach doe its simplicity (percutaneous transhepatic PVE [PTPE]) rather than the transileocolic approach. In this chapter, the details of the TIPE technique are described. Additionally, the advantages and disadvantages of TIPE in comparison to PTPE are discussed.

M. Makuuchi (✉)
Japanese Red Cross Medical Center,
4-1-22 Hiroo, Shibuya-ku, Tokyo 150-8935, Japan
e-mail: makuuchi_masatoshi@med.jrc.or.jp

15.1 Indications

Laboratory tests, including blood cell count, chemistry, and coagulation function must first be evaluated. Assessment of liver function in relation to remnant liver volume is also essential. We initially established an indication criteria of hepatectomy for other area.[2] When the resection area exceeds the criteria, PVE is indicated. The indication is limited to patients who are evaluated to be one grade above the criteria. For example, right PVE is carried out for patients with indocyanine green retention rate at 15 minutes (ICGR15) of 10–20% who require right hepatectomy. Then, Kubota et al.[3] presented that the liver volume to be resected (as evaluated by CT-volumetry) correlates with the actual

D.C. Madoff et al. (eds.), *Venous Embolization of the Liver*,
DOI 10.1007/978-1-84882-122-4_15,

resected liver volume, and they proposed criteria for the indications for PVE. Based on these criteria, we currently perform PVE in patients with an estimated remnant liver volume of no more than 40% of the total liver volume if the indocyanin green retention rate at 15 min (ICG R15) is less than 10%, and no more than 50% of the total liver volume if the ICG R15 is between 10% and 20%. Patients with ICG R15 greater than 20% are not indicated for major hepatic resection. In such instance, resection of one sector of right or left liver after PVE is indicated.

In patients with obstructive jaundice, majority of high volume centers routinely perform preoperative biliary drainage.[4-13] Physicians at several institutions are reluctant to perform biliary drainage because it increases the risk of cholangitis, postoperative liver failure and mortality.[14,15] In patients with hilar bile duct carcinoma where the right and the left hepatic ducts are separated cholangitis can be avoided by not performing cholangiography after biliary drainage except on the day before hepatic resection.[5] Biliary drainage of the future remnant liver is recommended at least for the following reasons. Because the Glisson sheath surrounds the portal veins and bile duct, biliary dilatation results in compression of the portal vein and decreased portal flow. Decompression of the biliary tract increases portal venous flow and enhances liver regeneration. Recent study has reported that bilirubin clearance and hypertrophy of the remnant liver is superior after biliary drainage of only the future liver remnant compared to that of the whole liver.[16] We, therefore, consider major hepatic resection only for patients with serum total bilirubin (T.Bil) value of 2.0 mg/dL or less.[1,17] In patients with obstructive jaundice, biliary drainage is performed first, and PVE is indicated only after the T.Bil value decreases to 5 mg/dL or less and the remnant liver volume is 50% or less to the total liver volume.[5] Imaging evaluations are also mandatory. Not only should the remnant liver volume be assessed, but the extent of the disease must also be carefully evaluated, especially in cases of biliary or gallbladder cancer with attention to hepatic artery or portal vein invasion or lymph node metastases. Although approach selection (transileocolic vs. percutaneous) may depend on institutional preferences, we believe that percutaneous approach is not appropriate in cases with giant or multiple bilateral liver tumors to avoid puncturing the tumor by an ipsilateral approach.

15.2 Techniques

15.2.1 Preparation

Indication for TIPE must be evaluated by volumetric analysis of the liver as well as liver function tests. The choice of embolization material is operator dependent. We prefer to use gelatin sponge mixed with contrast enhancement material and thrombin (Table 15.1). In addition, metallic coils of several kinds are used according to the diameter of the portal vein branches to be embolized. We routinely use a 5.2 Fr. catheter with a balloon (Selecon MP catheter II®, TERUMO Clinical Supply Co., Ltd., Gifu, Japan). There are several types of catheters with different curves, and an appropriate choice should be made for the embolization of each branch. We prefer to use catheter with two balloons with a hole on the tip and side holes between the two balloons.

15.2.2 Laparotomy and Catheter Insertion

Under general anesthesia, a laparotomy is performed with a pararectus skin incision to the right lower quadrant. An incision of approximately 10 cm in length is sufficient for the following procedures. The operator's right hand is inserted through the incision to search for peritoneal dissemination or other extrahepatic diseases. Careful palpation of the hepatoduodenal ligament is especially important in cases of cholangiocarcinoma with extensive infiltration around the hepatic hilum. After confirming that there is no peritoneal dissemination or tumor invasion around common and/or proper hepatic arteries that would jeopardize the surgery, following steps are performed.

The terminal portion of the ileum is extracted from the incision. One branch of the ileocolic vein is chosen. By dissecting the mesentery of the ileum, the branch is encircled with a 4-0 silk suture.[5] A 1-cm-long dissection along the selected vein is adequate. The vein is tapped with the index or the middle finger to dilate the vein and facilitate the puncture. One of the two to three branches conjugating to form the trunk of the ileocolic vein should be selected. Puncture of the marginal veins should be avoided because they are thin and a risk of injury during insertion of the sheath is high. An introducer 6 Fr. sheath is fixed in place (Fig. 15.1). A 5.2 Fr. catheter is inserted into the main trunk of the portal

Table 15.1 Contents of embolization material

Substance	Amount
Gelatin sponge powder	2 g
Diatrizoate sodium meglumine	40 mL
Gentamicin	40 mg
Thrombin	10,000 units

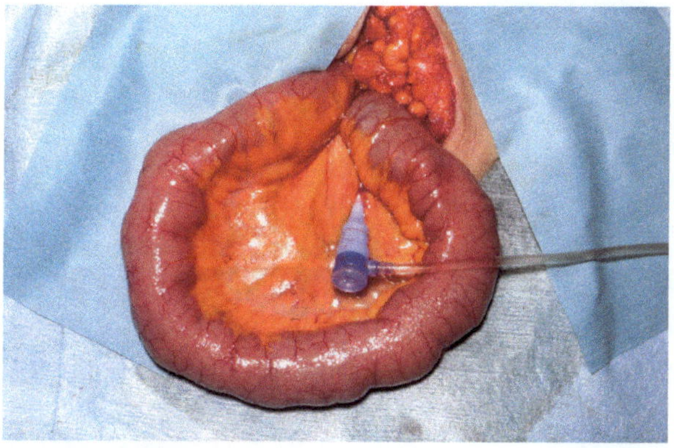

Fig. 15.1 Ileum extracted from the abdomen. A 5 Fr. introducer catheter is inserted from a branch of the ileocolic vein

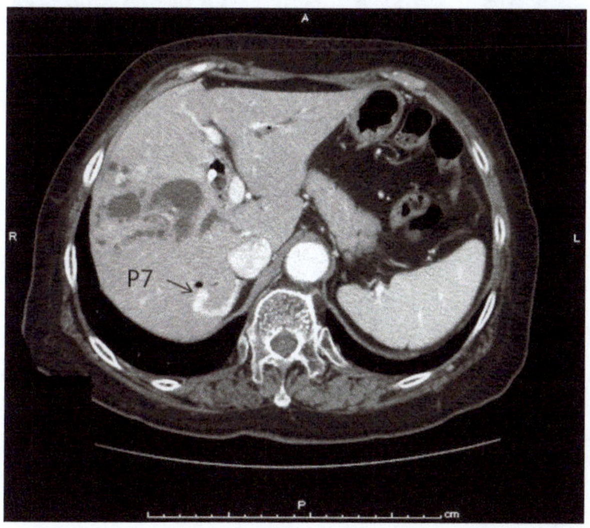

Fig. 15.2 Computed tomography image of a porto-venous shunt. Collateral vessel connecting the portal vein branch of segment 7 (P7, *arrow*) and the inferior vena cava is shown. Left bile ducts are drained

vein by guide wire manipulation. After the measurement of the portal vein pressure, portography is performed. Portography images must be carefully checked for the following features: (1) the anatomy of the portal vein branches, (2) tumor encasement of the main trunk or the major branches, and (3) the occurrence of a portovenous shunt (Fig. 15.2). Portovenous shunts are rare, but must be determined by Doppler ultrasound or CT-scan with contrast enhancement because the shunt must be embolized using coils before PVE. If the shunt cannot be occluded, PVE should be abandoned.

To precisely assess the anatomy, not only the usual anteroposterior (AP) images but also the right anterior oblique (RAO) images should be evaluated. In fact, RAO images facilitate accurate recognition of the right lateral portal vein branch; therefore, we usually embolize the lateral branch under fluoroscopic guidance along the RAO and then embolize the right paramedian branches.

15.2.3 Embolization

A balloon catheter is inserted selectively into the portal vein branch targeted for embolization. To prevent reflux of the embolic materials into the nonembolized liver, the catheter should be inserted into each tertiary branch to be embolized. The balloon of the catheter should be placed 1 cm distal to the origin of each branch. In right PVE, lateral branches are usually embolized first for the following reasons: First, the embolic materials are mixed with the contrast materials, making the specific gravity of the mixture is kept greater than that of the blood. Embolization of the paramedian branches increases the risk of reflux of the embolic materials. Second, the insertion of the catheter into the lateral branches is more difficult than insertion into the paramedian branches.

To minimize the risk of recanalization after PVE, we use coils in addition to embolic materials. Platinum coils are placed at the origin of each segmental branch, paying careful attention not to dislocate them to the proximal side. The segment 7 branches should first be embolized, followed by extraction of the catheter so that the trunk of the lateral branch is occluded by the balloon and the segment 6 branch is embolized. Paramedian branches are embolized after the embolization of the right lateral branch (Fig. 15.3). If the paramedian branch is embolized first, subsequent manipulation of the guide wire to embolize the lateral branches may result in incorporation of the embolic materials injected into the paramedian branch because the lateral branch usually bifurcates from the right trunk of the portal vein, making a tight curve, and the guide wire tends to proceed straight into the paramedian branch.

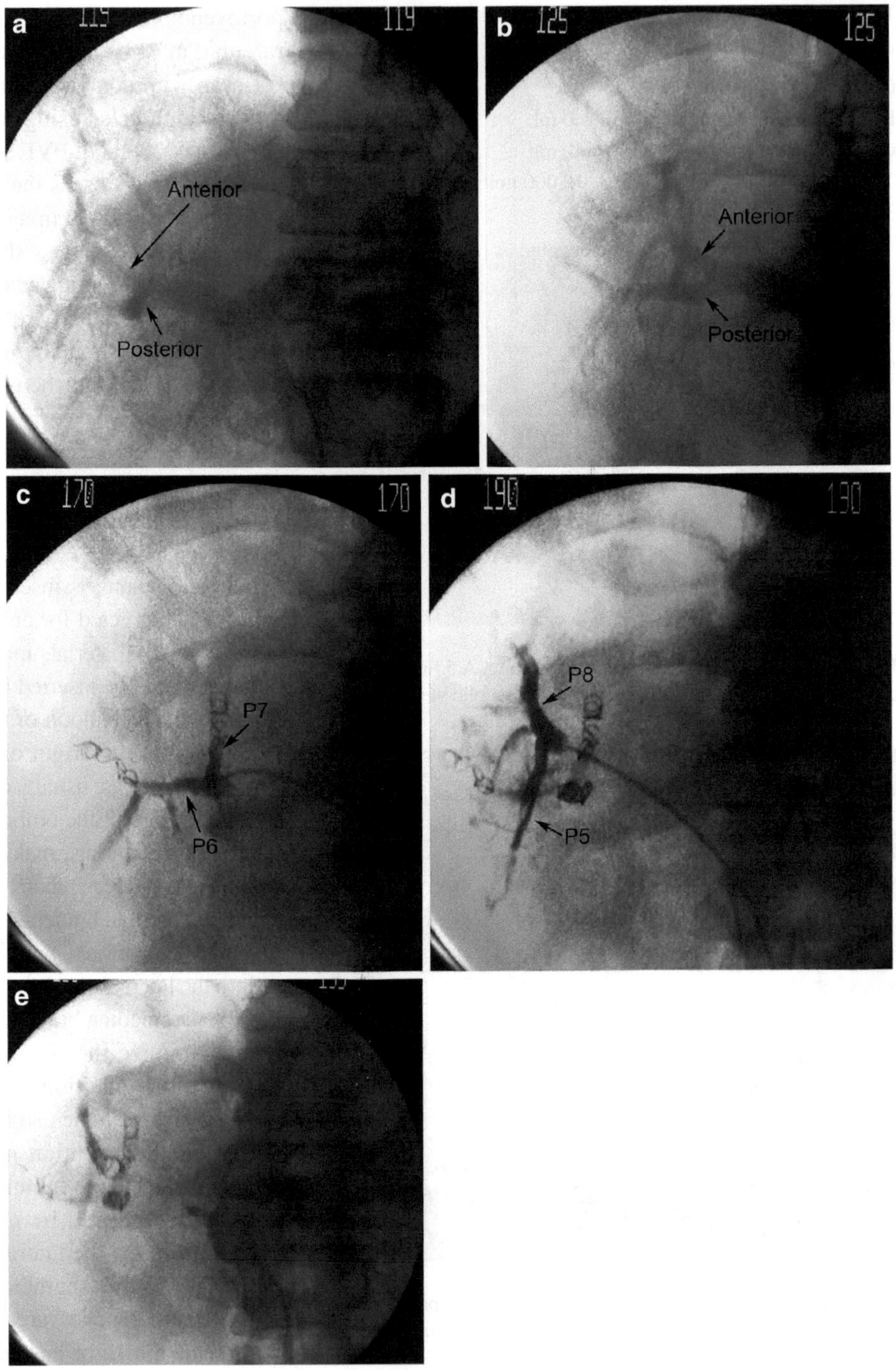

Fig. 15.3 Right portal vein embolization procedure. Portography of the anteroposterior view (**a**) and right anterior oblique view (**b**). Note that the origin of the lateral branch is more easily recognized with the right anterior oblique view compared to the anteroposterior view. Lateral branches are embolized first (**c**), followed by embolization of the paramedian branches (**d**). Coils are placed at the origin of each segmental branch (**e**). P7, P6, P8, and P5 indicate portal vein branches of segments 7, 6, 8, and 5, respectively

At each embolization, the embolic materials are injected slowly into the peripheral side tiding with the blood flow, then additional materials are injected after inflation of the balloon. Usually, 5–7 mL of embolic materials are used for each segmental or subsegmental branch. The balloon should be kept inflated for 3–5 min to prevent reflux of the materials into the nonembolized liver. Deflation of the balloon and extraction of the catheter should be done very slowly under radiographic guidance. In case of trifurcation pattern of portal vein anatomy, where the main trunk of right portal vein is absent, special attention should be paid to prevent the regurgitation of embolic materials to the left side. Tip of the catheter should be placed with some distance from the origin of lateral or paramedian branch to start the embolization. After completion of the embolization, the catheter is extracted to the proximal side, and both the embolic materials within the catheter lumen and 5 mL of blood are drawn. In cases that require embolization of the left liver, the catheter is inserted with the balloon located distal to the transverse portion of the left portal vein. The following procedures for embolization are the same as that for the right liver PVE.

15.2.4 Closure

After the completion of the embolization, catheter is extracted a little and the embolic materials within the catheter lumen must be sucked out before the catheter is extracted to the portal vein trunk. Portography is performed to confirm the efficacy of the embolization. Portal vein pressure is re-measured. Usually, an increase of 5–10 mmHg is expected. The vein used for insertion of the catheter is ligated at the time of the removal of the catheter and the introducer. The dissected mesentery is sutured. The omentum is placed on the intestine and the abdomen is closed.

15.2.5 After the Procedure

Doppler ultrasonography should be performed every day for the next few days following the procedure, to detect unembolized or recanalized portal vein branches. If such branches are detected, these branches are percutaneously punctured under the guidance of ultrasonography and embolized by ethanol injection.

Possible adverse events after PVE include pyrexia and abdominal pain. However, they are expected to be mild compared to those after transarterial embolization, and would usually subside within 3 days. Liver function tests (serum aspartate transaminase, alanine transaminase, bilirubin value) show only minimal changes, and in cases in which these values are elevated, they usually return to baseline levels within 1 week.[17]

15.3 Advantages and Disadvantages of TIPE Compared to PTPE

Primary advantage of TIPE is that peritoneal seeding and invasion of cholangiocarcinoma to the left side of the hepatoduodenal ligament can be detected. In such situation, PVE itself or the following unwanted laparotomy for radical resection may be avoided. Although portal vein embolization effectively enhances hypertrophy of the unembolized liver, it is not a curative treatment of the patient's disease. Therefore, safety becomes the primal concern. The incidence of adverse events induced by PVE is 3.6–12.8%.[18-20] Major complications include migration of the coils or embolization materials to the nonembolized liver, mechanical ileus, biliary peritonitis, and subcapsular hemorrhage. Among them, ileus is specific to transileocolic approach, whereas biliary peritonitis and hemorrhage are specific to percutaneous approach. Studies comparing these methods are limited, and PVE should be performed by the technique that is most commonly used at each institution. The major limitation of the transileocolic approach is that it requires general anesthesia and is more invasive than the percutaneously performed PVE.

There are however, several advantages to transileocolic PVE. First, in cases with multiple or large liver tumors, the transileocolic approach is preferable to prevent tumoral puncture. Second, from the viewpoint of catheter manipulation, the ipsilateral percutaneous approach requires more delicate maneuvering compared to the contralateral percutaneous approach or the transileocolic approach because the catheter would have to be passed through ramifications at a narrow angle (e.g., from the segment 5 portal vein branch to the segment 6 portal vein branch). Although catheter manipulation using the contralateral percutaneous approach is not technically complicated, the major disadvantage of this method is the risk of injury to the remnant liver including sudden perforation of the umbilical portion of the left portal vein during dissection of the umbilical fossa.

The disadvantages of ipsilateral approach includes technical difficulty in catheter manipulation and difficulty to perform completion portography.[21] A recent meta-analysis comparing the effects and adverse events between the transileocolic and percutaneous approaches showed that better regeneration is achieved when PVE is performed percutaneously. On the other hand, however, adverse events were more common and resection rates lower with the percutaneous approach. In this report, the transileocolic approach was recommended, especially in cases of gallbladder cancer because the percutaneous approach increased the risk of peritoneal dissemination during the procedure.[22] Other factors that might bias the results of the regeneration rate, however, such as underlying liver disease, types of embolization materials,[21] or timing of the volume evaluation after PVE,[20] were not considered. Shimura et al.[23] also pointed out the risk of peritoneal dissemination after percutaneous PVE, especially in patients with gall bladder cancer, although it is still not clear if PTPE itself is associated with the increased risk. Tsuge et al.[24] reported laparoscopic transileocolic PVE, which may be another option to avoid complications associated with puncture of the liver. This minimally invasive strategy may also allow for more accurate staging of the disease by laparoscopy or laparoscopic ultrasonography and contribute to reduce unnecessary PVE.

In this chapter, we have described, the techniques and the advantages and the disadvantages of the transileocolic approach to PVE. We must however, not forget that in PVE, priority must always be placed on safety rather than the completeness of the embolization.

References

1. Makuuchi M, Thai BL, Takayasu K, et al. Preoperative portal embolization to increase safety of major hepatectomy for hilar bile duct carcinoma: a preliminary report. *Surgery*. 1990; 107:521-527.
2. Makuuchi M, Kosuge T, Takayama T, Yamazaki S, Kakazu T, Miyagawa S, Kawasaki S. Surgery for small liver cancers. *Semin Surg Oncol*. 1993;9:298-304
3. Kubota K, Makuuchi M, Kusaka K, et al. Measurement of liver volume and hepatic functional reserve as a guide to decision-making in resectional surgery for hepatic tumors. *Hepatology (Baltimore, Md)*. 1997;26:1176-1181.
4. Todoroki T, Kawamoto T, Koike N, et al. Radical resection of hilar bile duct carcinoma and predictors of survival. *Br J Surg*. 2000;87:306-313.
5. Seyama Y, Kubota K, Sano K, et al. Long-term outcome of extended hemihepatectomy for hilar bile duct cancer with no mortality and high survival rate. *Ann Surg*. 2003;238:73-83.
6. Kawasaki S, Imamura H, Kobayashi A, Noike T, Miwa S, Miyagawa S. Results of surgical resection for patients with hilar bile duct cancer: application of extended hepatectomy after biliary drainage and hemihepatic portal vein embolization. *Ann Surg*. 2003;238:84-92.
7. Rea DJ, Munoz-Juarez M, Farnell MB, et al. Major hepatic resection for hilar cholangiocarcinoma: analysis of 46 patients. *Arch Surg*. 2004;139:514-523; discussion 23–5.
8. Kondo S, Hirano S, Ambo Y, et al. Forty consecutive resections of hilar cholangiocarcinoma with no postoperative mortality and no positive ductal margins: results of a prospective study. *Ann Surg*. 2004;240:95-101.
9. Hemming AW, Reed AI, Fujita S, Foley DP, Howard RJ. Surgical management of hilar cholangiocarcinoma. *Ann Surg*. 2005;241:693-699; discussion 9–702.
10. Dinant S, Gerhards MF, Rauws EA, Busch OR, Gouma DJ, van Gulik TM. Improved outcome of resection of hilar cholangiocarcinoma (Klatskin tumor). *Ann Surg Oncol*. 2006;13: 872-880.
11. Liu CL, Fan ST, Lo CM, Tso WK, Lam CM, Wong J. Improved operative and survival outcomes of surgical treatment for hilar cholangiocarcinoma. *Br J Surg*. 2006;93:1488-1494.
12. Baton O, Azoulay D, Adam DV, Castaing D. Major hepatectomy for hilar cholangiocarcinoma type 3 and 4: prognostic factors and longterm outcomes. *J Am Coll Surg*. 2007;204: 250-260.
13. Hasegawa S, Ikai I, Fujii H, Hatano E, Shimahara Y. Surgical resection of hilar cholangiocarcinoma: analysis of survival and postoperative complications. *World J Surg*. 2007;31: 1256-1263.
14. Hochwald SN, Burke EC, Jarnagin WR, Fong Y, Blumgart LH. Association of preoperative biliary stenting with increased postoperative infectious complications in proximal cholangiocarcinoma. *Arch Surg*. 1999;134:261-266.
15. Cherqui D, Benoist S, Malassagne B, Humeres R, Rodriguez V, Fagniez PL. Major liver resection for carcinoma in jaundiced patients without preoperative biliary drainage. *Arch Surg*. 2000;135:302-308.
16. Ishizawa T, Hasegawa K, Sano K, Imamura H, Kokudo N, Makuuchi M. Selective versus total biliary drainage for obstructive jaundice caused by a hepatobiliary malignancy. *Am J Surg*. 2007;193:149-154.
17. Miyagawa S, Makuuchi M, Kawasaki S, Kakazu T. Criteria for safe hepatic resection. *Am J Surg*. 1995;169:589-594.
18. Imamura H, Shimada R, Kubota M, et al. Preoperative portal vein embolization: an audit of 84 patients. *Hepatology*. 1999;29:1099-1105.
19. Di Stefano DR, de Baere T, Denys A, et al. Preoperative percutaneous portal vein embolization: evaluation of adverse events in 188 patients. *Radiology*. 2005;234:625-630.
20. Ribero D, Abdalla EK, Madoff DC, Donadon M, Loyer EM, Vauthey JN. Portal vein embolization before major hepatectomy and its effects on regeneration, resectability and outcome. *Br J Surg*. 2007;94:1386-1394.
21. Madoff DC, Abdalla EK, Gupta S, et al. Transhepatic ipsilateral right portal vein embolization extended to segment IV: improving hypertrophy and resection outcomes with spherical particles and coils. *J Vasc Interv Radiol*. 2005;16:215-225.
22. Abulkhir A, Limongelli P, Healey AJ, et al. Preoperative portal vein embolization for major liver resection: a meta-analysis. *Ann Surg*. 2008;247:49-57.
23. Shimura T, Suehiro T, Suzuki H, Okada K, Araki K, Kuwano H. Trans-ileocecal portal vein embolization as a preoperative treatment for right trisegmentectomy with caudate lobectomy. *J Surg Oncol*. 2007;96:438-441.
24. Tsuge H, Mimura H, Kawata N, Orita K. Right portal embolization before extended right hepatectomy using laparoscopic catheterization of the ileocolic vein: a prospective study. *Surg Laparosc Endosc*. 1994;4:258-263.

Contralateral Approach to Portal Vein Embolization

16

Pierre Bize, Nicolas Demartines, and Alban Denys

Abstract

Percutaneous transhepatic portal vein embolization can be done by an ipsilateral approach (i.e., the puncture of a peripheral right portal vein branch to embolize the right portal branches) or by a contralateral approach (i.e., the puncture of a left portal branch and the embolization of the right portal branches). The choice of the access route is based upon clinical and technical considerations as well as the experience of the operator with one technique or another. The access route influences the choice of the embolic material. This chapter presents the advantages, disadvantages, and results of the contralateral approach.

Keywords

Portal vein embolization • Contralateral approach to portal vein embolization • Future liver remnant • Liver embolization

Portal vein embolization can be done by an ipsilateral approach (i.e., the puncture of a peripheral right portal vein branch to embolize right portal branches) or by a contralateral approach (i.e., the puncture of the left portal branch and the embolization of the right portal branches). The choice of the access route is based on clinical and technical considerations as well as the experience of the operator with one technique or the other. The access route influences the choice of the embolic material.

A. Denys (✉)
Department of Radiology and Interventional Radiology, CHUV, University of Lausanne, CH-1011 Lausanne, Switzerland
e-mail: alban.denys@chuv.ch

16.1 Advantages of the Contralateral Approach

The contralateral approach has the advantage of antegrade catheterization of the right portal branches, without the sharp angulation that is usually encountered during ipsilateral embolization. The embolic agent is delivered in a prograde, free-flowing manner into the portal venous blood flow to all segments that need to be embolized (Fig. 16.1). Portograms can be obtained easily after or during the embolization procedure without the risk of dislodging the embolic material.[1] It also avoids potential tumor seeding that might occur when puncturing the tumor-containing right liver. This approach can also be easily combined with preoperative drainage of the FLR in patients with hilar cholangiocarcinoma who are candidates for surgical resection.

D.C. Madoff et al. (eds.), *Venous Embolization of the Liver*,
DOI 10.1007/978-1-84882-122-4_16, © Springer-Verlag London Limited 2011

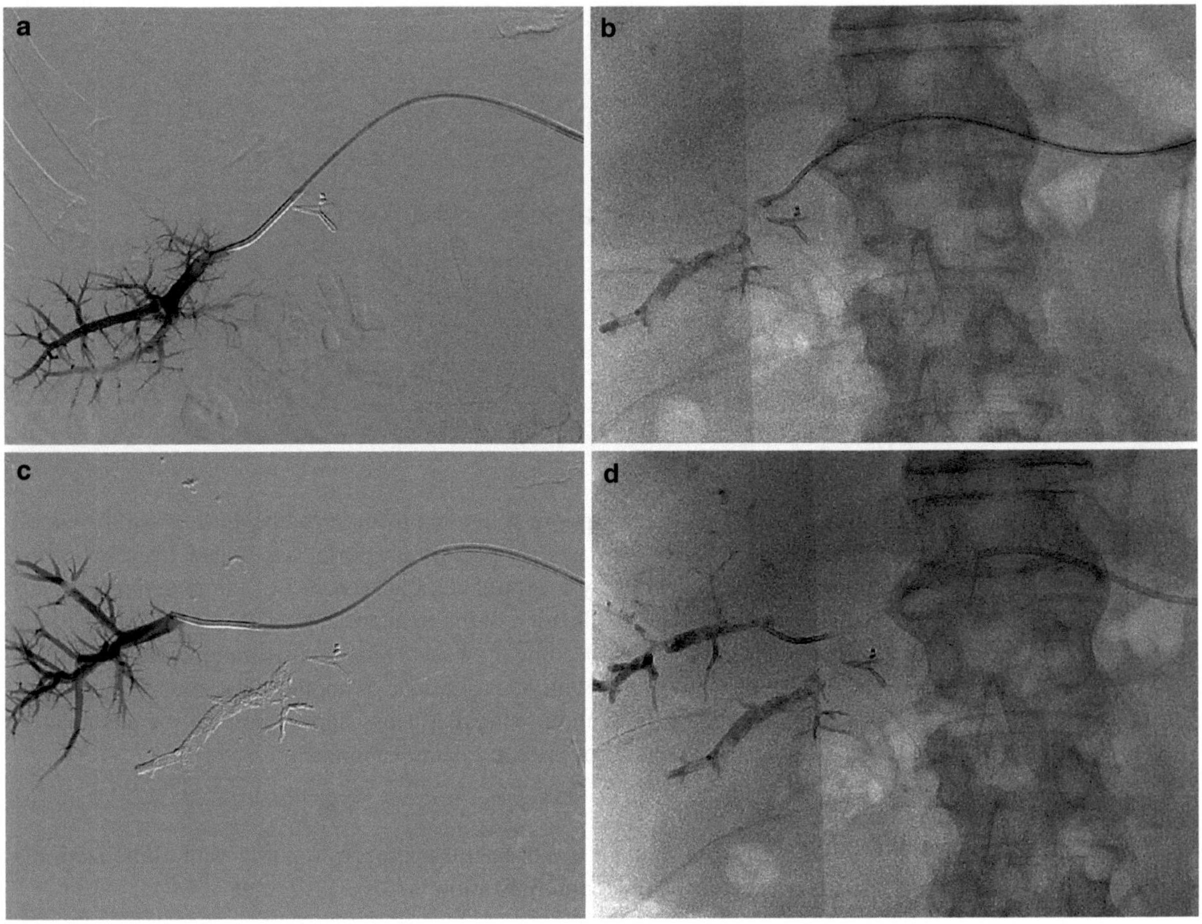

Fig. 16.1 Successive embolization of the right portal vein branches: (**a**) portal phlebography of segment 6 portal vein and (**b**) control after embolization with NCBA and Lipiodol. (**c**) Portal phlebography of segment 5 portal vein branch and (**d**) control after embolization with NCBA and Lipiodol. (Note the direct path of the catheter without angulation due to the contralateral access)

16.2 Disadvantages of the Contralateral Approach

The main disadvantage of this method is that the access is obtained through the future liver remnant (FLR) and any complication that might occur during the procedure can lead to damage of the FLR. In some cases, this damage can preclude future liver resection.[1] Furthermore, when segment 4 branch embolization is mandatory, catheterization may be tricky from the left side.

16.3 Embolization Method

We recommend performing the procedure under sedation or general anesthesia. A peripheral portal branch of the left portal vein is punctured under ultrasound (US) guidance, upstream of any branch bifurcation requiring embolization.[2] US allows us to identify the portal branch to be punctured and thus limits the need for multiple punctures. The portal vein of segment 3 is usually chosen because it is more anterior and easily located by US and allows access to segment 4 branches when needed. A puncture through the recess of Rex should be avoided as the peri-portal tissues are often thick and fibrotic in this area, making the Seldinger maneuver difficult. Access to segment 4 branches is more challenging due to the short distance and sharp angle between the access point and origin of segment 4 branches.

Contralateral approach is performed either using the Neff percutaneous access set (Cook, Bjaeverskov, Denmark) or using an 18-gauge echogenic-tipped needle (Chiba Biopsy Needle with Echogenic Tip, Angiotech, Gainesville, FL, USA) and a 0.035-in.

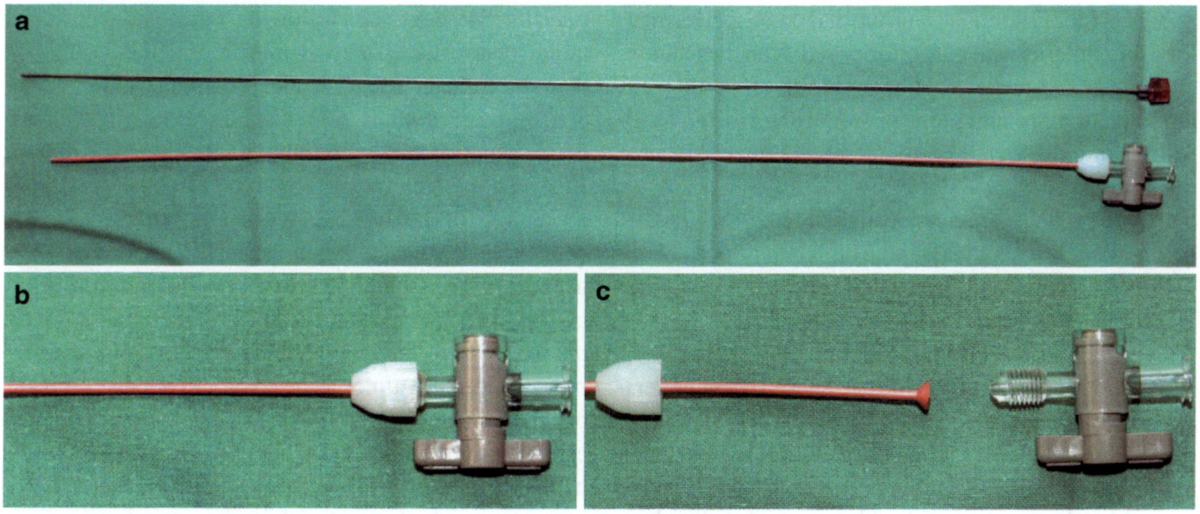

Fig. 16.2 (**a**) 5-Fr 40-cm Transhepatic Cholangiography Catheter (Cook, Bjaeverskov, Denmark)and 0.035-in. hydrophilic guidewire (Radifocus Guidewire, Terumo Europe, Leuven, Belgium) used for the delivery of *n*-butyl cyanoacrylate. (**b**, **c**) Showing detachable hub which allows flushing and multiple successive injections

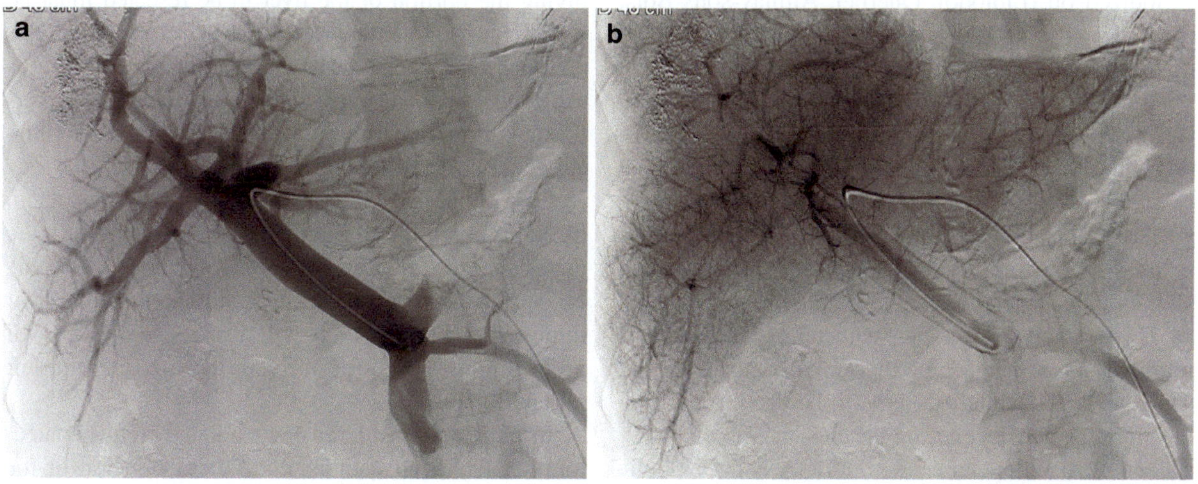

Fig. 16.3 Portography obtained through contralateral approach before right portal vein embolization: (**a**) portal phase and (**b**) parenchymal phase

hydrophilic guidewire (Radifocus Guidewire, Terumo Europe, Leuven, Belgium) (Fig. 16.2). Either a 5-Fr ring needle catheter or a 5-Fr introducer sheath is then placed in the portal system using the Seldinger technique. A standard polyethylene 5-Fr catheter is then inserted over the guidewire and placed at the splenomesenteric confluence to perform a portography. The anteroposterior position with 15° of the right anterior angulation allows better separation of the portal bifurcation. The portogram (Fig. 16.3) should allow detailed visualization of the portal system and recognition of any anatomical variants. The most frequent anatomical variant is joining of the right anterior portal vein with the left portal vein. New angiosystems allow volumetric acquisition during rotational acquisition and provide 3D views of the portal system. This may be helpful in case of an anatomical variant or in case of atypical portal embolization.[3-5] Care should be taken to localize segment 4 branches. The measurement of portal pressure should be done in every patient with chronic liver disease. Severe portal hypertension with a gradient over 12 mmHg is considered a relative contraindication to liver resection, making PVE not useful in this setting.[6]

Once the anatomical workup has been performed, the right anterior and posterior portal branches can be embolized. As with other techniques of portal vein embolization, the aim of the procedure is a distal, long-lasting embolization. Different embolic materials have been proposed.

Some products are not recommended:

- Gelfoam is associated with a high rate of portal vein recanalization and seems less efficient than other products.[1]
- Nonspherical polyvinyl alcohol particles have been used but are less efficient than more recent spherical particles.[7]
- The direct intraportal injection of alcohol has been described. Although efficient, it is hard to control and has been associated with severe complications (liver necrosis, portal vein thrombosis).[8]

The recommended products are[9]:

- The mixture of *n*-butyl cyanoacrylate (NBCA) and iodized oil (Lipiodol, Guerbet, Aulnay-sous-Bois, France) has been extensively described with good results and low morbidity.
- Spherical microparticles associated with coil embolization are used in North America and seem efficient, although less efficient than NBCA in animal studies.[10]
- The association of fibrin glue with iodized oil is used in Japan but needs special devoted 3-lumen balloon catheters that are available only in Asia.

The standard angiographic catheter used for the portography is exchanged for the embolization catheter. The choice of the catheter type to be used to perform the embolization depends on the chosen embolic material. In most European centers, NBCA is the embolic agent of choice. NBCA is a radiolucent liquid agent that polymerizes in ionic solutions. To perform embolization, NBCA is mixed with Lipiodol in a ratio of 1:1–1:3. Mixing NBCA with Lipiodol delays its polymerization and allows radiographic visualization of the embolic agent. By changing the NBCA/Lipiodol ratio, it is possible to adapt the polymerization time to individual and instant hemodynamic variations. The more the Lipiodol, the longer the polymerization time. This flexibility should allow distal and complete embolization in most situations. The NBCA/Lipiodol mixture is prepared in an insulin syringe immediately prior to the first embolization. The syringe is then connected to the embolization catheter with a three-way stopcock, and the embolic material is pushed with a nonionic solution (usually 5% dextrose) following the "sandwich technique": the volume of every injection should be smaller than the catheter's dead space. NBCA is usually delivered through a short 5-Fr catheter measuring 40 cm (Transhepatic Cholangiography Catheter needle, Cook, Bjaeverskov, Denmark). This type of catheter has the advantage of being easy to handle and provides a smaller dead space, which is especially important when using this type of embolic agent.[1] Furthermore, its hub can be disconnected and flushed easily allowing multiple successive injections (Fig. 16.2). This can be repeated as many times as necessary to obtain complete occlusion of the target vessel. If occlusion of the catheter by embolic material occurs, this can be addressed by passing a 0.035-in. guidewire gently in the catheter lumen to push the material in the embolized vessel under fluoroscopic guidance. We recommend careful flushing of the catheter and the hub between injections of NBCA to avoid occlusion. All portal branches supplying the portion of the liver to be resected must be embolized. Segmental branches are occluded one after the other until occlusion of the whole target segment is achieved. Supraselective embolization can be performed through a micro-catheter (Progreat, Terumo Europe, Leuven, Belgium) when needed.

Care should be taken to leave approximately 1 cm of the proximal main right portal vein free of embolic material as the inflammatory reaction caused by NCBA can make the surgical division and suture difficult or impossible (Fig. 16.4). It will also reduce the risk of propagation of right portal vein thrombus to the left portal branch.

In patients considered for extended right hepatectomy, it has been demonstrated that extension of the right liver embolization to segment 4 significantly improves the reactive hypertrophy of segments 2 and 3.[5] The embolization of segment 4 can be challenging as multiple branches supply this segment. These branches usually arise from the left portal branch, and the reflux of embolic material will result in the nontarget embolization of FLR and the potential complete occlusion of the portal vein. When it has to be done through a contralateral approach, segment 4 embolization can be performed after the embolization of the right liver. This usually allows a better depiction of segment 4 portal branches as they will become dilated and more apparent after right liver embolization. It will also diminish the risk of dislodging the embolic material during catheter exchange (Fig. 16.5). When

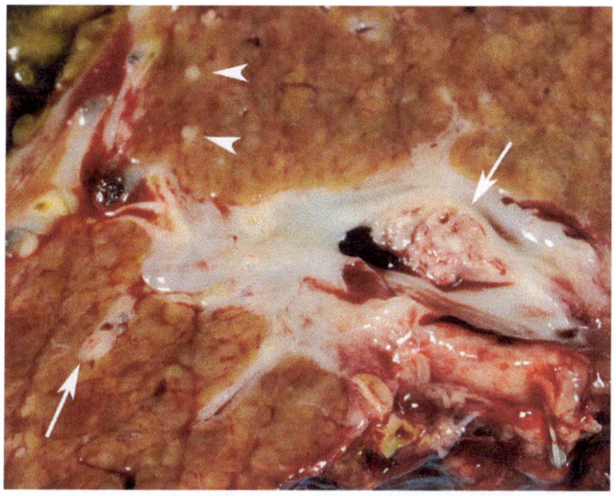

Fig. 16.4 Macroscopic view of embolic material in the right portal vein branches (*arrows*). There is an intense inflammatory reaction around the portal spaces. The inflammation around the portal spaces can be seen even in small order peripheral portal branches (*arrowheads*)

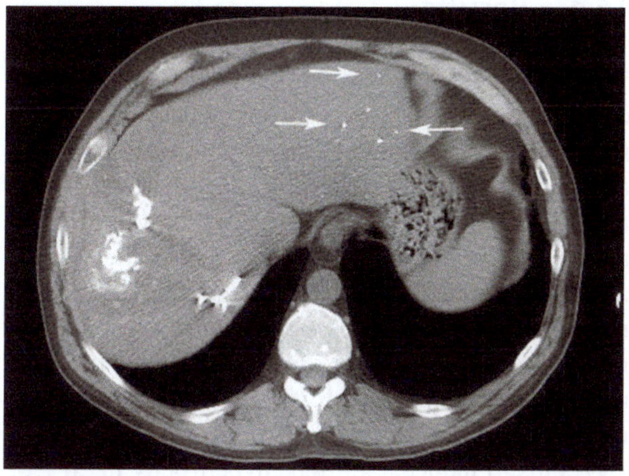

Fig. 16.5 CT scanner (without contrast media) performed 1 month after right portal vein embolization. There are small particles of embolic material located in the distal extremities of the left portal vein branches (*white arrows*). This migration probably occurred during catheter manipulation during the embolization procedure and did not have any negative influence on FLR hypertrophy

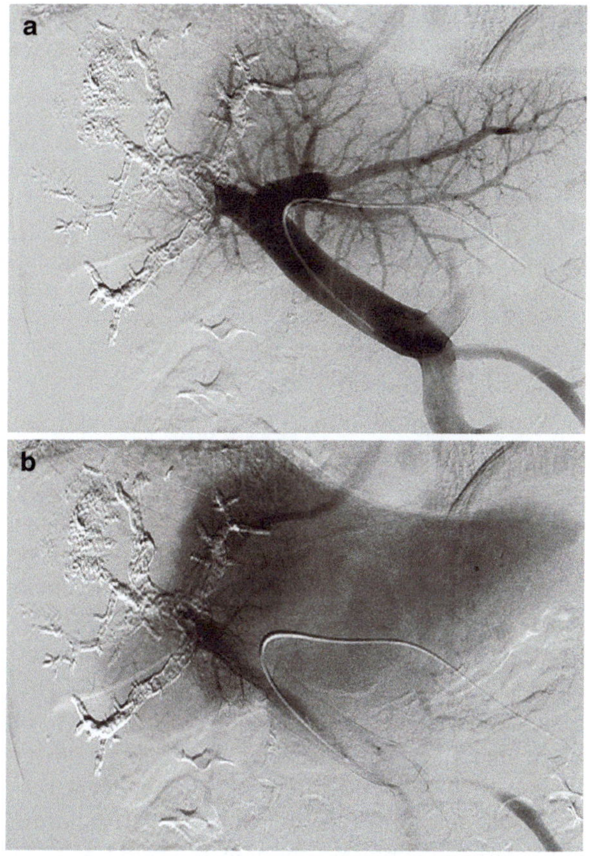

Fig. 16.6 Portography obtained though contralateral approach after the embolization of all right portal vein branches: (**a**) portal phase and (**b**) parenchymal phase. There is no contrast media flowing through the right portal vein branch and no parenchymal enhancement of the right liver

the anatomic configuration is such that there is a significant risk of reflux into the FLR, particles can be used to embolize segment 4 branches to diminish the consequences of potential reflux.[11]

Embolization should be done until complete stasis in the embolized branches and redistribution of the flow only to the FLR branches is achieved. A final portography is mandatory to verify this objective. A parenchymography should be visible only in the FLR (Fig. 16.6).

Complete embolization might be difficult to achieve, particularly in small portal branches. If the risk of potential reflux into branches of the FLR is judged to be too high, it might be better to leave some targeted branches patent rather than risk complete portal vein occlusion.

Final pressure measurement should be obtained at the end of the procedure in all patients with chronic liver disease in order to document the portal pressure increase, which is usually around 3 mmHg. At the end of the procedure, the catheter is removed without the embolization of the transhepatic tract. The puncture site is gently compressed for 5 min.

Table 16.1 FLR hypertrophy after portal vein embolization in normal and diseased liver

Author	Hypertrophy of FLR (%) in a normal liver	Hypertrophy of FLR (%) in a diseased liver	Hypertrophy of FLR (%) in all patients
Elias[20]			54
De Baere[21]			64
Roche[14]	83±58		
Vauthey[22]	36		
Azoulay[23]		46±24	
Farges[17]	44±19	35±28	
Di Stefano[11]	62	41	
Denys[16]		41±32	

When performed from the left side through the FLR, PVE can be easily combined with the percutaneous drainage of the left bile ducts in case of biliary obstruction such as in Klatskin tumor. The percutaneous drainage of the left bile ducts can be difficult or impossible from the right side in the case of a Bismuth type 3 or 4 hilar cholangiocarcinoma.

PVE can also be combined with the radiofrequency ablation (RFA) of metastasis located in the FLR. This association has been reported to avoid the growth of tumor located in the FLR after PVE.[12] Both procedures can be performed in the same treatment session: Both punctures (the insertion of the RFA needle and access to the portal vein branch) should be done before the RFA or PVE is initiated as the visibility of the targets (portal vein for PVE or tumor for RFA) can then be altered by artifacts.[1] Once both punctures are performed, RFA should be initiated first. This allows one to obtain a post-RFA portogram that will confirm the portal vein patency in the FLR before PVE is initiated.

16.3.1 Medication and Periprocedural Cure

The procedure can be done as an out-patient procedure, but many centers prefer to do it during a 2-day hospital stay. The procedure is done under intravenous sedation or general anesthesia. Antibiotics are not given as a standard of care[13] except in patients needing a simultaneous biliary procedure. Post PVE, some authors report mild to moderate abdominal pain in 20–30% of patients controlled by oral analgesia.[14]

Biological tests are not mandatory after the procedure. The prothrombin time remains above 70% of the baseline value. A slight elevation of AST and ALT with a peak increase up to threefold on day 3 after the procedure has been reported but without clinical significance.[14] Increases in the bilirubin level are insignificant. The use of pure alcohol as embolic material is associated with more severe abdominal pain and cytolysis.

16.4 Results

Technical success rate should be close to 100%. Rare cases of failures or of repeat procedures have been reported in the literature.[9,15] Resection rate should be around 85%. This rate may even decrease to 70% in the case of cirrhotic patients. Reasons for nonresection are tumor progression, overt peritoneal metastases, and the absence of hypertrophy (found in 20% of cirrhotic patients). In patients with liver metastases occurring in a normal liver, the increase of the FLR/TLV ratio is between 8% and 25%, and regeneration is nearly always observed after PVE. In cirrhotic patients, PVE fails to induce a left lobe hypertrophy in 20% of cases. The increase rate of the FLR/TLV ratio in this population is slightly lower (between 6% and 20%).

Recent studies have demonstrated that the factor that influences the regeneration most is the FLR/TLV ratio before PVE, which means that the smaller the left lobe, the more pronounced will be its regeneration.[16] Very small left lobes should not be considered as a contraindication for PVE. The degree of liver fibrosis has also been reported as an important factor influencing FLR regeneration in patients with chronic liver disease: All patients with normal liver develop FLR hypertrophy as compared to patients with chronic liver disease, only 86% of whom develop hypertrophy[17] (Table 16.1).

Table 16.2 Complications after portal vein embolization

	Reported rate (%)
Minor complications	
Abdominal pain	20
Fever	25
Nausea	2.5
Embolic material displaced into the future liver remnant	0.2
Major complications	
Liver abscess	0.3
Cholangitis	0.2
Main or left portal vein thrombosis	0.2
Subcapsular hematoma	0.2
Portal hypertension	0.1

16.5 Complications

In the hands of experienced teams, the complication rate is very low. The most frequently reported complications are pneumothorax, subcapsular hematoma, arterial pseudoaneurysm, and portal vein thrombosis. Other complications include hemobilia, liver abscesses, and transient liver insufficiency.[9,11,18,19] In terms of complications (Table 16.2), a rate of minor complications of 20–25% is acceptable. The rate of major complications should be below 5% and should not preclude further liver resection.

References

1. de Baere T, Denys A, Madoff DC. Preoperative portal vein embolization: indications and technical considerations. *Tech Vasc Interv Radiol*. 2007;10:67-78.
2. de Baere T, Roche A, Elias D, Lasser P, Lagrange C, Bousson V. Preoperative portal vein embolization for extension of hepatectomy indications. *Hepatology*. 1996;24:1386-1391.
3. Orth RC, Wallace MJ, Kuo MD. C-arm cone-beam CT: general principles and technical considerations for use in interventional radiology. *J Vasc Interv Radiol*. 2008;19:814-820.
4. Wallace MJ. C-arm computed tomography for guiding hepatic vascular interventions. *Tech Vasc Interv Radiol*. 2007;10:79-86.
5. Kishi Y, Madoff DC, Abdalla EK, et al. Is embolization of segment 4 portal veins before extended right hepatectomy justified? *Surgery*. 2008;144:744-751.
6. Bruix J, Castells A, Bosch J, et al. Surgical resection of hepatocellular carcinoma in cirrhotic patients: prognostic value of preoperative portal pressure. *Gastroenterology*. 1996;111:1018-1022.
7. Madoff DC, Abdalla EK, Gupta S, et al. Transhepatic ipsilateral right portal vein embolization extended to segment IV: improving hypertrophy and resection outcomes with spherical particles and coils. *J Vasc Interv Radiol*. 2005;16:215-225.
8. Shimamura T, Nakajima Y, Une Y, et al. Efficacy and safety of preoperative percutaneous transhepatic portal embolization with absolute ethanol: a clinical study. *Surgery*. 1997;121:135-141.
9. Abulkhir A, Limongelli P, Healey AJ, et al. Preoperative portal vein embolization for major liver resection: a meta-analysis. *Ann Surg*. 2008;247:49-57.
10. de Baere T, Denys A, Paradis V. Comparison of four embolic materials for portal vein embolization: experimental study in pigs. *Eur Radiol*. 2009;19:1435-1442.
11. Di Stefano DR, de Baere T, Denys A, et al. Preoperative percutaneous portal vein embolization: evaluation of adverse events in 188 patients. *Radiology*. 2005;234:625-630.
12. Elias D, Santoro R, Ouellet JF, Osmak L, de Baere T, Roche A. Simultaneous percutaneous right portal vein embolization and left liver tumor radiofrequency ablation prior to a major right hepatic resection for bilateral colorectal metastases. *Hepatogastroenterology*. 2004;51:1788-1791.
13. Madoff DC, Abdalla EK, Vauthey JN. Portal vein embolization in preparation for major hepatic resection: evolution of a new standard of care. *J Vasc Interv Radiol*. 2005;16:779-790.
14. Roche A, Lasser P, de Baere T, Elias D. Preoperative portal embolization: an effective means for inducing hypertrophy of the healthy liver and increasing indications for hepatic resection. *Chirurgie*. 1998;123:67-72. discussion 73.
15. Elias D, Ouellet JF, De Baere T, Lasser P, Roche A. Preoperative selective portal vein embolization before hepatectomy for liver metastases: long-term results and impact on survival. *Surgery*. 2002;131:294-299.
16. Denys A, Lacombe C, Schneider F, et al. Portal vein embolization with N-butyl cyanoacrylate before partial hepatectomy in patients with hepatocellular carcinoma and underlying cirrhosis or advanced fibrosis. *J Vasc Interv Radiol*. 2005;16:1667-1674.
17. Farges O, Belghiti J, Kianmanesh R, et al. Portal vein embolization before right hepatectomy: prospective clinical trial. *Ann Surg*. 2003;237:208-217.
18. Kodama Y, Shimizu T, Endo H, Miyamoto N, Miyasaka K. Complications of percutaneous transhepatic portal vein embolization. *J Vasc Interv Radiol*. 2002;13:1233-1237.
19. Abdalla EK, Hicks ME, Vauthey JN. Portal vein embolization: rationale, technique and future prospects. *Br J Surg*. 2001;88:165-175.
20. Elias D, Roche A, Vavasseur D, Lasser P. Induction of hypertrophy of a small left hepatic lobe by preoperative right portal embolization, preceding extended right hepatectomy. *Ann Chir*. 1992;46:404-410.
21. de Baere T, Roche A, Vavasseur D, et al. Portal vein embolization: utility for inducing left hepatic lobe hypertrophy before surgery. *Radiology*. 1993;188:73-77.
22. Vauthey JN, Chaoui A, Do KA, et al. Standardized measurement of the future liver remnant prior to extended liver resection: methodology and clinical associations. *Surgery*. 2000;127:512-529.
23. Azoulay D, Castaing D, Krissat J, et al. Percutaneous portal vein embolization increases the feasibility and safety of major liver resection for hepatocellular carcinoma in injured liver. *Ann Surg*. 2000;232:665-672.

The Ipsilateral Approach for Right PVE with or Without Segment 4

17

David C. Madoff

Abstract

Portal vein embolization (PVE) is now considered the standard of care to improve the safety for patients undergoing major hepatectomy with an anticipated small future liver remnant (FLR). PVE can induce contralateral liver hypertrophy in preparation for major liver resection and can be performed with various approaches. Which approach is chosen may be dependent on operator preference and on the type and extent of the subsequent resection. This chapter describes the transhepatic ipsilateral approach, an approach whereby access to the portal system is via the liver to be resected. The advantages and disadvantages of this approach will also be discussed.

Keywords

Embolization • Future liver remnant • Liver hypertrophy • Liver resection • Portal vein

Portal vein embolization (PVE) can be performed by any of three standard approaches: the intraoperative transileocolic venous approach, the transhepatic contralateral approach, and the transhepatic ipsilateral approach.[1] It is important to note that the approach to the portal vein is chosen at the discretion of the operator, and the decision may be based on multiple factors, including the extent of the embolization and surgery, the operator's preference for a specific embolic agent, the tumor burden within the liver, and the operator's level of experience with one technique over another.

D.C. Madoff
Division of Interventional Radiology, Department of Radiology, New York-Presbyterian Hospital/Weill Cornell Medical Center, 525 E 68th Street P-518, New York, NY 10065, USA
e-mail: dcm9006@med.cornell.edu

This chapter describes the technical aspects of performing PVE using the ipsilateral approach whether or not segment 4 embolization is also required.

17.1 Ipsilateral Technique

The percutaneous transhepatic ipsilateral approach was initially described by Nagino and colleagues[2] in the mid-1990s, and it is now utilized by many other researchers worldwide.[3-6] With this approach, portal venous access is obtained within the tumor-bearing liver (i.e., liver to be resected). A distinct advantage of the ipsilateral approach is that the future liver remnant (FLR) is not instrumented. Therefore, parenchymal injury from the percutaneous puncture, or left portal vein injury or thrombosis as a direct result of the catheterization is very unlikely. Furthermore, should

D.C. Madoff et al. (eds.), *Venous Embolization of the Liver*,
DOI 10.1007/978-1-84882-122-4_17, © Springer-Verlag London Limited 2011

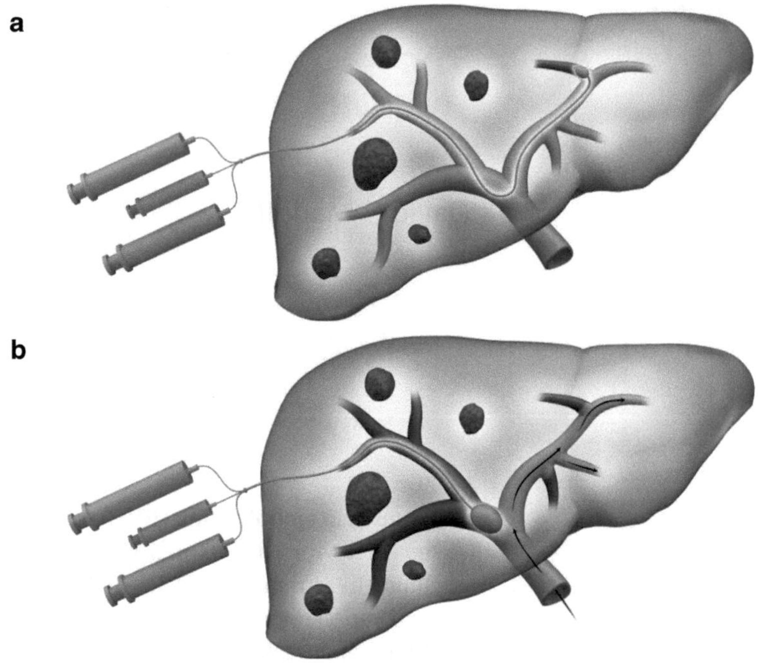

Fig. 17.1 Schematic representation of the ipsilateral approach for RPVE and segment 4 as described by Nagino and coworkers. Different balloon catheters are used for the antegrade embolization of segment 4 veins (**a**) and for the retrograde delivery of the embolic agent into the right portal system (**b**)

embolization of segment 4 be required, it allows for more straightforward catheterization of the segment 4 branches.

When planning the puncture, the anterior sector of the right portal vein is preferred over the posterior sector, since its use has been associated with a lower complication rate.[7] However, catheterization of the right portal venous branches can be challenging owing to the sharp angulation of the right portal veins from the ipsilateral approach. For this reason, reverse curve catheters or balloon occlusion catheters with multiple lumina are usually needed.[2-5]

In Nagino's original method, the right anterior sector portal vein is punctured using sonographic guidance, and a 6-Fr sheath is introduced into the right portal system.[2] To make this procedure feasible, the authors designed two types of 5.5-Fr triple-lumen balloon catheters. The first ("type 1") catheter was designed with one lumen connected to the balloon and two lumina connected to the tip (Fig. 17.1a). The second ("type 2") catheter had two separate lumina open proximal to the balloon (Fig. 17.1b). The balloons were used to prevent any backflow of embolic material. Both catheters had two separate lumina so that fibrin glue and iodized oil could be injected simultaneously. To facilitate hepatic resection, the authors advocated that a proximal right portal vein segment at least 1 cm in length remain patent. Depending on the portal vein anatomy, the need to spare the proximal right portal vein, and the utility of segment 4 embolization, type 1 or type 2 catheters were used for embolization. The type 1 catheter was used for embolization of branches distal to the catheter tip, whereas the type 2 catheter was used for embolization of branches proximal to the catheter tip, as mandated by each patient's portal vein anatomy.

In a more recent study, Gibo and colleagues[5] modified the technique described by Nagino by utilizing a four-lumen balloon catheter in eight patients. The authors recommended using this modified catheter because of its larger occlusion balloon and lumina, which allowed for safer and easier embolization using fibrin glue. Unfortunately, neither the original nor the modified catheters are presently available in the United States.

The ipsilateral approach is also advocated by Western operators. In the early 2000s, Madoff and colleagues reported on a technique using standard angiographic catheters that are commercially available worldwide[3,4] (Fig. 17.2). Under sonographic guidance, a 22-gauge Chiba needle (Neff Percutaneous Access Set; Cook Medical, Bloomington, IN) is used to puncture the distal branch of the right portal system.

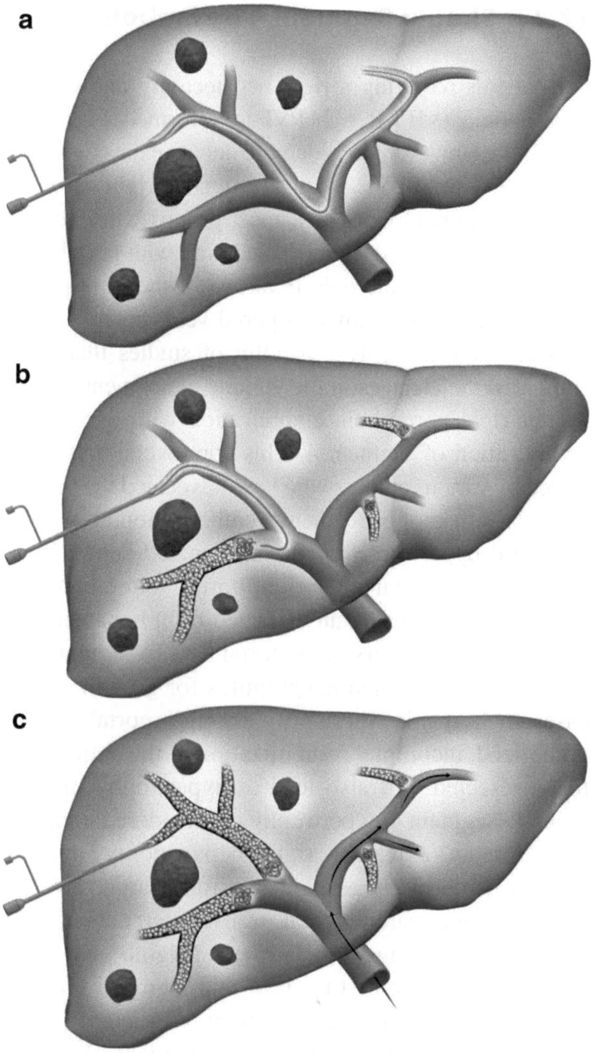

Fig. 17.2 Schematic representation shows the modification of the ipsilateral technique for RPVE extended to segment 4. (**a**) Placement of a 6-Fr vascular sheath into the right portal branch. An angled 5-Fr catheter is placed into the left portal system with the coaxial placement of a microcatheter into a segment 4 branch. Particulate embolization is performed, followed by the placement of coils until all the branches are occluded. (**b**) After segment 4 embolization is completely occluded, a 5-Fr reverse curve catheter is used for RPVE. (**c**) After embolization of the right and segment 4 portal veins is complete, the access tract is embolized with coils to prevent subcapsular hemorrhage

Subsequently, a 5- or 6-Fr vascular sheath is advanced over a guidewire into the right portal vein branch to aid with subsequent catheter manipulations and exchanges. Flush portography is performed with a 5-Fr angiographic flush catheter placed within the main portal vein. Anteroposterior and craniocaudal projections are obtained as needed to delineate the portal anatomy. Oblique views are not routinely used as these views may make understanding the anatomy more difficult due to the overlapping of the right portal veins with the segment 4 portal veins.

When embolization of the right portal vein is extended to segment 4, it is recommended by many that segment 4 embolization should be performed first.[4,8] This sequence is advocated due to the potential difficulty of exchanging catheters through a previously embolized right portal venous system and the possibility of dislodging embolic material from the right liver during the subsequent cannulation of the segment 4 portal veins. Furthermore, in the unlikely event that left portal vein thrombosis or injury occurs during segment 4 embolization, the procedure can be abandoned, and the patient may still remain a candidate for resection or future transcatheter therapies. Should a complication occur in the left liver following right portal vein embolization, the patient and the operator are left with few treatment options. Despite these issues, other operators suggest that performing embolization of the right portal system first may help with the catheterization of segment 4 portal veins due to the increased flow, especially when the branches are small and at difficult angulations.

At M. D. Anderson Cancer Center, segment 4 is usually embolized with a 3-Fr microcatheter placed coaxially through a selective 5-Fr angiographic catheter. Early in their experience, polyvinyl alcohol (PVA) particles ranging from 355 to 1,000 μm in diameter (Contour SE Microspheres, Boston Scientific) were the embolic agents of choice.[3] PVA was administered in a stepwise fashion: smaller particles (355–500 μm) were used first to occlude the distal branches, and larger particles (up to 1,000 μm) were used subsequently to occlude more proximally. Larger-sized particles were not used until the forward portal blood flow was considerably reduced. Additional embolization with the larger particles was then performed until near-complete stasis was achieved. Later, with the advent of spherical embolic agents, tris-acryl gelatin microspheres (EmboGold Microspheres, Biosphere Medical, Rockland, MA) became the embolic agents of choice.[4] The microspheres used in their study ranged from 100 to 700 μm in diameter and were administered in a stepwise fashion, similar to the method used for the PVA particles. After particulate embolization was complete, platinum microcoils were then placed within the proximal segment 4 branches to further reduce the portal blood inflow that could lead to recanalization.

For right portal vein embolization, the working 5-Fr catheter is then exchanged for a 5-Fr reverse curve catheter (Sos-2, Angiodynamics) to enable the delivery of the particulate embolic agent. These catheters are chosen for their ease of manipulation into the right portal branches, given the severe angulation of the right portal tree with the ipsilateral approach. As with segment 4 embolization, smaller particles are used first to occlude the distal, smaller portal branches, and the larger particles are used later to occlude the more proximal, larger branches. After near-complete stasis is achieved, 0.035- or 0.038-in. embolization coils (Gianturco, Cook Medical, Bloomington, IN) are placed within the secondary portal branches to further reduce the portal inflow that could lead to recanalization. A final portogram is obtained through the current 5-Fr catheter positioned within the main portal vein to assess the completeness of the embolization. The 5-Fr working catheter is not exchanged for the flush catheter for the final portogram so as not to dislodge the embolic material forward to the left portal system. At the completion of the procedure, the access tract is embolized with coils and/or gelfoam to minimize the risk of bleeding at the liver puncture site.

Overall, the ipsilateral approach is safe and effective for achieving FLR hypertrophy preoperatively. While disadvantages of the ipsilateral approach do exist, they are minor. As mentioned above, catheterization and embolization of the right portal vein branches may be challenging due to the severe angulations between right portal branches; however, this is rarely a problem when reverse curve catheters are used. Also, should catheters need to be exchanged, the exchange may need to take place through previously treated portal veins. However, if possible, the portal vein that was accessed should be embolized last. Considerable care should be used during catheter manipulations should they be needed. Finally, operators also need to be aware that the ipsilateral approach carries the risk of puncture through tumor tissues when multiple or large tumors are present, which could theoretically lead to bleeding or tumor seeding. Therefore, if these concerns do exist in a particular patient, the contralateral approach may be an option.

17.2 Should Segment 4 Be Embolized?

For patients requiring a right hepatectomy and have a small anticipated FLR, right PVE is performed (Figs. 17.3 and 17.4). However, considerable debate exists as to the optimal extent of PVE when an extended right hepatectomy is required.[9] Currently, most groups who prepare patients for extended right hepatectomy with portal vein embolization occlude only branches of the right portal vein and leave the segment 4 portal veins patent.[10,11] At present, there are only a handful of studies that have compared the changes in the volume of segments 2 and 3 after right portal vein embolization with or without embolization of segment 4. This controversy has been fueled by various authors who have advocated the benefit or the lack thereof of segment 4 embolization.

While hypertrophy of the anticipated future liver remnant does occur after right portal vein embolization, in patients where an extended right hepatectomy is required, full diversion of portal flow to segments 2, 3 ± 1 ensures the maximal stimulus for growth.[12-16] In cases such as this where only the right portal vein is embolized, incomplete embolization of the entire liver to be resected will also lead to hypertrophy of segment 4. Segment 4 hypertrophy is considered undesirable for an extended right hepatectomy due to increased morbidity associated with a larger area of intraoperative parenchymal transection across this hypertrophic segment.[12] Further, Nagino and colleagues[13] were the first to show that a greater left lateral bisegment hypertrophy occurs after right portal vein embolization extended to segment 4 (50% increase in FLR volume) than after only right portal vein embolization (31% increase, $P<.0005$). Recent studies have supported Nagino's conclusions without any increase in procedural-associated complications.[14,16] Because segment 4 embolization has been shown to be advantageous, the ipsilateral approach for right portal vein embolization extended to segment 4 has been further refined, and this has led to improved hypertrophy of the anticipated future liver remnant and operative outcomes.[4]

Another potential benefit of extending right portal vein embolization to include segment 4, from an oncological perspective, is that the entire tumor-bearing liver is systematically embolized (i.e., right portal vein embolization for right hepatectomy, right portal vein embolization extended to segment 4 for extended right hepatectomy) to reduce the risk of tumor growth that may result from increased portal blood flow and hepatotrophic factors.[17,18] A recent study from a large academic cancer center evaluated 112 patients where the entire tumor-bearing liver was systematically embolized and found no increase in the median tumor size during the waiting period.[17] However, tumor growth within the non-embolized liver has been discussed upon analysis of a very limited number of patients with primary and secondary liver tumors after right portal vein embolization alone (although no comparison to pre-embolization tumor growth rate was made so the true effect of portal vein embolization on tumor growth could not be proven).[19,20] At this time, the oncological effects of segment 4 embolization on tumor growth remain unclear. However, from the perspective of achieving better hypertrophy of the left lateral liver,

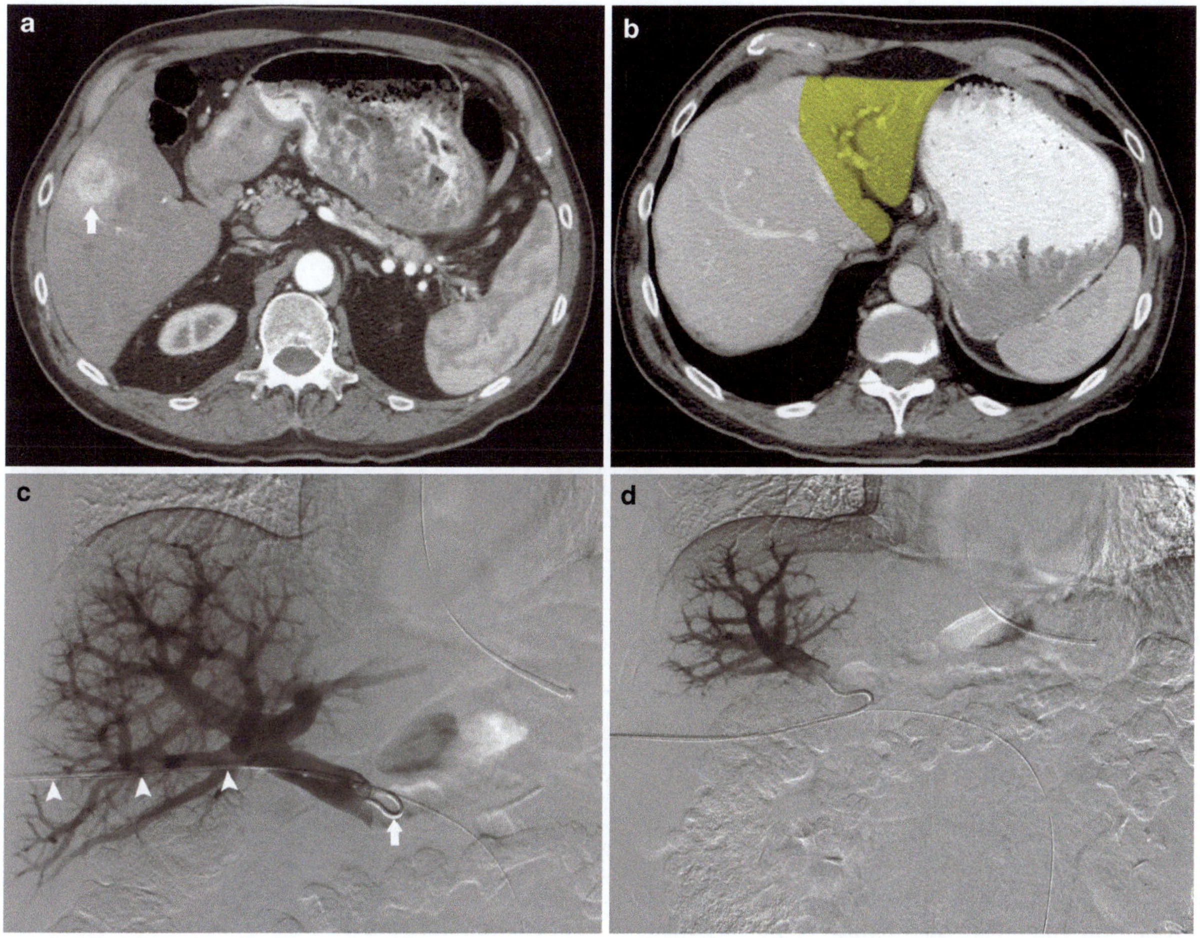

Fig. 17.3 A 69-year-old man with metastatic insulinoma to the right liver. He underwent an ipsilateral right portal vein embolization to induce hypertrophy of the left liver before right hepatectomy. (**a**) Contrast-enhanced CT scan obtained in the arterial phase shows a hypervascular mass in segment 6 of the liver (*arrow*). (**b**) Contrast-enhanced CT scan of the liver in the portal phase shows a small left liver with an FLR/TELV of 16% (*shaded area*). (**c**) Anteriorposterior flush portogram from the ipsilateral approach shows a 6-Fr vascular sheath (*arrowheads*) in a right portal vein branch and a 5-Fr flush catheter (*arrow*) in the main portal vein. (**d**) Contrast portography performed through a 5-Fr reverse curve catheter shows the catheterization of the segment 8 portal vein. (**e**) After coil embolization of the right anterior sector portal vein (*arrow*), the reverse curve catheter is now seen within the segment 7 portal vein. (**f**) Post-procedure anteroposterior flush portogram shows occlusion of the portal vein branches to segments 5–8 (*white arrows*) with continued patency of the vein supplying the left liver (*black arrow*). An *arrowhead* shows the subtracted contrast within a right portal vein branch overlying the left liver. (**g**) A later phase of portogram confirms persistent flow to the left liver (*arrows*). (**h**) Contrast-enhanced CT scan of the liver performed 1 month after RPVE shows hypertrophy of the left liver within the *shaded area* (FLR/TELV of 34%). The patient later underwent an uneventful right hepatectomy

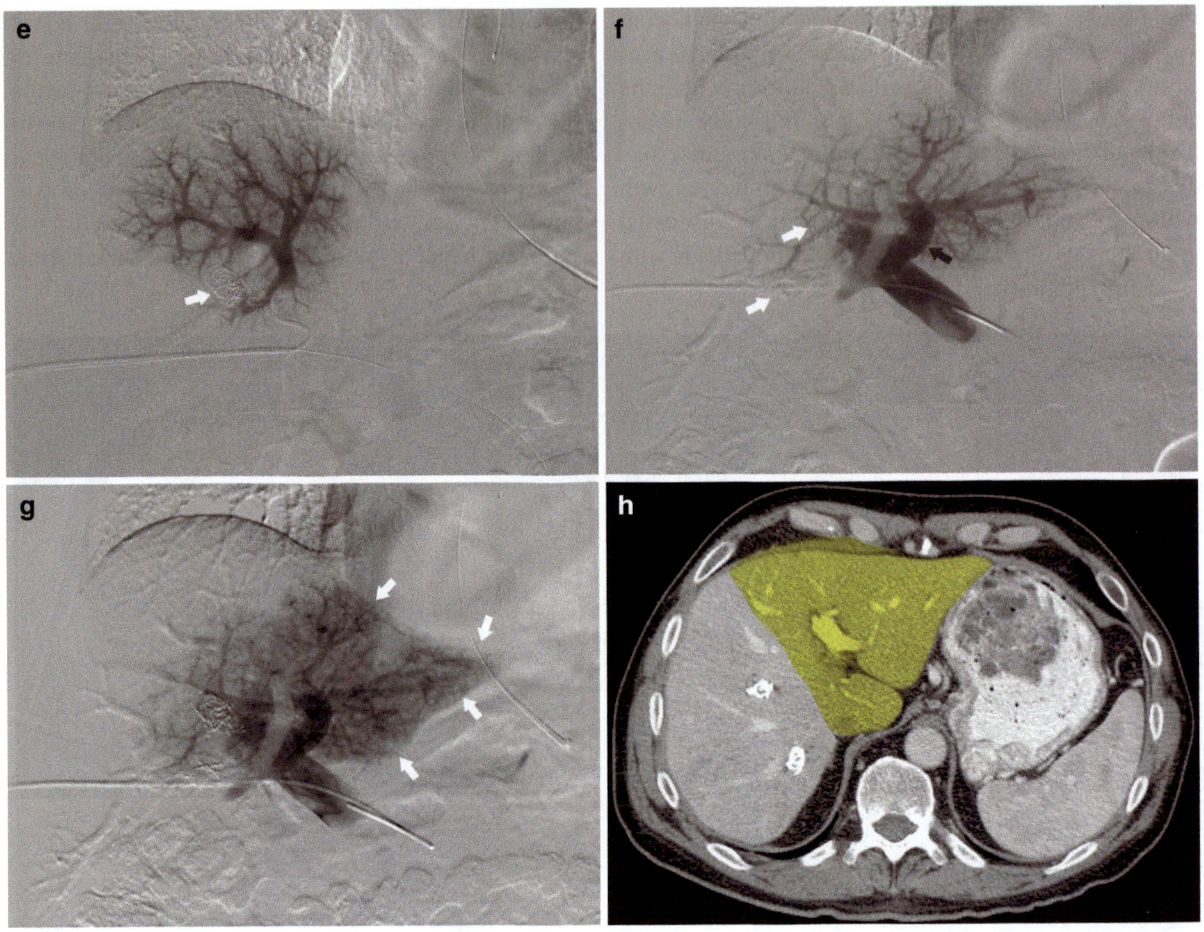

Fig. 17.3 (continued)

our approach at M. D. Anderson Cancer Center has been to perform right PVE extended to segment 4 whenever possible.

Despite the potential advantages described above, Capussotti and colleagues,[10] in 2005, reported similar FLR volume increases in patients treated with right portal vein embolization, whether or not segment 4 was also treated. In addition, they believe that extending right portal vein embolization to include segment 4 is theoretically associated with a higher risk of migration of embolization materials to left lateral portal vein branches and takes considerable technical expertise that may not be available at many centers. Therefore, because of this perceived risk of non-target embolization and their lack of evidence for improved hypertrophy, these authors concluded that embolization of segment 4 should not be routinely performed. This notion, however, has not been borne out in a study from an institution where right PVE and right PVE extended to segment 4 are performed[17] depending on the specific indications for performing the procedure.

17.3 Conclusion

Preoperative portal vein embolization is a safe and effective method of inducing hypertrophy of the anticipated future remnant liver before major hepatic resection. The percutaneous transhepatic ipsilateral approach is now becoming more widely used. However, there remains controversy as to whether or not right portal vein embolization should be extended to segment 4. Further study of this important topic will be necessary before definitive conclusions can be made.

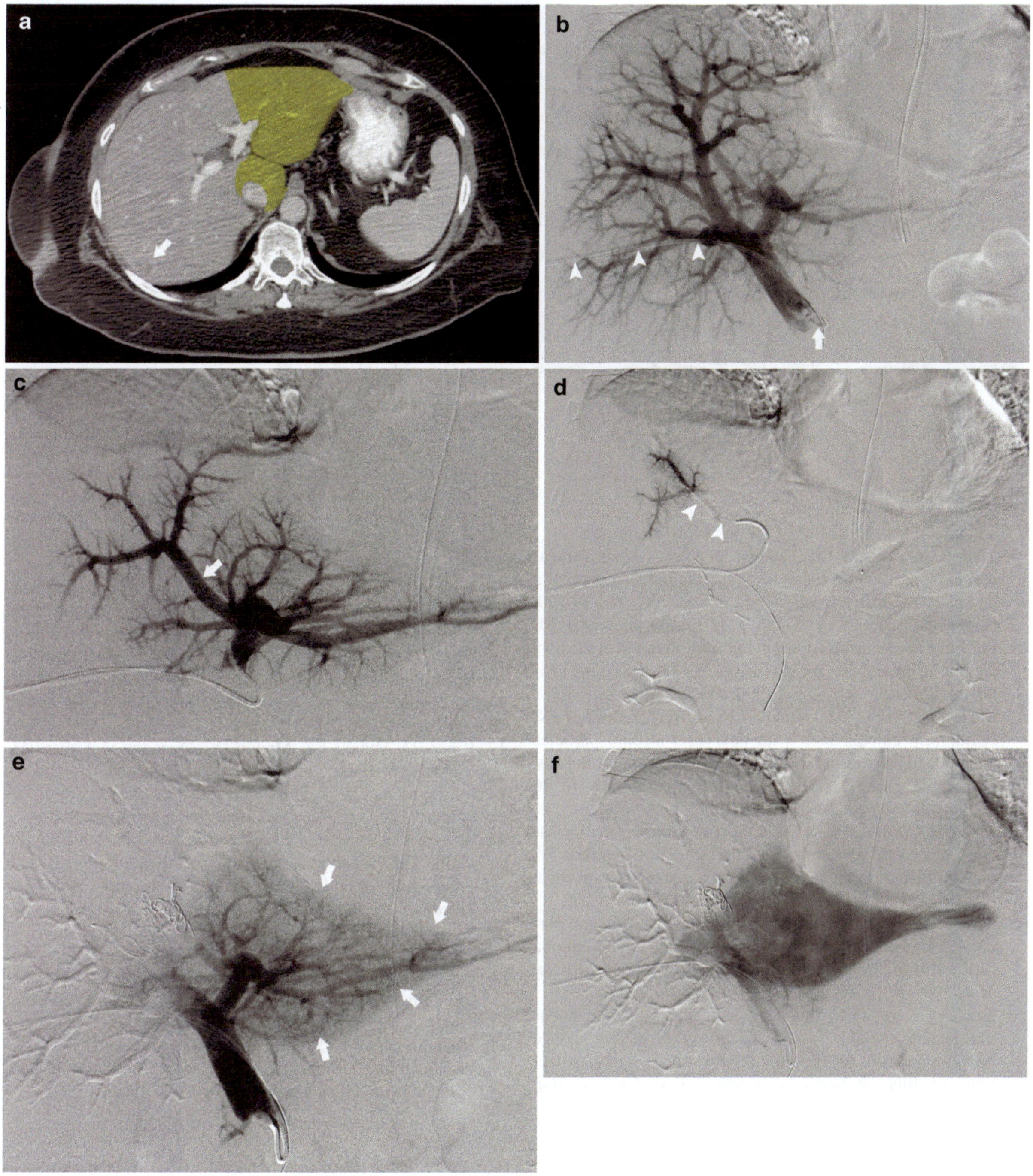

Fig. 17.4 A 66-year-old female with metastatic colorectal cancer to the right liver and segment 4 who had transhepatic ipsilateral RPVE extended to segment 4 with particles and coils prior to extended right hepatectomy. (**a**) Contrast-enhanced CT scan of the liver shows a mass in the right liver consistent with metastatic disease (*arrow*). CT volumetry was also performed, showing a small left lateral liver (*shaded area* – FLR/TELV of 15%). (**b**) Anteroposterior flush digital subtraction portogram shows a 6-Fr vascular sheath (*arrowheads*) in a right portal vein branch and a 5-Fr flush catheter (*arrow*) in the main portal vein. (**c**) Left portography via a 5-Fr reverse curve catheter shows a very prominent segment 4a portal vein branch (*arrow*). (**d**) A 3-Fr microcatheter (*arrowheads*) is shown within the segment 4a branch distally. (**e**) Post-procedure anteroposterior flush portogram shows occlusion of the portal vein branches to segments 4–8 with continued patency of the vein supplying the left lateral liver (*white arrows*). (**f**) A later phase of portogram confirms persistent flow to the left lateral liver. (**g**) Contrast-enhanced CT scan of the liver performed 1 month after RPVE extended to segment 4 shows hypertrophy of the left liver (*shaded area* – FLR/TELV of 25%). Coils (*arrows*) are seen in the access tract. The right liver also appears atrophic. The patient soon after underwent an uneventful extended right hepatectomy

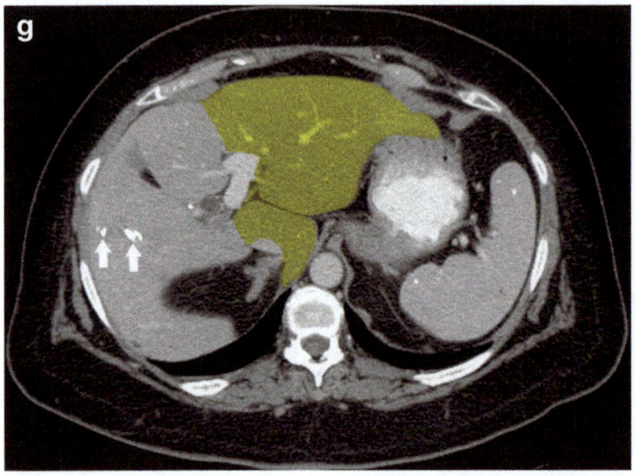

Fig. 17.4 (continued)

References

1. Madoff DC, Abdalla EK, Vauthey JN. Portal vein embolization in preparation for major hepatic resection: evolution of a new standard of care. *J Vasc Interv Radiol*. 2005;16:779-790.
2. Nagino M, Nimura Y, Kamiya J, Kondo S, Kanai M. Selective percutaneous transhepatic embolization of the portal vein in preparation for extensive liver resection: the ipsilateral approach. *Radiology*. 1996;200:559-563.
3. Madoff DC, Hicks ME, Abdalla EK, Morris JS, Vauthey JN. Portal vein embolization with polyvinyl alcohol particles and coils in preparation for major liver resection for hepatobiliary malignancy: safety and effectiveness–study in 26 patients. *Radiology*. 2003;227:251-260.
4. Madoff DC, Abdalla EK, Gupta S, et al. Transhepatic ipsilateral right portal vein embolization extended to segment IV: improving hypertrophy and resection outcomes with spherical particles and coils. *J Vasc Interv Radiol*. 2005;16:215-225.
5. Gibo M, Unten S, Yogi A, et al. Percutaneous ipsilateral portal vein embolization using a modified four-lumen balloon catheter with fibrin glue: initial clinical experience. *Radiat Med*. 2007;25:164-172.
6. Tsuda M, Kurihara N, Saito H, et al. Ipsilateral percutaneous transhepatic portal vein embolization with gelatin sponge particles and coils in preparation for extended right hepatectomy for hilar cholangiocarcinoma. *J Vasc Interv Radiol*. 2006;17:989-994.
7. Kodama Y, Shimizu T, Endo H, Miyamoto N, Miyasaka K. Complications of percutaneous transhepatic portal vein embolization. *J Vasc Interv Radiol*. 2002;13:1233-1237.
8. Madoff DC, Hicks ME, Vauthey JN, et al. Transhepatic portal vein embolization: anatomy, indications, and technical considerations. *Radiographics*. 2002;22:1063-1076.
9. van Gulik TM, van den Esschert JW, de Graaf W, et al. Controversies in the use of portal vein embolization. *Dig Surg*. 2008;25:436-444.
10. Capussotti L, Muratore A, Ferrero A, Anselmetti GC, Corgnier A, Regge D. Extension of right portal vein embolization to segment IV portal branches. *Arch Surg*. 2005;40: 1100-1103.
11. de Baere T, Roche A, Vavasseur D, et al. Portal vein embolization: utility for inducing left hepatic lobe hypertrophy before surgery. *Radiology*. 1993;188:73-77.
12. Nagino M, Nimura Y, Kamiya J, et al. Right or left trisegment portal vein embolization before hepatic trisegmentectomy for hilar bile duct carcinoma. *Surgery*. 1995;117:677-681.
13. Nagino M, Kamiya J, Kanai M, et al. Right trisegment portal vein embolization for biliary tract carcinoma: technique and clinical utility. *Surgery*. 2000;127:155-160.
14. Kishi Y, Madoff DC, Abdalla EK, et al. Is embolization of segment 4 portal veins before extended right hepatectomy justified? *Surgery*. 2008;144:744-751.
15. Broering DC, Hillert C, Krupski G, et al. Portal vein embolization vs. portal vein ligation for induction of hypertrophy of the future liver remnant. *J Gastrointest Surg*. 2002;6:905-913.
16. Mueller L, Hillert C, Möller L, Krupski-Berdien G, Rogiers X, Broering DC. Major hepatectomy for colorectal metastases: Is preoperative portal occlusion an oncological risk factor? *Ann Surg Oncol*. 2008;15:1908-1917.
17. Ribero D, Abdalla EK, Madoff DC, Donadon M, Loyer EM, Vauthey JN. Portal vein embolization before major hepatectomy and its effects on regeneration, resectability and outcome. *Br J Surg*. 2007;94:1386-1394.
18. de Graaf W, van den Esschert JW, van Lienden KP, van Gulik TM. Induction of tumor growth after preoperative portal vein embolization: Is it a real problem? *Ann Surg Oncol*. 2009;16:423-430.
19. Elias D, De Baere T, Roche A, Ducreux M, Leclere J, Lasser P. During liver regeneration following right portal embolization the growth rate of liver metastases is more rapid than that of the liver parenchyma. *Br J Surg*. 1999;86: 784-788.
20. Kokudo N, Tada K, Seki M, et al. Proliferative activity of intrahepatic colorectal metastases after preoperative hemihepatic portal vein embolization. *Hepatology*. 2001;34:267-272.

Complications of Portal Vein Embolization

18

Yoshihisa Kodama, Colette M. Shaw, and David C. Madoff

Abstract

Portal vein embolization (PVE) may be viewed as a tool used to improve the morbidity and mortality following major hepatectomy. While it is considered relatively safe, PVE is a complex procedure with potential complications. Adverse events may relate to the access approach or to the embolization procedure itself. Given that PVE is neither tumor-reductive nor does it guarantee hepatectomy, its technical and clinical success requires strict patient selection and careful pre-procedure planning. The aim of this chapter is to review the etiology, clinical presentation, and management of complications associated with this procedure.

Keywords

Portal vein embolization • Complications • Subcapsular hematoma • Pseudoaneurysm of hepatic artery • Hemothorax • Portal vein thrombus

While preoperative portal vein embolization (PVE) has been shown to be a safe and effective means of increasing the volume of the future liver remnant,[1-6] careful patient selection and pre-procedure planning are critical if complications are to be minimized and sufficient hypertrophy achieved. If the procedure fails or complications ensue that preclude surgery, then the patient's only chance for long-term survival may be lost. PVE operators need to be aware of the possible adverse events associated with the procedure and recognize the clinical signs early so that appropriate management can be implemented promptly. The Cardiovascular and Interventional Radiological Society of Europe (CIRSE) quality improvement guidelines for PVE recommend a minor complication rate of 20–25% and major complication rate less than 5% that does not preclude hepatectomy.[7] A 2008 meta-analysis of 37 PVE publications involving 1,088 patients in whom percutaneous and transileocolic PVE was performed reported a major complication rate of only 2.2%.[8]

Complications can be broadly divided into two categories: those related to the access approach and those related to the embolization of the targeted portal vein. PVE in the setting of chronic liver disease, neoadjuvant chemotherapy, and transcatheter arterial chemoembolization (TACE) are factors that can influence the rate and type of complication encountered.

Y. Kodama (✉)
Department of Radiology, Teine Keijinkai Medical Center, 1-12-1-40, Maeda, Teine-ku, Sapporo 006-8111, Japan
e-mail: ykodama@mud.biglobe.ne.jp

D.C. Madoff et al. (eds.), *Venous Embolization of the Liver*,
DOI 10.1007/978-1-84882-122-4_18,

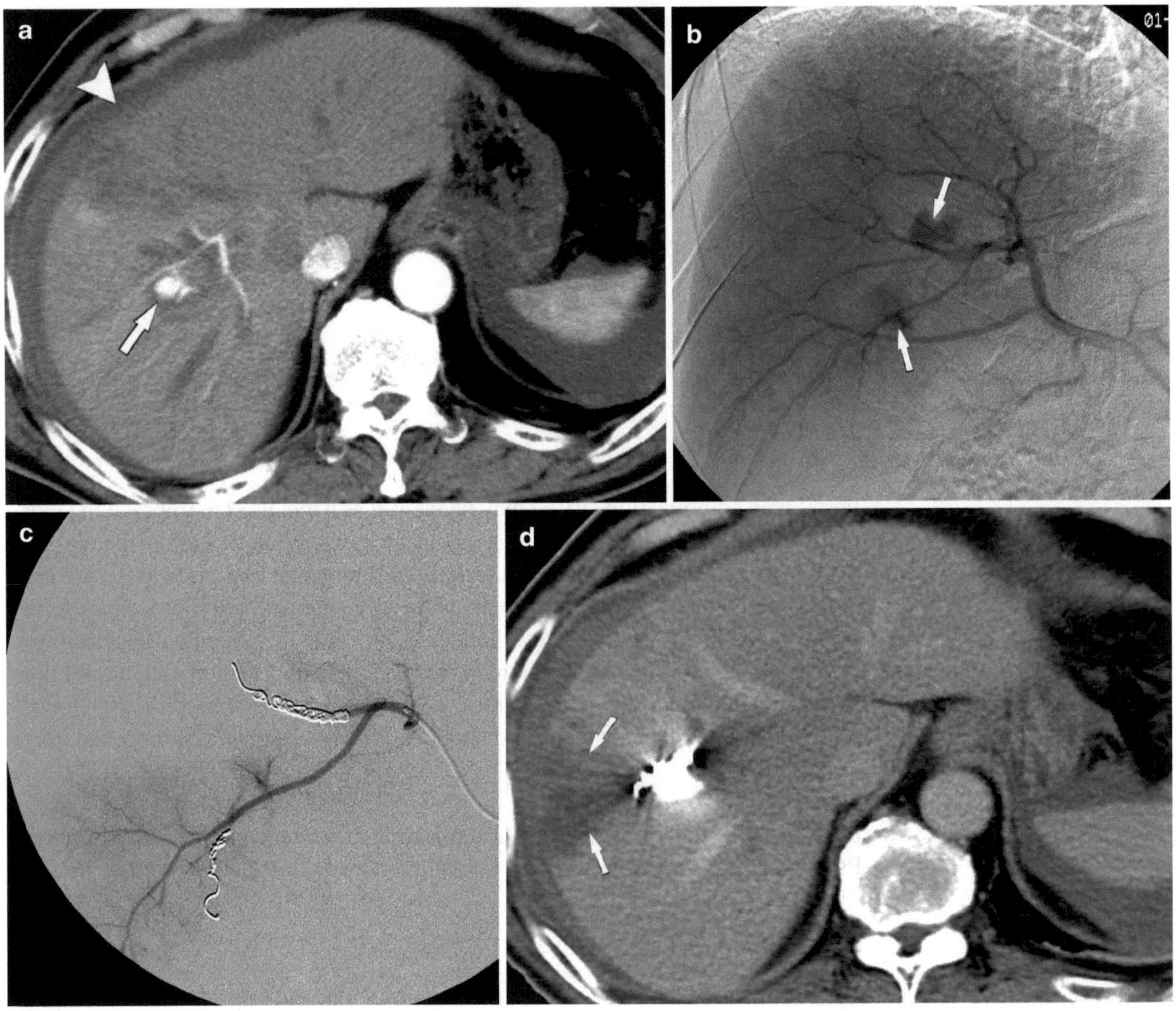

Fig. 18.1 PVE complicated by injury to the ipsilateral hepatic artery in a 72-year-old man diagnosed with cholangiocarcinoma. Percutaneous right PVE was performed via a right portal vein tributary. (**a**) CT abdomen arterial phase performed 2 days post procedure, revealed subcapsular hematoma (*arrowhead*) and pseudoaneurysm (*arrow*) in the right lobe. (**b**) Right hepatic arteriography demonstrated two focal areas of contrast extravasation consistent with pseudoaneurysms (*arrows*). (**c**) The pseudoaneurysms were successfully embolized with microcoils. (**d**) Follow-up CT abdomen portal venous phase showed no evidence of pseudoaneurysm but identified a wedge-shaped low-density area peripheral to the coils consistent with an infarct (*arrows*). The patient underwent extended right hepatectomy 27 days after PVE

18.1 Complications Related to Portal Vein Access

PVE may be performed percutaneously from an ipsilateral or contralateral transhepatic approach, a transjugular approach, or a trans-ileocolic approach. The latter is performed as an open surgical procedure. The approach adopted depends on the availability of interventional radiology services, operator preference, type of resection planned, extent of embolization, and type of embolic agent used.

The frequency of adverse events reported from experienced centers using a transhepatic approach ranges 9.114.9%.[9,10] Portal vein access can be acquired via the liver to be resected (ipsilateral) or via the future liver remnant (contralateral). Tissues that may be injured along the puncture route include the subcutaneous soft tissues, the pleura, and the liver parenchyma.

These complications usually manifest within a few days of the procedure and may be arterial, biliary, or pleural in origin.

Arterial injuries are the most serious and can involve an intercostal artery or a hepatic artery branch. Hepatic arteries run parallel to the portal veins, are smaller in diameter, and usually are not visible in normal B-mode ultrasound examination. Subcapsular and intrahepatic hematoma, pseudoaneurysm, and hemothorax are potential manifestations of an arterial injury (Fig. 18.1). Additional intervention is almost always needed, and thus, an arterial injury is categorized as a major complication. While abrupt changes in the vital signs, including a rapid and substantial drop in blood pressure and tachycardia, are clear-cut signs of acute hemorrhage, bleeding in a young patient may be less obvious. Acute confusion, right flank, epigastric or right shoulder pain, and progressive anemia are also possible indicators of hemorrhage. If an arterial injury is suspected, immediate resuscitative measures should be implemented. Once the patient is hemodynamically stable, a contrast-enhanced CT scan of the liver including arterial and portal venous phase imaging should be performed. The presence of a pseudoaneurysm warrants transarterial embolization to secure hemostasis. Subcapsular hematoma, even when not initially associated with a pseudoaneurysm, requires close clinical and imaging follow-up (Fig. 18.2). If the portal vein is punctured from a contralateral approach, a large subcapsular hematoma can compress the liver and possibly limit or prevent the hypertrophy of the future liver remnant. An arterial injury that requires transarterial embolization can compromise the blood supply to the remnant liver and render the patient unsuitable for surgery. If the arterial injury is within the ipsilateral liver, then transarterial embolization may cause hepatic infarction since the portal vein has already been embolized.

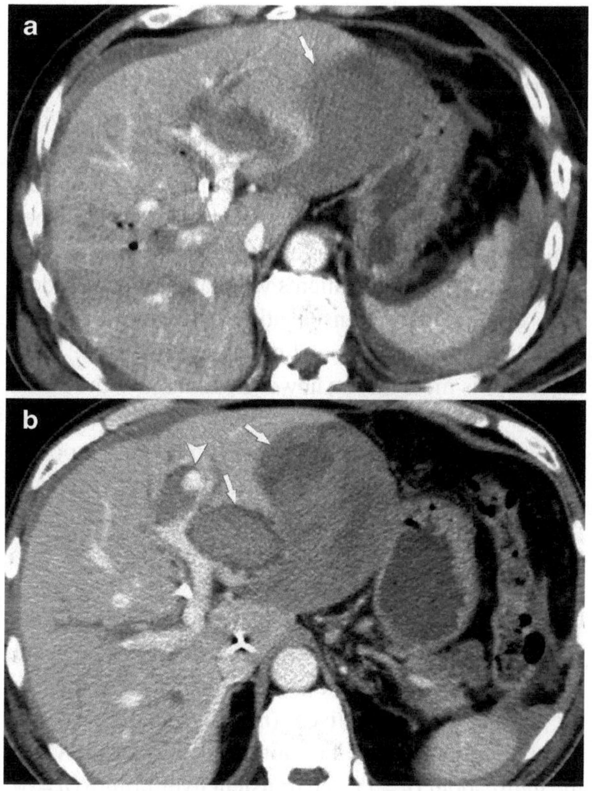

Fig. 18.2 Portal vein embolization from contralateral approach complicated by injury to the hepatic artery of the future liver remnant in a 61-year-old man diagnosed with carcinoma of the cystic duct. (**a**) Percutaneous PVE of the right lobe was performed via the umbilical portion of the left portal vein. Four hours after the procedure, the patient became hemodynamically unstable. CT of liver in the arterial phase revealed a large subcapsular hematoma (*arrow*). The patient was resuscitated with blood transfusions. (**b**) Follow-up CT of the abdomen in the arterial phase was performed 1 week after PVE and showed progressive subcapsular hematoma (*arrows*) and a pseudoaneurysm (*arrowhead*) of the left hepatic artery. Transcatheter arterial embolization was performed. This complication precluded the patient from undergoing a right hepatectomy

The bile duct is the third component of the portal triad. As the biliary radicals run alongside the portal vein, it is not uncommon for the bile duct to be inadvertently punctured. Despite this, biliary injury is rarely symptomatic or severe. Hemobilia and biliary leak are the commonest manifestations of bile duct injury. Hemobilia is usually self-limiting. If severe, embolization may be performed through the transhepatic track or by hepatic arteriography. Biliary drainage may be required to treat a biliary leak.

Pneumothorax and/or hemothorax can arise from pleural injury during a right transhepatic approach. Acute onset of chest pain, dyspnea, tachypnea, tachycardia, cyanosis, and absent breath sounds are some of the clinical symptoms and signs of pneumothorax. Confirmation and follow-up with chest radiograph should be performed. Although small pneumothoraces are often asymptomatic and subside without additional intervention, progressive pneumothorax or pneumothorax associated with new respiratory symptoms are an indication for chest tube placement. Changes in vital signs, progressive anemia, tachypnea, and/or decrease of percutaneous oxygen saturation are clinical signs of hemothorax. Diagnosis can be confirmed with CT study. Transcatheter arterial embolization of the intercostal artery may be required to restore hemodynamic stability.

In the United States, the ipsilateral transhepatic approach is commonly used. This technique, while technically challenging, avoids instrumentation and possible injury to the future liver remnant.[10-13] Potential complications include nontarget embolization when removing the reverse-curve catheter and hemorrhage and tumor seeding in patients with large tumor burden. The contralateral transhepatic approach was first described by Kinoshita and colleagues in 1986.[14] The trajectory is more direct; however, damage to the portal vein or liver parenchyma of the future liver remnant becomes a concern. Di Stefano and colleagues reported adverse events in 12.8% (24/188) of patients who underwent portal vein embolization via contralateral approach.[9] In 12 patients, additional treatment was required or the hospital stay was prolonged. Complications included complete portal vein thrombosis ($n=1$), inadvertent n-butyl-2-cyanoacrylate (NBCA) migration in the main left portal vein feeding the future remnant liver ($n=2$), hemoperitoneum ($n=1$), hemobilia ($n=1$), rupture of a metastasis into the gallbladder ($n=1$), and transient liver failure ($n=6$). Incidental findings included two cases of subcapsular hematoma located at the puncture site and 10 cases of migration of small NBCA fragments in the future remnant liver. A study by Kodama and colleagues reviewed 47 percutaneous PVE in 46 patients in which 11 were performed from the contralateral lobe.[10] An overall complication rate of 14.9% (7/47) was reported with no significant difference between ipsilateral and contralateral approaches. Adverse events included pneumothorax ($n=2$), subcapsular hematoma ($n=2$), arterial puncture ($n=1$), pseudoaneurysm ($n=1$), hemobilia ($n=1$), and PV thrombosis ($n=1$). Overall, complications were more frequent in the punctured lobe, thus, an ipsilateral transhepatic approach was recommended. Puncture of a posterior segment was associated with a significantly higher complication rate than the anterior segment ($P=0.04$). In cases in which the anterior segment cannot be visualized for puncture, the group recommended PVE via the lateral segment or transileocolic portal embolization.

There is limited experience with PVE performed via a transjugular approach. This technique may be considered in patients in whom a safe transhepatic trajectory cannot be identified or in whom hemostasis is a concern. A pilot study of 15 patients reported 100% technical success.[15] Eighty percent underwent hepatectomy. There were no significant complications. As with all percutaneous transjugular procedures, adverse events local to the puncture site include neck hematoma, accidental carotid puncture, transient Horner's syndrome, and transient dysphonia. Other potential complications include pneumothorax, cardiac arrhythmias, and damage to the liver parenchyma.

PVE via direct cannulation of the ileocolic vein is a technique sometimes used by surgeons.[16] This approach enables PVE to be performed during the resection of the primary tumor in patients with colorectal metastases in conjunction with staging laparoscopy or as part of a staged liver resection. In patients at risk for peritoneal carcinomatosis (e.g., gallbladder carcinoma), this finding at laparoscopy can eliminate the need for PVE and its potential complications. While portal vein ligation has not been shown to be superior to embolization and has similar complication rates, simultaneous embolization and ligation of the indicated portal vein branch during laparotomy has been performed in an effort to irreversibly occlude the portal vein tract in one lobe and to avoid nontarget embolization to the future liver remnant.[17] An open approach carries the risks associated with general anesthesia and laparotomy or laparoscopy. Damage to the ileocecal vein may result in ischemia of the terminal ileum. Given that the primary aim of PVE is not tumor reduction and technical success does not necessarily guarantee hepatic resection, PVE should be performed in the least invasive setting possible with minimum potential for complications.

18.2 Embolization-Related Complications

Adverse events specific to the embolization procedure include cholangitis, liver abscess, hepatic infarction, nontarget embolization and portal vein thrombosis, recanalization, and portal hypertension. While postembolization syndrome can occur after both arterial and venous embolization, it rarely manifests clinically after PVE. Side effects such as pain, fever, nausea, and vomiting are uncommon. Mild and transient liver dysfunction can occur. Transaminase levels may rise to less than three times the baseline 1–3 days after embolization and return to baseline within 7–10 days.[1,6,18,19] Hyperbilirubinemia is rare. A slight increase in white

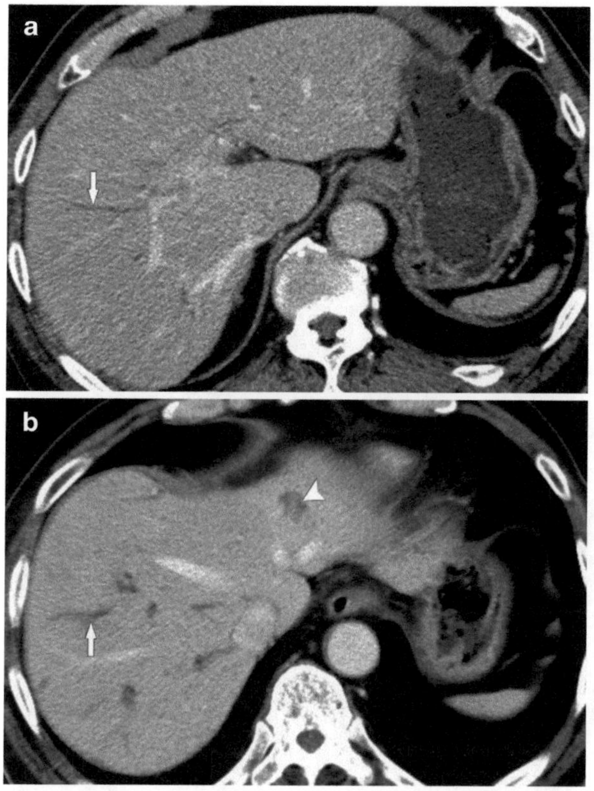

Fig. 18.3 PVE complicated by cholangitis and hepatic abscess in a 70-year-old man diagnosed with hilar cholangiocarcinoma. Percutaneous PVE of the right portal vein was performed via an ipsilateral approach through a right posterior portal vein tributary. (**a**) CT of the abdomen in the portal venous phase acquired prior to PVE showed slightly dilated intrahepatic bile ducts (*arrow*). Twelve days post-PVE, the patient developed symptoms and signs of cholangitis. (**b**) CT of the abdomen in the portal venous phase showed an abscess in the lateral segment of the left lobe (*arrowhead*) and increased biliary dilatation (*arrow*) within the right liver. The patient's symptoms resolved with the administration of antibiotics and biliary drainage. The patient underwent right hepatectomy 4 weeks following PVE

blood count and C-reactive protein are also frequent. Management is expectant. A prolonged abnormality raises the possibility of an underlying complication.

Cholangitis post-PVE most commonly arises from inadvertent puncture of an obstructed bile duct. Cholangitis can lead to biloma or abscess formation (Fig. 18.3). The classic presentation includes fever, jaundice, and right upper quadrant pain (Courvoisier's Triad). Bile leaks and abscesses can be easily detected by contrast-enhanced CT. These complications may be avoided by draining the biliary tree prior to PVE, and is particularly relevant to those with cholangiocarcinoma.[20] Without pre-procedural drainage, hyperbilirubinemia and biliary obstruction can also limit future remnant liver hypertrophy.[21] Prophylactic pre-procedural antibiotics may reduce post-PVE cholangitis and sepsis in those with segmental obstruction.

Hepatic infarction is a potential complication of simultaneous or sequential transarterial embolization followed soon after by PVE (Fig. 18.4). Once hepatic infarction occurs, the mainstay of treatment is supportive care. The CIRSE guidelines recommend a minimum of a 3-week delay between TACE and PVE.[7] In patients with hepatocellular carcinoma, TACE has been shown to successfully downstage disease.[22] It may be indicated prior to major hepatic resection to minimize disease progression and possibly to support hypertrophy of the future liver remnant in those who undergo PVE.[23,24] A retrospective review of 25 patients with HCC showed trans-arterial chemoembolization (TACE) following PVE to be safe with no major complications reported.[25] Ogata and colleagues compared outcomes in 36 patients diagnosed with hepatocellular carcinoma and liver cirrhosis in whom half underwent PVE alone and the other 18 underwent TACE followed by PVE. The latter was associated with greater hypertrophy in the future liver remnant and longer recurrence-free survival.[26]

Absolute ethanol is an effective embolic agent but less well-tolerated by patients. It can lead to considerable parenchymal destruction and necrosis, resulting in severe post-procedure pain.[18] NBCA can induce a marked peribiliary inflammatory reaction that can pose a technical challenge for the surgeon.[6,18] Recanalization post-PVE is most commonly associated with absorbable embolic agents, e.g., gelfoam.[1,6] If hypertrophy is inadequate, repeat PVE may be required.

One of the most serious complications of PVE is non-targeted portal vein thrombosis within the future liver remnant or complete occlusion of the main portal vein. This thrombosis may be the result of nontarget administration of the embolic agent or secondary to prolonged or traumatic catheter manipulation within the portal system. Migration of embolic material to the future liver remnant can occur with either ipsilateral or contralateral transhepatic approaches. Initial concerns relating to nontarget embolization of segments 2 and 3 when performing right PVE extended to segment 4 have not been substantiated by others.[27] Techniques developed to reduce the risk of nontarget embolization include the occlusion balloon catheter and the combined use of particulate embolic agents for distal

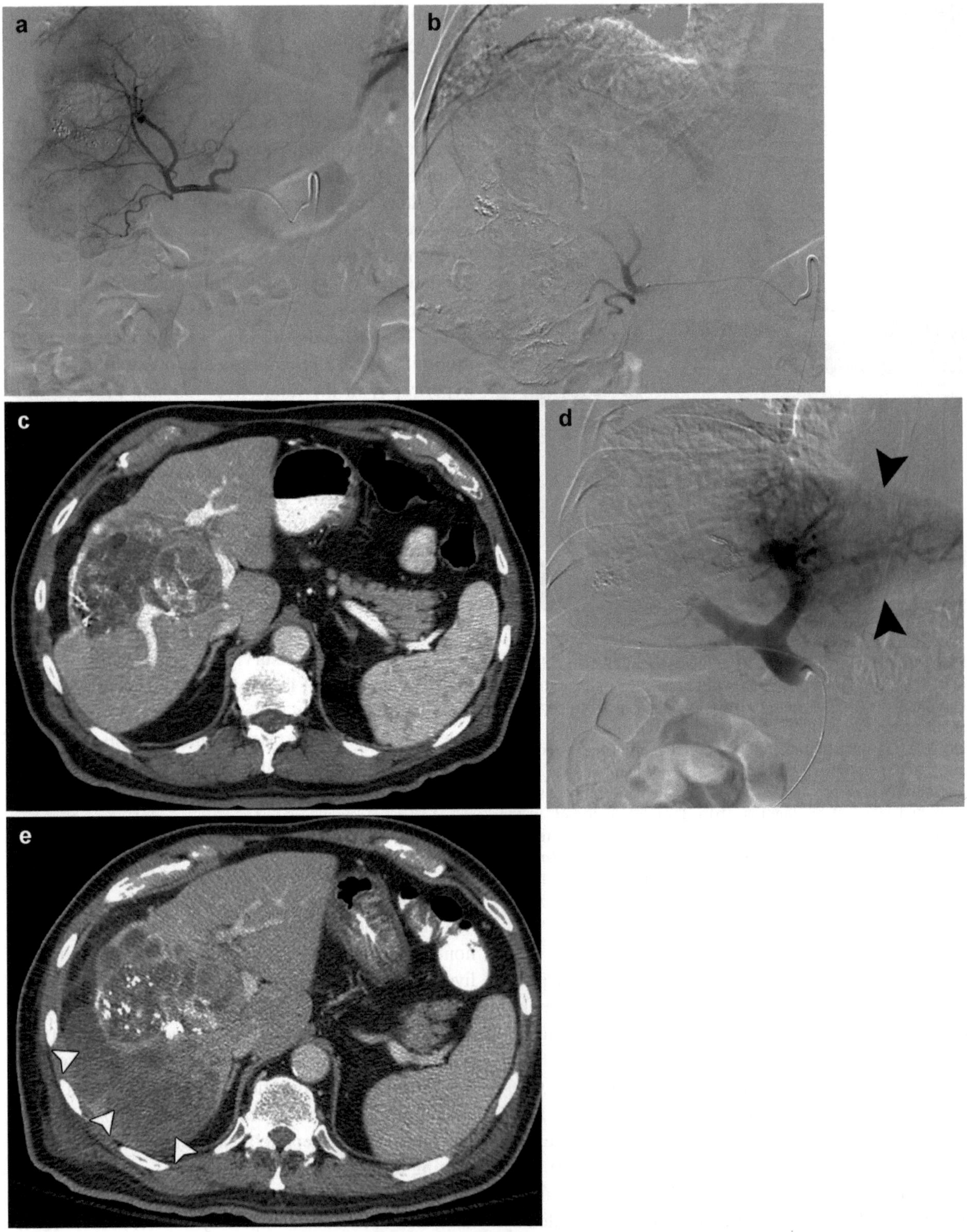
a
b
c
d
e

vein occlusion and coils for proximal vein occlusion. Di Stefano et al. reported nontarget embolization of NBCA in 12 of 188 PVE cases.[9] Ten were mild with no impact on hypertrophy of the future liver remnant. In two cases, the embolic material migrated into the main left portal vein feeding the future liver remnant. Both required portal vein angioplasty: one was successfully recanalized and the other was complicated by portal vein thrombosis. The incident was reported to have occurred toward the end of the procedure when only a few small branches remained patent and flow had significantly slowed. Abnormal portal vein flow dynamics has also been suggested as a factor contributing to nontarget embolization with NBCA in patients with chronic liver disease.[6]

There are numerous issues that can arise from portal vein thrombosis. If the thrombosis develops within the future liver remnant and persists for a prolonged period of time, hypertrophy may be impaired and atrophy may follow. Compromised blood flow to the future liver remnant could render the patient unsuitable for surgical resection. Thrombus extension from the targeted to the non-targeted portal vein is rare but can occur and can lead to complete portal occlusion.[12] If acute, fulminant liver failure and death can ensue. Nontarget portal thrombus can also occur in the punctured portal vein using the contralateral approach. If the thrombus within the vein is acute and low volume, the patient may be adequately treated with anticoagulation. If the thrombus is acute or subacute and extensive (i.e., within either the main portal vein or within the left portal vein), chemical thrombolysis with or without mechanical thrombectomy should be considered (Fig. 18.5). Of course, the use of these extreme measures will have a higher likelihood of success if the thrombus is acute and not associated with any nontarget embolic material. Portal vein thrombosis secondary to stasis within the portal vein trunk has been identified as the reason for higher complication rates following PVE in patients with chronic liver disease.

Clinical evidence of portal hypertension is a contraindication to PVE, but portal hypertension can also arise following PVE. In patients with cirrhosis, a portosystemic pressure gradient greater than 12 mmHg places the patient at major risk of perisurgical complications.[28,29] The CIRSE guidelines recommend measurement of the pre- and post-PVE portal pressure in patients with chronic liver disease. PVE should increase the gradient by approximately 3 mmHg.[7] At MD Anderson, a pre-embolization portal vein pressure greater than 20 mmHg in patients with chronic liver disease is worrisome for portal hypertension and may disqualify the patient from PVE. A dilemma arises when final portography demonstrates new portosystemic collaterals that may or may not be associated with a significant portal pressure increase. Embolization of these shunts may be performed in an attempt to maximize hepatopetal flow and minimize the risks of portal vein thrombosis and/or variceal hemorrhage (Fig. 18.6). How substantial increases in

Fig. 18.4 Portal vein embolization after chemoembolization complicated by hepatic infarction in a 71-year-old man diagnosed with hepatocellular carcinoma of the right lobe extending to segment 4. Multiple chemoembolizations via the right hepatic artery were performed. (**a**) Right hepatic arteriography showed hypervascular nodular enhancement, evidence of lipiodol deposition from previous chemoembolizations, and two hypovascular lesions in the superior aspect of the right lobe consistent with a previously treated disease. (**b**) Chemoembolization using doxorubicin, cisplatin, mitomycin-C, and lipiodol mix was administered from the right hepatic artery using a microcatheter. The vessels were embolized to stasis. (**c**) Two-week follow-up CT portal venous phase confirmed recent chemoembolization to the right lobe including the mass in segment 4 with heterogenous enhancement, focal areas of necrosis, and lipiodol deposition identified. The left portal vein and the right posterior portal vein were widely patent. The right anterior portal vein was encased by the tumor mass. (**d**) Portal vein embolization of the right lobe and segment 4 was performed 2 weeks after chemoembolization. The final portogram showed successful occlusion of the right portal vein and segment 4 portal veins with continued patency of the portal veins supplying the left lateral liver. (**e**) CT performed 4 days after PVE revealed diffuse hypodensity in the right lobe of the liver consistent with infarction (*arrowheads*). The study confirmed occlusion of the right portal vein and segment 4 portal veins. Segment 2 and 3 portal vein tributaries were widely patent

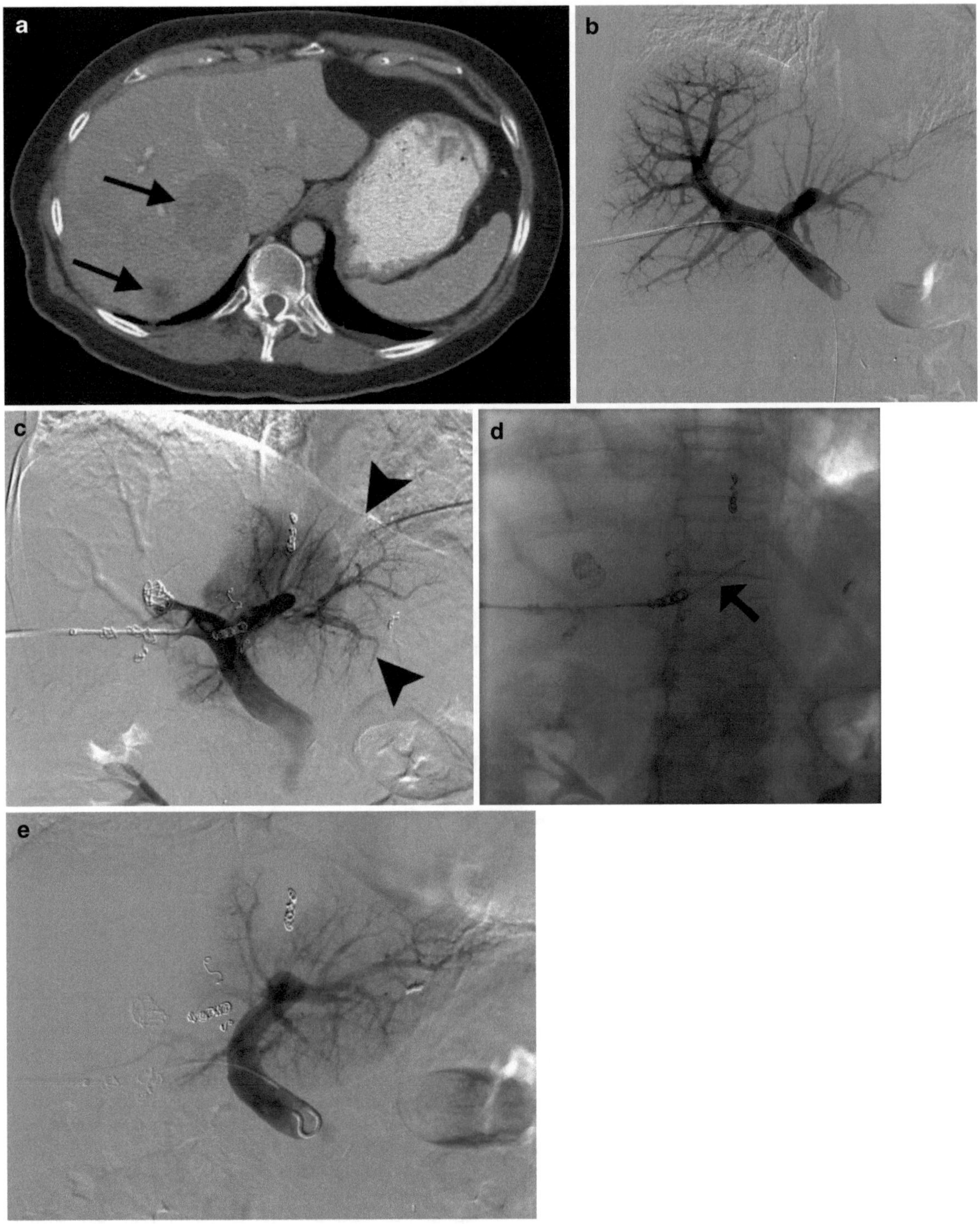

Fig. 18.5 Portal vein embolization complicated by portal thrombosis in a 79-year-old woman diagnosed with islet cell carcinoma. The patient developed liver metastases 3 years following a Whipple procedure. (**a**) CT abdomen portal venous phase demonstrated multiple liver masses (*arrows*) consistent with metastases and small future liver remnant. The patient underwent embolization of the right portal vein and segment 4 portal veins. (**b**) Normal pre-embolization portogram. (**c**) Post-embolization portogram showed acute thrombus within the left portal vein tributaries and heterogeneous parenchymal perfusion (*arrowheads*). (**d**) An infusion wire (*arrow*) was placed in the left portal vein for overnight thrombolysis using tissue plasminogen activator. (**e**) Follow-up portogram showed restoration of flow within the left portal venous system and successful occlusion of segment 4 and right liver portal veins. She underwent successful extended right hepatectomy 1 month after PVE

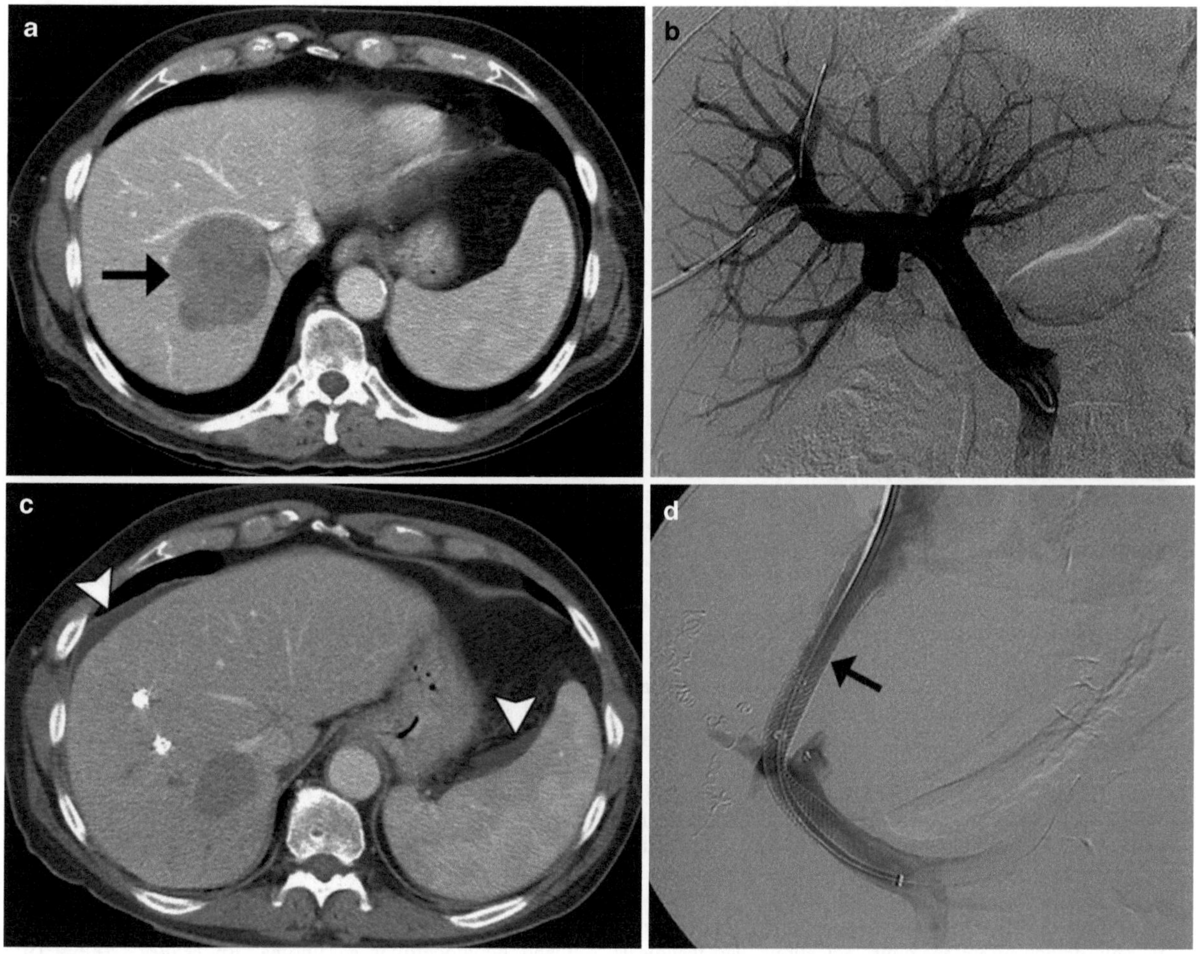

Fig. 18.6 Portal vein embolization complicated by portal hypertension in a 63-year-old man diagnosed with hepatocellular carcinoma. (**a**) CT abdomen in the portal venous phase demonstrated a mass involving the right lobe (*arrow*) and small future liver remnant. (**b**) The pre-embolization portogram showed no portosystemic collateral vessels. (**c**) Follow-up CT of the abdomen in the portal venous phase showed perihepatic and perisplenic ascites (*arrowheads*) and splenomegaly consistent with portal hypertension. (**d**) Patient required transjugular intrahepatic portosystemic shunt placement (*arrow*) for the treatment of recurrent variceal hemorrhage. The portosystemic pressure gradient dropped from 14 to 4 mmHg. The patient did not undergo hepatic resection

portal pressure after PVE relate to liver severity scores or post-operative morbidity is unclear.

18.3 Conclusion

The use of PVE prior to major hepatic resection in patients with both primary and secondary hepatic malignancies is supported by an abundance of retrospective data. Factors that may impact PVE complication rates include hyperbilirubinemia, biliary obstruction, chronic liver disease, the use of TACE in the same vascular distribution, and large tumor burden requiring extended or two-stage hepatectomy. Awareness of the various types of complications, how to avoid them, and how to manage them should they occur is essential to providing the best care possible for this patient population.

References

1. Makuuchi M, Thai BL, Takayasu K, et al. Preoperative portal embolization to increase safety of major hepatectomy for hilar bile duct carcinoma: a preliminary report. *Surgery*. 1990;107(5):521-527.
2. Abdalla EK, Barnett CC, Doherty D, Curley SA, Vauthey JN. Extended hepatectomy in patients with hepatobiliary malignancies with and without preoperative portal vein embolization. *Arch Surg*. 2002;137(6):675-680. discussion 680–681.

3. Abdalla EK, Hicks ME, Vauthey JN. Portal vein embolization: rationale, technique and future prospects. *Br J Surg*. 2001;88(2):165-175.
4. Azoulay D, Castaing D, Smail A, et al. Resection of nonresectable liver metastases from colorectal cancer after percutaneous portal vein embolization. *Ann Surg*. 2000;231(4):480-486.
5. Madoff DC, Abdalla EK, Vauthey JN. Portal vein embolization in preparation for major hepatic resection: evolution of a new standard of care. *J Vasc Interv Radiol*. 2005;16(6):779-790.
6. de Baere T, Roche A, Elias D, Lasser P, Lagrange C, Bousson V. Preoperative portal vein embolization for extension of hepatectomy indications. *Hepatology*. 1996;24(6):1386-1391.
7. Denys A, Bize P, Demartines N, Deschamps F, De Baere T. Quality improvement for portal vein embolization. *Cardiovasc Intervent Radiol*. 2010;33:452-456.
8. Abulkhir A, Limongelli P, Healey AJ, et al. Preoperative portal vein embolization for major liver resection: a meta-analysis. *Ann Surg*. 2008;247(1):49-57.
9. Di Stefano DR, de Baere T, Denys A, et al. Preoperative percutaneous portal vein embolization: evaluation of adverse events in 188 patients. *Radiology*. 2005;234:625-630.
10. Kodama Y, Shimizu T, Endo H, Miyamoto N, Miyasaka K. Complications of percutaneous transhepatic portal vein embolization. *J Vasc Interv Radiol*. 2002;13:1233-1237.
11. Madoff DC, Abdalla EK, Gupta S, et al. Transhepatic ipsilateral right portal vein embolization extended to segment IV: improving hypertrophy and resection outcomes with spherical particles and coils. *J Vasc Interv Radiol*. 2005;16(2 Pt 1):215-225.
12. Madoff DC, Hicks ME, Abdalla EK, Morris JS, Vauthey JN. Portal vein embolization with polyvinyl alcohol particles and coils in preparation for major liver resection for hepatobiliary malignancy: safety and effectiveness–study in 26 patients. *Radiology*. 2003;227(1):251-260.
13. Madoff DC, Hicks ME, Vauthey JN, et al. Transhepatic portal vein embolization: anatomy, indications, and technical considerations. *Radiographics*. 2002;22(5):1063-1076.
14. Kinoshita H, Sakai K, Hirohashi K, Igawa S, Yamasaki O, Kubo S. Preoperative portal vein embolization for hepatocellular carcinoma. *World J Surg*. 1986;10(5):803-808.
15. Perarnau JM, Daradkeh S, Johann M, Deneuville M, Weinling P, Coniel C. Transjugular preoperative portal embolization (TJPE) a pilot study. *Hepatogastroenterology*. 2003;50(51):610-613.
16. Shimura T, Suehiro T, Suzuki H, Okada K, Araki K, Kuwano H. Trans-ileocecal portal vein embolization as a preoperative treatment for right trisegmentectomy with caudate lobectomy. *J Surg Oncol*. 2007;96(5):438-441.
17. Wicherts DA, de Haas RJ, Andreani P, et al. Impact of portal vein embolization on long-term survival of patients with primarily unresectable colorectal liver metastases. *Br J Surg*. 2010;97(2):240-250.
18. Shimamura T, Nakajima Y, Une Y, et al. Efficacy and safety of preoperative percutaneous transhepatic portal embolization with absolute ethanol: a clinical study. *Surgery*. 1997; 121(2):135-141.
19. Imamura H, Shimada R, Kubota M, et al. Preoperative portal vein embolization: an audit of 84 patients. *Hepatology*. 1999;29(4):1099-1105.
20. Belghiti J, Ogata S. Preoperative optimization of the liver for resection in patients with hilar cholangiocarcinoma. *HPB*. 2005;7:252-253.
21. Fujii Y, Shimada H, Endo I, et al. Risk factors of posthepatectomy liver failure after portal vein embolization. *J Hepatobiliary Pancreat Sur*. 2003;10:226-232.
22. Chapman WC, Doyle MB, Stuart JE, et al. Outcomes of neoadjuvant transarterial chemoembolization to downstage hepatocellular carcinoma before liver transplantation. *Ann Surg*. 2008;248:617-625.
23. Nagino M, Kanai M, Morioka A, et al. Portal and arterial embolization before extensive liver resection in patients with markedly poor functional reserve. *J Vasc Interv Radiol*. 2000;11:1063-1068.
24. Lainas P, Boudechiche L, Osorio A, et al. Liver regeneration and recanalization time course following reversible portal vein embolization. *J Hepatol*. 2008;49:354-362.
25. Kang BK, Kim JH, Kim KM, et al. Transcatheter arterial chemoembolization for hepatocellular carcinoma after attempted portal vein embolization in 25 patients. *Am J Roentgenol*. 2009;193(5):W446-W451.
26. Ogata S, Belghiti J, Farges O, Varma D, Sibert A, Vilgrain V. Sequential arterial and portal vein embolizations before right hepatectomy in patients with cirrhosis and hepatocellular carcinoma. *Br J Surg*. 2006;93(9): 1091-1098.
27. Kishi Y, Madoff DC, Abdalla EK, et al. Is embolization of segment 4 portal veins before extended right hepatectomy justified? *Surgery*. 2008;144(5):744-751.
28. Bruix J, Castells A, Bosch J, et al. Surgical resection of hepatocellular carcinoma in cirrhotic patients: prognostic value of preoperative portal pressure. *Gastroenterology*. 1996;111(4):1018-1022.
29. Farges O, Malassagne B, Flejou JF, Balzan S, Sauvanet A, Belghiti J. Risk of major liver resection in patients with underlying chronic liver disease: a reappraisal. *Ann Surg*. 1999;229:210-215.

Hepatic Vein Embolization

19

Yonson Ku and Takumi Fukumoto

Abstract

Two major indications of hepatic vein embolization (HVE) have been identified to date. First, HVE can be performed to facilitate interlobar venous collateral formation prior to planned hepatectomies when predominant hepatic veins of the remnant liver are resected. HVE may also be indicated for cranial partial resection of the right lobe including the right hepatic vein trunk in patients with a malignant liver tumor in the Couinaud's segment VII and/or VIII. Second, HVE can be combined with portal vein embolization (PVE) as an adjunct treatment to increase future remnant liver volume in patients who had undergone PVE. The technique and materials are discussed.

Keywords

Hepatic vein embolization • Embolization of the hepatic vein • Portal vein embolization • Liver volume changes

19.1 Pathophysiological Background

The hepatic veins normally have an end-vein pattern of distribution, there being no communication between the same or different systems.[1-4] Therefore, pathological consequences of acute hepatic vein occlusion (HVO) differ depending on the extent of drainage area of the affected hepatic vein. Subtotal or total HVO results in a life-threatening sequence of events including cardiovascular circulatory failure, and liver failure. On the other hand, segmental HVO does not necessarily cause life threatening necrosis or atrophy of the liver if the involved liver segment remains in a range of 50–55% of total liver mass.[5-7]

Segmental HVO can be well tolerated through two major mechanisms.[6-12] In the early stage, retrograde flow in the portal vein from the affected liver segment to an unaffected segment functions as a means of hemodynamic compensation.[10-12] In the experimental setting, segmental hepatic vein ligation immediately increases portal venous pressure and it thereafter results in a prompt decrease to the baseline within 1 h.[13] Also, in the right lobe living donor liver transplantation, a reversed flow is ultrasonographically demonstrated immediately after reperfusion in the portal tributaries of the graft, which have drained into the middle hepatic vein in the donor.[14] These phenomena imply that the conversion of the portal tract to an outflow channel is rapidly established, and have an important role in

Y. Ku (✉)
Department of Surgery, Kobe University Graduate School of Medicine, 7-5-2 Kusunoki-cho, Chuo-ku, Kobe 650-0017, Japan
e-mail: yonson@med.kobe-u.ac.jp

D.C. Madoff et al. (eds.), *Venous Embolization of the Liver*,
DOI: 10.1007/978-1-84882-122-4_19, © Springer-Verlag London Limited 2011

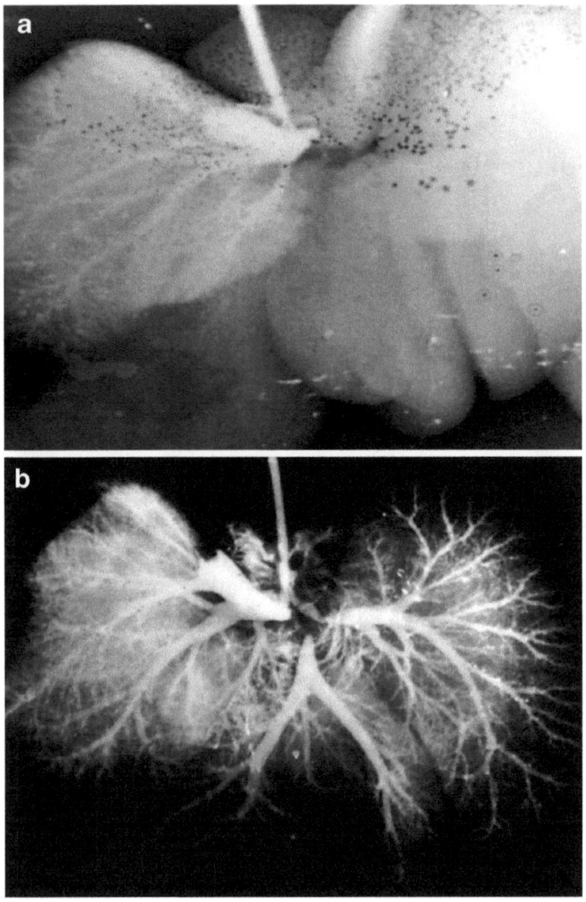

Fig. 19.1 Retrograde hepatic venographies after surgical hepatic vein ligation in beagles. (**a**) Hepatic venogram of the explanted liver taken immediately after ligation of the left hepatic vein. Note the lack of opacification of the entire left hepatic vein. (**b**) Hepatic venogram of the explanted liver taken 2 weeks after ligation of the left hepatic vein. A number of interlobar and interlobular collaterals were demonstrated between the patent and occluded hepatic veins

maintaining venous return from the affected segment in the acute stage of segmental HVO.

Another compensatory mechanism is intrahepatic venous collateral formation in the later stage of segmental HVO. Previous studies have shown that after hepatic veins are ligated, the liver is macroscopically not congestive at 2 weeks, and a number of interlobar and interlobular collaterals are radiographically demonstrated between the patent and occluded hepatic veins (Fig. 19.1).[6-9,13] Upon microscopic examination of the liver, bridging collaterals are seen within 2 weeks after HVE, and many thin-walled venous collaterals developed around the central venule. It has been shown that the affected liver segment recovers from congestion morphologically and functionally, as early as 7 days after segmental hepatic vein ligation.[9] Thus, adequate venous collaterals develop rapidly, and are established within 2 weeks in large animals including humans after segmental HVO.

19.2 Indications

Two major indications of hepatic vein embolization (HVE) have been identified to date. First, HVE can be performed to facilitate interlobar venous collateral formation prior to planned hepatectomies when predominant hepatic veins of the remnant liver are resected. The purposes of preoperative HVE are to spare normal liver parenchyma and to accomplish an adequate tumor clearance margin especially when there is a need to perform extended hepatectomies or when the patient has impaired liver function. Nagino et al.[15] successfully accomplished a left hepatic trisegmentectomy with combined resection of the right hepatic vein trunk after right hepatic vein embolization. HVE may also be indicated for cranial partial resection of the right lobe including the right hepatic vein trunk in patients with a malignant liver tumor in the Couinaud's segment VII and/or VIII. Preoperative HVE is likely a simple alternative to time-consuming hepatic vein reconstruction.[13,15,16]

Second, HVE can be combined with portal vein embolization (PVE) as an adjunct treatment to increase future remnant liver volume in patients who had undergone PVE. In this scenario, Hwang et al.[17] have recently reported a clinical pilot study of ipsilateral HVE after PVE in 12 patients who had shown limited liver regeneration after PVE awaiting right hepatectomy. This sequential treatment facilitates contralateral liver regeneration by inducing further damage to the embolized lobes. The additive increase of the future remnant liver volume with HVE after PVE was approximately 13% in nine patients with preplanned hepatectomies. These results strongly indicate the beneficial effects of HVE in the vicinity of technically demanding hepatectomies, and encourage further studies.

19.3 Technique and Embolic Materials

19.3.1 Experimental Basis

In contrast to hepatic arterial or portal vein embolization, HVE carries an inherent risk of dislodgement of

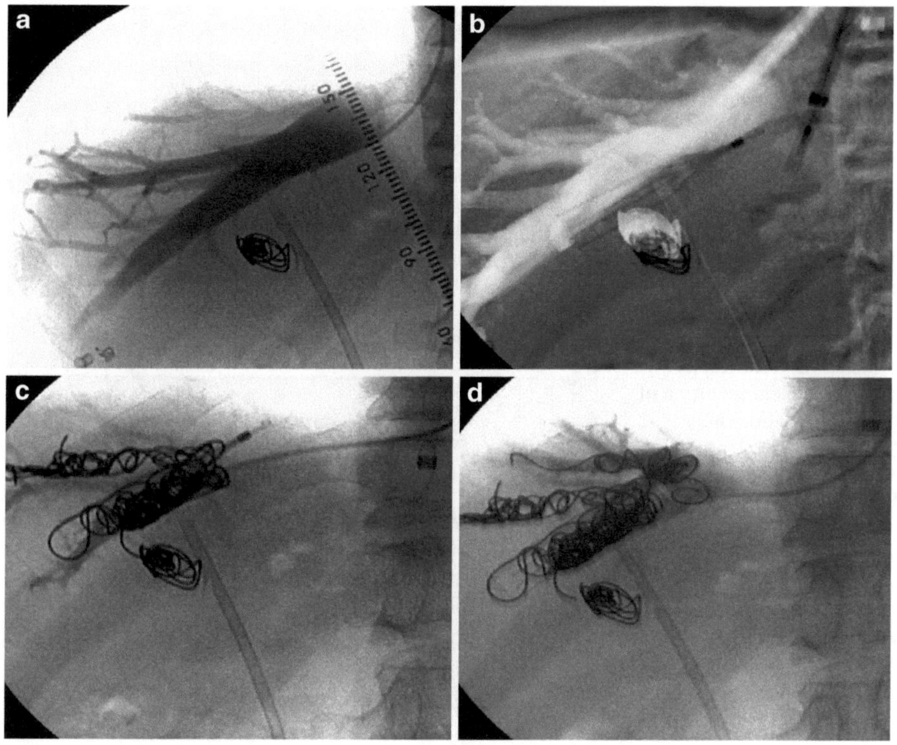

Fig. 19.2 The filter technique of right hepatic vein embolization using a retrievable vena cava filter. (**a**) The right internal jugular vein was punctured and right hepatic vein was selected using a guidewire. (**b**) A vena cava filter was inserted to prevent untoward coil migration. (**c**) The cobra catheter was advanced into the right hepatic vein and its main branches were embolized with multiple coils. (**d**) Contrast media was injected to confirm completeness of embolization (Courtesy of Dr. Hwang, Asan Medical Center, Seoul, South Korea)

embolic materials because of retrograde approach against the blood flow. Thus, the success of the HVE exclusively depends on establishing protective means to avoid this complication. In an experimental canine model, we used a balloon-tipped catheter to accomplish temporary occlusion of the ostia of the left hepatic vein when the embolic materials are released.[13] A standard 10-Fr introducer sheath was placed in the right external jugular vein through a small cut-down incision. An end-hole occlusion catheter size 8-Fr (Boston Scientific Japan Corp., Tokyo, Japan) with a 27 mm maximal diameter balloon at the distal end was passed via an introducer and advanced under fluoroscopic control to the inferior vena cava until the balloon was just above the hepatic veins. A temporary occlusion of the suprahepatic inferior vena cava was achieved by inflation of a 7–10 mL half strength contrast agent into the balloon of the catheter and a venogram was performed to obtain anatomic information on the hepatic veins. After deflating the balloon, the catheter was advanced under fluoroscopic guidance into the left hepatic vein, and the balloon was positioned as proximally as possible. When the desired position was reached, occlusion was achieved by inflating the balloon with a 3–4 mL half strength contrast agent. With the balloon in the optimal blocked position, the proximal left hepatic vein was embolized by delivering 3–4, 12-mm fiber-platinum coils (Target Therapeutics Inc., Fremont, USA). After the procedure, the introducer sheath was removed. It should be noted, however, that one of eight dogs had coils to be driven into the right atrium. The procedure of HVE has not been completely refined technically. Therefore further technical modifications should be required to avoid this critical complication of HVE in the human setting.

19.3.2 Clinical Application

To our knowledge, there have been two reports regarding clinical application of HVE. In one study, although the procedure of the HVE was not precisely described, two steel coils measuring 8 mm in diameter were used to accomplish embolization of the right hepatic vein (RHV).[15] In the other pioneering study with 12 patients, Hwang et al.[17] have elaborated the technique and outcome of HVE. In their initial approach (the filter technique, Fig. 19.2) the right internal jugular vein was punctured and a 9-Fr long sheath (Cook; Bloomington, IN, USA) was inserted. The RHV was selected using a 5-Fr cobra catheter

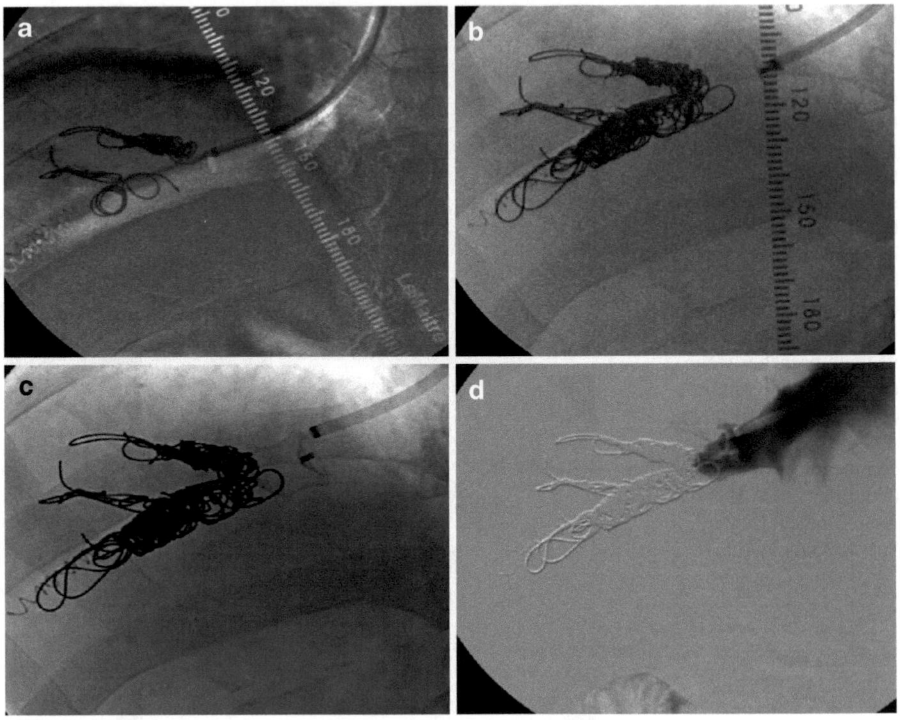

Fig. 19.3 The plugging technique of right hepatic vein embolization using a vascular plug. (**a**) After selection of the right hepatic vein, a vascular plug is placed first at the proximal right hepatic vein branch to prevent accidental migration of the coil. (**b**, **c**) Multiple embolization coils were inserted into the right hepatic vein branches through a catheter. (**d**) Venography shows complete occlusion of the right hepatic vein (Courtesy of Dr. Hwang, Asan Medical Center, Seoul, South Korea)

(Cook) and a 0.035-in. guide wire (Terumo; Tokyo, Japan). A 9-Fr sheath was inserted at the proximal portion of the RHV, followed by placement of either a Tulip filter (retrievable vena cava filter; Cook) or a Trap-Ease filter (Cordis; Miami, FL, USA) to prevent migration of deployed coils during embolization of the RHV. The cobra catheter was then advanced into the RHV and the main RHV branches were embolized with coils 8–12 mm in diameter (nester embolization coils; Cook). They experienced partial migration of the filter into the inferior vena cava in one of three patients.

Beginning on the fourth patient, they introduced a new technique using a vascular plug (the plug technique, Fig. 19.3); a 7-Fr sheath was inserted into the proximal RHV and a 5-Fr catheter was advanced deep into the RHV through different punctures at the right internal jugular vein. A vascular plug of 12–16 mm was placed at the proximal portion of RHV branches through the 7-Fr sheath to prevent accidental migration of the coils. Embolization coils were inserted into the RHV branches through the 5-Fr catheter. After complete embolization of all sizable RHV branches, both the 7-Fr sheath and the 5-Fr catheter were removed.

19.4 Clinical Outcomes

19.4.1 Liver Volume Changes Induced by HVE after PVE

Hwang et al. did not measure hepatic arterial flow rates before and after HVE.[17] However, morphologic changes of future liver remnant after HVE were presented, as shown in Figs. 19.4 and 19.5. Density changes in the embolized liver segments on post-HVE CT indicated a decreasing hepatic arterial flow (Fig. 19.4). As to the effect of HVE and PVE on liver volume changes, future remnant liver volume to total liver volume before PVE was approximately 35%, which increased to 44% when combined with HVE, indicating that HVE after PVE reduced the liver resection rate by 9%.

19.4.2 Liver Damage and Complications

The most common histological findings in the acute phase of HVE were centrilobular congestion and scattered areas of focal parenchymal hemorrhage.[6,8] Thereafter in a few weeks many central venules

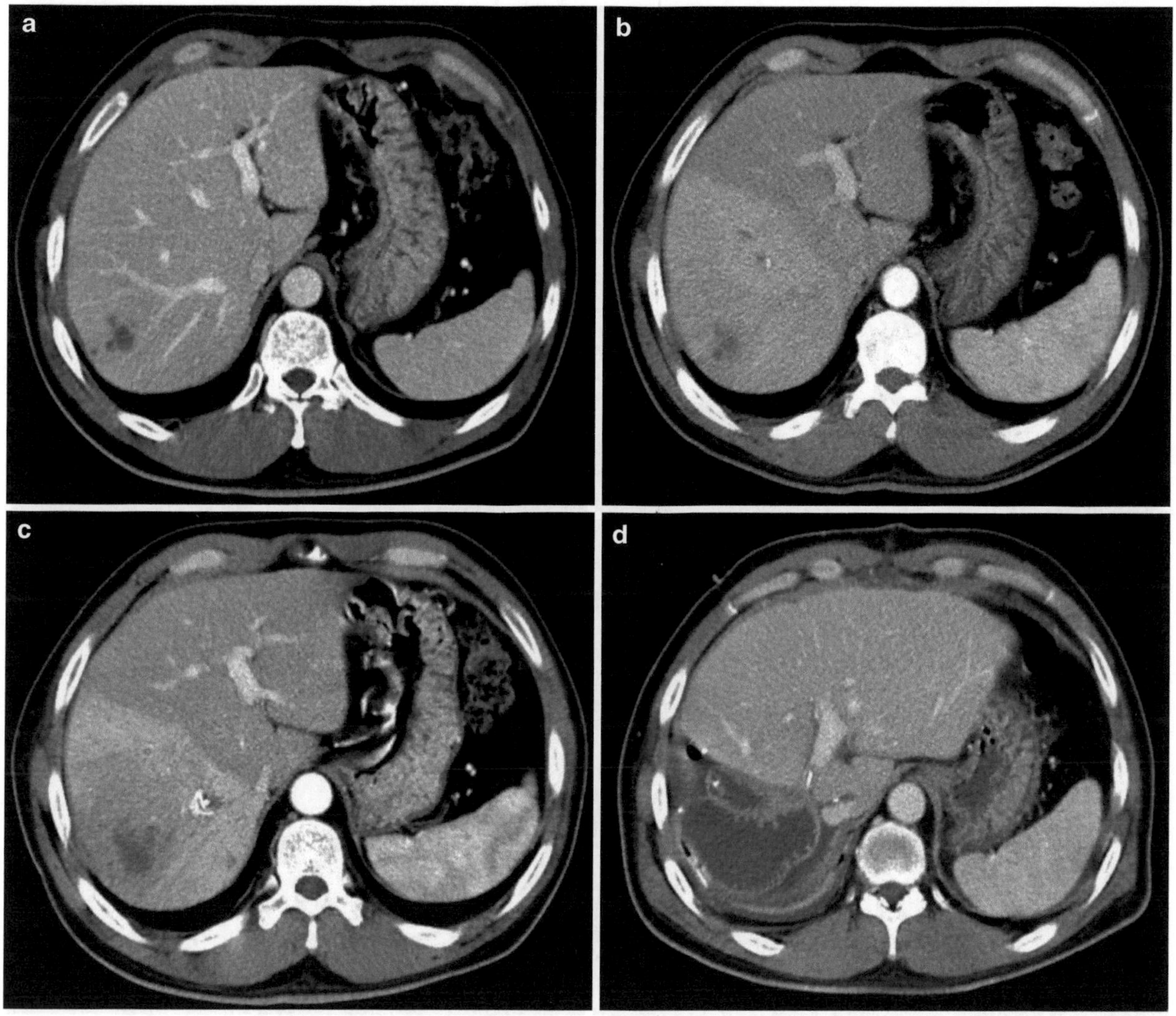

Fig. 19.4 Serial CT scan follow-up in a patient with intrahepatic cholangiocarcinoma. Morphological changes of future remnant liver are shown before PVE (**a**), 8 days after PVE (**b**), 14 days after HVE (**c**), and 7 days after right hepatectomy (**d**) (Courtesy of Dr. Hwang, Asan Medical Center, Seoul, South Korea)

became moderately dilatated with intimal thickening, and surrounded by a number of venous collaterals in the adjacent liver.[5-8] Both experimentally and clinically, these histological findings were reflected to transient increases of serum aspartate and alanine aminotransferase activities early after HVE. Biochemical derangements caused by HVE were almost similar to what was seen after PVE.[17] Although mild abdominal pain, low grade fever, and nausea were observed in some patients, no serious adverse effects were reported in two clinical trials.[15,17] Of further note, patients with preoperative HVE showed some more bleeding from dilated intrahepatic venous collaterals during hepatic parenchymal transection.[17] Based on these observations, HVE is reasonably a safe procedure comparable to PVE when the risk of migration of embolic materials to the heart or lung is prevented.

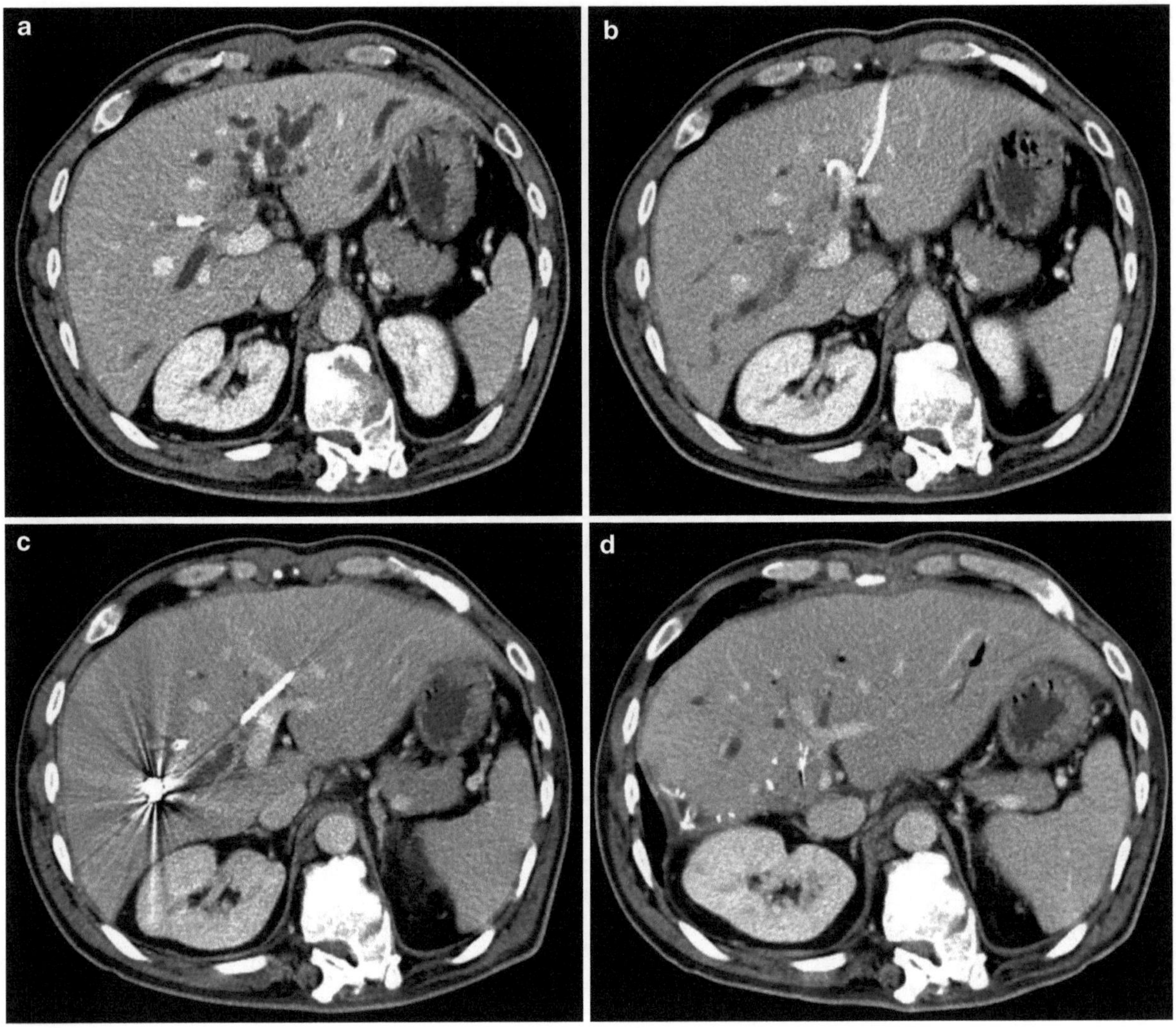

Fig. 19.5 Serial CT scan follow-up in a patient with hilar cholangiocarcinoma. Morphological changes of future remnant liver are shown before PVE (**a**), 14 days after PVE (**b**), 15 days after HVE (**c**), and 7 days after right hepatectomy (**d**) (Courtesy of Dr. Hwang, Asan Medical Center, Seoul, South Korea)

References

1. Elias H, Petty D. Gross anatomy of the blood vessels and ducts within the human liver. *Am J Anat*. 1952;90:59-111.
2. Goldsmith NA, Woodburne RT. The surgical anatomy pertaining to liver resection. *Surg Gynecol Obstet*. 1957;105: 310-318.
3. Hales MR, Allan JS, Hall EM. Injection corrosion studies of normal and cirrhotic livers. *Am J Pathol*. 1959;35:909-941.
4. Gibson JB. The hepatic veins in man and their sphincter mechanisms. *J Anat*. 1959;93:368-379.
5. Winternitz MG. The effect of occlusion of the various hepatic vessels upon the liver. *Bull Johns Hopkins Hosp*. 1911;22:396-404.
6. Widmann WD, Hales MR, Greenspan RH. The effects of hepatic vein occlusions. *Am J Pathol*. 1962;41:439-454.
7. Ou QJ, Hermann RE. Hepatic vein ligation and preservation of liver segments in major resections. *Arch Surg*. 1987;122: 1198-1200.
8. Maetani S. Experimental obstruction of left hepatic vein in dogs. I. Histopathological changes and gross vascular alterations. *Arch Jap Chir*. 1965;34:216-221.
9. Kaman J, Cerveny C. Die Bildung intrahepataler Kollateralen nach verschieden lokalisiertem Verschlub der Lebervenen beim Schwein. *Acta Anat*. 1971;80:481-503.
10. Gross FS, Raffucci FL, Toon RW, Wangensteen OH. Effect of complete hepatic vein ligation on portal pressures and ascites formation in dogs with porta-caval shunts. *Proc Soc Exp Biol Med*. 1953;82:505-509.

11. Elias H, Sokol A. Dependence of the lobular architecture of the liver on the porto-hepatic blood pressure gradient. *Anat Rec*. 1953;115:71-85.
12. Child CG, McDonough EF Jr, DesRochers GC. Reversal of hepatic venous circulation in dogs. *Proc Soc Exp Biol Med*. 1958;99:596-598.
13. Ku Y, Tominaga M, Sugimoto T, et al. Preoperative hepatic venous occlusion for partial hepatectomy combined with segmental resection of the major hepatic vein. *Br J Surg*. 2002;89:63-69.
14. Sano K, Makuuchi M, Miki K, et al. Evaluation of hepatic venous congestion: proposed indication criteria for hepatic vein reconstruction. *Ann Surg*. 2002;236:241-247.
15. Nagino M, Yamada T, Kamiya J, Uesaka K, Arai T, Nimura Y. Left hepatic trisegmentectomy with right hepatic vein resection after right hepatic vein embolization. *Surgery*. 2003;133:580-582.
16. Nakamura S, Sakaguchi S, Hachiya T, et al. Significance of hepatic vein reconstruction in hepatectomy. *Surgery*. 1993;114: 59-64.
17. Hwang S, Lee SG, Ko GY, et al. Sequential preoperative ipsilateral hepatic vein embolization after portal vein embolization to induce further liver regeneration in patients with hepatobiliary malignancy. *Ann Surg*. 2009;249:608-616.

Part IV

Clinical Outcomes

Clinical Outcomes for Hepatocellular Carcinoma

20

Stéphane Zalinski and Jacques Belghiti

Abstract

Hepatocellular carcinoma (HCC) patients with >3 cm and/or multiple lesions can only expect a prolonged survival if they are eligible for a surgical treatment, e.g., resection or liver transplantation. Liver transplantation is the best option as it cures both the HCC and the underlying disease and is therefore associated with a better disease-free survival than resection. Yet, liver transplantation is selectively indicated because of graft shortage and is being offered to a limited number of patients with the best oncological prognosis, those entering the Milan criteria. Liver resection in the setting of chronic liver disease is a risky procedure, which calls for a stringent selection and preparation of the patients before surgery. Besides the stage of the tumor, the selection process is mainly based on the evaluation of the liver function reserve and the liver volume. When the patients are not good candidates for a surgical treatment, transarterial chemoembolization (TACE) is the treatment of choice. Because TACE is associated with a longer survival than symptomatic treatment in palliative cares, TACE has been used as a neoadjuvant treatment before surgery in order to reduce the recurrence rate. To date, no data support its use prior to surgery in patients deemed resectable up-front, but by downsizing the tumor in good responders, nonresectable patients may become resectable. In patients with a borderline liver function, portal vein embolization (PVE) is used to increase the future liver remnant volume without compromising the prognosis. Although there is some theoretical reason to use PVE cautiously in HCC patients, published data indicates that PVE offers an extension of the indication of liver resection for HCC. Finally, to counterbalance the potential side effects of PVE in the setting of HCC, it was thought to use a sequential arterioportal approach as both procedures may be synergistic. TACE may enhance the impact of PVE on regeneration and PVE may enhance the anticancer effect of TACE. There are very few series evaluating this sequence and none are prospective but, to date, it seems to be the best preoperative option before liver resection in HCC patients.

J. Belghiti (✉)
Department of Hepato-Pancreato-Biliary Surgery and Liver Transplantation, Beaujon Hospital, Clichy, France
e-mail: jacques.belghiti@bjn.aphp.fr

D.C. Madoff et al. (eds.), *Venous Embolization of the Liver*,
DOI 10.1007/978-1-84882-122-4_20, © Springer-Verlag London Limited 2011

Keywords

Hepatocellular carcinoma • Liver transplantation • Transarterial chemoembolization • Liver function reserve • Chronic liver disease

Owing to the increasing incidence of chronic liver disease (CLD) related to viral infection, particularly to HCV, and to the increasing prevalence of metabolic syndrome, the number of patients diagnosed with hepatocellular carcinoma (HCC) is rising.[1] The most effective curative treatment of HCC relies on surgery, and the patients may only expect a prolonged survival if they are eligible for liver transplantation (LT) or liver resection (LR). LT, which represents the best treatment option for patients with CLD and limited tumors, has a considerable advantage over LR as it also cures underlying liver disease and is, therefore, associated with a lower recurrence rate than liver resection, which may reach 80% at 5 years.[2-5] Although the vast majority of patients considered for LT have early stages of carcinoma fulfilling the Milan criteria,[6] the shortage of grafts results in a long waiting period. Tumor development during the waiting period may be associated with tumor progression and vascular invasion, which is a strong factor of postoperative recurrence and is associated with a poor prognosis.[7,8] Besides, tumor progression while the patients are on the waiting list may result in a high dropout rate. Therefore, local treatment of the tumor including transarterial chemoembolization (TACE) can be used before transplantation. In addition, TACE can be utilized to downstage HCC from United Network for Organ Sharing (UNOS) T3 to T2, allowing LT. [9]

Liver resection may be used as a definitive treatment option or as a bridge treatment in patients waiting for transplantation.[10] Up to 90% of HCC develops in a cirrhotic liver, and the main limitations of liver resection include (1) the risk of postoperative liver insufficiency, thus, limiting the number of patients being deemed resectable and (2) a high rate of recurrence in the remnant diseased liver among those undergoing resection.[11] The decision for surgical resection of HCC relies on a balance between the need to remove the neoplasic tissue while retaining sufficient liver parenchyma to ensure a satisfactory postoperative liver function. Indeed, liver resection in the setting of advanced liver disease is associated with an increased morbidity and mortality that may overcome its oncologic benefit. The poor functional reserve and the high risk of postoperative liver insufficiency are correlated to the size of the liver remnant.[12] Consequently, the evaluation of the severity of the liver disease and the liver functional reserve is pivotal in the preoperative workup. In those patients with compensated cirrhosis and an insufficient liver remnant, portal vein embolization (PVE) is used to trigger a preoperative hypertrophy of the liver remnant with excellent results.[13,14]

As mentioned previously, intrahepatic recurrence rate following liver resection for HCC is over 60%, which represents its main limitation over LT.[2,3,5] In order to improve the recurrence rate following liver resection for HCC, many strategies have been attempted. To date, despite intensive efforts made in clinical research, no adjuvant or neoadjuvant systemic therapy has been shown to improve the prognosis after liver resection for HCC. TACE has been used by many centers to improve the recurrence rate, but the current literature reports conflicting results and no convincing evidence supports its routine use alone before liver resection.

Finally, TACE may also be used in combination with PVE as a sequential arterioportal embolization. Indeed, preparation of the patients before liver resection is two-sided and aims at improving oncologic results while limiting the risk of postoperative liver dysfunction. The patients may either be operated up-front, following a preoperative transarterial chemoembolization or a preoperative portal vein embolization, or, as recently reported, following a sequential arterioportal embolization. In this chapter, we will review each strategy and evaluate the rationale for a sequential approach.

20.1 Rationale for the Use of TACE Before Liver Transplantation for Hepatocellular Carcinoma

LT is currently an established therapy for small, early stage HCC (UNOS T2)[6] in patients with cirrhosis but requires, in most cases, a long waiting period. Tumor development during the waiting period may be associated with vascular invasion and tumor growth, which may result in a high dropout rate or be associated with a higher recurrence rate among transplanted patients. Therefore, local treatment of the tumor, including transarterial chemoembolization (TACE), has been used before transplantation aiming at improving survival, reducing the drop-out rate, and expanding the selection criteria for a selected group of patients with HCC beyond the Milan criteria at presentation. Initial series reporting on this strategy of neoadjuvant TACE before LT were deceiving. Although TACE induced complete tumor necrosis in some patients, there are no convincing arguments showing that this treatment reduces the rate of dropout before LT nor improves the survival after LT. In 2006, Lesurtel et al. have performed a review of the literature aiming at assessing the impact of transarterial chemoembolization as a neoadjuvant therapy before orthotopic liver transplantation in order to spread evidence based recommendations.[15] The authors found no convincing evidence among published series to support the use of TACE before LT. In particular, no series could clearly demonstrate a survival advantage and a lower dropout rate from the waiting list among patients undergoing pre-transplantation TACE as compared to those being transplanted up-front. Finally, the authors did not find data supporting its routine use to expand selection criteria for LT. This latter point has been subsequently challenged by other reports.[9,16]

Chapman et al.[9] have evaluated the outcomes of downstaging patients with advanced HCC with TACE to allow eligibility for LT. Seventy-six (37.6%) patients with American Liver Tumor Study group stage III/IV HCC were potential transplant candidates if downstaging was achieved by TACE based on follow-up imaging findings (RECIST criteria). Overall, 18 (23.7%) patients had adequate downstaging to qualify for LT under the Milan criteria. Radiologic response was partial and stable, and tumor progression was observed in 27 (35.5%), 22 (29%), and 27 (35.5%). Seventeen of seventy-six (22.4%) patients who met other qualifications underwent LT after successful downstaging (13/38 stage III; 4/38 stage IV). Explant review demonstrated 28 identifiable tumors in which post-TACE necrosis was greater than 90% in 21 (75%). At a median of 19.6 months (range 3.6–104.7), 16/17 (94.1%) patients who underwent LT were alive. Based on their findings, the authors concluded that in highly selected patients with stage III/IV HCC being downstaged to the Milan criteria with TACE, LT was associated with excellent midterm disease-free and overall survival similar to stage II HCC.

Aiming at expending the selection criteria for LT, many strategies have been assessed as neoadjuvant therapy to downstage the HCC in patients otherwise ineligible based on UNOS criteria (HCC staged T2). Among these strategies, transarterial radioembolization (TARE) has been compared to TACE with promising results.[16] In a study reported by Lewandowski et al., 86 patients treated with either TACE ($n=43$) or TARE with Yttrium-90 microspheres (TARE-Y90; $n=43$) were compared. Median tumor size was similar in both groups. Partial response rates favored TARE-Y90 (61%) versus TACE (37%). Downstaging to UNOS T2 was achieved in 31% of TACE and 58% of TARE-Y90 patients, and event-free survival was significantly greater in the TARE-Y90 group (17.7 vs. 7.1 months, $p=0.0017$). Overall survival favored TARE-Y90 compared to TACE. Although the authors agreed that their results may be subject to methodological bias, they concluded that TARE-Y90 may better downstage HCC from UNOS T3 to T2 than TACE.

As new techniques evolve and are being refined, they are being associated with promising results. Yet, data provided in the current literature are scarce and need further confirmation by prospective controlled studies in order to define a consensual approach.

20.2 Results of Liver Resection for Hepatocellular Carcinoma After TACE

Many strategies aiming at lowering the recurrence rate post liver resection have been attempted. Among these strategies, chemotherapy has been delivered either as a systemic option or selectively. Series reporting on the impact of preoperative TACE on the prognosis are conflicting (Table 20.1). [17-28]

Although the liver blood supply is mainly venous with 80% of the inflow supplying the liver coming from the portal system, the hepatic artery is the only blood supply to HCC, which rationalize the use of the hepatic artery to deliver locoregional treatment in HCC patients. Given the benefit of TACE in nonresectable patients as compared to palliative therapy and supportive cares,[29] it has been evaluated as a neoadjuvant option,

Table 20.1 Selection of series reporting outcomes following liver resection for HCC following transarterial chemoembolization

Authors	Year	Type	*n*	Morbidity (%)	Mortality (%)	Disease-free survival	Degree of necrosis	Actuarial survival
Zhou et al.[17]	2009	RCT	52 (TACE)	32	0	5 yrs 12.8%	–	5 yrs 30.7%
			56 (Control)	21	0	5 yrs 8.9%	–	5 yrs 21.1%
Gerunda et al.[26]	2000	Prospective	20 (TACE)	–	0	5 yrs 57%	–	5 yrs 43%
			20 (Control)	–	0	5 yrs 21%	–	5 yrs 38%
Majno et al.[22]	1997	Retrospective	49 (TACE)	–	4	5 yrs 29%	–	–
			27 (Control)	–	7	5 yrs 11%	–	–
Luo et al.[23]	2002	Retrospective	62 (TACE)	3.2	0	–	–	–
			64 (Control)	0	0	–	–	–
Paye et al.[32]	1998	Retrospective	24 (TACE)	–	12.5	3 yrs 33%	–	–
			24 (Control)	–	8.3	3 yrs 32%	–	–
Harada et al.[25]	1996	Retrospective	105 (TACE)	–	4.7	5 yrs 30%	–	5 yrs 53%
			35 (Control)	–	2.8	5 yrs 29%	–	5 yrs 46%
Sasaki et al.[20]	2006	Retrospective	109 (TACE)	–	17.4	5 yrs 19%	–	5 yrs 29%
			126 (Control)	–	4.8	5 yrs 22%	–	5 yrs 49%
Choi et al.[27]	2007	Retrospective	120 (TACE)	23.3	2.5	5 yrs 51%	–	–
			153 (Control)	24.8	0.6	5 yrs 47%	–	–
Wu et al.[19]	1995	RCT	24 (TACE)	20.8	4.1	5 yrs 20%	–	5 yrs 32%
			28 (Control)	25	7.1	5 yrs 42%	–	5 yrs 60%

TACE transarterial chemoembolization, *RCT* randomized controlled trial

prior to liver resection, to improve the prognosis.[17-28] The rationale for such an approach was to reduce tumor size, induce tumor necrosis, and prevent from tumor cell dissemination during surgery. Several clinical studies have reported conflicting results, and no conclusion can be drawn based on the current literature. Because published studies are retrospective and heterogeneous, there is actually no convincing evidence to support its routine use before liver resection in patients with resectable disease at presentation.

The first series reporting on the impact of preoperative transarterial chemoembolization have been published in the late 1980s.[24,28,30,31] These series did not bring enough results due to the study design and small cohort samples to draw firm conclusions, and mainly failed to demonstrate a favorable impact on postoperative outcomes. We have reported our experience in a retrospective study[32] in which we compared outcomes following liver resection for HCC between patients undergoing a preoperative TACE ($n=24$) or not ($n=24$). Although one of the rationale for performing a preoperative TACE is tumor shrinkage, we did not confirm a reduction in tumor size following TACE, but the mean tumor size was >5 cm, and other authors have reported a correlation between tumor size and the degree of necrosis.[33] Although we found a higher rate of tumor necrosis on pathological examination of the resected specimen among patients who underwent preoperative TACE, no impact was found on the rate of tumor encapsulation, vascular invasion, and the presence of daughter nodules. Although a higher degree of tumor necrosis may be thought to positively impact on the oncologic prognosis,[25] it has also been suggested that partial necrosis could be associated with a loss of adhesion between cancer cells, which may enhance tumoral cell dislodgment during liver mobilization, and therefore early recurrences.[34,35] One of our findings may be concordant with this theory as disease-free survival was not superior in the group of patients undergoing liver resection following TACE ($33\% \pm 12\%$ vs. $32\% \pm 12\%$) at 3 years, and it may counterbalance the potential favorable impact that tumor necrosis could have on prognosis. Finally, as previously reported by others,[19,36] up to 88% of the patients who underwent a preoperative TACE were found to have inflammatory pediculitis, perihepatic adhesions, or arterial thrombosis, which led to an increased difficulty of the surgical procedure in these patients.

Luo et al.[23] have reviewed 126 patients among whom 62 underwent a preoperative TACE. The authors did not report on long-term prognosis but also found increased surgical difficulties, longer operative time, and increased blood loss when liver resection was performed after TACE as compared to up-front liver resection. Although retrospective, our series were concordant with other studies reporting that the preoperative use of TACE had no influence on the oncological prognosis.[17,19,20,25,27,28]

Harada et al.[25] reviewed 140 patients, among whom 105 underwent a preoperative TACE. They reported a high rate of complications following TACE, which negatively impact on the delay between TACE and resection. Although postoperative morbimortality was comparable among groups, TACE did not influence the overall and disease-free survival. More significantly, Sasaki et al.[20] even reported a worse 5-year overall survival when liver resection was preceded by TACE (28.6% vs. 50.6%), preoperative TACE being an independent predictor of poor outcomes in a multivariate model in combination with preoperative aspartate alanine aminotransferase elevation and microscopic portal invasion. Based on these observations, the authors concluded that TACE should be avoided in patients with resectable HCC at presentation.

One of the main limitations of retrospective series comparing the influence of a preoperative TACE before liver resection for HCC relies on a major selection bias. Indeed, it is often noted in these series that the two populations of patients being compared are not strictly comparable with a tendency to perform TACE in patients with more advanced disease. Consequently, definitive conclusions regarding long-term prognosis cannot be made. A prospective randomized trial provides the most statistically significant conclusion. Gerunda et al.[26] have reported in a prospective series a clear benefit of preoperative TACE before liver resection for HCC based on an improved disease-free survival in this subgroup of patients, 57% vs. 21% at 5 years. Yet, the authors have also reported a higher rate of postoperative liver failure in those patients receiving a preoperative TACE, which highlights the potential adverse impact of TACE in patients with diseased liver and, thus an impaired functional reserve. Furthermore, the treatment allocation was based on the patients' home site and not randomized, which may negatively impact on the power of the study.

The most significant study with the best design and statistical power has recently been published by Zhou et al.[17] In this work, 108 patients with resectable HCC ≥ 5 cm were randomly assigned to undergo liver resection with ($n = 52$) or without ($n = 56$) a preoperative TACE and the follow-up was prospective. First, the authors highlight the side effect of preoperative liver function, as 10% could not be resected following TACE because of extrahepatic disease or liver failure. Consequently, the resection rate was diminished among the TACE, and a longer operative procedure was noted because of increased surgical difficulties due to local adherence and inflammation following TACE. Yet, it did not translate into an increased postoperative morbidity nor did it increase the postoperative mortality. Finally, both disease-free and overall survival were similar, demonstrating that in their series, TACE had no influence on the prognosis following liver resection for HCC in patients deemed resectable at presentation.

Taken together, the role of preoperative TACE in resectable HCC cannot be recommended routinely as (1) it may further deteriorate the hepatic functional reserve and, thus, negatively impact on the postoperative outcomes in patients with chronic liver disease, (2) many series have shown increased surgical difficulties following TACE mainly due to a subsequent local inflammation and (3) it has no proven influence on the long-term prognosis. TACE may be discussed in non resectable or border line resectable patients because of a small FLR. Indeed, in good responders, tumors shrinkage following TACE may render these patients resectable, providing that they become elligible for a function sparing resection. In patients responding to TACE and experiencing a significant downsizing of the tumor, TACE may be a useful tool to expand the resection rate.[22,37] Finally, the use of arterial embolization may also be considered as an adjuvant option (i.e., postoperatively) and promising results have been reported in one prospective controlled trial showing an improved overall and disease-free survival with the use of adjuvant intra-arterial radioembolization (^{131}I-lipiodol) after curative resection of HCC.[38]

20.3 Results of Liver Resection for Hepatocellular Carcinoma Following a Preoperative Portal Vein Embolization

As the majority of HCC develop on a cirrhotic liver, one of the main limitations is a poor functional reserve and an inadequate liver remnant that may cause ineligibility for liver resection in patients otherwise good

Table 20.2 Selection of series reporting outcomes of liver resection for HCC after a preoperative portal vein embolization

Authors	Year	Type	*n*	Morbidity (%)	Mortality (%)	Disease-free survival	Actuarial survival
Wakabayashi et al.[47]	2001	Retrospective	26 (PVE)	–	11.5	5 yrs 40%	5 yrs 46%
			43 (Control)	–	3.5	5 yrs 46%	5 yrs 53%
Azoulay et al.[52]	2000	Retrospective	10 (PVE)	55	0	5 yrs 21%	5 yrs 44%
			19 (Control)	57	0	5 yrs 17%	5 yrs 53%
Tanaka et al.[48]	2000	Retrospective	33 (PVE)		3	5 yrs 33%	5 yrs 50%
			38 (Control)		5	5 yrs 20%	5 yrs 25%
Palavecino et al.[44]	2009	Retrospective	21 (PVE)	24	0	5 yrs 56%	5 yrs 72%
			33 (Control)	36	18	5 yrs 49%	5 yrs 54%
Seo et al.[45]	2007	Retrospective	32 (PVE)	19	0	5 yrs 37%	5 yrs 72%

PVE portal vein embolization

candidates on an oncologic standpoint. If the FLR is too small, the regenerative capacity is being outbalanced by the functional parenchyma loss with an inadequation of the immediate postoperative functional needs and by the regenerative capacity of the liver.[39] Liver failure represents the main cause of death after liver resection in the setting of cirrhosis, and the patients must be stringently selected and prepared before liver resection.

Portal vein embolization has been routinely applied to clinical practice by Makuuchi et al. in an intent to improve the safety of liver resection in patients with small liver remnant.[40] The rationale for such an approach was to hypotrophy the segments to be resected subsequently to the occlusion of their portal branches with a compensatory hypertrophy of the segment to remain after resection. This strategy has been shown to improve the safety of major liver resection, which consequently led to an extension of the indications of liver resections.[41] The functional reserve is correlated to the volume of liver parenchyma,[42] and its aim was to render nonresectable patients, because of an insufficient liver remnant, resectable. Yet, Makuuchi described the use of preoperative PVE in patients with biliary cancer, and many authors were initially reluctant for its use in HCC patients.

The reason for such a limited use of PVE in HCC patients was multifold. First, as mentioned above, HCCs are mainly fed by a branch of hepatic artery, and portal (branch) occlusion leads to a compensatory increase in the arterial flow in the HCC-feeding artery which may trigger an increase in the size of the tumor that may become nonresectable. Second, in patients with cirrhosis, it was thought to be a potential cause of liver decompensation and decrease of the functional reserve. Finally, regenerative ability of diseased liver is known to be impaired, and therefore its impact on liver regeneration was suspected to be dismal. Besides, in cirrhotic patients, arteriovenous shunts are frequent, which may further limit the efficacy of preoperative PVE. Taken together, authors did not recommend this technique in HCC patients.

Although the impact of preoperative PVE has been reported with good results in patients with biliary cancer or colorectal liver metastases,[43] its evaluation on long-term prognosis in HCC patients is scarce (Table 20.2).[44-52] The concept of using PVE to extend liver resection indications in HCC patients has been initially reported by Kinoshita et al.[50] Tanaka et al.[48] have evaluated the impact of preoperative PVE on long-term prognosis and found no difference in recurrence rates between patients being resected with or without a preoperative PVE. This lack of difference on long-term prognosis despite the theoretical pro-carcinogenic effect of PVE was thought to be related to the fact that portal occlusion may prevent from tumor dissemination in the portal system, which may counterbalance other factors. The main finding was the efficacy of PVE to improve the prognosis in patients with an impaired liver function, permitting an extension of the indications of liver resection. Although postoperative mortality was similar between groups, the cumulative survival was worse among patients with an Indocyanine Green retention rate at 15 min ($ICGR_{15}$)≥13% undergoing a right hepatectomy without a preoperative PVE. An analysis of this survival curve clearly illustrates that this difference is mainly related to an increased number of death during the first year post liver resection, which is likely

Table 20.3 Series of patients undergoing liver resection for HCC after a sequential arterioportal embolization

Authors	Year	Type	*n*	Morbidity (%)	Mortality (%)	Disease-free survival	Degree of necrosis	Actuarial survival
Ogata et al.[55]	2006	Retrospective	18 (TACE+PVE)	39	–	5 yrs 37%		–
			18 (PVE)	56	–	5 yrs 19%		–
Aoki et al.[53]	2004	Retrospective	17 (TACE+PVE)	24	0	5 yrs 47%		5 yrs 56%

to be related to a delayed postoperative liver failure than early recurrences. In this specific subgroup of patients, the lack of preoperative PVE was an independent factor of poor prognosis. Wakabayashi et al.[47] have subsequently confirmed the lack of impact on long-term prognosis of PVE after liver resection for HCC, but the authors have also highlighted that it may be helpful to increase the resectability rate.

Outcomes following liver resection for HCC following a preoperative PVE have been recently reported by the MD Anderson Cancer Center group in a small retrospective series, with good results. Preoperative PVE was associated with a significant decrease in postoperative mortality in the group of patients undergoing liver resection after PVE whereas mortality was 18% among patients operated upfront. Although not statistically significant, 5-year survival rate was 72% in the PVE group and 54% in the non-PVE group. Finally, the authors did not find an increased recurrence rate in patients undergoing preoperative PVE as DFS were comparable (5 years, 56% for the PVE group and 49% for the non-PVE group; $p=0.38$). Based on their results, the authors concluded that the use of PVE before liver resection for HCC was an efficient technical tool to improve immediate postoperative outcomes without compromising the oncologic results.

20.4 Sequential Preoperative Arterioportal Embolization Before Liver Resection for Hepatocellular Carcinoma

Although there are some theoretical limits for the use of preoperative PVE before liver resection for HCC as described above, published data support favorable outcome. It has been suggested that it may be even more efficient when used in combination with TACE, both procedures being theoretically synergistic. The rationale for this sequential approach is that TACE may suppress arteriovenous shunt, thus, enhancing the effect of PVE and increasing the rate of hypertrophy; a combination of arterioportal embolization may increase the rate of tumor necrosis, but the use of such a sequential approach may be limited by an increased rate of parenchymal damaged in the embolized liver. Series reporting outcomes following a sequential arterioportal embolization are summarized in Table 20.3.

Aoki et al. were the first to perform a comparative study comparing the sequential approach with TACE+PVE or PVE alone before major resections in cirrhotic patients. As previously reported by this team, indication for PVE was based on a combined evaluation of the future liver remnant and on the $ICGR_{15}$.[54] The authors aimed to evaluate the tolerance of the liver following a dual arterioportal embolization and its impact on postoperative outcomes and long-term prognosis. The follow-up following the TACE and PVE was assessed by biological liver function tests. The authors have reported a significant increase in portal venous pressure before and after PVE but without clinical significance. AST, ALT, and total bilirubin increased significantly after TACE and PVE but returned to baseline values within 2 weeks, and five (30%) experienced a complication after PVE. PVE was performed after a median interval of 9 days after TACE. Volumetric evaluation of the FLR showed a significant increase, and the AFP decreased significantly. Only one patient experienced a deterioration of liver function and could not be operated. A major liver resection could be carried out in 16 patients (94%). Postoperative morbidity was 25% and mortality was nil. Pathological examination of the resected specimen showed a necrosis >70% in 75% of the population. In this report, the authors have illustrated that a sequential TACE and PVE before major liver resection was feasible and safe, with a good outcome and a high tumor necrosis rate, which may be associated with a better prognosis.

This sequential strategy had been subsequently evaluated by Ogata et al.[55] in a retrospective comparative series, which assessed outcomes following liver resection for HCC following portal vein embolization of a sequential arterioportal approach. Overall, 36 patients were included (PVE: 18; TACE + PVE: 18). A longer delay was observed between both procedures as TACE preceded PVE by 3–4 weeks in Ogata's series, whereas the median delay was 9 days in Aoki's study. This longer delay may be associated with a better tolerance of the cirrhotic liver to ischemia, and postoperative course seemed to be better after a 3- to 4-week delay than after 9 days.[53,55,56] The main finding of this study was a significantly increased rate of hypertrophy of the FLR after TACE + PVE as compared to PVE alone. The rate of complete tumor necrosis was 83% among the patients who had undergone a sequential approach, and disease-free survival was significantly increased.

These two series fully support the use of a sequential approach among patients with a limited function reserve if they are planning to undergo a major liver resection for HCC. Indeed, it fully supports the rationale of such an approach as liver hypertrophy and tumor necrosis are significantly increased after TACE + PVE rather than PVE alone. Both series illustrate that a sequential embolization is safe even in patients with HCC, provided that they have a compensated cirrhosis. Besides, it increases the hypertrophy rate, and it may be used even in nonresectable patients as they may become resectable, and thus, indications for liver resection in such patients may be extended with such a strategy. Interestingly, a high rate of tumor necrosis is observed following the sequential approach, which may also support the oncologic rationale of such approach.

The reasons for such a high rate of tumor necrosis probably rely on the occlusion of arteriovenous shunt and on the need for HCC of a patent portal flow after TACE. Also, disease-free survival was increased after TACE + PVE in Ogata's paper, and these results need to be further confirmed with further studies. Although TACE is now widely accepted as the treatment of choice in the case of unresectable HCC[29], it leads to around 50% of complete tumor necrosis, whereas this rate is over 80% after sequential arterioportal embolization. Our experience is that of an 83% complete tumor necrosis rate after a sequential arterioportal approach.[55] Aoki et al.[53] have reported a necrosis rate >70% in 12/17 (71%). Yamakado et al.,[57] who have evaluated the long-term efficacy of TACE combined with transportal ethanol injection (TPEI) in a series of 26 patients with unresectable HCC, observed a complete tumoral necrosis in 78% and a promising 1, 3, and 5-year survival rates of 87%, 72%, and 51%, respectively. A rare but interesting case remain this of patients not being operated despite a preoperative PVE or TACE+PVE. Indeed, it is usually admitted that a PVE should contraindicate a subsequent TACE, leaving these patients without any treatment option and therefore a poor prognosis. This dogma may be revisited in selected cases, as some cases of arterial embolization following a PVE have been reported[58,59] with good tolerance and excellent outcomes (Fig. 20.1). Given these results, it appears that new fields of clinical research have to be explored, and the role and rationale of a sequential arterioportal embolization in patients with unresectable HCC remain to be defined by further studies.

20.5 Conclusion

Surgery, which remains the gold standard to treat HCC patient, can be used in combination with endovascular treatment. When transplantation is considered, TACE can be used as a first option in patients beyond the selection criteria, aiming at downstaging the disease and, in good responders, expanding the selection criteria. Patients fulfilling the selection criteria may benefit from TACE as a bridge treatment on the waiting list to avoid tumor progression and therefore being dropped out. When partial resection is considered, preoperative TACE can be used in selected patients in order to downsize the tumor in view of a function sparing resection or to render unresectable patients resectable. In patients with chronic liver disease, a major resection should always be preceded by a volume modulation using PVE. Sequential arterioportal embolization is safe, well tolerated, and induces an efficient regeneration, which is associated with improved outcomes following liver resection. Besides, it represents a good selection tool before liver resection as it tests the liver's regenerative capacity. Finally, this sequential strategy may even represent a valuable therapeutic option if the patient is not resected. Further prospective studies are needed to better define the best combination of surgical and radiological treatments in terms of survival.

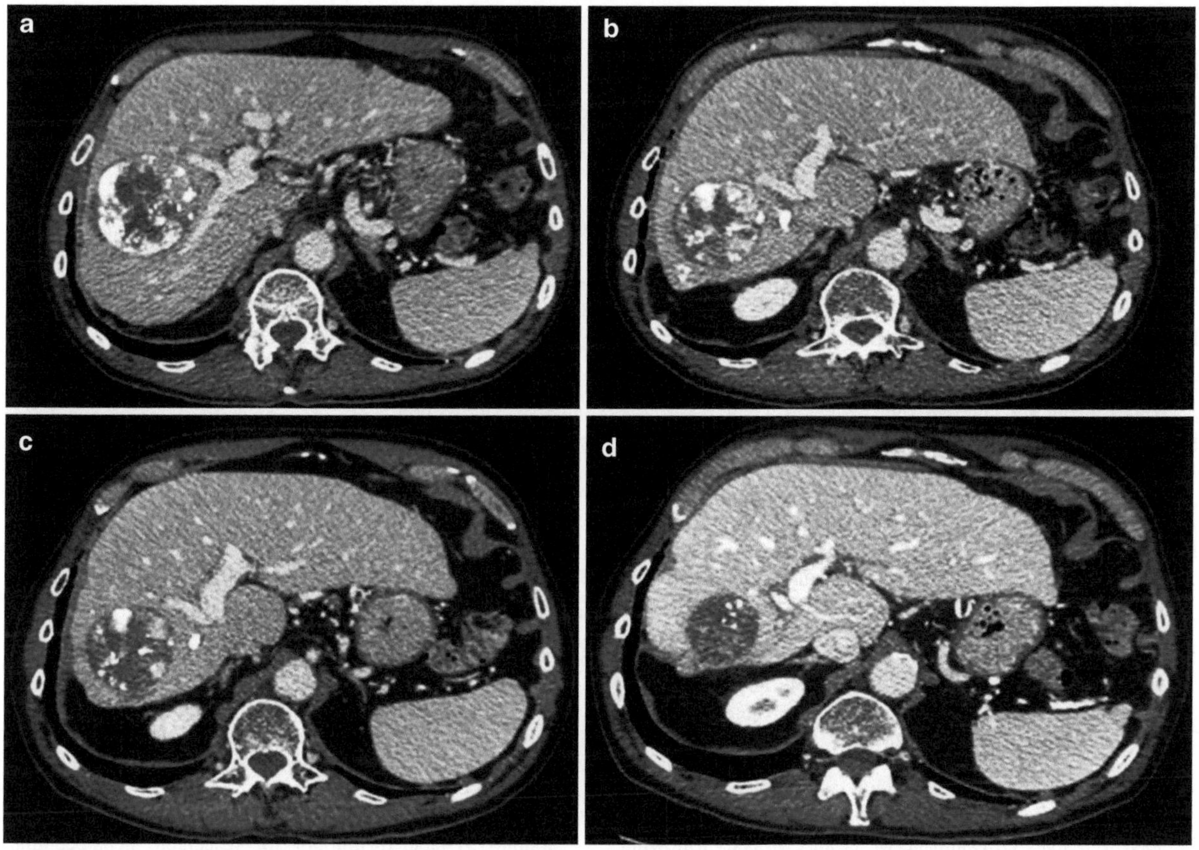

Fig. 20.1 An 84-year-old man with normal liver function was diagnosed with a 9-cm hepatocellular carcinoma arising in a background of hepatitic C cirrhosis. Alfa-foeto-protein was normal. He underwent a sequential arterioportal embolization within a 3-week delay. (**a**, **b**) An enhanced computed tomography performed after the first TACE and 1 month after PVE. Although a right hepatectomy was initially planned, he did not undergo liver resection because of his medical condition. A second TACE was then performed (**c**). The patient is still alive with an excellent tumor response after 22 months of follow-up (**d**)

References

1. Bosch FX, Ribes J, Diaz M, et al. Primary liver cancer: worldwide incidence and trends. *Gastroenterology*. 2004;127:S5-S16.
2. Belghiti J, Panis Y, Farges O, et al. Intrahepatic recurrence after resection of hepatocellular carcinoma complicating cirrhosis. *Ann Surg*. 1991;214:114-117.
3. Nagasue N, Uchida M, Makino Y, et al. Incidence and factors associated with intrahepatic recurrence following resection of hepatocellular carcinoma. *Gastroenterology*. 1993;105: 488-494.
4. Takayasu K, Wakao F, Moriyama N, et al. Postresection recurrence of hepatocellular carcinoma treated by arterial embolization: analysis of prognostic factors. *Hepatology*. 1992;16:906-911.
5. Nonami T, Isshiki K, Katoh H, et al. The potential role of postoperative hepatic artery chemotherapy in patients with high-risk hepatomas. *Ann Surg*. 1991;213:222-226.
6. Mazzaferro V, Regalia E, Doci R, et al. Liver transplantation for the treatment of small hepatocellular carcinomas in patients with cirrhosis. *N Engl J Med*. 1996;334:693-699.
7. Okada S, Shimada K, Yamamoto J, et al. Predictive factors for postoperative recurrence of hepatocellular carcinoma. *Gastroenterology*. 1994;106:1618-1624.
8. Vauthey JN, Lauwers GY, Esnaola NF, et al. Simplified staging for hepatocellular carcinoma. *J Clin Oncol*. 2002;20:1527-1536.
9. Chapman WC, Majella Doyle MB, Stuart JE, et al. Outcomes of neoadjuvant transarterial chemoembolization to downstage hepatocellular carcinoma before liver transplantation. *Ann Surg*. 2008;248:617-625.
10. Belghiti J, Cortes A, Abdalla EK, et al. Resection prior to liver transplantation for hepatocellular carcinoma. *Ann Surg*. 2003;238:885-892. discussion 892–883.
11. Belghiti J. Resection of hepatocellular carcinoma complicating cirrhosis. *Br J Surg*. 1991;78:257-258.
12. Kubota K, Makuuchi M, Kusaka K, et al. Measurement of liver volume and hepatic functional reserve as a guide to

decision-making in resectional surgery for hepatic tumors. *Hepatology*. 1997;26:1176-1181.
13. Abulkhir A, Limongelli P, Healey AJ, et al. Preoperative portal vein embolization for major liver resection: a meta-analysis. *Ann Surg*. 2008;247:49-57.
14. Truty MJ, Vauthey JN. Uses and limitations of portal vein embolization for improving perioperative outcomes in hepatocellular carcinoma. *Semin Oncol*. 2010;37:102-109.
15. Lesurtel M, Mullhaupt B, Pestalozzi BC, et al. Transarterial chemoembolization as a bridge to liver transplantation for hepatocellular carcinoma: an evidence-based analysis. *Am J Transplant*. 2006;6:2644-2650.
16. Lewandowski RJ, Kulik LM, Riaz A, et al. A comparative analysis of transarterial downstaging for hepatocellular carcinoma: chemoembolization versus radioembolization. *Am J Transplant*. 2009;9:1920-1928.
17. Zhou WP, Lai EC, Li AJ, et al. A prospective, randomized, controlled trial of preoperative transarterial chemoembolization for resectable large hepatocellular carcinoma. *Ann Surg*. 2009;249:195-202.
18. Zhang Z, Liu Q, He J, et al. The effect of preoperative transcatheter hepatic arterial chemoembolization on disease-free survival after hepatectomy for hepatocellular carcinoma. *Cancer*. 2000;89:2606-2612.
19. Wu CC, Ho YZ, Ho WL, et al. Preoperative transcatheter arterial chemoembolization for resectable large hepatocellular carcinoma: a reappraisal. *Br J Surg*. 1995;82:122-126.
20. Sasaki A, Iwashita Y, Shibata K, et al. Preoperative transcatheter arterial chemoembolization reduces long-term survival rate after hepatic resection for resectable hepatocellular carcinoma. *Eur J Surg Oncol*. 2006;32:773-779.
21. Paye F, Farges O, Dahmane M, et al. Cytolysis following chemoembolization for hepatocellular carcinoma. *Br J Surg*. 1999;86:176-180.
22. Majno PE, Adam R, Bismuth H, et al. Influence of preoperative transarterial lipiodol chemoembolization on resection and transplantation for hepatocellular carcinoma in patients with cirrhosis. *Ann Surg*. 1997;226:688-701. discussion 701–683.
23. Luo YQ, Wang Y, Chen H, et al. Influence of preoperative transcatheter arterial chemoembolization on liver resection in patients with resectable hepatocellular carcinoma. *Hepatobiliary Pancreat Dis Int*. 2002;1:523-526.
24. Hwang TL, Chen MF, Lee TY, et al. Resection of hepatocellular carcinoma after transcatheter arterial embolization. Reevaluation of the advantages and disadvantages of preoperative embolization. *Arch Surg*. 1987;122:756-759.
25. Harada T, Matsuo K, Inoue T, et al. Is preoperative hepatic arterial chemoembolization safe and effective for hepatocellular carcinoma? *Ann Surg*. 1996;224:4-9.
26. Gerunda GE, Neri D, Merenda R, et al. Role of transarterial chemoembolization before liver resection for hepatocarcinoma. *Liver Transpl*. 2000;6:619-626.
27. Choi GH, Kim DH, Kang CM, et al. Is preoperative transarterial chemoembolization needed for a resectable hepatocellular carcinoma? *World J Surg*. 2007;31:2370-2377.
28. Nagasue N, Galizia G, Kohno H, et al. Adverse effects of preoperative hepatic artery chemoembolization for resectable hepatocellular carcinoma: a retrospective comparison of 138 liver resections. *Surgery*. 1989;106:81-86.
29. Llovet JM, Bruix J. Systematic review of randomized trials for unresectable hepatocellular carcinoma: chemoembolization improves survival. *Hepatology*. 2003;37:429-442.
30. Monden M, Okamura J, Sakon M, et al. Significance of transcatheter chemoembolization combined with surgical resection for hepatocellular carcinomas. *Cancer Chemother Pharmacol*. 1989;23(Suppl):S90-S95.
31. Shimamura Y, Gunven P, Takenaka Y, et al. Combined peripheral and central chemoembolization of liver tumors. Experience with lipiodol-doxorubicin and gelatin sponge (L-TAE). *Cancer*. 1988;61:238-242.
32. Paye F, Jagot P, Vilgrain V, et al. Preoperative chemoembolization of hepatocellular carcinoma: a comparative study. *Arch Surg*. 1998;133:767-772.
33. Shim JH, Kim KM, Lee YJ, et al. Complete necrosis after transarterial chemoembolization could predict prolonged survival in patients with recurrent intrahepatic hepatocellular carcinoma after curative resection. *Ann Surg Oncol*. 2010;17:869-877.
34. Adachi E, Matsumata T, Nishizaki T, et al. Effects of preoperative transcatheter hepatic arterial chemoembolization for hepatocellular carcinoma. The relationship between postoperative course and tumor necrosis. *Cancer*. 1993;72: 3593-3598.
35. Liou TC, Shih SC, Kao CR, et al. Pulmonary metastasis of hepatocellular carcinoma associated with transarterial chemoembolization. *J Hepatol*. 1995;23:563-568.
36. Yu YQ, Xu DB, Zhou XD, et al. Experience with liver resection after hepatic arterial chemoembolization for hepatocellular carcinoma. *Cancer*. 1993;71:62-65.
37. Lau WY, Ho SK, Yu SC, et al. Salvage surgery following downstaging of unresectable hepatocellular carcinoma. *Ann Surg*. 2004;240:299-305.
38. Lau WY, Lai EC, Leung TW, et al. Adjuvant intra-arterial iodine-131-labeled lipiodol for resectable hepatocellular carcinoma: a prospective randomized trial-update on 5-year and 10-year survival. *Ann Surg*. 2008;247:43-48.
39. Garcea G, Maddern GJ. Liver failure after major hepatic resection. *J Hepatobiliary Pancreat Surg*. 2009;16:145-155.
40. Makuuchi M, Thai BL, Takayasu K, et al. Preoperative portal embolization to increase safety of major hepatectomy for hilar bile duct carcinoma: a preliminary report. *Surgery*. 1990;107:521-527.
41. de Baere T, Roche A, Elias D, et al. Preoperative portal vein embolization for extension of hepatectomy indications. *Hepatology*. 1996;24:1386-1391.
42. Yigitler C, Farges O, Kianmanesh R, et al. The small remnant liver after major liver resection: How common and how relevant? *Liver Transpl*. 2003;9:S18-S25.
43. Hemming AW, Reed AI, Howard RJ, et al. Preoperative portal vein embolization for extended hepatectomy. *Ann Surg*. 2003;237:686-691. discussion 691–683.
44. Palavecino M, Chun YS, Madoff DC, et al. Major hepatic resection for hepatocellular carcinoma with or without portal vein embolization: perioperative outcome and survival. *Surgery*. 2009;145:399-405.
45. Seo DD, Lee HC, Jang MK, et al. Preoperative portal vein embolization and surgical resection in patients with hepatocellular carcinoma and small future liver remnant volume: comparison with transarterial chemoembolization. *Ann Surg Oncol*. 2007;14:3501-3509.
46. Chik BH, Liu CL, Fan ST, et al. Tumor size and operative risks of extended right-sided hepatic resection for hepatocellular carcinoma: implication for preoperative portal vein embolization. *Arch Surg*. 2007;142:63-69. discussion 69.

47. Wakabayashi H, Ishimura K, Okano K, et al. Is preoperative portal vein embolization effective in improving prognosis after major hepatic resection in patients with advanced-stage hepatocellular carcinoma? *Cancer*. 2001;92:2384-2390.
48. Tanaka H, Hirohashi K, Kubo S, et al. Preoperative portal vein embolization improves prognosis after right hepatectomy for hepatocellular carcinoma in patients with impaired hepatic function. *Br J Surg*. 2000;87:879-882.
49. Lee KC, Kinoshita H, Hirohashi K, et al. Extension of surgical indications for hepatocellular carcinoma by portal vein embolization. *World J Surg*. 1993;17:109-115.
50. Kinoshita H, Sakai K, Hirohashi K, et al. Preoperative portal vein embolization for hepatocellular carcinoma. *World J Surg*. 1986;10:803-808.
51. Sugawara Y, Yamamoto J, Higashi H, et al. Preoperative portal embolization in patients with hepatocellular carcinoma. *World J Surg*. 2002;26:105-110.
52. Azoulay D, Castaing D, Krissat J, et al. Percutaneous portal vein embolization increases the feasibility and safety of major liver resection for hepatocellular carcinoma in injured liver. *Ann Surg*. 2000;232:665-672.
53. Aoki T, Imamura H, Hasegawa K, et al. Sequential preoperative arterial and portal venous embolizations in patients with hepatocellular carcinoma. *Arch Surg*. 2004;139:766-774.
54. Makuuchi M, Kosuge T, Lygidakis NJ. New possibilities for major liver surgery in patients with Klatskin tumors or primary hepatocellular carcinoma—an old problem revisited. *Hepatogastroenterology*. 1991;38:329-336.
55. Ogata S, Belghiti J, Farges O, et al. Sequential arterial and portal vein embolizations before right hepatectomy in patients with cirrhosis and hepatocellular carcinoma. *Br J Surg*. 2006;93:1091-1098.
56. Yamakado K, Takeda K, Matsumura K, et al. Regeneration of the un-embolized liver parenchyma following portal vein embolization. *J Hepatol*. 1997;27:871-880.
57. Yamakado K, Nakatsuka A, Tanaka N, et al. Long-term follow-up arterial chemoembolization combined with transportal ethanol injection used to treat hepatocellular carcinoma. *J Vasc Interv Radiol*. 1999;10:641-647.
58. Zalinski S, Scatton O, Randone B, et al. Complete hepatocellular carcinoma necrosis following sequential porto-arterial embolization. *World J Gastroenterol*. 2008;14:6869-6872.
59. Wallace MJ, Ahrar K, Madoff DC. Chemoembolization of the liver after portal vein embolization: report of three cases. *J Vasc Interv Radiol*. 2008;19:1513-1517.

21 Clinical Outcomes for Biliary Tract Cancer

Yukihiro Yokoyama and Masato Nagino

Abstract

Surgical treatment for biliary tract cancer is challenging. Biliary cancer originating from the perihilar region is especially difficult to treat, due to anatomical complexity at the hepatic hilus. However, in the past few decades there have been dramatic advancements with regard to diagnosis, surgical technique, and perioperative patients' management for biliary tract cancer. These advancements have not only decreased the rate of postoperative morbidity and mortality but have also improved patients' survival. The standard surgical procedure for hilar cholangiocarcinoma comprises major hepatectomy combined with caudate lobectomy and extrahepatic bile duct resection. This means that surgeons must overcome the complications accompanying this highly invasive surgery. In this regard, the innovation of portal vein embolization has substantially contributed to a decrease in the risk of major hepatectomy.

Keywords

Biliary tract cancer • Cancer of the biliary tract • Management of biliary tract cancer • Hilar cholangiocarcinoma • Hepatectomy • Portal vein embolization

Surgical treatment for biliary tract cancer is challenging. To completely remove the tumor, it is often necessary to perform major hepatectomy, caudate lobectomy, or pancreatoduodenectomy[1] depending on longitudinal tumor extension along the bile duct. Due to the thin nature of the bile duct wall, cancer occurring in the biliary tract also easily invades adjacent vessels, such as the portal vein and the hepatic artery. In such cases, combined resection and reconstruction of these vessels are necessary[2]; these procedures render surgery for biliary tract cancer even more difficult.

Surgical treatment for the biliary cancer originating from the perihilar region is especially difficult due to anatomical complexity at the hepatic hilus. Since hilar cholangiocarcinoma was recognized as a distinct disease by Klatskin[3] and Altemeiter,[4] many surgeons have attempted to treat this challenging disease through surgery. As a result, there have been dramatic advancements in the past few decades with regard to diagnosis, surgical technique, and perioperative patient management. These advancements have not only decreased the rate of postoperative morbidity and mortality but have also improved patient survival.[5-7]

M. Nagino (✉)
Division of Surgical Oncology, Department of Surgery, Nagoya University Graduate School of Medicine, 65 Tsurumai-cho, Showa-ku, Nagoya, Aichi, 466-8550, Japan
e-mail: nagino@med.nagoya-u.ac.jp

D.C. Madoff et al. (eds.), *Venous Embolization of the Liver*,
DOI 10.1007/978-1-84882-122-4_21, © Springer-Verlag London Limited 2011

Advancements in peri-surgical management of biliary tract cancer include (1) a sophisticated drainage technique for biliary obstruction,[8,9] (2) accurate diagnosis by various advanced diagnostic modalities,[10-13] (3) an improved surgical technique based on a deeper understanding of the perihilar surgical anatomy,[14-17] (4) careful perioperative patients' management,[18,19] and (5) development of adjuvant therapy,[20] and others. The innovation represented by portal vein embolization (PVE) increased the safety of major hepatectomy and substantially contributed to a decrease in postoperative complications.[21-23]

Each improvement enhanced not only the treatment of biliary tract cancer, but also treatment of other liver diseases, such as hepatocellular carcinoma and colorectal liver metastasis, which are generally considered relatively easier diseases to manage than biliary tract cancer. Nevertheless, the surgical outcome for biliary tract cancer is still unsatisfactory and may still be improved. Further advancement in perioperative patient management may improve the outcome for the surgical treatment of biliary tract cancer, especially cases requiring major hepatectomy such as perihilar cholangiocarcinoma. This section discusses the historical shift in the style of surgical approach for biliary tract cancer and recent advancements in surgical outcome. Future possibilities for surgical treatment will also be discussed.

21.1 History of Surgical Treatment for Biliary Tract Cancer with a Focus on Hilar Cholangiocarcinoma

Among biliary tract cancers, hilar cholangiocarcinoma is the most difficult to treat. Since the earliest report of hilar cholangiocarcinoma by Klatskin,[3] a surgical approach has been the only way to achieve long-term survival with this disease.[24,25] Therefore, surgeons have invested much effort to improve the accuracy of diagnosis, understand variable anatomy at the hepatic hilus, and improve perioperative patient management.

In a report by Bismuth et al. in 1990s, resection for hilar cholangiocarcinoma was possible in only a small proportion of patients.[26] In this study, the microscopic curative resection rate was unsatisfactorily low (10/23, 43%), probably due to a high rate of local excision without hepatic resection. The rate of curative resection may be much lower in patients undergoing local resection as compared to patients undergoing aggressive hepatic resection.[27] Hilar cholangiocarcinoma easily invades the biliary branches of the caudate lobe because most of the biliary branches from this segment merge into the right or left hepatic duct at the hepatic hilus. Therefore, a combination of caudate lobectomy with extrahepatic bile duct resection was necessary to ensure a safe surgical margin. However, the caudate lobe sits in the dorsal part of the liver and is adjacent to the inferior vena cava, hepatic vein, and hepatic hilus. Therefore, the resection of only the caudate lobe required a meticulous surgical technique, a longer operation time, and involved greater intraoperative blood loss. The procedure is like "digging a tunnel" in the liver, even though the volume of removed liver after caudate lobectomy was only 3–5% of the total liver volume. Furthermore, hilar cholangiocarcinoma that originated in the hepatic hilus easily extends to the right or left hepatic duct or even to the subsegmental branch of the intrahepatic bile duct. In such cases, caudate lobectomy is not sufficient, and combined major hepatectomy was necessary to completely remove the tumor.

Consequently, the standard surgical procedure for hilar cholangiocarcinoma has shifted from the local excision or caudate lobectomy with extrahepatic bile duct resection to the major hepatectomy combined with caudate lobectomy and extrahepatic bile duct resection. Even for nodular or infiltrating Bismuth type I or II hilar cholangiocarcinomas, survival was better in patients who underwent right hepatectomy with caudate lobectomy rather than in those who underwent other types of less invasive surgery.[28] In a case with severely extended tumor in the longitudinal direction along the bile duct, pancreatoduodenectomy combined with major hepatectomy is necessary to completely remove the tumor.[29] This means that surgeons had to simultaneously overcome the complications accompanying these highly invasive surgeries, which are sometimes fatal for patients.[25,30] However, several recent advancements in peri-surgical patient management in major hepatectomy, including portal vein embolization (PVE), have enabled us to perform this highly invasive surgery with much less risk than before.

21.2 Recent Progress with regard to Surgical Outcome

As the surgical procedure for hilar cholangiocarcinoma shifted to a more aggressive approach, the surgical outcome has also changed, especially in high volume centers.[5-7] Surgical outcome of hilar cholangiocarcinoma used to be unsatisfactory. In 1996, Nakeeb et al. reported their experience in the treatment of cholangiocarcinoma over the past two decades (from 1973 to 1995) in the Johns Hopkins Medical Institutions.[31] For 196 perihilar cholangiocarcinomas, the respectability was 56%; the 5-year survival rate and median survival were 11% and 19 months, respectively. The report by Madariaga et al. in 1998 showed their 14-year experience with 62 consecutive patients with hilar cholangiocarcinoma.[32] In this study, postoperative morbidity and mortality were considerably high (32% and 14%, respectively). Nevertheless, the survival rate was not satisfactory: 79% at 1 year, 39% at 3 year, and only 8% at 5 years. The median survival rate was 24 months. The report by Iwatsuki et al. on the authors' treatment experience with hilar cholangiocarcinoma between 1981 and 1996 also showed a similar survival rate after hepatic resection; the 5-year survival rate was 9%.[33]

However, since around the year 2000, surgical outcome for hilar cholangiocarcinoma has substantially improved in many institutions. Ito et al. analyzed their surgical experience for 69 patients with hilar cholangiocarcinoma by comparing an earlier era (1985–1994) and a recent era (1995–2006).[5] In the recent era, resectability rates improved compared to the past era (69% vs. 17%). Median survival in the patients with R0 resection was significantly longer (65 months) than in those with R1 or R2 resection (16 months). Ito et al. concluded that concomitant hepatic resection was associated with improved survival and a slower rate of hepatic recurrence. Sano et al. analyzed 126 patients after major hepatobiliary resection for hilar cholangiocarcinoma in a single center and compared the group from the early period (1980–1999, 63 patients) to the group from the late period (2000–2004, 63 patients).[6] Their results showed that the mortality rate improved from 7.9% in the early period to 0% in the late period. The rate of major morbidity (15/63 vs. 6/63, $P<0.031$) and length of hospital stay (74.4 vs. 29.0, $P<0.001$) were also improved in the late period as compared with the early period. Dinant et al. have also applied an extensive surgical approach in treating hilar cholangiocarcinoma in recent years.[7] In this study, a total of 99 consecutive patients underwent resection for hilar cholangiocarcinoma from 1988 to 2003. The authors divided the term in three 5-year time periods: periods (1) (1988–1993; $n=45$), (2) (1993–1998; $n=25$), and (3) (1998–2003; $n=29$). The proportion of margin-negative resections increased considerably in the recent periods (13% in period 1 to 59% in period 3) and this has resulted in improved survival without significantly affecting postoperative morbidity or mortality.

All of these improvements are likely due to multiple factors, including improvement in preoperative diagnosis, increased rate of major hepatectomy in the treatment of biliary cancer performed with a safe surgical margin (due to the contribution of PVE), and improvements in peri-surgical management.

21.3 Surgical Outcome of Biliary Tract Cancer: Nagoya Experience

We have been treating many patients with perihilar cholangiocarcinoma in our institution (Division of Surgical Oncology, Nagoya University Graduate School of Medicine) since the beginning of the 1980s. Simultaneously, we have been performing PVE for many patients before major hepatectomy for perihilar cholangiocarcinoma. Here we present our recent data for the surgical treatment of perihilar cholangiocarcinomas that require preoperative PVE.

Among 606 hepatectomies performed for biliary cancer in our institution from 1991 to 2008, 314 hepatectomies (52%) were performed after PVE. The surgical outcomes for these patients (except for one patient who revealed ICG excretory defect) were analyzed.

In principle, PVE was indicated when a future liver remnant was estimated to be less than 40% (therefore, resection rate is ≥60%). In jaundiced patients, PVE was not performed until the serum total bilirubin concentrations had decreased to at least <5 mg/dL following biliary drainage.[34] All PVEs were performed by the ipsilateral approach, in which the portal vein was accessed by ultrasound-guided puncture of the portal vein to be embolized.[22,34,35] From 1991 to 2000, fibrin glue mixed with iodized oil was used as the embolic material. After 2001, absolute ethanol with embolization steel coils was used because the Prefectural Insurance System prohibited the use of fibrin glue. In our data, there was no difference between the two different embolic materials in either the effectiveness or the post-procedure complication rate.

Table 21.1 shows the clinical characteristics of 313 patients. PVE was performed for the cases of major hepatectomy, including right trisectionectomy ($n=36$), left trisectionectomy ($n=74$), right hepatectomy

Table 21.1 Clinical characteristics of 313 patients included in this study

Age	
Range	25–83
Mean	64.6±9.7
Gender	
Male (%)	175 (56)
Female (%)	138 (44)
Diagnosis	
Cholangiocarcinoma (%)	235 (75)
Gallbladder carcinoma (%)	78 (25)
Type of hepatectomy[a]	
Right trisectionectomy (%)	36 (11.5)
Left trisectionectomy (%)	74 (23.6)
Right hepatectomy (%)	202 (64.5)
Central bisegmentectomy (%)	1 (0.3)
Combined resection	
Portal vein resection and reconstruction (%)	111 (35.5)
Hepatic artery resection and reconstruction (%)	29 (9.3)
Pancreatoduodenectomy (%)	77 (24.5)
Liver volume by CT volumentry (mL)	1078 ± 226
Proportion of FLR (%)	42.7 ± 7.9
Plasma disappearance rate of indocyanine green (ICGK)	0.158 ± 0.030
Plasma disappearance rate of indocyanine green for future liver remnant (ICGK-F)	0.067 ± 0.017

[a]All hepatectomies except for three right hepatectomies were combined with caudate lobectomy

(n=202), and central bisegmentectomy (n=1). PVE was not indicated for the patients who would undergo left hepatectomy, because in these patients, the volume of the future liver remnant (FLR) was sufficiently large. We routinely performed the test for plasma disappearance rate of the indocyanine green (ICGK) and computed tomography (CT) volumetry to assess the capacity of the future liver remnant with regard to both volume and function. Using these two indices, we calculated future liver remnant ICGK (ICGK-F) by multiplying the proportion of future liver remnant and ICGK, as a useful predictor for the functional reserve of the liver after hepatectomy. We considered ICGK-F 0.05 as a critical cutoff value in predicting postoperative mortality, as shown in our previous study.[36] The average ICGK-F for 313 patients with PVE was 0.067 (range 0.027–0.122).

In general, patients underwent CT within 3 weeks after PVE. In four patients, additional transcatheter arterial embolization (TAE) was performed due to insufficient volume increase in the non-embolized lobe. The calculated volume of the embolized lobe decreased from 683±169 cm^3 (range, 341–1,283 cm^3) before PVE to 570±154 cm^3 (range, 252–1,153 cm^3) after PVE (P<0.0001), whereas the volume of the non-embolized lobe increased from 375±123 cm^3 (range, 103–800 cm^3) before PVE to 469±124 cm^3 (range, 238–854 cm^3) after PVE (P<0.0001) (Fig. 21.1). The atrophy ratio of the embolized lobe was 71%±21% (range, 27–170%), whereas the hypertrophy ratio of the non-embolized lobe was 129%±24% (range, 88–271%). The average atrophy ratio in patients ≥70 years of age was significantly higher than that in patients with <70 years of age, although there was no difference in the hypertrophy ratio between these two groups. Gender, presence of diabetes, maximum preoperative serum total bilirubin ≥10 mg/dL, history of cholangitis, and low ICGK clearance rate (<0.125) did not affect volume dynamics after PVE (Table 21.2).

In the 313 hepatectomized patients, we experienced 21 postoperative deaths (non-survivors). The clinical characteristics and the trigger of death for these patients are described in Table 21.3. Among the 21 non-survivors, the ICGK-F was <0.05 in eight patients (38%), the operation time was ≥10 h in 19 patients (90%), and the intraoperative blood loss was ≥2,000 mL in 16 patients (76%). Infectious complications, intra-abdominal bleeding, and portal vein thrombosis were the major triggers of death, although most of the patients finally experienced hepatic failure with serum total bilirubin levels ≥10 mg/dL.

Among the preoperative variables, the proportion of patients with gallbladder cancer, diabetes, and ICGK-F <0.05 was significantly higher among the non-survivors than among the survivors (Table 21.4). Among the intraoperative variables, the proportions of patients with an operation time ≥600 min, blood loss ≥2,000 mL, or use of allogeneic blood transfusion were significantly higher in the non-survivors than in the survivors (Table 21.5). With multivariate analysis including all the factors that showed a significant difference, the significant factors in predicting postoperative mortality remained the type of disease, presence of diabetes, and ICGK-F <0.05 (odds ratio: type of disease, 3.16; diabetes, 7.41; ICGK-F <0.05, 4.98) (Table 21.6).

In our department, as in other high volume institutions, there has been a significant increase in the number

Fig. 21.1 Changes in liver volume of the embolized lobe and the non-embolized lobe before and after portal vein embolization (PVE)

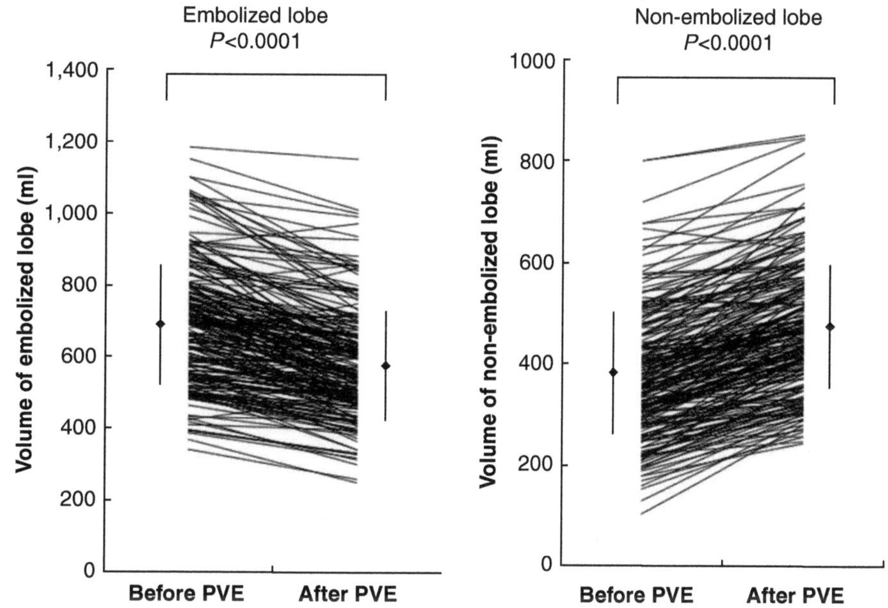

Table 21.2 Potential factors affecting atrophy and hypertrophy ratio after PVE

	No.	Atrophy ratio of the embolized lobe (%)	*P* value	Hypertrophy ratio of the nonembolized lobe (%)	*P* value
Gender					
Male	175	71±23	0.521	129±22	0.841
Female	138	72±19		130±26	
Age≥70					
Yes	109	75±21	0.039	132±28	0.136
No	204	69±21		128±21	
Diabetes					
Present	33	73±22	0.716	132±22	0.462
Absent	280	71±21		129±24	
Maximum T-Bil≥1 0 mg/dL					
Yes	81	71±20	0.748	126±22	0.124
No	232	72±22		131±24	
History of cholangitis					
Yes	55	71±21	0.700	129±23	0.862
No	258	72±25		129±27	
ICGK <0.125					
Yes	127	71±21	0.107	126±19	0.354
No	186	77±24		130±24	

of major hepatectomies for biliary tract cancer in recent years, and postoperative morbidity and mortality have dramatically improved. Therefore, we re-analyzed our data by separating the term from 1991 to 2000 (the former period) and the term from 2001 to 2008 (the latter period). The proportions of patients with operation time ≥600 min, blood loss ≥2,000 mL, or allogeneic blood transfusion were also significantly lower in the latter period, even though in recent years we have been performing more aggressive surgery, such as combined hepatic artery resection and reconstruction for the cases with suspected arterial invasion

Table 21.3 Clinical characteristics of 21 patients who died postoperatively

Year of operation	Gender	Age	ICGK-F	Type of disease	Performed operation	PV-R	Operation time (min)	Blood loss (mL)	Tigger of death
1991	M	72	0.039	GBC	R2	No	807	2,969	Pneumonia
1991	M	67	0.084	GBC	R2	No	1,020	17,114	Intra-abdominal bleeding
1995	M	75	0.027	GBC	R2+PD	No	915	9,100	Intra-abdominal abscess[a]
1995	M	67	0.058	BDC	R2	No	640	2,803	Intra-abdominal bleeding
1995	F	70	0.056	GBC	R2+PD	No	1,055	4,922	Cardiac failure
1997	M	67	0.031	BDC	R3	No	840	1,750	Sepsis, intestinal bleeding
1997	F	60	0.070	GBC	R2+PD	Yes	1,115	3,263	MRSA sepsis
1998	M	80	0.041	BDC	R2	No	595	2,069	MRSA cholangitis
1998	M	71	0.048	GBC	R2+PD	Yes	940	7,037	Pneumonia, hemoptysis
1998	M	74	0.067	BDC	L3	Yes	835	3,594	Sepsis, intestinal bleeding
1999	F	76	0.077	BDC	R3	Yes	775	1,531	Intra-abdominal bleeding, sepsis
1999	M	72	0.046	GBC	R2	Yes	725	1,404	MRSA sepsis
2000	F	62	0.063	GBC	R2	Yes	635	2,056	MRSA sepsis
2002	F	55	0.071	GBC	R2+PD	Yes	730	3,156	Intra-abdominal abscess[b]
2004	M	71	0.038	GBC	R2	Yes	935	10,835	Intra-abdominal abscess and bleeding[b]
2004	F	56	0.083	GBC	R2+PD	Yes	1,095	5,955	Intra-abdominal abscess and bleeding[b]
2005	F	68	0.061	BDC	R2+PD	Yes	805	1,834	Intra-abdominal abscess
2005	M	60	0.069	BDC	R2+PD	No	790	1,726	PV thrombosis
2006	F	64	0.049	BDC	R2	No	800	3,669	PV thrombosis
2007	F	78	0.057	BDC	R2	Yes	571	2,386	PV thrombosis
2008	F	77	0.059	GBC	R2+PD	Yes	791	8,502	PV thrombosis

R2 resection of the segment 1, 5, 6, 7, 8; *R3* resection of the segment 1, 4, 5, 6, 7, 8; *L3* resection of the segment 1, 2, 3, 4, 5, 8; *PD* pancreaticoduodenectomy; *PV thrombosis* portal veinous thrombosis; *MRSA* methicillin-resistant staphylococcus aureus; *GBC* gallbladder cancer; *BDC* bile duct cancer; *PV-R* portal vein resection and reconstruction

[a]Due to anastomotic leakage

[b]Due to pancreatic fistula

Table 21.4 Univariate analysis of preoperative variables associated with postoperative mortality

	Survivors (*N*=292)		Nonsurvivors (*N*=21)		
Variables	*N*	(%)	*N*	(%)	*P* value
Age					
≥70	98	(34)	11	(52)	0.098
Gender					
Male	164	(56)	11	(52)	0.821
Type of disease					
BDC	226	(77)	9	(43)	0.001
GBC	66	(23)	12	(57)	
Diabetes					
Yes	26	(9)	8	(38)	0.001
Maximum T-Bil≥10 mg/dL					
Yes	75	(26)	8	(38)	0.306
History of cholangitis					
Yes	51	(17)	4	(19)	0.772
ICGK					
<0.125	34	(12)	5	(24)	0.160
ICGK-F					
<0.05	40	(14)	8	(38)	0.007

BDC bile duct cancer; *GBC* gallbladder cancer

Table 21.5 Univariate analysis of intraoperative variables associated with postoperative mortality

	Survivors (*N*=292)		Nonsurvivors (*N*=21)		
Variables	*N*	(%)	*N*	(%)	*P* value
Extent of liver resection					
≥60%	106	(36)	10	(48)	0.351
Combined portal vein resection					
Yes	99	(34)	12	(57)	0.056
Combined hepatic artery resection					
Yes	29	(10)	0	(–)	0.238
Combined pancreatoduodenectomy					
Yes	68	(23)	9	(43)	0.063
Operation time					
≥600 min	183	(63)	19	(90)	0.009
Blood loss					
≥2,000 mL	140	(48)	16	(76)	0.013
Allogeneic blood transfusion					
Yes	121	(41)	14	(67)	0.038

by the cancer. Nevertheless, the rates of postoperative death, infectious complications, and postoperative hepatic failure were significantly lower in the latter period as compared to the former period (Table 21.7). Moreover, the 5-year survival rate was significantly higher in the latter group as compared with the former group (43% vs. 20%, $P<0.001$) (Fig. 21.2). These results indicated that improved perioperative patient management including PVE enabled us to perform more aggressive surgery for biliary tract cancer. This strategy not only contributed to a decrease in postoperative morbidity and mortality but also to prolong patient survival.

21.4 Future Plans

There has been a dramatic advancement in the surgical treatment for hilar cholangiocarcinoma in the past few decades. In this regard, patients with perihilar

Table 21.6 Multiple logistic regression analysis of variables associated with mortality

Variables	Odds ratio	95% confidence interval	*P* value
Type of disease			
GBC	3.16	1.17–8.51	0.023
Diabetes			
Yes	7.41	2.43–22.59	<0.001
ICGK-F			
<0.05	4.98	1.67–14.91	0.004
Operation time			
≥600 min	3.60	0.65–19.90	0.142
Blood loss			
≥2,000 mL	1.76	0.48–6.46	0.397
Allogeneic BT			
Yes	1.27	0.41–3.99	0.681

BT blood transfusion

cholangiocarcinoma, even in advanced stages, apparently benefit from surgery, although it may be highly invasive for the patient. Performing PVE for a case that needs major hepatectomy may be one of the most effective strategies. Nevertheless, there are several questions that need to be addressed in the future including: (1) the necessity and safety of hepatopancreatoduodenectomy to completely remove cancer, (2) the necessity and safety of combined vascular resection and reconstruction (especially for the hepatic artery), (3) the extent of lymph node dissection (Is paraaortic lymph node dissection necessary?), and (4) the method of preoperative evaluation of the future liver remnant. The number of incidents of hilar cholangiocarcinoma is now increasing year by year. However, the actual

Table 21.7 Comparison of the clinical variables between the patients in the former and latter period

	Former period 1991–2000 (*N*=101)		Latter period 2001–2008 (*N*=212)		
Variables	*N*	(%)	*N*	(%)	*P* value
Age					
≥70	30	30	79	37	0.206
Gender					
Male	52	51	123	58	0.330
Extent of liver resection					
≥60%	45	45	71	33	0.062
ICGK					
<0.125	14	14	25	12	0.586
ICGK-F					
<0.05	17	17	31	15	0.618
Combined PV resection					
Yes	34	34	77	36	0.705
Combined HA resection					
Yes	1	1	28	13	<0.001
Combined PD					
Yes	24	24	53	25	0.889
Operation time					
≥600 min	82	81	120	57	<0.001
Blood loss					
≥2,000 mL	65	64	91	43	<0.001
Allogeneic BT					
Yes	65	64	70	33	<0.001
Postoperative death					
Yes	13	13	8	4	0.006
Infectious complications					
Yes	70	69	71	33	<0.001
Hepatic failure					
Yes	31	31	20	9	<0.001

PV portal vein; *HA* hepatic artery

Fig. 21.2 Survival curves for the patients who underwent major hepatectomy after PVE (surgeries performed without PVE were excluded). The patients were separated in the former period (1991–2000) and the latter period (2001–2008)

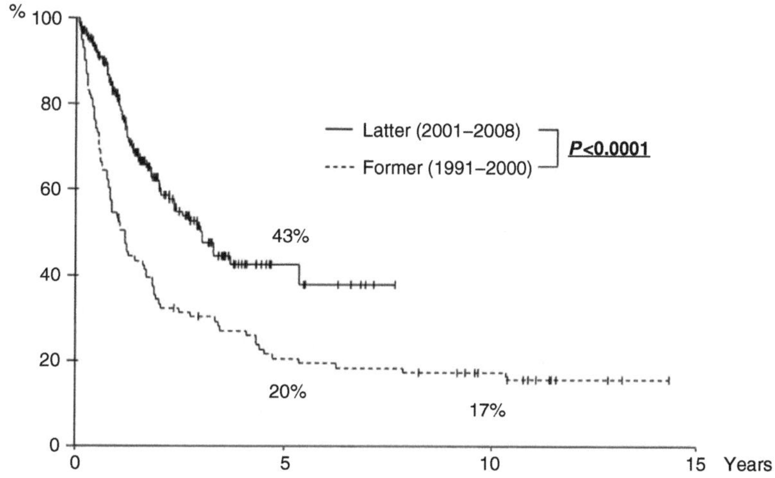

Numbers at risk

Latter (2001–2008)	212	9	
Former (1991–2000)	101	19	11

number of surgeries performed in a single institution is still not very high. Therefore, multi-institutional or international collaboration is necessary to perform well-controlled studies to answer these questions.

References

1. Nimura Y, Hayakawa N, Kamiya J, et al. Hepatopancreatoduodenectomy for advanced carcinoma of the biliary tract. *Hepatogastroenterology*. 1991;38:170-175.
2. Ebata T, Nagino M, Kamiya J, et al. Hepatectomy with portal vein resection for hilar cholangiocarcinoma: audit of 52 consecutive cases. *Ann Surg*. 2003;238:720-727.
3. Klatskin G. Adenocarcinoma of the hepatic duct at its bifurcation within the porta hepatis. An unusual tumor with distinctive clinical and pathological features. *Am J Med*. 1965;38:241-256.
4. Altemeier WA, Gall EA, Zinninger MM, et al. Sclerosing carcinoma of the major intrahepatic bile ducts. *AMA Arch Surg*. 1957;75:450-460; discussion 460-451.
5. Ito F, Agni R, Rettammel RJ, et al. Resection of hilar cholangiocarcinoma: concomitant liver resection decreases hepatic recurrence. *Ann Surg*. 2008;248:273-279.
6. Sano T, Shimada K, Sakamoto Y, et al. Changing trends in surgical outcomes after major hepatobiliary resection for hilar cholangiocarcinoma: a single-center experience over 25 years. *J Hepatobiliary Pancreat Surg*. 2007;14:455-462.
7. Dinant S, Gerhards MF, Rauws EA, et al. Improved outcome of resection of hilar cholangiocarcinoma (Klatskin tumor). *Ann Surg Oncol*. 2006;13:872-880.
8. Nimura Y. Preoperative biliary drainage before resection for cholangiocarcinoma (Pro). *HPB (Oxford)*. 2008;10:130-133.
9. Nagino M, Takada T, Miyazaki M, et al. Preoperative biliary drainage for biliary tract and ampullary carcinomas. *J Hepatobiliary Pancreat Surg*. 2008;15:25-30.
10. Unno M, Okumoto T, Katayose Y, et al. Preoperative assessment of hilar cholangiocarcinoma by multidetector row computed tomography. *J Hepatobiliary Pancreat Surg*. 2007;14: 434-440.
11. Sugiura T, Nishio H, Nagino M, et al. Value of multidetector-row computed tomography in diagnosis of portal vein invasion by perihilar cholangiocarcinoma. *World J Surg*. 2008;32:1478-1484.
12. Nimura Y. Staging cholangiocarcinoma by cholangioscopy. *HPB (Oxford)*. 2008;10:113-115.
13. Senda Y, Nishio H, Oda K, et al. Value of multidetector row CT in the assessment of longitudinal extension of cholangiocarcinoma—correlation between MDCT and microscopic findings. *World J Surg*. 2009;33(7):1459-1467.
14. Nimura Y. Radical surgery: vascular and pancreatic resection for cholangiocarcinoma. *HPB (Oxford)*. 2008;10:183-185.
15. Nimura Y. Radical surgery of left-sided klatskin tumors. *HPB (Oxford)*. 2008;10:168-170.
16. Jonas S, Benckert C, Thelen A, et al. Radical surgery for hilar cholangiocarcinoma. *Eur J Surg Oncol*. 2008;34: 263-271.
17. Hidalgo E, Asthana S, Nishio H, et al. Surgery for hilar cholangiocarcinoma: the Leeds experience. *Eur J Surg Oncol*. 2008;34:787-794.
18. Sugawara G, Nagino M, Nishio H, et al. Perioperative synbiotic treatment to prevent postoperative infectious complications in biliary cancer surgery: a randomized controlled trial. *Ann Surg*. 2006;244:706-714.
19. Kamiya S, Nagino M, Kanazawa H, et al. The value of bile replacement during external biliary drainage: an analysis of intestinal permeability, integrity, and microflora. *Ann Surg*. 2004;239:510-517.
20. Nakeeb A, Pitt HA. Radiation therapy, chemotherapy and chemoradiation in hilar cholangiocarcinoma. *HPB (Oxford)*. 2005;7:278-282.
21. Makuuchi M, Thai BL, Takayasu K, et al. Preoperative portal embolization to increase safety of major hepatectomy for

hilar bile duct carcinoma: a preliminary report. *Surgery*. 1990;107:521-527.
22. Nagino M, Nimura Y, Kamiya J, et al. Right or left trisegment portal vein embolization before hepatic trisegmentectomy for hilar bile duct carcinoma. *Surgery*. 1995;117:677-681.
23. Abdalla EK, Barnett CC, Doherty D, et al. Extended hepatectomy in patients with hepatobiliary malignancies with and without preoperative portal vein embolization. *Arch Surg*. 2002;137:675-680; discussion 680-671.
24. Launois B, Campion JP, Brissot P, et al. Carcinoma of the hepatic hilus. Surgical management and the case for resection. *Ann Surg*. 1979;190:151-157.
25. Blumgart LH, Hadjis NS, Benjamin IS, et al. Surgical approaches to cholangiocarcinoma at confluence of hepatic ducts. *Lancet*. 1984;1:66-70.
26. Bismuth H, Nakache R, Diamond T. Management strategies in resection for hilar cholangiocarcinoma. *Ann Surg*. 1992; 215:31-38.
27. Miyazaki M, Ito H, Nakagawa K, et al. Aggressive surgical approaches to hilar cholangiocarcinoma: Hepatic or local resection? *Surgery*. 1998;123:131-136.
28. Ikeyama T, Nagino M, Oda K, et al. Surgical approach to bismuth Type I and II hilar cholangiocarcinomas: audit of 54 consecutive cases. *Ann Surg*. 2007;246:1052-1057.
29. Ebata T, Nagino M, Nishio H, et al. Right hepatopancreatoduodenectomy: improvements over 23 years to attain acceptability. *J Hepatobiliary Pancreat Surg*. 2007;14: 131-135.
30. Miyazaki M, Itoh H, Ambiru S, et al. Radical surgery for advanced gallbladder carcinoma. *Br J Surg*. 1996;83: 478-481.
31. Nakeeb A, Pitt HA, Sohn TA, et al. Cholangiocarcinoma. A spectrum of intrahepatic, perihilar, and distal tumors. *Ann Surg*. 1996;224:463-473; discussion 473-465.
32. Madariaga JR, Iwatsuki S, Todo S, et al. Liver resection for hilar and peripheral cholangiocarcinomas: a study of 62 cases. *Ann Surg*. 1998;227:70-79.
33. Iwatsuki S, Todo S, Marsh JW, et al. Treatment of hilar cholangiocarcinoma (Klatskin tumors) with hepatic resection or transplantation. *J Am Coll Surg*. 1998;187:358-364.
34. Nagino M, Nimura Y, Kamiya J, et al. Selective percutaneous transhepatic embolization of the portal vein in preparation for extensive liver resection: the ipsilateral approach. *Radiology*. 1996;200:559-563.
35. Nagino M, Kamiya J, Kanai M, et al. Right trisegment portal vein embolization for biliary tract carcinoma: technique and clinical utility. *Surgery*. 2000;127:155-160.
36. Nagino M, Kamiya J, Nishio H, et al. Two hundred forty consecutive portal vein embolizations before extended hepatectomy for biliary cancer: surgical outcome and long-term follow-up. *Ann Surg*. 2006;243:364-372.

Clinical Outcomes for Liver Metastases

22

Daria Zorzi, Yuky Hayashi,
and Jean-Nicolas Vauthey

Abstract

Liver resection is associated with prolonged survival in patients with colorectal liver metastases. Unfortunately, only 15–25% of patients with colorectal liver metastases are candidates for surgery at the time of diagnosis of the metastatic disease. To date, the definition of resectability of colorectal liver metastases is based on complete resection and preservation of sufficient future liver remnant (FLR). In patients with unresectable colorectal liver metastases, portal vein embolization (PVE) induces hypertrophy of the FLR and allows safe liver resection. The safety and the usefulness of this procedure have been evaluated in large series of patients with colorectal liver metastases. Depending on the quality of the liver parenchyma, portal vein embolization is recommended for patients whose standardized FLR is less than 20% in normal liver, less than 30% in case of hepatic injury, and less than 40% in case of fibrosis or cirrhosis. The role of PVE has not been specifically evaluated in patients with metastases from other malignancies (neuroendocrine tumor or noncolorectal nonneuroendocrine liver metastases). However, the indications for PVE are dictated by the volume of the FLR and the quality of liver parenchyma, and the guidelines provided for colorectal liver metastases also apply to other types of liver metastases.

Keywords

Colorectal liver metastases • Neuroendocrine tumor liver metastases • Hepatic resection • Liver metastases

22.1 Colorectal Liver Metastases

Colorectal adenocarcinoma is the second leading cause of cancer-related death in the United States. The liver is the most common site for hematogenous metastasis from colorectal cancers. The 20–25% of patients are found to have synchronous colorectal liver metastasis (CLM),[1,2] and 35–55% of patients with colorectal cancer develop hepatic metastasis during the course of their disease.[3] Without any treatment, the median survival of CLM patients is approximately 6 months.[2,4] On the other hand, 20–35% of patients with metastatic colorectal cancers has the liver as the only site of metastatic disease and the 5 year overall survival rate after hepatic resection is reported to be up to 58%.[5-8] Moreover, the 10 year disease free survival rate after

J.-N. Vauthey (✉)
Liver Service, Department of Surgical Oncology, The University of Texas M.D. Anderson Cancer Center, 1515 Holcombe Boulevard, Unit 444, Houston, TX 77030, USA
e-mail: jvauthey@mdanderson.org

D.C. Madoff et al. (eds.), *Venous Embolization of the Liver*,
DOI 10.1007/978-1-84882-122-4_22, © Springer-Verlag London Limited 2011

Table 22.1 Changing paradigm in criteria of irresectability in patient with CLM

Traditional criteria	Contemporary criteria
Four or more metastases	Inability to perform R0 resection
Size >5 cm	
Bilateral disease	
Surgical margin <1 cm	Histologically positive margin
Extrahepatic disease	Inability to resect all detectable disease
Clinicopathologic prognostic scoring systems, predatin modern chemotherapy	Disease progression on modern chemotherapy in patients with more than three metastases

Adapted from Ribero et al.[58] with permission

hepatic resection is reported to be at 25%.[8] Hepatic resection for CLM remains the only treatment that has curative potential. The progress of workup methods, systemic chemotherapy, and innovative surgical techniques has now enabled the patients to undergo potentially curative treatment.

22.1.1 Surgical Candidates

Previously, surgical indication for CLM focused on the morphologic characteristics of the tumor and the absence of extrahepatic disease. Four or more liver metastases with each nodule >5 cm in diameter, bilateral disease, and surgical margin <1 cm were reported as negative prognostic factors after hepatic resection[9-11] and were contraindications for surgery. Extrahepatic disease was also considered as a criterion of irresectability. Nowadays, the focus of the current criteria is shifting towards resection of all metastases with negative histologic margins while preserving sufficient functional hepatic parenchyma which is more than 20–30% of the total estimated liver volume in a normal liver.[3,12-14] Even with extrahepatic disease, selected patients are expected to be offered curative resection (Table 22.1).

22.1.2 Tumor Number

In patients with solitary CLM, Aloia et al. report 92% of local recurrence-free, 50% of disease-free, and 71% of overall survival at 5 years.[15] While the patients with multiple or bilateral metastases have been considered to be contraindicated for hepatic resection, Kokudo et al. demonstrated however, a 5-year survival rate of approximately 50% in the patients with four or more liver tumors and did not show a significant difference from the patients with three or fewer tumors.[14] Similar results were reported in patients with a negative surgical margin.[16] Weber et al. also showed that even patients with 9–20 tumors can reach long-term survival, although the actuarial 5-year survival decreased as the number of tumors increased.[17] The number of tumors is no longer a contraindication for hepatic resection.

22.1.3 Surgical Margin

Previously, a 10-mm negative tumor margin for hepatic resection of CLM was recommended, and it was related to better disease-free survival.[18,19] Recent articles demonstrate that the width of surgical margin is not a significant prognostic factor in patient survival[20] or risk of recurrence.[21] In a multicenter study of 557 patients, margin status was classified as a positive, 1–4 mm, 5–9 mm, or 10 mm or more.[6] The 5-year survival rate was 17.1% for patients with a positive margin, compared with 63.8% for patients with negative margin, and the width of the negative surgical margin did not affect the survival rate or recurrence risk. Only the presence of a positive surgical margin (R1) was associated with an increased risk of recurrence (11%) and an inferior survival rate (Fig. 22.1).

22.1.4 Extra Hepatic Metastasis

Several reports have shown that long-term prognosis can be expected after surgical resection of both isolated hepatic and pulmonary colorectal metastasis, and that the 5-year survival can reach approximately 30%.[22-24] Other extrahepatic metastases sites, including hepatic pedicle lymph node metastasis, peritoneal implants, and distant organ metastasis have a very poor prognosis, and are usually contraindications for surgical treatment. On the other hand, Elias et al. showed that the 5-year survival for patients with any kind of resectable extrahepatic disease (e.g., lymph node, peritoneum, lung, and so on) reached 28%.[25]

The prevalence of regional hepatic lymph node involvement in CLM has been reported to be from 3% to 33%.[26] In a systematic review of 15 studies, authors

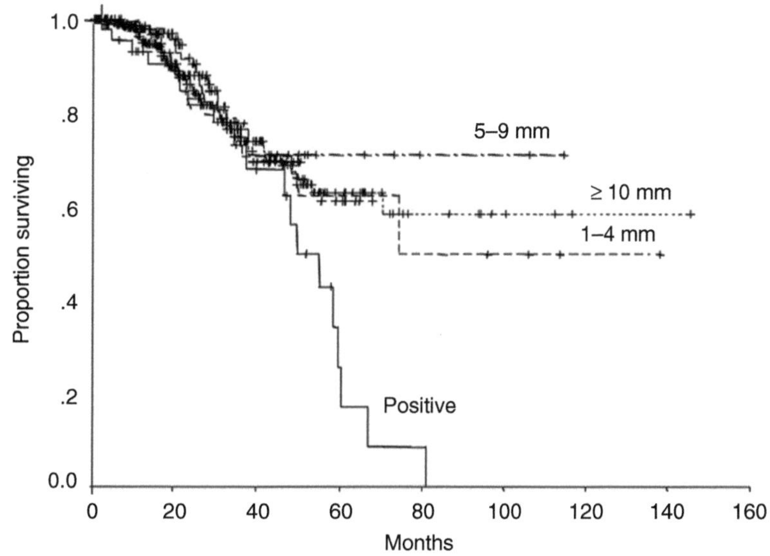

Fig. 22.1 Postresection margin width and overall survival. (From Pawlik et al.[6] with permission)

concluded that there are few 5-year survivors after liver resection for CLM involving the hepatic lymph nodes, regardless of lymph node dissection.[27] However, a prospective study showed that survival rate in patients with hepatic pedicle lymph node in area 1 (hepatoduodenal ligament and retropancreatic portion) was significantly higher than in patients with area 2 involvement (common hepatic artery and celiac axis) after surgery with lymph node dissection.[26,28] Another retrospective study, comparing prognosis of the patient with or without resectable extrahepatic disease, also demonstrated that the hilar lymph node involvement was not associated with an unfavorable prognosis, and even the resection of localized peritoneal implants may benefit patient survival.[29] Moreover, according to the findings of a review of CLM patients with extrahepatic metastasis,[30] the lymph node dissection in the presence of macroscopic metastasis in the hepatic pedicle can be expected to result in a 5-year survival of 5–12%, and the patients with peritoneal metastasis have a potential to get an acceptable survival if the disease can be eradicated.

Because the number of patients included in the studies is very small, surgical treatment is still controversial in regard to CLM patients with extrahepatic metastasis, and a multidisciplinary treatment including chemotherapy is mandatory. In well selected patients, however, extrahepatic metastasis is no longer a contraindication to hepatectomy if a margin negative resection can be achieved.

22.1.5 Perioperative Results

Liver resection is a well-established procedure that can be performed with mortality rates of less than 5%, large centers now quoting rates close to 0%.[31] The most powerful determinants of poor outcome after liver resection are intraoperative bleeding, requirement for perioperative blood transfusions, insufficient remnant liver, and development of postoperative infections. Indeed, these conditions can lead to hepatic failure, which although it occurs in fewer than 5% of cases can have devastating consequences.[32] Optimal patient selection, meticulous intraoperative technique, and careful postoperative management are thus essential to minimize surgical complications.

22.1.6 Long-Term Survival

The main predictors of recurrence in major published series of liver resection for colorectal metastases are reported in Table 22.2. Despite expanding indications for resection of colorectal metastases, the overall 5-year survival is now reported to be as high as 58% in single and multi-institutional studies.[33] The factors with the greatest influence on survival are margin status, stage of the primary colon tumor, preoperative CEA level, size, and number of hepatic lesions, and presence or absence of extrahepatic disease.

Table 22.2 Predictors of recurrence and long-term survival after resection for colorectal liver metastases

Author, year	R1 status	Synchronous presentation	Primary nodes +	Size of metastases	Number of metastases	Preoperative CEA	Extrahepatic disease	Pathologic response	5-Year survival
Gayowski, 1994[131]	+	+	+	–	+	–	+		32%
Scheele, 1995[132]	+	+	+	+	–	–	–		40%
Nordlinger, 1996[133]	+	+	+	+	+	+			28%
Jaeck, 1997[134]	+	+	+	+	+	+	–		26%
Jamison, 1997[135]	–			–	–				32%
Jenkins, 1997[136]	+			–	–		+		25%
Elias, 1998[137]	+	+	–	–	–	–	–		28%
Ambiru, 1999[138]	+	–	+		+	+			23%
Fong, 1999[11]	+		+		+	+	+		46%
Minagawa, 2000[10]	–		–	–	+	–	–		38%
Figueras, 2001[139]	+	–			+	+	+		53%
Choti, 2002[140]	+	–	–	–	+	+			58%
Fernandez, 2004[141]		–	–	–	+	–			58%
Abdalla, 2004[33]	+	–		+	+				58%
Pawlik, 2005[6]	+	–	–	+	+	+			58%
Blazer, 2008[34]								+	56% major response 75% complete response

CEA carcino-embryonic antigen

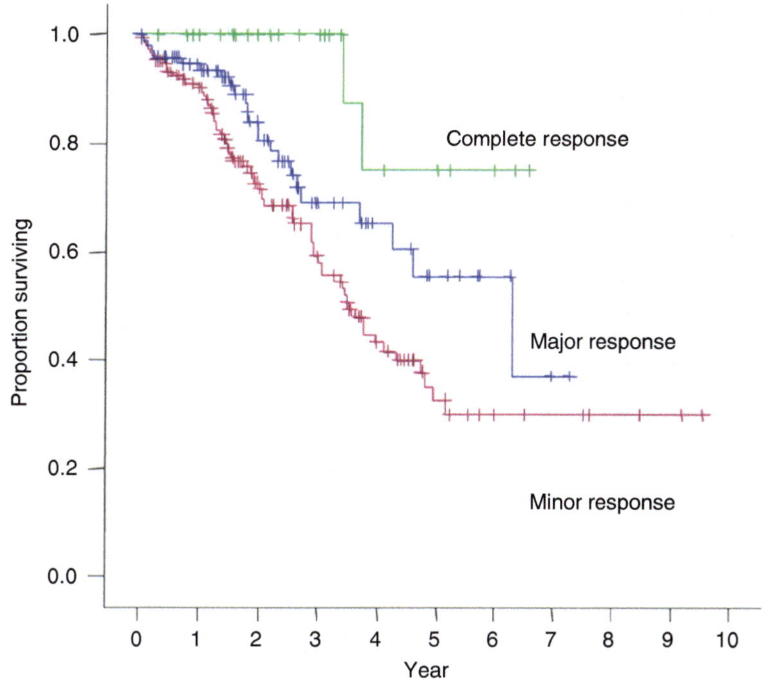

Fig. 22.2 Overall survival curves according to the degree of Pathologic Response. (From Blazer[34] with permission)

Surgical margin status is an important factor that influences long-term survival. Historically, a margin less than 1 cm was considered suboptimal. However, a recent study by Pawlik et al.[6] showed that the width of resected margin (1–10 mm) did not affect local recurrence or survival, and indeed only the presence of a positive surgical margin (R1) was associated with an increased risk of recurrence and inferior survival (Fig. 22.1). Thus, patients with an anticipated surgical margin of less than 1 cm based on preoperative imaging or intraoperative findings should still undergo resection as long as a negative margin is achievable.

More recently, a study from MD Anderson Cancer Center found a new predictor of survival in the era of preoperative systemic chemotherapy (Table 22.2). Pathologic response of tumor to chemotherapy along with a positive margin, and not the commonly used predictors of recurrence, predicts survival in patients with colorectal liver metastases treated preoperatively with systemic chemotherapy.[34] Pathologic response was evaluated according to the man percentage of residual cancer cells and classified in three subsets: complete response (no residual cancer cell remaining), major response (1–49% residual cancer cell remaining), and minor response (≥50% residual cancer cell remaining). Cumulative 1-, 3-, and 5-year overall survival rates by response were as follows: complete response, 100%, 100%, and 75%; major response, 95%, 69%, and 56%; and minor response, 91%, 58%, and 33%, respectively. The survival differences between complete and major responses ($P = 0.037$) and between major and minor responses ($P = 0.028$) were both statistically significant by log-rank test[34] (Fig. 22.2).

22.1.7 Expanding the Criteria to Improve Resectability

Several strategies are available to render initially unresectable colorectal liver metastases resectable. The advances made by chemotherapy have been the major determinant of new therapeutic approaches for primarily unresectable patients. Previously, patients with unresectable hepatic colorectal metastases were treated with palliative chemotherapy, and almost no such patients achieved prolonged survival.[35] Recently, advances in chemotherapy have permitted resection in some patients with initially unresectable metastases.

22.1.8 Preoperative Systemic Chemotherapy

Over a decade ago, 5-fluorouracil (5-FU) was the sole chemotherapy used for CLM and yielded response rates of 20% with no improvement in survival. However,

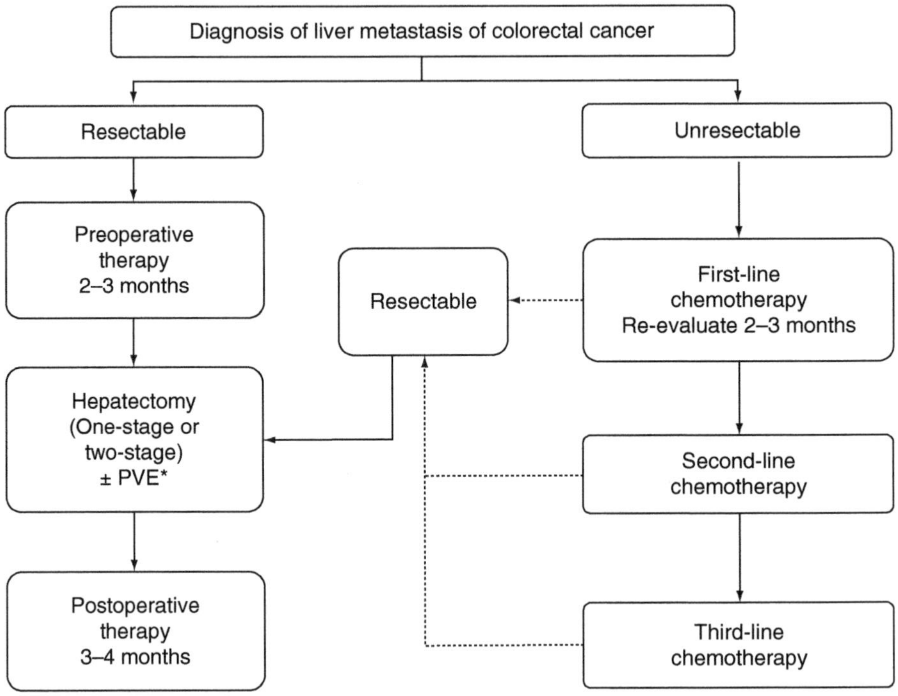

Fig. 22.3 Evolving treatment algorithm for patients with mCRC involving multidisciplinary collaboration. Patients initially considered resectable may go directly to surgery or may have preoperative therapy first. In the initially unresectable group, a multidisciplinary team approach is necessary to assess patient's resectability status and transfer potentially resectable patients to the resectable group

advances in chemotherapeutic agents and delivery have changed the treatment of CLM dramatically. The introduction of oxaliplatin and irinotecan to the chemotherapeutic armamentarium has resulted in response rates of over 50% and in the conversion of unresectable metastases to resectable in up to 38% of patients.[35,36] Moreover, the advent of monoclonal antibodies has augmented response rates to upwards of 80%.[37,38] Effective modern chemotherapy allows not only the downsizing of liver disease but also the treatment of systemic disease to reduce the chance of distant failure. Another benefit of preoperative systemic treatment is the identification of patients whose disease progresses on chemotherapy and who would not benefit from surgery. Finally, response to chemotherapy can guide postoperative treatment. Many groups, including our own, use preoperative chemotherapy for patients with resectable and unresectable liver metastases (Fig. 22.3).[39]

Recently, Nordlinger et al.[40] published the results from a randomized study of perioperative oxaliplatin-based chemotherapy for patients with up to four resectable metastases: patients were randomly assigned to receive surgery alone or to receive six cycles of chemotherapy given both before and after surgery. The authors showed that perioperative chemotherapy reduced the risk of progression-free survival events at 3 years. The absolute increase in 3-year progression free survival rate, with the addition of perioperative chemotherapy, was 9% in patients who had resection, from 33% to 42%, showing a significant ($P=0.025$) benefit of administering chemotherapy.

The extent of resection after downsizing with chemotherapy remains problematic. In a study by Benoist et al., 55 of 66 (83%) tumors that had complete radiographic response after neoadjuvant therapy demonstrated persistent macroscopic or microscopic disease or early recurrence.[41] In patients who have complete radiographic response to neoadjuvant therapy, outcome and patterns of recurrence are ill-defined. Until conclusive evidence is available, hepatic resection should be performed on the basis of prechemotherapy imaging to encompass the area initially involved by tumor.

22.1.8.1 Safety of Hepatectomy After Chemotherapy

The effect of perioperative chemotherapy on postoperative morbidity and mortality is controversial. Irinotecan and 5-FU are associated with hepatic steatosis, while oxaliplatin induces sinusoidal obstruction.[42,43] Nonetheless, most series show that perioperative morbidity and mortality are not higher after hepatectomy following neoadjuvant chemotherapy than after de novo

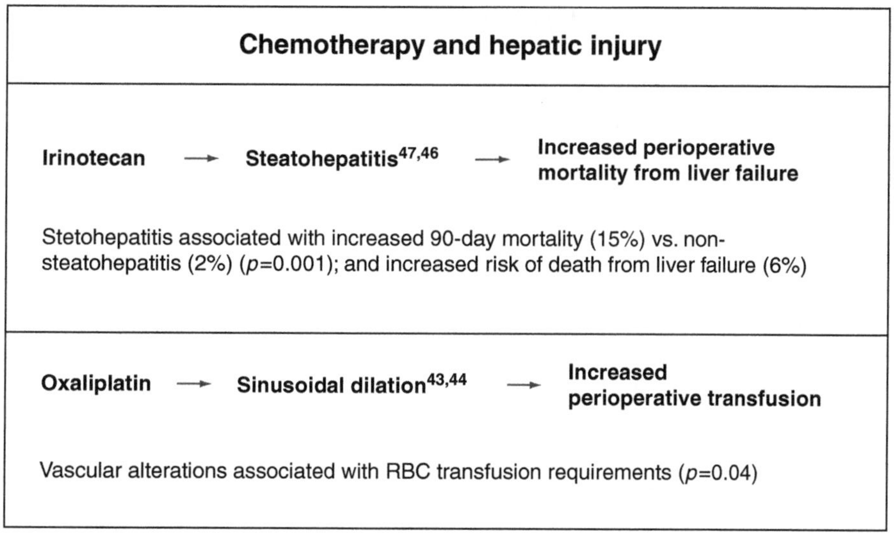

Fig. 22.4 Chemotherapy-induced hepatotoxicity and clinical outcome

resection, provided the duration of chemotherapy is less than six cycles.[44,45] In a study from the MD Anderson Cancer Center of 248 patients who received neoadjuvant chemotherapy and 158 who did not, oxaliplatin was associated with sinusoidal dilation (19% vs. 2%), which did not affect the postoperative complication rate.[46] On the other hand, irinotecan was associated with steatohepatitis (20% vs. 4%), irrespective of body mass index (BMI), but more pronounced in patients with a higher BMI. Patients with steatohepatitis had increased postoperative mortality, and the authors cautioned against using irinotecan-based therapies in patients with known steatosis or steatohepatitis. In patients with suspected steatosis on preoperative imaging, laparoscopy before laparotomy is advisable, to directly evaluate the liver, with biopsies as indicated.

In general, hepatic resection should be performed as soon as CLM become resectable. Preoperative chemotherapy results in damage to the liver that may increase morbidity and mortality after hepatic resection (Fig. 22.4).[45-47]

22.1.8.2 Biologic Agents

Bevacizumab, a monoclonal antibody against vascular endothelial growth factor (VEGF), has resulted in increased response rate in patients with stage IV colorectal cancer and improved progression-free survival. However, the critical role of VEGF in liver regeneration has raised concerns regarding impaired liver regeneration after preoperative administration of bevacizumab. Recent studies show that bevacizumab can be administrated safely before hepatectomy. A study from Memorial Sloan–Kettering Cancer Center compared 32 patients who underwent hepatectomy after bevacizumab with a matched set of controls and found no increase in morbidity.[48] The authors recommend 6–8 weeks after the last dose of bevacizumab as the optimal time interval between bevacizumab administration and hepatic resection. Another study from MD Anderson Cancer Center analyzed the addition of bevacizumab to oxaliplatin-based chemotherapy and found that bevacizumab improved the pathologic response to chemotherapy, demonstrated by a lower percentage of residual viable tumor cells in liver metastases.[49] Moreover, bevacizumab was found to have a protective effect from oxaliplatin-induced sinusoidal injury. The antiangiogenic effects of bevacizumab have raised concerns regarding potential effects on bleeding, wound healing, and liver regeneration. A recent study from the MD Anderson Cancer Center reported that the addition of bevacizumab to chemotherapy before portal vein embolization did not impair liver regeneration.[50]

Cetuximab, a chimeric monoclonal antibody against epidermal growth factor receptor, has been shown to have activity as a single agent and to exert synergistic activity in combination with cytotoxic chemotherapy. A French study[51] showed that combination therapy with cetuximab increases resectability rates without increasing operative mortality or liver injury. Specific cetuximab-associated pathologic features were not identified, and potential hepatotoxic effects of cetuximab remain unknown.

22.1.9 Portal Vein Embolization

There are some patients considered marginal candidates for resection based on a small future liver remnant volume. In such patients, preoperative portal vein embolization (PVE) is a safe, minimally invasive procedure which leads to an ipsilateral hepatic atrophy and compensatory contralateral hypertrophy.[52-54] In a study comparing patients with a normal underlying liver who underwent extended hepatectomy with or without preoperative PVE, patients with standardized future liver remnant (sFLR) of ≤20% had a complication rate of 50%, versus 13% complication rate in patients with sFLR >20%.[55] Among patients who receive extensive chemotherapy prior to hepatectomy, liver injuries can compromise liver regeneration and postoperative recovery. In such patients, resection can be safely performed with an sFLR volume of at least 30%.[56,57] Moreover, in patients with severe hepatic fibrosis or cirrhosis, PVE is indicated when the sFLR is ≤40% of total liver volume (TLV).

Hypertrophy of the remnant liver follows a nonlinear kinetic profile. The FLR volume significantly increased in the first 3 weeks after PVE, after that, the growth rate reached a plateau phase of minimal regeneration. A slower rate of liver regeneration continued in the following months.[58] Thus, 3–4 weeks should be considered as the optimum time interval to assess the hypertrophy response to PVE. In addition, Ribero et al. demonstrated that a degree of hypertrophy of ≤5% had been associated with increases in liver-related major complications after hepatectomy.[58]

Contraindications to PVE include portal hypertension, tumor extension to the FLR or portal vein, coagulopathy that cannot be corrected, biliary dilatation in the FLR, and renal failure.

22.1.10 Synchronous Metastasis

Several investigators have recommended delayed hepatic resection for synchronous CLM.[59,60] After delaying hepatic resection for 3–6 months, occult metastasis may become evident, and patients who benefit from hepatic resection can be more accurately selected. Others reported no significant difference between simultaneous and delayed hepatectomy in overall survival rate and less complications after simultaneous colon resection and minor hepatectomy, compared to a delayed hepatectomy, but simultaneous major hepatectomy (more than three segments) increased mortality and morbidity.[32,61-63] In such patients, systemic therapy before hepatectomy is recommended. In the study of Allen et al.[64] comparing patients with synchronous CLM undergoing delayed hepatectomy with or without preoperative chemotherapy, authors suggested that the response to preoperative chemotherapy might be a prognostic indicator of survival, although the 5-year survival was similar between the two groups.

22.1.11 Conclusions

Even in the patients with higher risk of recurrence, only surgical resection for CLM can expect long-term survival results than other treatments. The current goal of hepatic resection is to resect all metastasis disease with negative histological margins. After resection, the 5-year overall survival rate in selected patients reaches 58%, thanks to the progress of preoperative imaging, surgical techniques, and systemic chemotherapy. A multidisciplinary team approach management is nowadays mandatory for patients with CLM.

22.2 Neuroendocrine Liver Metastases

Neuroendocrine tumors (NETs) include a group of carcinomas arising from neuroendocrine cells dispersed throughout the body. These tumors are indolent growing and metastasize primarily to the liver. At the time of diagnosis, the 40% of patients already had liver metastasis.[65-67] The majority of the neuroendocrine metastases to the liver are from small intestine carcinoids or pancreatic endocrine tumors.[68] Carcinoid tumors usually arise from the small bowel, lung, and bronchi, less often in the appendix, and very rarely in the pancreas. Pancreatic endocrine tumors are known as islet cell carcinoma and produce insulin, glucagon, gastrin, and vasoactive intestinal peptide. The major functioning endocrinopathies associated with pancreatic neuroendocrine tumors and their frequency of malignancy are insulinoma (10%), gastrinoma (50%), glucagonoma (70%), somatostatinoma (80%), GREoma (30%), VIPoma (40%), ACTHoma or CRHoma (100%), and PTHoma (100%).[69]

Symptoms include flushing, diarrhea, bronchospasm with breathlessness and wheezing, and right-sided heart failure. However, the severity of symptoms is not always correlated with the extent of tumor growth. Patients with high tumor burden can remain asymptomatic for years, while others with minimal disease can suffer all the symptoms of the carcinoid syndrome. Carcinoid liver metastases rarely lead to rapid liver dysfunction and failure and are often associated with a long, indolent disease course.

The best treatment for patients with hepatic NETs metastasis remains controversial and should always remain within the domain of the multidisciplinary team. In selected patients, surgical resection of hepatic metastasis may prolong survival.[65]

22.2.1 Hepatic Resection

Surgical resection of liver NETs metastasis has prolonged survival and resulted in long-term relief of symptoms in selected patients. The mortality rate of 1.2% and major morbidity rate of 15%[70] show that surgery can be performed safely in patients with liver metastasis for NETs. The use of PVE in patients candidate for resection of advanced NET metastases has not been specifically evaluated. From a clinical perspective, provided adequate control of hormonal manifestation, PVE can be safely performed if indicated based on the calculation of the FLR (<20% TLV in normal liver). However, benefits and risk of the procedure as well as the subsequent resectability of the patient have to be carefully evaluated because prior PVE in nonresected patients represents a relative contraindication to hepatic arterial embolization which is an adequate treatment of unresectable patients. The 5-year overall survival rates after hepatic resection were reported at 60–85%.[71-76] Even if the resection cannot be a curative surgery, resection of ≥90% of the tumor volume is significantly associated with extended survival compared to resection of < 90% of the tumor volume.[70,74] The negative prognostic indicators for survival after operation have been assessed by several authors and include size of metastasis >3 cm, pancreatic origin, poorly differentiated carcinoma, and presence of extrahepatic disease.[66,71,75] On the other hand, the 5-year survival rate of the patients with unresectable liver metastasis was reported only at 30%.[77]

Excellent palliation of hormonal symptoms from hepatic metastasis of NETs is also achieved with resection. Almost 100% of patients with such symptoms can get amelioration and 70–80% of them have complete relief.[73-75,78] Cytoreduction of more than 90% of tumor volume resulted in an improved, not only survival, but also symptomatic relief when compared with other therapy including hepatic arterial embolization and medical therapy.[68,75]

Liver transplantation is advocated as a treatment for patients with extensive liver only NETs metastases that are unresectable or failed medical treatment. There have been some recent improvements in operative mortality for this procedure in carefully selected patients with 5-year survival ranging from 36% to 67%.[79,80]

22.2.2 Hepatic Arterial Embolotherapy

Surgical resection of the NET liver metastasis is possible in 10% of patients or less. Transcatheter arterial embolization (TAE) and transcatheter arterial chemoembolization (TACE) are alternative treatments for patients not candidates for hepatic resection. TAE is based on the principle that tumors receive blood supply exclusively from the hepatic artery and has reported good results in controlling hormonal symptoms and reducing tumor size. Gupta et al.[81] demonstrated that patients with carcinoid tumors had better outcomes than patients with pancreatic islet cell carcinomas when they were treated with TAE or TACE. Although the complete response is rare and 5-year survival is about 30%, 50–80% of patients with liver metastasis from carcinoids can obtain radiological response, and 60–90% of patients report improved symptoms.[81-85] Chemotherapy agents used during TACE include doxorubicin,[86] streptozotocin,[87] or combinations of cytotoxic regimens with Yttrium-90 resin microspheres for radioembolization.[88,89]

Almost all patients experienced some kinds of postembolization syndrome (fever, nausea, vomiting, abdominal pain, and elevated liver enzyme level).[82] Major complications, such as hepatorenal syndrome and severe infection, are reported to occur in 10% of the patients after embolization.[81-83]

22.2.3 Systemic Therapy

Somatostatin inhibits a variety of physiological functions in the gastrointestinal tract, including gastrointestinal motility and the secretion of pancreatic and intestinal hormones such as insulin, glucagon, secretin, and vasoactive intestinal polypeptide (VIP).[90] Somatostatin analogs are the initial treatment for control of hormone-mediated symptoms. Two analogs, octreotide and lanreotide, are widely used now. Octreotide is an intermediate-acting somatostatin analog which can be administered subcutaneously every 6–12 h. It gives a complete or partial relief from hormonal symptoms in 50–80% of patients and also gives biochemical response in 70% of patients with NETs.[90-93] Recently, Octreotide LAR has also been shown to significantly lengthen the time to tumor progression compared with placebo in patients with functionally active and inactive metastatic midgut neuroendocrine tumors.[94] Lanreotide is a long-acting somatostatin analog which can lower the number of injections required to control NETs. Common side effects of somatostatine analog include nausea, abdominal cramps, loose stools, mild steatorrhea, and flatulence.[90] These symptoms are dose-dependent but usually improve within the first few of treatment.

Interferon-α has also been used in the treatment of carcinoid tumors. It is effective in controlling hormonal syndromes in more than 50% of patients and has high antitumor activity than somatostatin.[68] However, interferon-α is more toxic than somatostatin analogs.[93]

Although some nonrandomized trials showed that there is an additive effect in the combination group, it has not yet been clearly defined whether the combined use of interferon-α and somatostatin f is clinically more effective than the single use.[91]

Recently, the targeted biological therapies (e.g., bevacizumab) are also reported to be effective with the carcinoid patients.[95] Experimental studies provide arguments that mTOR inhibitors could inhibit proliferation of neuroendocrine tumor cell lines and could be effective agents for the treatment of these patients.[96] Cytotoxic chemotherapy has had only limited success in the treatment of advanced NETs. The Eastern Cooperative Oncology Group (ECOG) performed a randomized study of doxorubicin+fluorouracil (DOX/FU) compared with streptozocin+fluorouracil (STZ/FU) in advanced carcinoid tumors.[97] In this study, there was no difference in response rates (15.9% and 16%) and progression-free survival (4.5 and 5.3 months). STZ/FU group had longer median survival than DOX/FU group (24.3 and 15.7 months). The same regimens are used in the patients with advanced pancreatic islet cell carcinomas with no proven effect.[98,99]

22.2.4 Conclusion

More evidences are needed to define the ideal treatment for NETs liver metastases. Many published data demonstrated that the hepatic resection is associated with both survival and symptom improvement in patients with liver only NETs metastasis. In most cases, however, this type of neoplasm remains incurable. Multidisciplinary approach including TAE and systemic treatment is necessary to palliate syndromes or prolong time without symptoms for better quality of life. In patients with NET liver metastases, the indications for PVE are based on the quality of the liver parenchyma and the volume of the FLR, the same as CLM. The potential further need for hepatic transarterial therapies (TAE or radioembolization) underscores the importance of the pretreatment assessment evaluating the benefits and the risk of PVE. Prior PVE is a relative contraindication for transarterial therapies if the nonembolized liver has not been resected.

22.3 Noncolorectal, Nonneuroendocrine Liver Metastases

There is now considerable evidence for long-term survival after resection of colorectal and neuroendocrine liver metastasis. In contrast, survival rates of patients with noncolorectal and nonneuroendocrine liver metastasis still remain low, and the role of resection of such liver metastasis is unknown.

Several recent studies have shown outcomes after hepatic resection of noncolorectal and nonneuroendocrine liver metastasis.[76,100-104] The most common primary sites of resected liver metastasis were from breast cancer, gastrointestinal tumor, melanoma, and renal cancer. They reported that the overall survival and disease-free survival at 5 years after resection is approximately 40% and 25%, respectively, with 2% or less mortality rate and 20–30% morbidity rate. Different outcomes depended on the primary tumor sites.

22.3.1 Breast Cancer

In clinical studies, liver metastasis is found in 20–30% of patients with metastatic breast cancer.[75,105,106] Liver metastases tend to be considered as the sign of dissemination because the systemic malignancy should first pass the pulmonary circulation. Actually, only 5% of metastatic breast cancers have the liver as the sole site of metastasis.[107] Combination of cytotoxic regimens, especially anthracycline and/or taxan-containing regimens were shown to produce higher response rates and longer durations of response and survival than the single agent therapy.[108] However, median overall survival of metastatic breast cancer is 20–25 months, and time to progression is 8–14 months even with those regimens.[107,109-111]

Recent studies suggest that hepatectomy is beneficial for selected patients with isolated liver metastases, and it can be performed with low risk and offers a chance of long-term survival. 5-year survival rate is 20–40% with a median survival of 30–40 months.[112-115]

22.3.2 Sarcoma

The most common histology of the patients with sarcoma liver metastasis is gastrointestinal stromal tumor (GIST) and leiomyosarcoma. Approximately 70% of patients with gastrointestinal sarcomas will develop hepatic metastasis.[116,117] Complete resection of the sarcoma liver metastasis is the only potentially curative treatment with postoperative 5 year overall survival of 30%.[118,119]

Currently, imatinib mesylate is the first-line therapy for unresectable or metastatic GIST, and response rate reaches 68%.[120] However, complete response is rare and some patients with GIST develop resistance to imatinib.[121] The multidisciplinary approach is necessary for patients with liver metastasis from GIST, and hepatectomy should be considered when complete resection is possible.

22.3.3 Melanoma

Hepatic metastasis is diagnosed in about 10–20% of patients with distant metastatic melanoma (Stage IV). Especially for ocular melanoma, up to 40% of patients have hepatic metastasis at presentation. The prognosis of the patients with hepatic melanoma metastases is dismal, with median survival of 4 months and 5-year overall survival of 3%.[122,123]

Dacarbazine, which is the only drug approved by the US Food and Drug Administration (FDA) for treatment of melanoma, has only 10–20% of response rate and less than 2% of 5-year survival.[124] Most clinical trials of combined chemotherapy which adds vinca alkaloid, cisplatin, or tamoxifen to decarbazine failed to demonstrate an advantage over decarbazine single-use.[125] Some reports showed that biochemotherapy, the combination of chemotherapy and biologic response modifiers, such as interferon and interleukin-2, produced response rates of 50–60%, complete remission rates of 10–20%, and a median survival of 11–12 months.[125] However, toxicity is higher than other therapies.

In selected patients, hepatic resection is the potentially curative option with reported median survival of 28 months and 5-year survival of 29%.[126] Moreover, Pawlik et al. reported that patients with a primary ocular melanoma have a significantly better prognosis than those with primary cutaneous melanoma.[127] Since most patients will experience disease recurrence, resection should be performed as a part of a multidisciplinary approach.

22.3.4 Other

There are few reports of surgical resection of the patients with other malignant tumors metastatic to the liver. About 10% of patients with renal cancer develop to the liver metastasis. The median survival of 14 patients after hepatectomy was reported to be 26 months with a survival rate of 26% at 3 years.[128]

Liver metastases are also common in patients with squamous cell carcinoma (SCC). In a multicenter study of metastatic SCC to the liver,[129] which primary sites include anal, head/neck, lung, and esophagus, authors reported that the overall median survival after hepatic resection was 22.3 months and 5-year overall survival was 20.5%.

Liver metastasis from gastric cancer is frequently accompanied by peritoneal dissemination and rarely considered as a surgical indication. However, more than 3-year survival has been reported after curative resection of metachronous liver metastasis from distal gastric cancer was reported.[130]

22.4 Conclusion

Hepatic resection for metastasis from noncolorectal and nonneuroendocrine carcinoma is safe and can offer long term survival in selected patients. Recurrence within 1 year of treatment of the primary tumor and positive surgical resection margin has been found to be highly predictive of poor outcome regardless of the primary sites. In patients with noncolorectal non-NET liver metastases, the indications for PVE are based on the quality of the liver parenchyma and the volume of the FLR. However, the preoperative assessment must carefully evaluate the benefits and risks of PVE as some of these patients may fail the resection strategy and require further locoregional liver-directed therapies.

References

1. Almersjo O, Bengmark S, Hafstrom L. Liver metastases found by follow-up of patients operated on for colorectal cancer. *Cancer*. 1976;37(3):1454-1457.
2. Bengmark S, Hafstrom L. The natural history of primary and secondary malignant tumors of the liver. I. The prognosis for patients with hepatic metastases from colonic and rectal carcinoma by laparotomy. *Cancer*. 1969;23(1):198-202.
3. Pawlik TM, Choti MA. Surgical therapy for colorectal metastases to the liver. *J Gastrointest Surg*. 2007;11(8):1057-1077.
4. Havlik R et al. Results of resection for hilar cholangiocarcinoma with analysis of prognostic factors. *Hepatogastroenterology*. 2000;47(34):927-931.
5. Fong Y et al. Liver resection for colorectal metastases. *J Clin Oncol*. 1997;15(3):938-946.
6. Pawlik TM et al. Effect of surgical margin status on survival and site of recurrence after hepatic resection for colorectal metastases. *Ann Surg*. 2005;241(5):715-722; discussion 722-724.
7. Ito H et al. Effect of postoperative morbidity on long-term survival after hepatic resection for metastatic colorectal cancer. *Ann Surg*. 2008;247(6):994-1002.
8. Gruner BA et al. Hepatocellular carcinoma in children associated with Gardner syndrome or familial adenomatous polyposis. *J Pediatr Hematol Oncol*. 1998;20(3):274-278.
9. Minagawa M et al. Simplified staging system for predicting the prognosis of patients with resectable liver metastasis: development and validation. *Arch Surg*. 2007;142(3):269-276.
10. Minagawa M et al. Extension of the frontiers of surgical indications in the treatment of liver metastases from colorectal cancer: long-term results. *Ann Surg*. 2000;231(4):487-499.
11. Fong Y et al. Clinical score for predicting recurrence after hepatic resection for metastatic colorectal cancer: analysis of 1001 consecutive cases. *Ann Surg*. 1999;230(3):309-318; discussion 318-321.
12. Curley SA et al. Surgical treatment of colorectal cancer metastasis. *Cancer Metastasis Rev*. 2004;23(1-2):165-182.
13. Charnsangavej C et al. Selection of patients for resection of hepatic colorectal metastases: expert consensus statement. *Ann Surg Oncol*. 2006;13(10):1261-1268.
14. Kokudo N et al. Surgery for multiple hepatic colorectal metastases. *J Hepatobiliary Pancreat Surg*. 2004;11(2):84-91.
15. Aloia TA et al. Solitary colorectal liver metastasis: resection determines outcome. *Arch Surg*. 2006;141(5):460-466; discussion 466-467.
16. Imamura H et al. Single and multiple resections of multiple hepatic metastases of colorectal origin. *Surgery*. 2004;135(5): 508-517.
17. Weber SM et al. Survival after resection of multiple hepatic colorectal metastases. *Ann Surg Oncol*. 2000;7(9):643-650.
18. Cady B et al. Surgical margin in hepatic resection for colorectal metastasis: a critical and improvable determinant of outcome. *Ann Surg*. 1998;227(4):566-571.
19. Steele G Jr et al. A prospective evaluation of hepatic resection for colorectal carcinoma metastases to the liver: Gastrointestinal Tumor Study Group Protocol 6584. *J Clin Oncol*. 1991;9(7):1105-1112.
20. Kokudo N et al. Genetic and histological assessment of surgical margins in resected liver metastases from colorectal carcinoma: minimum surgical margins for successful resection. *Arch Surg*. 2002;137(7):833-840.
21. Bodingbauer M et al. Size of surgical margin does not influence recurrence rates after curative liver resection for colorectal cancer liver metastases. *Br J Surg*. 2007;94(9): 1133-1138.
22. Miller G et al. Outcomes after resection of synchronous or metachronous hepatic and pulmonary colorectal metastases. *J Am Coll Surg*. 2007;205(2):231-238.
23. Pfannschmidt J, Dienemann H, Hoffmann H. Surgical resection of pulmonary metastases from colorectal cancer: a systematic review of published series. *Ann Thorac Surg*. 2007;84(1):324-338.
24. Headrick JR et al. Surgical treatment of hepatic and pulmonary metastases from colon cancer. *Ann Thorac Surg*. 2001;71(3):975-979; discussion 979-980.
25. Elias D et al. Hepatic and extrahepatic colorectal metastases: when resectable, their localization does not matter, but their total number has a prognostic effect. *Ann Surg Oncol*. 2005;12(11):900-909.
26. Jaeck D et al. Significance of hepatic pedicle lymph node involvement in patients with colorectal liver metastases: a prospective study. *Ann Surg Oncol*. 2002;9(5):430-438.
27. Rodgers MS, McCall JL. Surgery for colorectal liver metastases with hepatic lymph node involvement: a systematic review. *Br J Surg*. 2000;87(9):1142-1155.
28. Jaeck D. The significance of hepatic pedicle lymph nodes metastases in surgical management of colorectal liver metastases and of other liver malignancies. *Ann Surg Oncol*. 2003;10(9):1007-1011.
29. Ishizawa T et al. Neither multiple tumors nor portal hypertension are surgical contraindications for hepatocellular carcinoma. *Gastroenterology*. 2008;134(7):1908-1916.
30. Yang YY, Fleshman JW, Strasberg SM. Detection and management of extrahepatic colorectal cancer in patients with resectable liver metastases. *J Gastrointest Surg*. 2007;11(7): 929-944.
31. Imamura H et al. One thousand fifty-six hepatectomies without mortality in 8 years. *Arch Surg*. 2003;138(11):1198-1206; discussion 1206.
32. Mullen JT et al. Hepatic insufficiency and mortality in 1,059 noncirrhotic patients undergoing major hepatectomy. *J Am Coll Surg*. 2007;204(5):854-862; discussion 862-864.
33. Abdalla EK et al. Recurrence and outcomes following hepatic resection, radiofrequency ablation, and combined resection/ablation for colorectal liver metastases. *Ann Surg*. 2004;239(6):818-825.

34. Blazer DG 3rd et al. Pathologic response to preoperative chemotherapy: a new outcome end point after resection of hepatic colorectal metastases. *J Clin Oncol.* 2008;26(33):5344-5351; discussion 825-827.
35. Giacchetti S et al. Long-term survival of patients with unresectable colorectal cancer liver metastases following infusional chemotherapy with 5-fluorouracil, leucovorin, oxaliplatin and surgery. *Ann Oncol.* 1999;10(6):663-669.
36. Adam R et al. Rescue surgery for unresectable colorectal liver metastases downstaged by chemotherapy: a model to predict long-term survival. *Ann Surg.* 2004;240(4):644-657; discussion 657-658.
37. Hurwitz H et al. Bevacizumab plus irinotecan, fluorouracil, and leucovorin for metastatic colorectal cancer. *N Engl J Med.* 2004;350(23):2335-2342.
38. Wicherts DA, de Haas RJ, Adam R. Bringing unresectable liver disease to resection with curative intent. *Eur J Surg Oncol.* 2007;33(suppl 2):S42-S51.
39. Kopetz S, Vauthey JN. Perioperative chemotherapy for resectable hepatic metastases. *Lancet.* 2008;371(9617):963-965.
40. Nordlinger B et al. Perioperative chemotherapy with FOLFOX4 and surgery versus surgery alone for resectable liver metastases from colorectal cancer (EORTC Intergroup trial 40983): a randomised controlled trial. *Lancet.* 2008;371(9617):1007-1016.
41. Benoist S et al. Complete response of colorectal liver metastases after chemotherapy: Does it mean cure? *J Clin Oncol.* 2006;24(24):3939-3945.
42. Peppercorn PD et al. Demonstration of hepatic steatosis by computerized tomography in patients receiving 5-fluorouracil-based therapy for advanced colorectal cancer. *Br J Cancer.* 1998;77(11):2008-2011.
43. Rubbia-Brandt L et al. Severe hepatic sinusoidal obstruction associated with oxaliplatin-based chemotherapy in patients with metastatic colorectal cancer. *Ann Oncol.* 2004;15(3):460-466.
44. Aloia T et al. Liver histology and surgical outcomes after preoperative chemotherapy with fluorouracil plus oxaliplatin in colorectal cancer liver metastases. *J Clin Oncol.* 2006;24(31):4983-4990.
45. Karoui M et al. Influence of preoperative chemotherapy on the risk of major hepatectomy for colorectal liver metastases. *Ann Surg.* 2006;243(1):1-7.
46. Vauthey JN et al. Chemotherapy regimen predicts steatohepatitis and an increase in 90-day mortality after surgery for hepatic colorectal metastases. *J Clin Oncol.* 2006;24(13):2065-2072.
47. Kleiner DE et al. Design and validation of a histological scoring system for nonalcoholic fatty liver disease. *Hepatology.* 2005;41(6):1313-1321.
48. D'Angelica M et al. Lack of evidence for increased operative morbidity after hepatectomy with perioperative use of bevacizumab: a matched case-control study. *Ann Surg Oncol.* 2007;14(2):759-765.
49. Ribero D et al. Bevacizumab improves pathologic response and protects against hepatic injury in patients treated with oxaliplatin-based chemotherapy for colorectal liver metastases. *Cancer.* 2007;110(12):2761-2767.
50. Zorzi D et al. Chemotherapy with bevacizumab does not affect liver regeneration after portal vein embolization in the treatment of colorectal liver metastases. *Ann Surg Oncol.* 2008;15(10):2765-2772.
51. Adam R et al. Hepatic resection after rescue cetuximab treatment for colorectal liver metastases previously refractory to conventional systemic therapy. *J Clin Oncol.* 2007;25(29):4593-4602.
52. Abulkhir A et al. Preoperative portal vein embolization for major liver resection: a meta-analysis. *Ann Surg.* 2008;247(1):49-57.
53. Mueller L et al. Major hepatectomy for colorectal metastases: Is preoperative portal occlusion an oncological risk factor? *Ann Surg Oncol.* 2008;15(7):1908-1917.
54. Giraudo G et al. Preoperative contralateral portal vein embolization before major hepatic resection is a safe and efficient procedure: a large single institution experience. *Surgery.* 2008;143(4):476-482.
55. Abdalla EK et al. Extended hepatectomy in patients with hepatobiliary malignancies with and without preoperative portal vein embolization. *Arch Surg.* 2002;137(6):675-680; discussion 680-681.
56. Covey AM et al. Combined portal vein embolization and neoadjuvant chemotherapy as a treatment strategy for resectable hepatic colorectal metastases. *Ann Surg.* 2008;247(3):451-455.
57. Abdalla EK et al. Improving resectability of hepatic colorectal metastases: expert consensus statement. *Ann Surg Oncol.* 2006;13(10):1271-1280.
58. Ribero D et al. Portal vein embolization before major hepatectomy and its effects on regeneration, resectability and outcome. *Br J Surg.* 2007;94(11):1386-1394.
59. Bismuth H, Castaing D, Traynor O. Resection or palliation: priority of surgery in the treatment of hilar cancer. *World J Surg.* 1988;12(1):39-47.
60. Lambert LA, Colacchio TA, Barth RJ Jr. Interval hepatic resection of colorectal metastases improves patient selection. *Arch Surg.* 2000;135(4):473-479; discussion 479-480.
61. Minagawa M et al. Selection criteria for simultaneous resection in patients with synchronous liver metastasis. *Arch Surg.* 2006;141(10):1006-1012; discussion 1013.
62. Tanaka K et al. Outcome after simultaneous colorectal and hepatic resection for colorectal cancer with synchronous metastases. *Surgery.* 2004;136(3):650-659.
63. Martin R et al. Simultaneous liver and colorectal resections are safe for synchronous colorectal liver metastasis. *J Am Coll Surg.* 2003;197(2):233-241; discussion 241-242.
64. Allen PJ et al. Importance of response to neoadjuvant chemotherapy in patients undergoing resection of synchronous colorectal liver metastases. *J Gastrointest Surg.* 2003;7(1):109-115; discussion 116-117.
65. Chamberlain RS et al. Hepatic neuroendocrine metastases: Does intervention alter outcomes? *J Am Coll Surg.* 2000;190(4):432-445.
66. Panzuto F et al. Prognostic factors and survival in endocrine tumor patients: comparison between gastrointestinal and pancreatic localization. *Endocr Relat Cancer.* 2005;12(4):1083-1092.
67. Insa A et al. Prognostic factors predicting survival from first recurrence in patients with metastatic breast cancer: analysis of 439 patients. *Breast Cancer Res Treat.* 1999;56(1):67-78.
68. Madoff DC et al. Portal vein embolization: a preoperative approach to improve the safety of major hepatic resection. *Curr Med Imaging Rev.* 2006;2(4):385-404.

69. Gumbs AA et al. Review of the clinical, histological, and molecular aspects of pancreatic endocrine neoplasms. *J Surg Oncol*. 2002;81(1):45-53; discussion 54.
70. Sarmiento JM et al. Surgical treatment of neuroendocrine metastases to the liver: a plea for resection to increase survival. *J Am Coll Surg*. 2003;197(1):29-37.
71. Cho CS et al. Histologic grade is correlated with outcome after resection of hepatic neuroendocrine neoplasms. *Cancer*. 2008;113(1):126-134.
72. Touzios JG et al. Neuroendocrine hepatic metastases: Does aggressive management improve survival? *Ann Surg*. 2005;241(5):776-783; discussion 783-785.
73. Norton JA et al. Morbidity and mortality of aggressive resection in patients with advanced neuroendocrine tumors. *Arch Surg*. 2003;138(8):859-866.
74. Knox CD et al. Survival and functional quality of life after resection for hepatic carcinoid metastasis. *J Gastrointest Surg*. 2004;8(6):653-659.
75. Clark GM et al. Survival from first recurrence: relative importance of prognostic factors in 1,015 breast cancer patients. *J Clin Oncol*. 1987;5(1):55-61.
76. Elias D et al. Resection of liver metastases from a noncolorectal primary: indications and results based on 147 monocentric patients. *J Am Coll Surg*. 1998;187(5):487-493.
77. Chen H et al. Isolated liver metastases from neuroendocrine tumors: Does resection prolong survival? *J Am Coll Surg*. 1998;187(1):88-92; discussion 92-93.
78. Musunuru S et al. Metastatic neuroendocrine hepatic tumors: resection improves survival. *Arch Surg*. 2006;141(10):1000-1004; discussion 1005.
79. Florman S et al. Liver transplantation for neuroendocrine tumors. *J Gastrointest Surg*. 2004;8(2):208-212.
80. Frilling A et al. Liver transplantation for patients with metastatic endocrine tumors: single-center experience with 15 patients. *Liver Transpl*. 2006;12(7):1089-1096.
81. Gupta S et al. Hepatic arterial embolization and chemoembolization for the treatment of patients with metastatic neuroendocrine tumors: variables affecting response rates and survival. *Cancer*. 2005;104(8):1590-1602.
82. Ho AS et al. Long-term outcome after chemoembolization and embolization of hepatic metastatic lesions from neuroendocrine tumors. *AJR Am J Roentgenol*. 2007;188(5):1201-1207.
83. Bloomston M et al. Hepatic artery chemoembolization in 122 patients with metastatic carcinoid tumor: lessons learned. *J Gastrointest Surg*. 2007;11(3):264-271.
84. Lemaire E et al. Functional and morphological changes in the pancreatic remnant following pancreaticoduodenectomy with pancreaticogastric anastomosis. *Br J Surg*. 2000;87(4):434-438.
85. Rothenberg ML et al. Superiority of oxaliplatin and fluorouracil-leucovorin compared with either therapy alone in patients with progressive colorectal cancer after irinotecan and fluorouracil-leucovorin: interim results of a phase III trial. *J Clin Oncol*. 2003;21(11):2059-2069.
86. Roche A et al. Trans-catheter arterial chemoembolization as first-line treatment for hepatic metastases from endocrine tumors. *Eur Radiol*. 2003;13(1):136-140.
87. Lladó L et al. A prognostic index of the survival of patients with unresectable hepatocellular carcinoma after transcatheter arterial chemoembolization. *Cancer*. 2000;88(1):50-57.
88. Abdalla EK et al. Treatment of large and advanced hepatocellular carcinoma. *Ann Surg Oncol*. 2008;15(4):979-985.
89. King J et al. Radioembolization with selective internal radiation microspheres for neuroendocrine liver metastases. *Cancer*. 2008;113(5):921-929.
90. Weiss L et al. Haematogenous metastatic patterns in colonic carcinoma: an analysis of 1541 necropsies. *J Pathol*. 1986;150(3):195-203.
91. Fazio N et al. Interferon-alpha and somatostatin analog in patients with gastroenteropancreatic neuroendocrine carcinoma: Single agent or combination? *Ann Oncol*. 2007;18(1):13-19.
92. Welin SV et al. High-dose treatment with a long-acting somatostatin analogue in patients with advanced midgut carcinoid tumours. *Eur J Endocrinol*. 2004;151(1):107-112.
93. Schnirer II, Yao JC, Ajani JA. Carcinoid—a comprehensive review. *Acta Oncol*. 2003;42(7):672-692.
94. Rinke A et al. Placebo-controlled, double-blind, prospective, randomized study on the effect of octreotide LAR in the control of tumor growth in patients with metastatic neuroendocrine midgut tumors: a report from the PROMID Study Group. *J Clin Oncol*. 2009;27(28):4656-4663.
95. Yao JC et al. Targeting vascular endothelial growth factor in advanced carcinoid tumor: a random assignment phase II study of depot octreotide with bevacizumab and pegylated interferon alpha-2b. *J Clin Oncol*. 2008;26(8):1316-1323.
96. Grozinsky-Glasberg S et al. Octreotide and the mTOR inhibitor RAD001 (everolimus) block proliferation and interact with the Akt-mTOR-p70S6K pathway in a neuro-endocrine tumour cell Line. *Neuroendocrinology*. 2008;87(3):168-181.
97. Sun W et al. Phase II/III study of doxorubicin with fluorouracil compared with streptozocin with fluorouracil or dacarbazine in the treatment of advanced carcinoid tumors: Eastern Cooperative Oncology Group Study E1281. *J Clin Oncol*. 2005;23(22):4897-4904.
98. McCollum AD et al. Lack of efficacy of streptozocin and doxorubicin in patients with advanced pancreatic endocrine tumors. *Am J Clin Oncol*. 2004;27(5):485-488.
99. Cheng PN, Saltz LB. Failure to confirm major objective antitumor activity for streptozocin and doxorubicin in the treatment of patients with advanced islet cell carcinoma. *Cancer*. 1999;86(6):944-948.
100. Adam R et al. Hepatic resection for noncolorectal nonendocrine liver metastases: analysis of 1,452 patients and development of a prognostic model. *Ann Surg*. 2006;244(4):524-535.
101. Rees M et al. Evaluation of long-term survival after hepatic resection for metastatic colorectal cancer: a multifactorial model of 929 patients. *Ann Surg*. 2008;247(1):125-135.
102. Harrison LE et al. Hepatic resection for noncolorectal, nonneuroendocrine metastases: a fifteen-year experience with ninety-six patients. *Surgery*. 1997;121(6):625-632.
103. Earle SA et al. Hepatectomy enables prolonged survival in select patients with isolated noncolorectal liver metastasis. *J Am Coll Surg*. 2006;203(4):436-446.
104. Weitz J et al. Partial hepatectomy for metastases from noncolorectal, nonneuroendocrine carcinoma. *Ann Surg*. 2005;241(2):269-276.
105. Wyld L et al. Prognostic factors for patients with hepatic metastases from breast cancer. *Br J Cancer*. 2003;89(2):284-290.

106. Zinser JW et al. Clinical course of breast cancer patients with liver metastases. *J Clin Oncol.* 1987;5(5):773-782.
107. Er O et al. Clinical course of breast cancer patients with metastases limited to the liver treated with chemotherapy. *Cancer J.* 2008;14(1):62-68.
108. Hortobagyi GN. Developments in chemotherapy of breast cancer. *Cancer.* 2000;88(12 suppl):3073-3079.
109. Nabholtz JM et al. Docetaxel and doxorubicin compared with doxorubicin and cyclophosphamide as first-line chemotherapy for metastatic breast cancer: results of a randomized, multicenter, phase III trial. *J Clin Oncol.* 2003;21(6):968-975.
110. Jassem J et al. Doxorubicin and paclitaxel versus fluorouracil, doxorubicin, and cyclophosphamide as first-line therapy for women with metastatic breast cancer: final results of a randomized phase III multicenter trial. *J Clin Oncol.* 2001;19(6):1707-1715.
111. Madoff DC et al. Management of TIPS-related refractory hepatic encephalopathy with reduced Wallgraft endoprostheses. *J Vasc Interv Radiol.* 2003;14(3):369-374.
112. Adam R et al. Is liver resection justified for patients with hepatic metastases from breast cancer? *Ann Surg.* 2006;244(6):897-907; discussion 907-908.
113. Sakamoto Y et al. Hepatic resection for metastatic breast cancer: prognostic analysis of 34 patients. *World J Surg.* 2005;29(4):524-527.
114. Lubrano J et al. Liver resection for breast cancer metastasis: Does it improve survival? *Surg Today.* 2008;38(4): 293-299.
115. Elias D et al. An attempt to clarify indications for hepatectomy for liver metastases from breast cancer. *Am J Surg.* 2003;185(2):158-164.
116. DeMatteo RP et al. Two hundred gastrointestinal stromal tumors: recurrence patterns and prognostic factors for survival. *Ann Surg.* 2000;231(1):51-58.
117. Ng EH, Pollock RE, Romsdahl MM. Prognostic implications of patterns of failure for gastrointestinal leiomyosarcomas. *Cancer.* 1992;69(6):1334-1341.
118. Pawlik TM et al. Results of a single-center experience with resection and ablation for sarcoma metastatic to the liver. *Arch Surg.* 2006;141(6):537-543; discussion 543-544.
119. DeMatteo RP et al. Results of hepatic resection for sarcoma metastatic to liver. *Ann Surg.* 2001;234(4):540-547; discussion 547-548.
120. Blanke CD et al. Long-term results from a randomized phase II trial of standard- versus higher-dose imatinib mesylate for patients with unresectable or metastatic gastrointestinal stromal tumors expressing KIT. *J Clin Oncol.* 2008;26(4):620-625.
121. Antonescu CR et al. Acquired resistance to imatinib in gastrointestinal stromal tumor occurs through secondary gene mutation. *Clin Cancer Res.* 2005;11(11):4182-4190.
122. Martinez SR et al. The utility of estrogen receptor, progesterone receptor, and Her-2/neu status to predict survival in patients undergoing hepatic resection for breast cancer metastases. *Am J Surg.* 2006;191(2):281-283.
123. Rothbarth J et al. Isolated hepatic perfusion with high-dose melphalan for the treatment of colorectal metastasis confined to the liver. *Br J Surg.* 2003;90(11):1391-1397.
124. Ahmann DL et al. Complete responses and long-term survivals after systemic chemotherapy for patients with advanced malignant melanoma. *Cancer.* 1989;63(2):224-227.
125. O'Day SJ, Kim CJ, Reintgen DS. Metastatic melanoma: chemotherapy to biochemotherapy. *Cancer Control.* 2002; 9(1):31-38.
126. Rose DM et al. Surgical resection for metastatic melanoma to the liver: the John Wayne Cancer Institute and Sydney Melanoma Unit experience. *Arch Surg.* 2001;136(8):950-955.
127. Pawlik TM et al. Hepatic resection for metastatic melanoma: distinct patterns of recurrence and prognosis for ocular versus cutaneous disease. *Ann Surg Oncol.* 2006;13(5):712-720.
128. Laurent A et al. Controlling tumor growth by modulating endogenous production of reactive oxygen species. *Cancer Res.* 2005;65(3):948-956.
129. Pawlik TM et al. Liver-directed surgery for metastatic squamous cell carcinoma to the liver: results of a multicenter analysis. *Ann Surg Oncol.* 2007;14(10):2807-2816.
130. Zacherl J et al. Analysis of hepatic resection of metastasis originating from gastric adenocarcinoma. *J Gastrointest Surg.* 2002;6(5):682-689.
131. Gayowski TJ et al. Experience in hepatic resection for metastatic colorectal cancer: analysis of clinical and pathologic risk factors. *Surgery.* 1994;116(4):703-710.
132. Scheele J et al. Resection of colorectal liver metastases. *World J Surg.* 1995;19(1):59-71.
133. Nordlinger B et al. Surgical resection of colorectal carcinoma metastases to the liver. A prognostic scoring system to improve case selection, based on 1568 patients. Association Francaise de Chirurgie. *Cancer.* 1996;77(7):1254-1262.
134. Jaeck D et al. Long-term survival following resection of colorectal hepatic metastases. Association Francaise de Chirurgie. *Br J Surg.* 1997;84(7):977-980.
135. Jamison RL et al. Hepatic resection for metastatic colorectal cancer results in cure for some patients. *Arch Surg.* 1997;132(5):505-510.
136. Jenkins LT et al. Hepatic resection for metastatic colorectal cancer. *Am Surg.* 1997;63(7):605-610.
137. Elias D et al. Results of 136 curative hepatectomies with a safety margin of less than 10 mm for colorectal metastases. *J Surg Oncol.* 1998;69(2):88-93.
138. Ambiru S et al. Hepatic resection for colorectal metastases: analysis of prognostic factors. *Dis Colon Rectum.* 1999;42(5):632-639.
139. Figueras J et al. Clinical study of 437 consecutive liver resections. *Med Clin (Barc).* 2001;117(2):41-44.
140. Choti MA et al. Trends in long-term survival following liver resection for hepatic colorectal metastases. *Ann Surg.* 2002;235(6):759-766.
141. Fernandez FG et al. Five-year survival after resection of hepatic metastases from colorectal cancer in patients screened by positron emission tomography with F-18 fluorodeoxyglucose (FDG-PET). *Ann Surg.* 2004;240(3):438-447.

Part V

Additional Strategies for Resection and Embolization

Nontraditional Resection Including the Two-Stage Hepatectomy

23

Elie Oussoultzoglou, Daniel Jaeck, Edoardo Rosso, and Philippe Bachellier

Abstract

Liver surgery can only be offered to approximately 20% of patients with colorectal liver metastases, provided that the primary tumor is controlled. Currently, a selected subgroup of the remaining 80% of the patients, who were initially considered as unresectable and were assigned to receive palliative chemotherapy, may benefit from liver surgery and often require a multidisciplinary approach in order to achieve a curative liver resection. This multidisciplinary approach may also use additional methods such as radiofrequency, portal vein embolization, and downsizing or conversion chemotherapy. The combination of these different therapies resulted in the development of nontraditional liver resection techniques including the so-called two-stage hepatectomy procedure. The aim of these strategies is to achieve a complete tumoral resection in a curative intent, to increase safely the indications of liver resection for patients presenting with initially unresectable liver metastases, and to offer to them similar results in term of short- and long-term outcome to that observed in patients with initially resectable liver metastases.

Keywords

Liver resection for colorectal liver metastases • Colorectal liver metastases • Portal vein embolization • Two-stage hepatectomy

Liver resection for colorectal liver metastases is recognized as the only curative treatment offering a chance of long-term survival.[1-4] Based on advances in knowledge of liver anatomy and preoperative imaging, better selection of candidates for surgery, improvement in surgical techniques including intraoperative ultrasound, progress in anesthesia, and refinements in pre- and postoperative care, elective liver resection can be performed today with low mortality (<5%) and acceptable morbidity (<20%) rates.[5] However, there are many papers reporting a 0% mortality for liver resection. Five percent is for HCCs, and the mortality for metastasis is lower. Furthermore, the decisive progress accomplished by chemotherapy,[6-9] especially during the last decade, resulted in the improvement of survival rates, particularly in patients presenting with colorectal liver metastases which are currently close to 40% at 5 years.[5]

However, liver surgery can only be offered to approximately 20% of patients with colorectal liver metastases, provided that the primary tumor is

D. Jaeck (✉)
Centre de Chirurgie Viscérale et de Transplantation, Hôpital de Hautepierre, Université Louis Pasteur, Hôpitaux Universitaires de Strasbourg, Avenue Molière, Strasbourg 67200, France
e-mail: daniel.jaeck@chru-strasbourg.fr

D.C. Madoff et al. (eds.), *Venous Embolization of the Liver*,
DOI 10.1007/978-1-84882-122-4_23, © Springer-Verlag London Limited 2011

controlled.[2,3,10] Currently, a selected subgroup of the remaining 80% of the patients, who were initially considered as unresectable and assigned to receive palliative chemotherapy, may benefit from liver surgery and often require a multidisciplinary approach in order to achieve a curative liver resection. This multidisciplinary approach may also use additional methods such as radiofrequency, portal vein embolization, and downsizing or conversion chemotherapy. The combination of these different therapies resulted in the development of nontraditional liver resection techniques including the so-called two-stage hepatectomy procedure. The aim of these strategies is to achieve a complete tumoral resection in a curative intent, to increase safely the indications of liver resection for patients presenting with initially unresectable liver metastases, and to offer to them similar results in term of short- and long-term outcome to that observed in patients with initially resectable liver metastases.

23.1 Limits of Liver Surgery

In some patients, liver resection cannot be technically feasible or contraindicated because of the high risk of postoperative liver failure. Among them, the number, size, and bilobar distribution of liver metastases and the insufficient future remnant liver volume constitute the main obstacle for liver resection. While the topography of liver metastases (unilobar or bilobar distribution) has not yet been definitively demonstrated to affect overall or disease-free survival,[11-15] a higher postoperative mortality rate (9.1%) was reported in patients undergoing liver resection for bilobar liver metastases.[16] This increased mortality rate is mainly due to the occurrence of postoperative liver failure which represents the leading cause of death after a major liver resection.[17,18] Currently, these patients were reconsidered with an increasing interest as potential candidates for safe curative resection. Indeed, postoperative liver failure is determined by two factors including a small remnant liver volume and a poor quality of liver parenchyma. A close correlation between the future remnant liver volume and the occurrence of postoperative complications has been already demonstrated.[19] Therefore, in case of technically resectable liver metastases independent of the resection margins,[20,21] an adequate functional liver volume needs to be preserved in order to minimize the risk of lethal postoperative liver failure.

23.2 Portal Vein Embolization

Makuuchi et al. underlined that fatal liver failure did not occur after major liver resection when the portal branch of the resected hemiliver was previously occluded.[22] A median hypertrophy of the liver remnant of around 42% follows a preoperative portal vein embolization in patients presenting with initially unresectable colorectal liver metastases due to a too small liver remnant volume (<30% of the functional total liver volume).[23] The use of this procedure has progressively been extended in order to increase the resectability rate of colorectal liver metastases.[19,23-27] However, the benefit of portal vein embolization has not yet been demonstrated by a randomized controlled trial. Indeed, available data in the literature showed that a right hepatectomy could be achieved safely without a need for a preoperative portal vein embolization in patients with normal underlying liver parenchyma[28] while an extended hepatectomy may benefit from a preoperative portal vein embolization, particularly when the estimated remnant liver volume is less than 25%.[19] Furthermore, it has been suggested to raise the volumetric safety threshold up to 40% in patients heavily treated with systemic chemotherapy (Fig. 23.1)[29,30] or to prolong the liver regeneration interval after portal vein embolization by delaying liver resection in patients with an injured liver.[31,32] This prolonged interval allows the injured livers to reach an adequate hypertrophy as its regeneration time is longer compared to normal liver parenchyma.[32,33] Recently, a possible carcinologic advantage of preoperative portal vein embolization has been highlighted among patients presenting with unilobar colorectal liver metastases and who had undergone a right hepatectomy with and without preoperative portal vein embolization.[4] Indeed, the multivariate analysis showed that preoperative portal vein embolization, neoadjuvant chemotherapy, and single liver metastasis were significantly associated with a decreased rate of intrahepatic recurrences. The retrograde portal dissemination, which is commonly observed with hepatocellular carcinoma, is schematically represented in Fig. 23.2. Therefore, preoperative portal vein embolization may reduce intrahepatic tumoral shedding by intraluminal occlusion of the peripheral portal branches. However, this hypothesis needs further randomized studies with the quantification of the circulating tumoral cells to be confirmed. When metastases preoperatively unknown are discovered through IOUS, inspection, or palpation, they may be removed.[34]

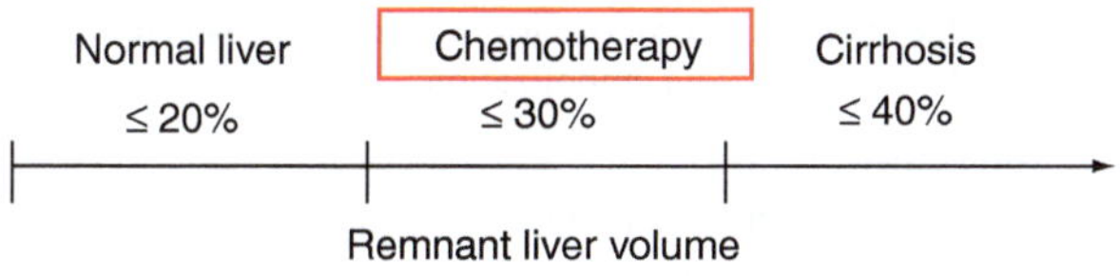

Fig. 23.1 Indication for portal vein embolization before major liver resection: safety criteria. Correlation between liver volume (%) and quality of the underlying nontumoral liver parenchyma

Table 23.1 Technique of portal vein embolization adopted in our institution

Radiologic approach
Percutaneous contralateral transhepatic approach
4-Fr catheter
Portal pressure monitoring (before and after PVE)
Proximal branches : Histoacryl+Lipiodol injection
Distal portal branches occluded by adsorbable particles (Embosphères®)

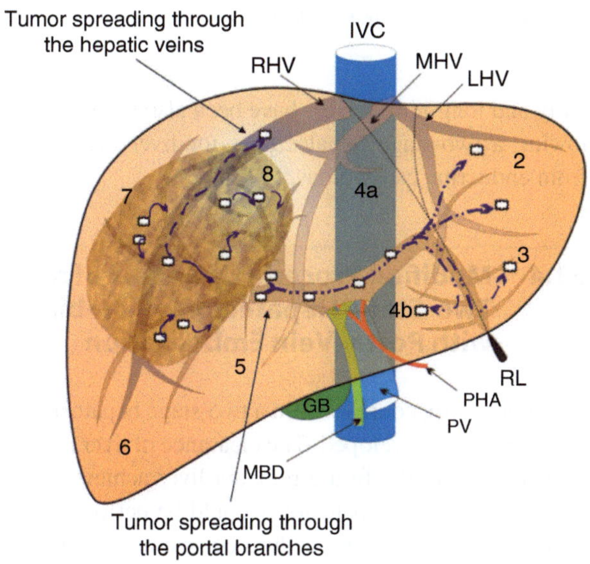

Fig. 23.2 Retrograde portal dissemination hypothesis: representative schema of tumoral cells spreading in a patient presenting with colorectal right liver metastases. Two pathways are illustrated: (1) following the normal hepatic outflow through the hepatic veins and (2) retrogradely through the portal branches with potential intrahepatic satellite nodules. *IVC* inferior vena cava, *RHV* right hepatic vein, *MHV* middle hepatic vein, *LHV* left hepatic vein, *GB* gallbladder, *MBD* main biliary duct, *PV* portal vein, *PHA* proper hepatic artery, *RL* round ligament

23.3 Two-Stage Hepatectomy Procedure Combined with Portal Vein Embolization

The main drawback of preoperative portal vein embolization is the risk of growth of liver metastases located in the nonembolized hemiliver[35-37] as a result of the hepatotrophic growth factors reaching the liver by the splenoportal venous flow. Moreover, the growth of liver metastases in the future remnant nonembolized hemiliver seems to be faster and of greater amplitude than the hypertrophy of the nontumoral liver parenchyma.[37] Subsequently, progression of metastases in the future remnant liver following portal vein embolization may withdraw the option for a curative surgery. Therefore, resection of liver metastases in the future remnant liver should be ideally performed before portal vein embolization during a first-stage hepatectomy, leaving the liver metastases in the hemiliver which will be embolized after postoperative recovery.[27,38] Often, the left hemiliver is selected to be cleared from the metastases and the right portal vein to be embolized. Therefore, the aim of the first-stage hepatectomy is to perform a full excision of the liver metastases in the future remnant liver. Then, a preoperative right portal vein embolization is performed percutaneously 2–4 weeks later under ultrasound guidance. The technique of portal vein embolization is summarized in Table 23.1. In our experience, a contralateral approach was used (Fig. 23.3).[31] Liver hypertrophy is measured by a three-dimensional CT scan. After 46–84% of liver mass resection, the remaining liver doubled within 2–3 weeks,[39] and after portal vein embolization, 93.5% of the patients reached an adequate compensatory liver hypertrophy within 4–8 weeks.[40] It has been also advocated that the functional gain is probably more rapid and of greater amplitude than the volume gain.[41] The volume of the future remnant liver should be at least equal to 30% of the total functional liver volume in patients without any underlying liver disease and 40% in those presenting injured liver parenchyma.[23,42] This higher cutoff is based on series evaluating neoadjuvant chemotherapy, which is known to be a risk factor for postoperative liver failure.[43,44] A second-stage hepatectomy can then be performed safely to achieve a curative-intent liver resection. This second-stage liver

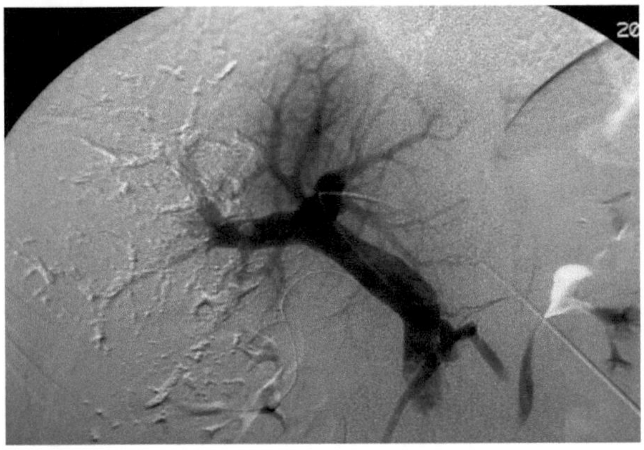

Fig. 23.3 Percutaneous portogram showing a contralateral left hepatic approach for a right portal vein embolization

Table 23.2 Selection criteria for a two-stage hepatectomy combined with portal vein embolization

Inclusion criteria
1. Patients with multiple bilobar colorectal liver metastases
2. Left hemiliver clearance feasible (first-stage hepatectomy)
3. Left hepatic vein non-invaded
4. Left pedicle non-invaded
5. FLR volume <30% (before right PVE)
Exclusion criteria
1. Obstructive jaundice (bilirubin > 50 μmol/L)
2. ICG-15 >20%
3. Nonresectable extrahepatic disease

resection is often a right hepatectomy or sometimes, a right hepatectomy extended to the segment IV. This strategy called "two-stage hepatectomy combined with portal vein embolization" was designed to limit the risk of disease progression in the nonembolized hemiliver and to avoid the occurrence of postoperative liver failure. Two main factors are keys for the success of a two-stage hepatectomy. They include a careful patient selection (Table 23.2) and an adequate use of the new chemotherapies (oxaliplatin, irinotecan, bevacizumab, and erbitux). Portal vein embolization after the first-stage hepatectomy may accelerate the liver regeneration process and may also allow to achieve earlier the second-stage liver resection which consists in a curative resection. The expected benefit of chemotherapy between the two hepatectomies is to avoid disease progression. However, it is currently recognized that chemotherapy is associated with increased perioperative morbidity, particularly in patients undergoing major liver resection.[42,44] Furthermore, chemotherapy administered between the two hepatectomies may inhibit the expected liver regeneration following portal vein embolization. For this reason, in our practice, chemotherapy is delayed at least 3 weeks after portal vein embolization to avoid inhibition of liver regeneration during its critical period. In our series,[27,38] as well as in others,[45-47] the reported 3-year survival ranged from 45% to 47% with a median survival of 18–35 months which is similar to the results reported in patients with initially resectable liver metastases. The short- and long-term results of these series focusing on two-stage hepatectomies for initially unresectable multiple and bilobar colorectal liver metastases are shown in Table 23.3. Satisfactory early and long-term results have been also reported following a two-stage hepatectomy for liver metastases from endocrine carcinomas.[48]

23.4 Modified Procedures as Part of a Two-Stage Hepatectomy Combined with Portal Vein Embolization

Alternative procedures within a two-stage hepatectomy have been also developed. The clearance of liver metastases located in the future remnant liver achieved during the first-stage hepatectomy could be performed by a minimally invasive procedure consisting in percutaneous radiofrequency ablation or by microwave ablation.[49] However, a percutaneous approach may overlook either small metastases in the future remnant liver or extrahepatic disease including peritoneal carcinomatosis and locoregional recurrence of the primary tumor, which can be easily detected during laparotomy. Furthermore, in patients presenting with synchronous colorectal liver metastases, the clearance of liver metastases located in the future remnant liver can be also performed during a laparoscopic approach performed in order to resect the primary colorectal tumor.

Finally, there is an alternative to portal vein embolization in order to induce hypertrophy of the future remnant liver. Indeed, a percutaneous portal vein embolization can be replaced either by an intraoperative portal branch ligature – first reported in 1975 for hepatocellular carcinoma[50] – of the tumorous lobe which can be performed at the time of the first-stage hepatectomy[47,51,52] or by direct intraoperative exposure of an ileocolic vein which allows to embolize the portal vein.[22,53] However, the risk of postoperative liver failure still exists

Table 23.3 Short- and long-term results after a two-stage hepatectomy of the reported series and of our own experience

Authors	No. of patients	PVE	Chemotherapy	Mortality (%)	Morbidity (%)	3-year survival (%)
Togo	11/11	±	±	0	18	45
Adam	31/45	±	+	6.5	48	47
Jaeck	45/56	+	±	0	53	46

by combining simultaneously during the same laparotomy a clearance of one hemiliver from tumoral deposits and a contralateral portal vein occlusion.

23.5 Two-Stage Hepatectomy Procedure Without Portal Vein Embolization

Preoperative portal embolization is not routinely necessary in patients with multiple and bilobar liver metastases which were scheduled for a planned two-stage hepatectomy procedure. Indeed, a longer waiting period, during which chemotherapy is administered to avoid disease progression, may allow adequate compensatory hypertrophy of the nonembolized nontumorous hemiliver leading to a second-stage hepatectomy to be performed without the need of a preoperative portal vein embolization.[45] In brief, during the first-stage hepatectomy, a resection of the largest number of liver metastases is performed, regardless of their distribution in the right or left hemiliver. The retained liver metastases at the first-stage hepatectomy will be treated by a subsequent liver resection in a second-stage hepatectomy scheduled after a period of liver regeneration without preoperative portal vein embolization. During this regeneration period, patients are routinely treated with chemotherapy. To avoid the occurrence of postoperative liver failure, even after the first- or the second-stage hepatectomy, the anatomical and functional integrity of at least 30–40% of the nontumoral liver parenchyma should be preserved. The results of this strategy are close to those obtained after liver resection for initially resectable metastatic colorectal cancer.[45] However, it should be underlined that higher rates of specific postoperative complications and even occurrence of inhospital mortality were registered compared to those reported after a two-stage hepatectomy routinely combined with preoperative portal vein embolization. This may be related to the fact that the second-stage hepatectomy carries the same risks, with a complex repeat hepatectomy in an area with adhesions and postoperative modifications.

23.6 Ex Vivo Liver Resection

Despite of the major advances in surgical techniques, most of the patients with colorectal liver metastases still are unresectable. Indeed, resection using conventional techniques is often hazardous and even impossible due to the size, location, and proximity or involvement of major vascular pedicles. In such cases, an ex vivo liver resection, first described by Pichlmayr in 1988,[54] may offer, in selected patients, an option for a curative treatment.[55] In brief, in this technique, the liver is partially or completely explanted from the patient, following a protective hypothermia obtained by perfusion of a cytoprotective solution with additional cooling of the liver surface in order to prolong the ischemic tolerance during liver resection. A bloodless liver transection can then be performed, allowing a complex reconstruction of the hepatic veins and/or portal pedicles. Then, the liver is reimplanted in the patient.

Three different approaches for ex vivo liver resection[56-58] have been reported: (1) "in situ" liver resection and crossclamping without dissection of major vessels, (2) "ante situm" resection with dissection of the suprahepatic inferior vena cava only, and (3) "ex situ" resection with complete removal of the liver from the body and resection on bench procedure. All three approaches require complete mobilization of the liver, hypothermic perfusion, and the use of veno-venous bypass.

The largest series currently available in the literature reported eight cases of ex vivo resection for colorectal liver metastases with postoperative morbidity and mortality rates of 87% and 25%, respectively, and one long-term survivor at 30 months.[55]

Ex vivo liver resection should be considered as the ultimate surgical option in the treatment of an otherwise unresectable tumor. However, the potential benefit of such an aggressive approach is counterbalanced by the high morbidity and mortality rates. Therefore, ex vivo liver resection should be limited to carefully selected patients and should be performed exclusively in specialized centers with skill experience in conventional liver surgery and liver transplantation.

23.7 Liver Resection for Colorectal Liver Metastases Associated with Major Vascular Resection

Ill-located colorectal liver metastases may require, in a curative intent, the resection/reconstruction of the portal vein bifurcation, of the inferior vena cava, and/or of the hepatocaval confluence. To achieve safely this kind of nontraditional liver resection, it is mandatory to preserve an adequate volume of the future remnant liver with an optimal liver inflow and outflow. This can only be achieved with appropriate vascular reconstruction. Several short series have reported major hepatectomy for colorectal liver metastases combined with major vascular resection/reconstruction.[59-63] Even if firm recommendations cannot be drawn, it seems interesting to underline that patients scheduled for an additional vascular resection/reconstruction combined with major liver resection should be carefully selected before operation as postoperative morbidity and mortality rates seem higher than after a standard major hepatectomy, and the increased perioperative risk associated with the procedure should be balanced with the eventual benefits.

23.8 Radiofrequency and Trans-metastasis Liver Resection

Radiofrequency thermocoagulation or ablation has been proposed as a new modality of treatment for liver tumors[64] and has contributed to the development of a new technique of liver transection.[65] In this technique, a Cool-tip® radiofrequency electrode (Radionics Inc., Burlington, MA, USA) is inserted along the transection plane serially 1–2 cm apart, and radiofrequency energy is applied for 1–2 min to create overlapping areas of coagulated tissue, followed by transection of the coagulated liver using a simple scalpel.

Another innovative method of liver resection, combining conventional liver resection techniques and radiofrequency destruction, has been developed.[66,67] This technique may be useful for patients ineligible for curative surgery due to the presence of one or more liver metastases lying in the "ideal" plane of hepatectomy; therefore, they require a wider or extended hepatic resection which is considered as unsafe due to the presence of a too small future remnant liver. In such circumstances, a trans-metastasis liver transection immediately following the radiofrequency destruction enables to perform a curative-intent resection in patients with bilateral, unresectable colorectal liver metastases, when the only possible resection plane passes through liver metastases. In brief, during the operation, all colorectal liver metastases in the future remnant liver are ablated by radiofrequency and the liver transection plane is conducted, passing through a trans-metastasis ablated zone. Such technique should be considered only in selected patients with otherwise unresectable colorectal liver metastases. Elias et al.[66] reported a series of patients with multiple bilobar colorectal liver metastases treated with this procedure, showing the feasibility and efficacy of this approach. The mortality and morbidity rates were 7.6% and 24%, respectively. Postoperative recurrence rate at the site of trans-metastasis hepatectomy was nil after a median follow-up of 19.4 months. Radiofrequency ablation of small metastatic deposits (<3 cm) has been also associated with resection of larger nodules in order to achieve a curative procedure, avoiding lethal postoperative liver failure. Curley et al. reported a median overall survival of 37 months in patients with colorectal liver metastases considered as unresectable for cure.[68] However, a single institutional retrospective report showed that recurrences after radiofrequency ablation are more frequent than those observed in patients undergoing liver resection.[69] Currently, as no randomized studies comparing radiofrequency ablation and liver resection are available, radiofrequency ablation cannot be considered as curative. This fact allows to consider all surgical approaches using radiofrequency as nontraditional procedures.

23.9 Radiofrequency-Assisted Liver Transection (Habib Device)

In a preliminary study ($n=15$) of segmental or wedge resections reported by Weber et al.,[65] the intraoperative blood loss was reduced, and no complications such as bile leak were observed. However, one potential disadvantage of this technique is the amount of parenchyma in the remnant liver which is sacrificed. Moreover, the major concern still remains the possible thermal injury to the hilar structures and hepatic veins when using this technique for major liver resection.[70] This technique has not been compared with conventional techniques of liver transection. Recently, an in-line radiofrequency device consisting of multiple parallel radiofrequency probes has been specifically developed for liver transection. This device has been shown to reduce bleeding compared with CUSA in a preliminary pilot study.[71] However, the role of this device in hepatic resection has to be validated in the future.

In conclusion, selected patients considered as unresectable because of extensive multiple and bilobar colorectal liver metastases can be treated by a two-stage hepatectomy to achieve a complete resection of the tumoral deposits. This strategy justifies leaving the metastases in place during the first-stage hepatectomy, provided that a complete removal of liver metastases could be obtained during a second-stage liver resection. The rationale of this staged liver resection is to minimize the risk of liver failure. In patients for whom a staged liver resection is planned, preoperative evaluation should indicate that complete resection of the metastatic disease can be achieved, respecting an adequate amount of viable and functional liver remnant. However, approximately one-fourth of the patients will experience a failure of the strategy as there is a risk of patient dropout due to disease progression occurring between the two liver resections. However, when feasible, a two-stage hepatectomy should be attempted regardless of the number and the size of liver metastases in order to achieve a complete resection with tumor-free margins. A preoperative portal vein embolization accelerates the process, but a two-stage hepatectomy can also be achieved in selected cases without portal vein embolization. Chemotherapy administration between the two hepatectomies needs further evaluation. Finally, other multidisciplinary innovations, including radiofrequency and complex vascular reconstruction procedures, have been demonstrated to be useful in selected patients, but the increased rates of disease recurrence and of perioperative morbidity and mortality remain an obstacle to extend the indications of such nontraditional liver resections.

References

1. Hughes KS, Simon R, Songhorabodi S, et al. Resection of the liver for colorectal carcinoma metastases: a multi-institutional study of patterns of recurrence. *Surgery*. 1986;100(2):278-284.
2. Nordlinger B, Jaeck D, Guiguet M, et al. Surgical resection of hepatic metastases. Multicentric retrospective study by the French Association of Surgery. In: Nordlinger B, Jaeck D, eds. *Treatment of Hepatic Metastases of Colorectal Cancer*. Paris: Springer; 1992:129-146.
3. Fong Y, Fortner J, Sun RL, et al. Clinical score for predicting recurrence after hepatic resection for metastatic colorectal cancer: analysis of 1001 consecutive cases. *Ann Surg*. 230;3:309-318. discussion 318–321.
4. Oussoultzoglou E, Bachellier P, Rosso E, et al. Right portal vein embolization before right hepatectomy for unilobar colorectal liver metastases reduces the intrahepatic recurrence rate. *Ann Surg*. 2006;244(1):71-79.
5. Simmonds PC, Primrose JN, Colquitt JL, et al. Surgical resection of hepatic metastases from colorectal cancer: a systematic review of published studies. *Br J Cancer*. 2006; 94(7):982-999.
6. Folprecht G, Grothey A, Alberts S, et al. Neoadjuvant treatment of unresectable colorectal liver metastases: correlation between tumour response and resection rates. *Ann Oncol*. 2005;16(8):1311-1319.
7. Hurwitz H, Fehrenbacher L, Novotny W, et al. Bevacizumab plus irinotecan, fluorouracil, and leucovorin for metastatic colorectal cancer. *N Engl J Med*. 2004;350(23):2335-2342.
8. Nordlinger B, Sorbye H, Glimelius B, et al. Perioperative chemotherapy with FOLFOX4 and surgery versus surgery alone for resectable liver metastases from colorectal cancer (EORTC Intergroup trial 40983): a randomised controlled trial. *Lancet*. 2008;371(9617):1007-1016.
9. Portier G, Elias D, Bouche O, et al. Multicenter randomized trial of adjuvant fluorouracil and folinic acid compared with surgery alone after resection of colorectal liver metastases: FFCD ACHBTH AURC 9002 trial. *J Clin Oncol*. 2006;24(31): 4976-4982.
10. Minagawa M, Makuuchi M, Torzilli G, et al. Extension of the frontiers of surgical indications in the treatment of liver metastases from colorectal cancer: long-term results. *Ann Surg*. 2000;231(4):487-499.
11. Doci R, Gennari L, Bignami P, et al. One hundred patients with hepatic metastases from colorectal cancer treated by resection: analysis of prognostic determinants. *Br J Surg*. 1991;78(7):797-801.
12. August DA, Sugarbaker PH, Ottow RT, et al. Hepatic resection of colorectal metastases. Influence of clinical factors and adjuvant intraperitoneal 5-fluorouracil via Tenckhoff catheter on survival. *Ann Surg*. 1985;201(2):210-218.
13. Nordlinger B, Guiguet M, Vaillant JC, et al. Surgical resection of colorectal carcinoma metastases to the liver. A prognostic scoring system to improve case selection, based on 1568 patients. Association Francaise de Chirurgie. *Cancer*. 1996;77(7):1254-1262.
14. Scheele J, Stangl R, Altendorf-Hofmann A, Gall FP. Indicators of prognosis after hepatic resection for colorectal secondaries. *Surgery*. 1991;110(1):13-29.
15. Younes RN, Rogatko A, Brennan MF. The influence of intraoperative hypotension and perioperative blood transfusion on disease-free survival in patients with complete resection of colorectal liver metastases. *Ann Surg*. 1991;214(2): 107-113.
16. Bolton JS, Fuhrman GM. Survival after resection of multiple bilobar hepatic metastases from colorectal carcinoma. *Ann Surg*. 2000;231(5):743-751.
17. Balzan S, Belghiti J, Farges O, et al. The "50–50 criteria" on postoperative day 5: an accurate predictor of liver failure and death after hepatectomy. *Ann Surg*. 2005;242(6):824-828. discussion 828–829.

18. Mullen JT, Ribero D, Reddy SK, et al. Hepatic insufficiency and mortality in 1,059 noncirrhotic patients undergoing major hepatectomy. *J Am Coll Surg*. 2007;204(5):854-862. discussion 862–864.
19. Abdalla EK, Barnett CC, Doherty D, et al. Extended hepatectomy in patients with hepatobiliary malignancies with and without preoperative portal vein embolization. *Arch Surg*. 2002;137(6):675-680. discussion 680–681.
20. Kokudo N, Miki Y, Sugai S, et al. Genetic and histological assessment of surgical margins in resected liver metastases from colorectal carcinoma: minimum surgical margins for successful resection. *Arch Surg*. 2002;137(7):833-840.
21. de Haas RJ, Wicherts DA, Flores E, et al. R1 resection by necessity for colorectal liver metastases: Is it still a contraindication to surgery? *Ann Surg*. 2008;248(4):626-637.
22. Makuuchi M, Thai BL, Takayasu K, et al. Preoperative portal embolization to increase safety of major hepatectomy for hilar bile duct carcinoma: a preliminary report. *Surgery*. 1990;107(5):521-527.
23. Azoulay D, Castaing D, Smail A, et al. Resection of nonresectable liver metastases from colorectal cancer after percutaneous portal vein embolization. *Ann Surg*. 2000;231(4):480-486.
24. Hemming AW, Reed AI, Howard RJ, et al. Preoperative portal vein embolization for extended hepatectomy. *Ann Surg*. 2003;237(5):686-691. discussion 691–693.
25. Elias D, Ouellet JF, De Baere T, et al. Preoperative selective portal vein embolization before hepatectomy for liver metastases: long-term results and impact on survival. *Surgery*. 2002;131(3):294-299.
26. Vauthey JN, Chaoui A, Do KA, et al. Standardized measurement of the future liver remnant prior to extended liver resection: methodology and clinical associations. *Surgery*. 2000;127(5):512-519.
27. Jaeck D, Oussoultzoglou E, Rosso E, et al. A two-stage hepatectomy procedure combined with portal vein embolization to achieve curative resection for initially unresectable multiple and bilobar colorectal liver metastases. *Ann Surg*. 2004;240(6):1037-1049. discussion 1049–1051.
28. Farges O, Belghiti J, Kianmanesh R, et al. Portal vein embolization before right hepatectomy: prospective clinical trial. *Ann Surg*. 2003;237(2):208-217.
29. Kubota K, Makuuchi M, Kusaka K, et al. Measurement of liver volume and hepatic functional reserve as a guide to decision-making in resectional surgery for hepatic tumors. *Hepatology*. 1997;26(5):1176-1181.
30. Yigitler C, Farges O, Kianmanesh R, et al. The small remnant liver after major liver resection: How common and how relevant? *Liver Transpl*. 2003;9(9):S18-S25.
31. Giraudo G, Greget M, Oussoultzoglou E, et al. Preoperative contralateral portal vein embolization before major hepatic resection is a safe and efficient procedure: a large single institution experience. *Surgery*. 2008;143(4):476-482.
32. Yamanaka N, Okamoto E, Kawamura E, et al. Dynamics of normal and injured human liver regeneration after hepatectomy as assessed on the basis of computed tomography and liver function. *Hepatology*. 1993;18(1):79-85.
33. Yokoyama Y, Nagino M, Nimura Y. Mechanisms of hepatic regeneration following portal vein embolization and partial hepatectomy: a review. *World J Surg*. 2007;31(2):367-374.
34. Kawasaki S et al. Resection for multiple metastatic liver tumors after portal embolization. *Surgery*. 1994;115:674.
35. Slooter GD, Marquet RL, Jeekel J, Ijzermans JN. Tumour growth stimulation after partial hepatectomy can be reduced by treatment with tumour necrosis factor alpha. *Br J Surg*. 1995;82(1):129-132.
36. Picardo A, Karpoff HM, Ng B, et al. Partial hepatectomy accelerates local tumor growth: potential roles of local cytokine activation. *Surgery*. 1998;124(1):57-64.
37. Elias D, De Baere T, Roche A, et al. During liver regeneration following right portal embolization the growth rate of liver metastases is more rapid than that of the liver parenchyma. *Br J Surg*. 1999;86(6):784-788.
38. Jaeck D, Bachellier P, Nakano H, et al. One or two-stage hepatectomy combined with portal vein embolization for initially nonresectable colorectal liver metastases. *Am J Surg*. 2003;185(3):221-229.
39. Joyeux H, Collet H, Saint-Aubert B, et al. Computed gamma-tomographic estimation of a hepatic weight index during liver regeneration. *Gastroentérol Clin Biol*. 1984;8 (6–7):507-511.
40. de Baere T, Roche A, Elias D, et al. Preoperative portal vein embolization for extension of hepatectomy indications. *Hepatology*. 1996;24(6):1386-1391.
41. Uesaka K, Nimura Y, Nagino M. Changes in hepatic lobar function after right portal vein embolization. An appraisal by biliary indocyanine green excretion. *Ann Surg*. 1996;223(1): 77-83.
42. Elias D, Lasser P, Rougier P, et al. Frequency, technical aspects, results, and indications of major hepatectomy after prolonged intra-arterial hepatic chemotherapy for initially unresectable hepatic tumors. *J Am Coll Surg*. 1995;180(2):213-219.
43. Karoui M, Penna C, Amin-Hashem M, et al. Influence of preoperative chemotherapy on the risk of major hepatectomy for colorectal liver metastases. *Ann Surg*. 2006;243(1):1-7.
44. Nakano H, Oussoultzoglou E, Rosso E, et al. Sinusoidal injury increases morbidity after major hepatectomy in patients with colorectal liver metastases receiving preoperative chemotherapy. *Ann Surg*. 2008;247(1):118-124.
45. Adam R, Laurent A, Azoulay D, et al. Two-stage hepatectomy: a planned strategy to treat irresectable liver tumors. *Ann Surg*. 2000;232(6):777-785.
46. Shimada H, Tanaka K, Masui H, et al. Results of surgical treatment for multiple (> or =5 nodules) bi-lobar hepatic metastases from colorectal cancer. *Langenbecks Arch Surg*. 2004;389(2):114-121.
47. Togo S, Nagano Y, Masui H, et al. Two-stage hepatectomy for multiple bilobular liver metastases from colorectal cancer. *Hepatogastroenterology*. 2005;52(63):913-919.
48. Kianmanesh R, Sauvanet A, Hentic O, et al. Two-step surgery for synchronous bilobar liver metastases from digestive endocrine tumors: a safe approach for radical resection. *Ann Surg*. 2008;247(4):659-665.
49. Lygidakis NJ, Singh G, Bardaxoglou E, et al. Two-stage liver surgery for advanced liver metastasis synchronous with colorectal tumor. *Hepatogastroenterology*. 2004;51(56):413-418.
50. Honjo I, Suzuki T, Ozawa K, et al. Ligation of a branch of the portal vein for carcinoma of the liver. *Am J Surg*. 1975;130(3):296-302.
51. Broering DC, Hillert C, Krupski G, et al. Portal vein embolization vs. portal vein ligation for induction of hypertrophy of the future liver remnant. *J Gastrointest Surg*. 2002;6(6):905-913. discussion 913.

52. Kianmanesh R, Farges O, Abdalla EK, et al. Right portal vein ligation: a new planned two-step all-surgical approach for complete resection of primary gastrointestinal tumors with multiple bilateral liver metastases. *J Am Coll Surg*. 2003;197(1):164-170.
53. Imamura H, Shimada R, Kubota M, et al. Preoperative portal vein embolization: an audit of 84 patients. *Hepatology*. 1999;29(4):1099-1105.
54. Pichlmayr R, Bretschneider HJ, Kirchner E, et al. Ex situ operation on the liver. A new possibility in liver surgery. *Langenbecks Arch Chir*. 1988;373(2):122-126.
55. Lodge JP, Ammori BJ, Prasad KR, Bellamy MC. Ex vivo and in situ resection of inferior vena cava with hepatectomy for colorectal metastases. *Ann Surg*. 2000;231(4):471-479.
56. Raab R, Schlitt HJ, Oldhafer KJ, et al. Ex-vivo resection techniques in tissue-preserving surgery for liver malignancies. *Langenbecks Arch Surg*. 2000;385(3):179-184.
57. Hemming AW, Chari RS, Cattral MS. Ex vivo liver resection. *Can J Surg*. 2000;43(3):222-224.
58. Gruttadauria S, Marsh JW, Bartlett DL, et al. Ex situ resection techniques and liver autotransplantation: last resource for otherwise unresectable malignancy. *Dig Dis Sci*. 2005; 50(10):1829-1835.
59. Hemming AW, Reed AI, Langham MR, et al. Hepatic vein reconstruction for resection of hepatic tumors. *Ann Surg*. 2002;235(6):850-858.
60. Hemming AW, Reed AI, Langham MR Jr, et al. Combined resection of the liver and inferior vena cava for hepatic malignancy. *Ann Surg*. 2004;239(5):712-719. discussion 719–721.
61. Azoulay D, Andreani P, Maggi U, et al. Combined liver resection and reconstruction of the supra-renal vena cava: the Paul Brousse experience. *Ann Surg*. 2006;244(1):80-88.
62. Ohwada S, Hamada K, Kawate S, et al. Left renal vein graft for vascular reconstruction in abdominal malignancy. *World J Surg*. 2007;31(6):1215-1220.
63. Yamamoto H, Nagino M, Kamiya J, et al. Surgical treatment for colorectal liver metastases involving the paracaval portion of the caudate lobe. *Surgery*. 2005;137(1):26-32.
64. Poon RT, Ng KK, Lam CM, et al. Learning curve for radiofrequency ablation of liver tumors: prospective analysis of initial 100 patients in a tertiary institution. *Ann Surg*. 2004; 239(4):441-449.
65. Weber JC, Navarra G, Jiao LR, et al. New technique for liver resection using heat coagulative necrosis. *Ann Surg*. 2002; 236(5):560-563.
66. Elias D, Manganas D, Benizri E, et al. Trans-metastasis hepatectomy: results of a 21-case study. *Eur J Surg Oncol*. 2006;32(2):213-217.
67. Ouellet JF, Pessaux P, Pocard M, Elias D. Transmetastasis curative liver resection immediately following radiofrequency destruction. *J Surg Oncol*. 2002;81(2):108-110.
68. Curley SA, Izzo F, Delrio P, et al. Radiofrequency ablation of unresectable primary and metastatic hepatic malignancies: results in 123 patients. *Ann Surg*. 1999;230(1):1-8.
69. Abdalla EK, Vauthey JN, Ellis LM, et al. Recurrence and outcomes following hepatic resection, radiofrequency ablation, and combined resection/ablation for colorectal liver metastases. *Ann Surg*. 2004;239(6):818-825. discussion 825–827.
70. Navarra G, Spalding D, Zacharoulis D, et al. Bloodless hepatectomy technique. *HPB (Oxford)*. 2002;4(2):95-97.
71. Haghighi KS, Wang F, King J, et al. In-line radiofrequency ablation to minimize blood loss in hepatic parenchymal transection. *Am J Surg*. 2005;190(1):43-47.

24 Preoperative Portal Vein Embolization Strategy for Complex Liver Resection

Thierry de Baere

Abstract

Portal vein embolization (PVE) is part of the standard of care to prepare extended liver resections when the future remnant liver is too small and induces the risk of postoperative liver insufficiency. PVE is most often reported before right or right extended hepatectomy but can be used in the preparation of any type of liver surgery including the most atypical ones. Such atypical PVE requires excellent collaboration between surgeons and interventional radiologists to precisely determine the segment that will be resected and consequently which will require embolization. Excellent quality pre-PVE imaging, namely CTAP 3D reconstruction, will greatly help in better defining the access route to the portal system and facilitate catheterization of all target segments for embolization. Due to the usual complexity of catheterization, oblique view and at best 3D rotational angiography will greatly help the completion of atypical PVE. When complex liver resections include preoperative radiofrequency ablation (RFA) in the future remnant liver (FRL), RFA zone including safety margins must be taken into account during preoperative volumetry to avoid an overestimation of the FRL volume. RFA can be used at the time of PVE to treat tumor located in the FRL and thus avoid potential growth in the waiting period between PVE and surgery.

Keywords

Portal vein embolization • Liver resection • Imaging in preoperative portal vein embolization • Radiofrequency ablation

24.1 Introduction

Liver resection is the only curative therapeutic modality for liver tumors. Consequently, if the liver is the only site of neoplastic disease, liver resection should be proposed when it is considered safe and feasible. In patients in whom the only contraindication to hepatic resection is insufficient FRL, preoperative portal vein embolization (PVE) of the portal branches feeding the liver segment to be resected must be advised. PVE redistributes portal blood flow to the branches of the FRL. This portal blood flow, which is rich in hepatotrophic substance,[1] induces hypertrophy of the unembolized liver segments of the FRL, thereby authorizing the planned hepatectomy. PVE was first described in 1986 in Japan.[2] During

T. de Baere
Department of Interventional Radiology, Institut Gustave Roussy, 114 rue Edouard Vaillant, 94805 Villejuif, France
e-mail: debaere@igr.fr

D.C. Madoff et al. (eds.), *Venous Embolization of the Liver*,
DOI 10.1007/978-1-84882-122-4_24,

the early 1990s, PVE was reported in Japan and France.[3-5] Today, PVE is a standard of care.[6] It is used in cirrhotic and noncirrhotic, with different thresholds according to the underlying liver disease. Usually an FRL below 25% of the TLV is an indication for PVE in noncirrhotic liver. What defined an insufficient volume of future remnant liver might vary slightly according to different teams. A recent report demonstrated that in noncirrhotic patient with normal liver function, an FRL value below 26.5% predicted postoperative liver dysfunction with 66.7% sensitivity, 97.1% specificity, 50% positive predictive value, and 98.5% negative predictive value.[7] In patients with impaired liver function secondary to neoadjuvant chemotherapy or cholestasis (bilirubin >2 mg/100 mL), postoperative liver dysfunction was correlated with an FRL value below 31.05% which predicted postoperative liver dysfunction with 75% sensitivity, 79.1% specificity, 25% positive predictive value, and 97.1% negative predictive value.[7]

24.2 Atypical Liver Resection and PVE

Most of the hepatectomies performed are right hepatectomies (resection of segments V, VI, VII, and VIII) or extended right hepatectomies (resection of segments IV, V, VI, VII, and VIII). Consequently, PVE is reported almost exclusively to prepare the liver for right or right hepatectomies extended or not to segment IV.[8-11] The resections of segments II, III, and IV are less frequent due to the fact that metastases are most often located to the right part of the liver, and that the right liver or right liver lobe provide usually large enough FRL to allow for left or left extended hepatectomy without the need for PVE. Consequently, few reports of PVE in left or left extended hepatectomies exists, even if use of PVE has been reported in left trisegmentectomy in a limited number of cases.[11,12] Other hepatic resections, often called atypical hepatectomies, are even less frequent due to the technical challenge. However, such atypical hepatectomy will sometimes be associated with the resection of large volume of healthy liver parenchyma, consequently, with a small volume of FRL than can be hypertrophied preoperatively with PVE. The more extended atypical resection reported until today is probably a resection of all liver segments except segments V and VI, therefore resecting the three major hepatic veins. To date, this type of surgical procedure has been reported in only five patients to treat five hepatocellular carcinomas,[13-15] one metastasis from colorectal cancer,[16] and one metastasis from a germ cell carcinoma.[17] This surgical procedure is possible when a large inferior hepatic vein is depicted on CT. Such a vein is found on CT in 21–47% of patients[18,19] and is reported to measure more than 5 mm in 8% of CT,[18,19] and more than 4 mm in 27% of cadaveric studies,[20] and it is important to report that it allows such extended resections. Moreover, such complex and extended hepatectomy which will often leave a small FRL in place is an illustration of a very atypical resection that can be prepared or rendered possible by PVE (Fig. 24.1).

24.2.1 Indication, Volumetry, Principle

24.2.1.1 Indication

When an atypical hepatectomy is technically feasible, able to resect all tumors, and safe, hepatic surgeons and interventional radiologists must define together the segments to be resected in order to perform liver volumetry to evaluate the ratio FRL to total liver volume (TLV). From the results of this volumetric evaluation, status of liver function, and the thresholds of their own institution, they will decide if there is a need for preoperative PVE.

24.2.1.2 Volumetry

Even if volumetric measurement with CT reconstruction has been reported to have 5% variability,[21] volumetry to predict FRL after an atypical hepatectomy will be more complicated and probably more prone to errors. Indeed, the need for volume calculation of numerous separate volumes induces the risk of cumulative errors and possible errors at each single measurement. A volumetric study before a right or a left hepatectomy (whether it is extended or not) requires measurement of the three different volumes (FRL, tumor, total liver), whereas a complex resection, such as before a central hepatectomy with an FRL split into two parts, requires measurement of additional volumes. For example, in case of a central hepatectomy resecting segments IV, V, and VIII, separate volumetric measurements of the left lobe (segments II and III), segment I, and the right posterior segments (segments VI and VII) will be needed to determine the volume of the FRL. Moreover, another cause of increase in error in measurement is that the anatomical landmarks required to delineate some liver segments are difficult to evidence on CT, especially when they are in the axial planes (e.g. distinguishing segment V and VI from segments VII and VIII), notably in the axial plane.

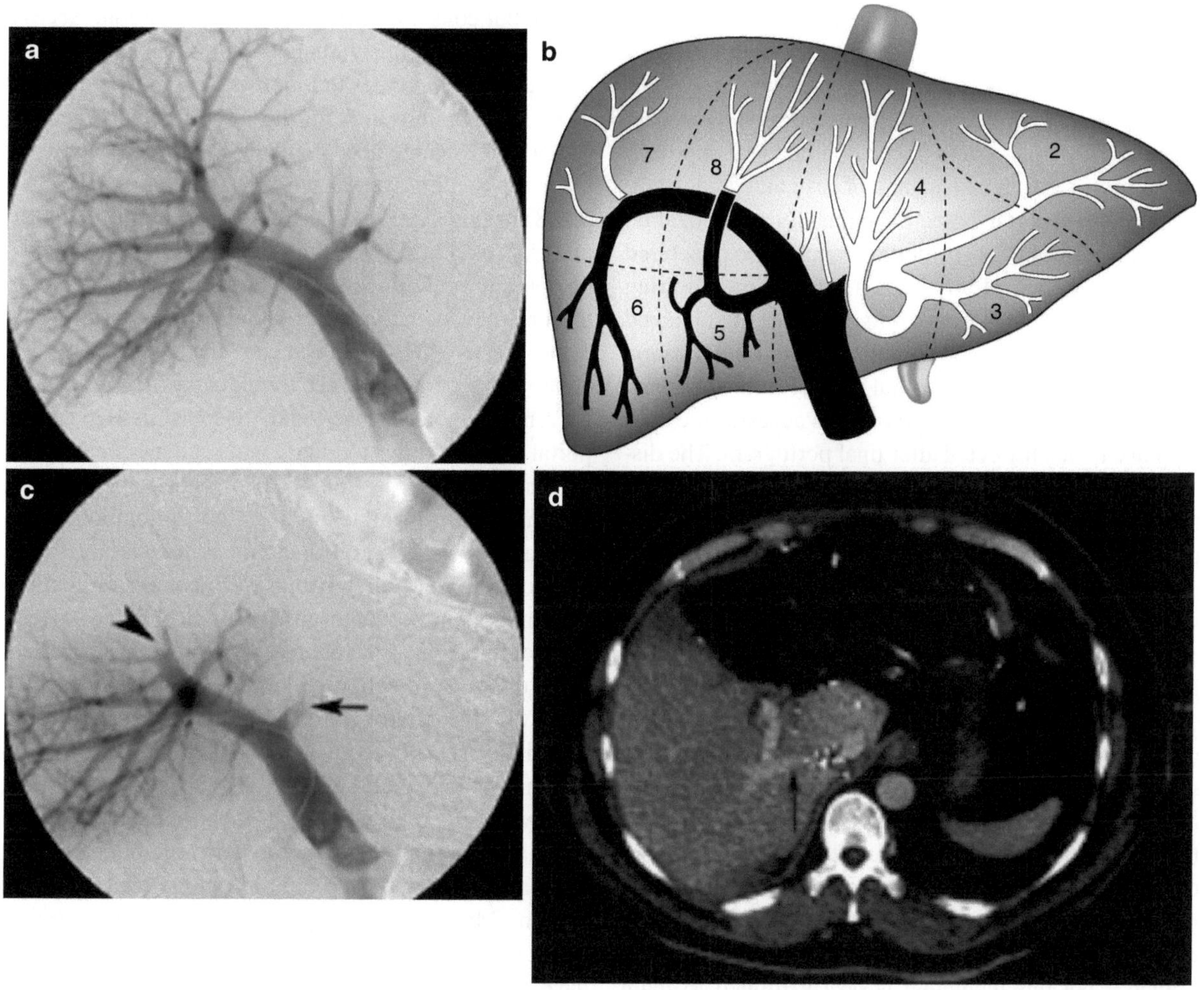

Fig. 24.1 (**a**) Portography in the anteroposterior projection obtained after insertion of a 5-French catheter through a portal branch of the FRL (segment VI). Note that the left liver demonstrates poor parenchymography due to large metastases in this part of the organ. (**b**) Schematic drawing of the planned PVE according to a hepatectomy scheduled to resect all liver segments except segments V and VI. Branches of the liver to be resected and thus targeted for embolization are in *gray*, branches of the FRL are in *black*. (**c**) Portogram obtained after PVE demonstrates complete occlusion of all portal branches except segments V and VI, including occlusion of left portal branch (*arrow*) and branch to segments VII and VIII (*arrowhead*). (**d**) CT scan obtained after liver resection shows the small remnant liver with the right inferior hepatic vein (*arrow*) which render the resection possible

24.2.1.3 Principle

PVE performed to prepare atypical hepatectomies must follow the same rules of embolization procedure of any PVE procedure with the goal to embolize all portal branches feeding the liver planned to be resected. However, in the same manner that these atypical liver resections are usually technically more challenging than a right or right extended hepatectomy, the PVE will be more challenging due to the frequent need for more numerous selective catheterizations, several sites of embolization, and various imaging projections to guide catheterization and embolization of liver segments that are sometimes difficult to differentiate in the anteroposterior projection usually.

24.2.2 Technique

24.2.2.1 Access Route

Atypical PVE does not escape from the debate between ipsilateral or contralateral access with the known advantages of both accesses, which are summarized below.

The contralateral approach is performed by accessing the portal venous system via the future remnant liver FRL. This approach is sometimes preferred to ipsilateral approach to avoid puncturing tumors on the access route to the portal system.[22] The contralateral approach has in most cases the advantage of easy antegrade catheterization of portal branches target for embolization without sharp angles. The portal branch to be punctured must be upstream of any branch bifurcation requiring embolization. A final portogram can be easily obtained to evaluate the extent and completeness of embolization without the risk of potential embolic dislodgment because the portal branch used for the access route does not have to be obstructed after final portogram. The disadvantage of the contralateral approach is that the FRL is traversed and any damage to the FRL can potentially preclude the planned surgery. The ipsilateral approach is performed by accessing the portal venous branches within the tumor-bearing liver, which is the liver to be resected. The main advantage of the ipsilateral approach is that it avoids puncturing through healthy FRL parenchyma. The ipsilateral approach carries the theoretical risk of puncture through tumor tissue when multiple or very large tumors are present thereby leading to a risk of tumor seeding. Such seeding has never been reported but it is difficult to evidence and to differentiate from occurrence of new tumors after surgery. Some teams are performing PVE downstream of a balloon occlusion catheter placed at the origin of the main right portal branch,[23] but this technique is nearly limited to main right portal branch embolization and difficult to apply to atypical PVE due to the difficulties to navigate a balloon catheter through the tortuous way to reach these small branches. Transjugular access has been reported but pertains to atypical PVE because of the need for multiple and sometimes complex catheterization. During atypical PVE, catheterization maneuvers will be numerous, usually more numerous than in standard right or extended right PVE, and the physician must approach the portal vein through the route that will favorize the easiest catheterization and good quality final portogram. This choice can be greatly helped by the study of pre-PVE CT with 3D reconstruction. In our experience, we most often used the contralateral approach.

24.2.2.2 Technique

Atypical PVE procedures usually last longer than right or extended right PVE due the complexity of catheterization which might prone to use general anesthesia, but conscious sedation is a valid option. Access to the portal system is obtained with ultrasound-guided percutaneous puncture that allows to achieve puncture of the branch chosen from the 3D CT reconstruction. Either an 18-gauge needle and a 0.035-in guidewire or a micropuncture system with a 20-gauge needle and 0.018-in guidewire can be used according to operator preferences. Placement of an introducer sheet depends on operator preferences. It can be useful when clogging the catheter, namely, when using cyanoacrylate. The drawback is that an introducer sheath will slightly enlarge the puncture tract through the liver. Then, a 5-French catheter is inserted to place its tip to the main portal trunk in order to obtain an excellent quality portogram with the injection of 20 cm^3 non ionic contrast medium at a flow rate of 5 cm^3/s. Pre-embolization evaluation of the portal anatomy is mandatory to be able to perform accurately any PVE, but this evaluation is even more important in case of atypical PVE. Indeed, differently from a standard right or right extended PVE, oblique projection will often be needed for atypical PVE. Pre-embolization imaging of the liver and especially MDCT acquisition and multiplanar reconstruction obtained at the portal venous phase will be of great value in order to define in advance the best choice for C-arm angulation in order to perform oblique protogram and to use it during fluoroscopic-guided catheterization. Most of the time, when the right posterior segment portal branches (segments VI and VII) will have to be occluded and the right anterior segments (segments V and VIII) will have to be left opened, or vice versa, an oblique anteroposterior (45° or more) angulation of the C-arm will be able to obtain a portogram able to differentiate the best branches feeding the right anterior from the branches feeding the right posterior segments. The choice between right or left angulation has to be determined from the 3D reconstruction even if in most of cases a right oblique will be preferred. Indeed, it is nearly impossible in an anteroposterior projection to differentiate these two segments. Most of the anatomical views represent the right posterior segments projection external to the right anterior segments, but anatomical view corresponds to a liver placed on a table and thus in a slight right anterior-oblique projection. In clinical practice on the anteroposterior projection of a portogram, the right posterior segments can project medial, lateral, or superimposed to the right anterior segments. If portal branches to the right liver lobe have to be differentiated from segment

IV branches, a slight right anteroposterior angulation might be helpful. In some instances, segment IV branches will project on the main right portal branch, and right anterior oblique angulation will help the operator to evaluate completeness of the embolization (Fig. 24.2). If the left branches to segments II and III have to be differentiated from segment IV, an anteroposterior projection is usually fine, but a slight left anterior angulation might be helpful.

Today, cone beam CT 3D rotational angiography or MDCT portography obtained in the interventional room after placement of the catheter in the portal trunk can provide 3D and multiplanar anatomy of the portal system. Such acquisition at the beginning of the procedure can be very helpful to define and understand the portal anatomy before starting the embolization (Figs. 24.2 and 24.3). It will guide the choice of C-arm angulation to obtain the best projection during

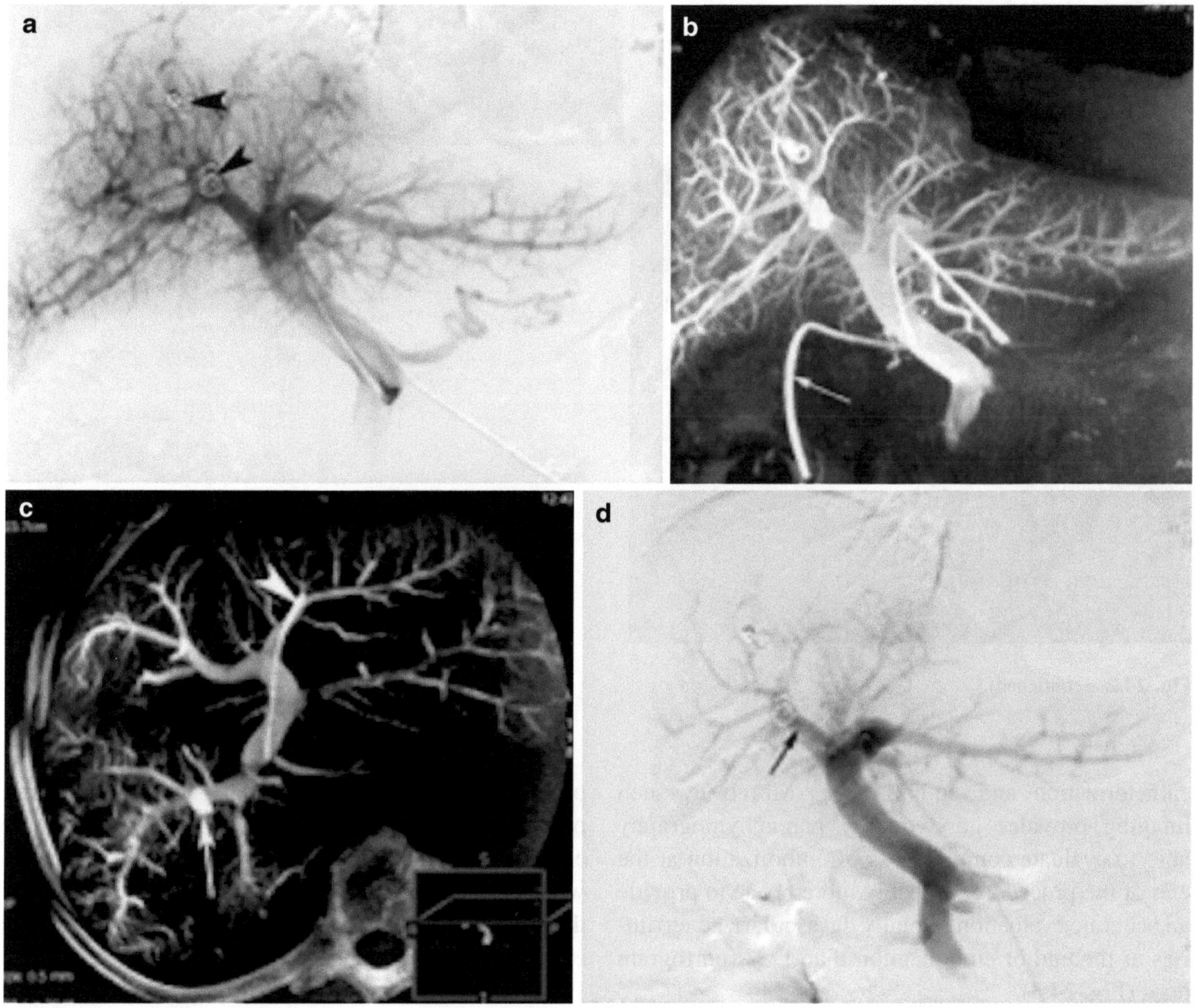

Fig. 24.2 (**a**, **b**) Anteroposterior portography and 3D rotational portogram obtained after insertion of a 5-French catheter through a portal branch of the FRL (segment III). Note that the right portal branches remain patent despite previous PVE performed in another center with coils (*arrowheads*). (**c**) Axial reconstructions from 3D rotational angiography demonstrated the coil (*arrow*) in a patent portal branch and access of the catheter through segment III portal branch (*arrowhead*). (**d**) Portogram obtained after PVE of branches to the right liver seems to show still patent branches (*arrow*) to the right liver. (**e**) Oblique right anterior projection portogram demonstrates that the branches seen in (**d**) projecting on the right liver were branches for segment IV (*arrow*), and shows the stump of the completely occluded right portal branch (*arrowhead*). Right oblique anterior (**f**) and right oblique anteroinferior (**g**) views of the 3D rotational portogram obtained before PVE can easily help to study anatomy and understand spatial location of segment IV branch (*arrow*)

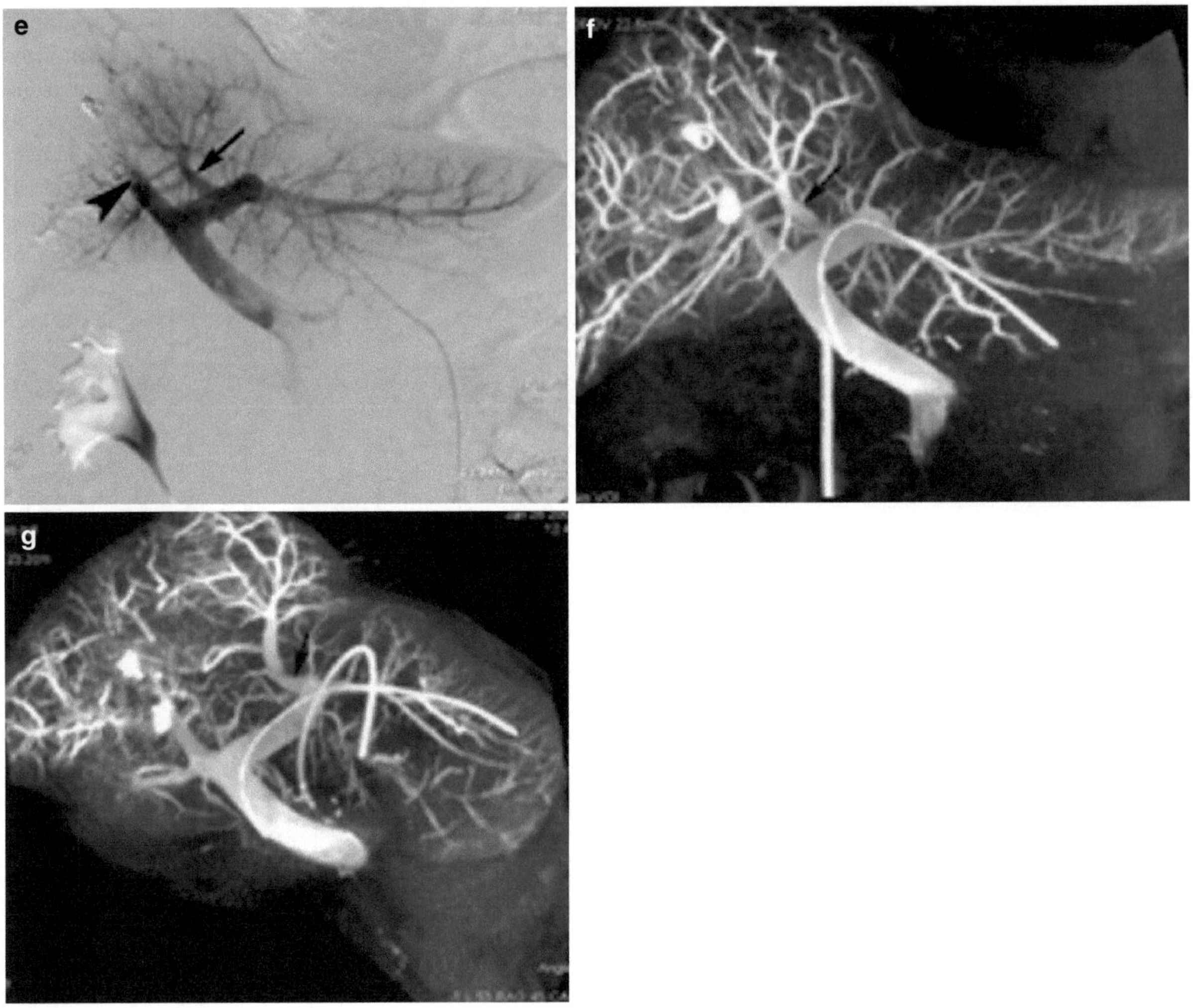

Fig. 24.2 (continued)

catheterization and embolization. Moreover, such imaging provides good quality parenchymography able to evaluate completeness of embolization at the end of the procedure, probably more prone to provide an accurate evaluation of really devascularized territories at the end of embolization than DSA portogram does (Fig. 24.3).

Selective catheterization of the branches targeted for embolization is usually obtained with a 5-French catheter. A C-curve or cobra-shaped catheter is used when contralateral access is performed. Reverse-curved catheters are usually useful when ipsilateral approach is used. The targeted segmental portal veins are embolized one after the other under constant fluoroscopic surveillance. Microcatheter can be used when particulate embolization material is injected but are poorly compatible with used of NBCA. Complete embolization of the targeted portal branches is assessed with direct portography at the completion of the procedure. Then, the 5-French catheter is retrieved without embolization of the puncture track.

24.2.2.3 Embolic Material

In our experience, we used a mixture of n-butyl-cyanoacrylate (NBCA) (Braun, Melsungen, Germany) and iodized oil (Lipiodol, André Guerbet, Aulnay-sous-Bois, France) with a ratio of 1:1 to 1:2 as the main embolic agent used. Successive 0.2–0.5 cm^3 aliquots of the mixture are injected with abundant flushing of the catheter with a 5% glucose solution between each injection using a three-way stopcock. Embolization is flow-guided through a single lumen 5-French catheter without any occlusion balloon catheter or microcatheter. Particulate embolization material can be used and have been reported in numerous studies. Spherical particles are preferable to noncalibrated PVA because it provides larger hypertrophy.[9] Most of the team used initial embolization with 300–500 μm particles followed by 500–700 μm and then coil ligation of the proximal part of the portal branches. A large amount of particles will be usually needed, with up to 20 vials of embolic material needed. Proximal ligations are easy to obtain during right PVE, but probably more complex and risky when several separate branches have to be occluded during atypical PVE. In addition, when using coils or other proximal embolization devices, it is advisable to leave unembolized approximately 1 cm of the proximal trunk to facilitate the

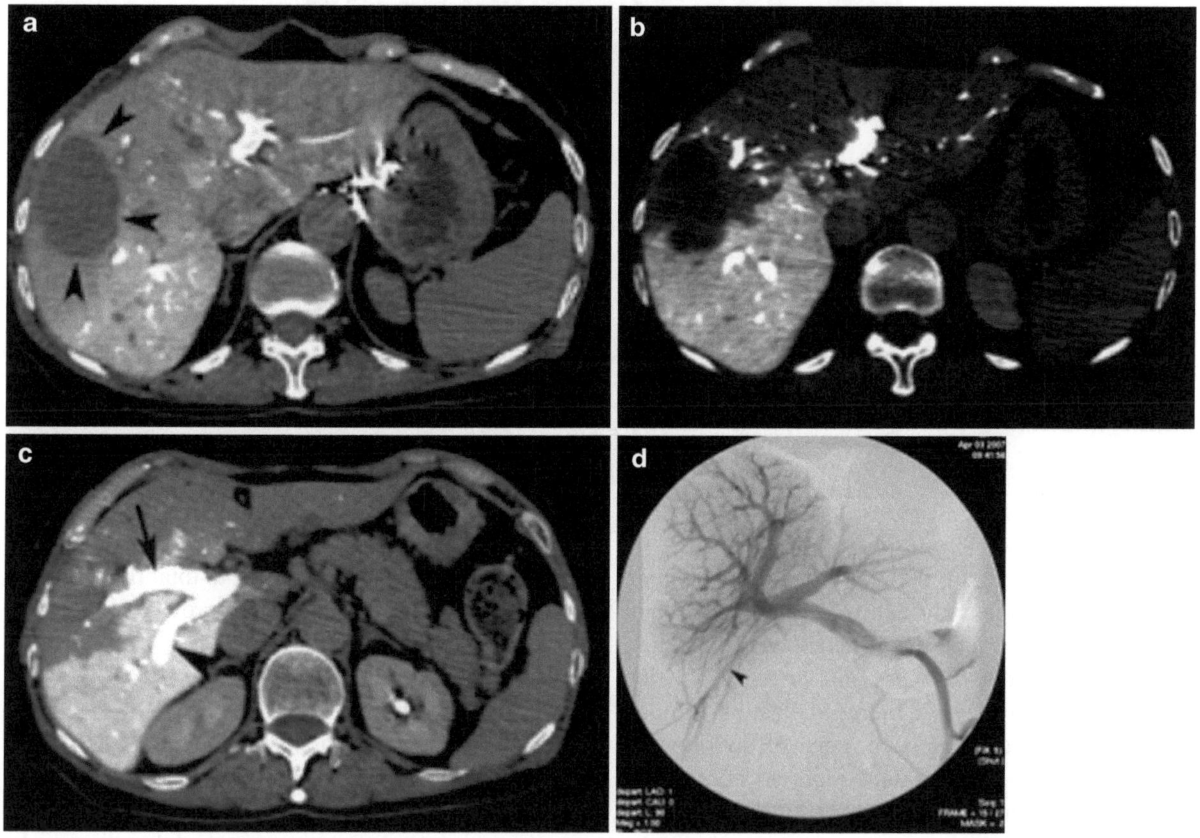

Fig. 24.3 (**a**, **b**) CT portograms obtained before and after PVE with injection through a catheter placed in the portal trunk in a patient schedule to have resection of all liver segment except right posterior segment (Couinaud's segments VI and VII). (**a**) Notice the absence of enhancement of the liver metastasis before PVE (*arrowheads*). After PVE, (**b**) only right posterior segments are enhanced. (**c**) CT portograms obtained after PVE at a lower level than (**a**) and (**b**) shows the embolized portal branch for right anterior segments (Couinaud's segments V and VIII) (*arrow*), and non-embolized branch for right posterior (*arrowhead*). (**d**) Portogram in the anteroposterior projection does not allow to differentiate the right anterior from the right posterior branches. Notice the access obtained through segment VI (*arrowhead*). (**e**) The 3D reconstruction from CT portography allows comprehensive understanding of the anatomy which demonstrated a replaced right anterior segment branch (*arrow*) to the left branch. This is the most common anatomical variant in portal vein. The catheter is seen entering through segment VI branch (*arrowhead*). (**f**) A left oblique portogram projection with C-arm angulation decided from the 3D reconstruction allows to differentiate the right anterior (*arrow*) from the right posterior branch (*arrowhead*). (**g**) Portogram obtained in the same projection after PVE demonstrates complete occlusion of the right anterior branch (*arrow*). (**h**) 3D CT portography obtained after PVE shows occlusion with cast of cyanoacrylate and cyanoacrylet in distal branches of the left portal branch (*black arrow*) and the right anterior portal branch (*arrowhead*), while opacification of the remaining right posterior branch is clearly seen (*white arrow*)

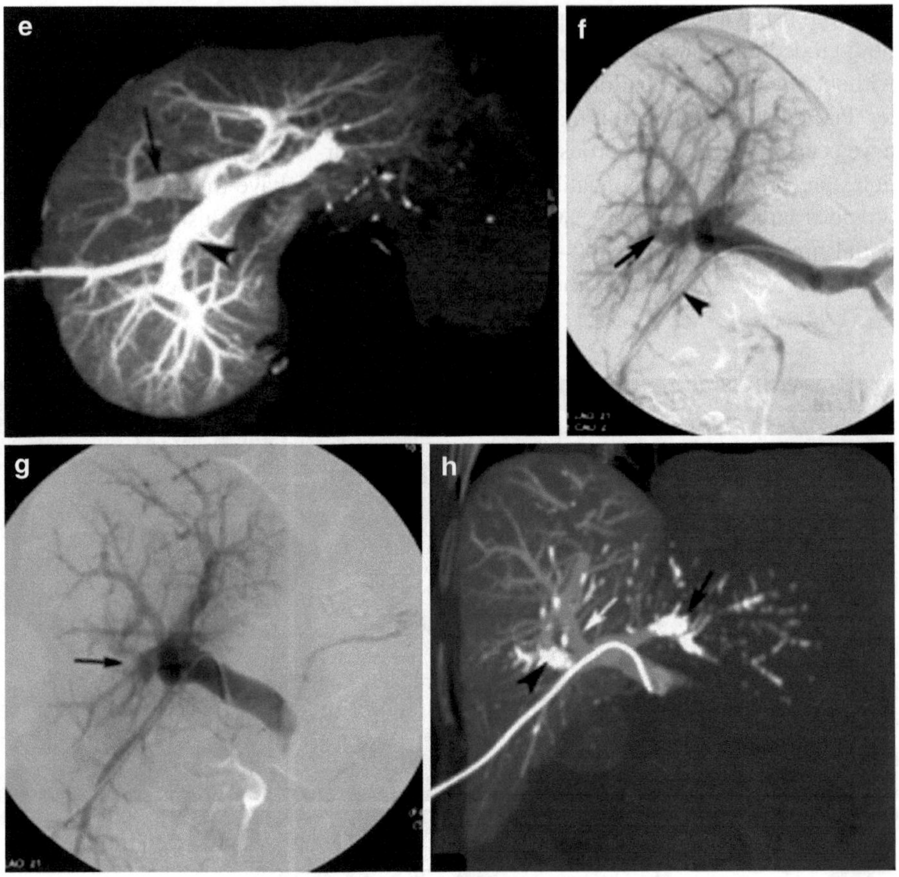

Fig. 24.3 (continued)

division and suture of portal vein during surgery. Furthermore, it might reduce the risk of propagation of right portal vein thrombus in the neighboring branches. At last, it is not advised to use only proximal ligation with coils due to the risk of recanalization through coils (Fig. 24.2) and the occurrence of arterioportal shunting[24] or portoportal shunts reported after proximal surgical ligation.[25]

24.3 Results

In our experience, atypical PVEs were always performed by an interventional radiologist with more than 10 years of experience and lasted 45–115 min (Mean ± SD = 76 ± 26), which is longer than a right PVE. Post embolization liver biology changes were the same as usually reported after PVE with an increase by two- to threefold in ASAT and ALAT, and no changes in bilirubin level, but we have no experience in atypical PVE in cirrhotic patients.

In patients with an initial FRL to total liver volume ratio of 17:38%, atypical PVE provided 49 ± 25% hypertrophy of the FRL after 32 days. Hypertrophy was sufficient to allow for surgery in 88% of case. However this 49% rate of hypertrophy was significantly lower than that obtained in the 101 other PVEs targeting the right liver or the right liver and segment IV in our series which was 74 ± 52%. We do not know exactly why such differences occurred, but they could be linked to less complete occlusion due to a more technically challenging embolization. Possibly, less accurate CT volumetry could be another explanation, as discussed earlier.

24.4 Radiofrequency Ablation and PVE

Recent advances in treatment of liver cancer include the use of local tumor ablation techniques, which can be used percutaneously or preoperatively. Radiofrequency ablation (RFA) is the most commonly used one and will be the only one discussed in this manuscript, excluding cryotherapy, microwaves ablation, electroporation, and ethanol injection, that can anyhow be used in the same type of combination than RFA. Percutaneous RFA produced excellent local tumor control in small tumors and survival close to surgery in small size paucinodular tumors.[26] Preoperative RFA is most often used in combination with surgical resection, where resection addresses the larger tumors while RFA is used for smaller ones that cannot be resected, thus located in the remnant liver. Another use of preoperative RFA is liver resection through metastases previously ablated with radiofrequency.[27]

Both percutaneous RFA and preoperative can be combined with PVE. Preoperative RFA extends the possibilities of liver surgery and consequently the indications to perform PVE. Percutaneous RFA can be combined with PVE in the same procedure to avoid growth of metastases that will be left in the non-embolized liver.

24.4.1 Preoperative RFA After PVE

Preoperative RFA will induce a loss of functional liver in the FRL, corresponding to the margin of ablation around the targeted tumor(s). Consequently, when one or several tumors are planned to be ablated with radiofrequency during surgery, it is mandatory than volumetric evaluation of the FRL to take into account the volume(s) of the metastase(s) to be ablated with the tumor volume and additional safety margin(s) according to the type of ablation that will be performed. These volumes must be subtracted from the volume of FRL in order to avoid overestimation of the FRL and postoperative liver insufficiency.

24.4.2 Percutaneous RFA Combined with PVE

Percutaneous RFA can be used in combination with PVE to target small liver metastases located in the FRL, while there is no interest in performing RFA for small metastases located in the liver planned to be resected. The rationale for performing RFA for metastases located in the FRL is that if a metastasis is left in place in the FRL during the waiting period between RFA and surgery, this tumor will benefit from portal flow diversion and might grow rapidly during FRL regeneration, then precluding or complicating liver surgery. The growth rate of tumor remaining in the unembolized liver after PVE (tumor scheduled for wedge resection or radiofrequency ablation combined with the hepatectomy) is reported to be 1.0–15.6 faster than the growth rate of the unembolized liver.[28] Even if it is difficult to know whether PVE increases the growth rate of tumor in unembolized liver or if this growth is due to the natural history of the tumor, it is in the clinician's interest to destroy tumor in the FRL at the time of PVE to avoid further tumor growth that might preclude surgery a few weeks later. PVE combined with radiofrequency ablation has been reported to be a useful association to avoid growth of residual tumor in the FRL after PVE.[29] Both procedures can be performed safely and efficiently at the same time. From a technical standpoint, both punctures (radiofrequency probe insertion, access to the portal system) have to be performed before ablation or embolization because visibility of the targets to puncture under ultrasound (tumor for ablation and portal branches for PVE) can be altered by artifacts due to portal vein embolization or RFA. After both punctures have been done, RFA is performed in the FRL first in order to obtain at the completion of RFA a portogram that allows confirmation that no damage has occurred in the portal system of the FRL before starting PVE. If PVE is performed before RFA and damages the left portal vein, there will be a risk of complete portal vein obstruction. Because liver resection is most often performed a few weeks after PVE, no evaluation of the efficacy of RFA will be possible at the time of surgery. Consequently, RFA should be done at the time of PVE only if the chances of success of RFA are high, which includes small size tumor less than 2–3 cm in diameter that can be easily targeted and seen under ultrasound guidance. Indeed, incomplete ablation will induce the surgeon to leave in place active tumor at the time of surgery. In case of doubtful technical quality of RFA, the ablated zone must be resected at the time of surgery if possible.

24.5 Limitation of PVE in Complex Liver Resections

The aim of PVE is to embolize all portal branches feeding the liver planned to be resected according to the planned surgery, and this principle remains true when performing atypical PVE. However, atypical PVE will be more challenging due to the frequent need for more numerous sites of embolization, and will increase the risk of inadvertent embolization of nontarget portal branches when compare with right PVE. Physician must keep in mind that inadvertent embolization to the FRL is potentially more harmful to the patient than incomplete embolization of portal branch feeding the liver to be resected. Indeed, a reflux to the nontarget branch carries the risk of complete portal obstruction, or complete obstruction of the FRL portal system that will cancel any possibility of surgery. On the other hand, incomplete embolization might lower hypertrophy in the FRL but will probably not preclude surgery. Consequently, the operator must choose the embolic material with the lower risk of reflux and not embolized a branch which carries high risk of reflux towards the portal branches of the FRL. To which extent PVE can be used to prepare complex atypical liver resection remains to be explored according to technical possibilities of surgeons and interventional radiologists. It is noteworthy that the degree of hypertrophy is inversely proportional to the volume of the initial FRL,[30] which means that theoretically, PVE can be proposed even for initially very small FRL which are the one that will hypertrophy the most. A technical limitation to PVE is to be able to catheterize the branches feeding the liver segments to be resected, and regarding this point, PVE of segment I is nearly impossible and never reported to our knowledge.

24.6 Conclusion

PVE can be tailored to any type of hepatectomy according to what is planned by surgeons, even in the case of atypical hepatectomy with initially very small FRL. 3D imaging greatly helps in the understanding of the portal anatomy and consequently the achievement of PVE before an atypical hepatectomy. Inadvertent embolization of a branch to the FRL being one of the most severe complications of PVE, great care must be taken to avoid it.

References

1. Starzl T, Francavilla A, Halgrimson C. The origin, hormonal nature, and action of hepatotrophic substances in portal venous blood. *Surg Gynecol Obstet*. 1973;137:179-199.
2. Kinoshita H, Sakai K, Hirohasji K, Igawa S, Yamasaki O, Kubo S. Preoperative portal vein embolization for hepatocellular carcinome. *World J Surg*. 1986;10:803-808.
3. de Baere T, Roche A, Vavasseur D, Therasse E. Portal vein embolisation: utility for inducing left hepatic lobe hypertrophy before surgery. *Radiology*. 1993;188:73-77.
4. Makuuchi M, Le Thai B, Takayasu K, et al. Preoperative portal embolization to increase safety of major hepatectomy for hilar bile duct carcinoma: a preliminary report. *Surgery*. 1990;107:521-527.
5. Nagino M, Nimura Y, Kamiya J, et al. Changes in hepatic lobe volume in biliary tract cancer patients after right portal vein embolization. *Hepatology*. 1995;21:434-439.
6. Madoff DC, Abdalla EK, Vauthey JN. Portal vein embolization in preparation for major hepatic resection: evolution of a new standard of care. *J Vasc Interv Radiol*. 2005;16:779-790.
7. Ferrero A, Vigano L, Polastri R, et al. Postoperative liver dysfunction and future remnant liver: where is the limit? Results of a prospective study. *World J Surg*. 2007;31:1643-1651.
8. de Baere T, Roche A, Elias D, Lasser P, Lagrange C, Bousson V. Preoperative portal vein embolization for extension of hepatectomy indications. *Hepatology*. 1996;24:1386-1391.
9. Madoff DC, Abdalla EK, Gupta S, et al. Transhepatic ipsilateral right portal vein embolization extended to segment IV: improving hypertrophy and resection outcomes with spherical particles and coils. *J Vasc Interv Radiol*. 2005;16:215-225.
10. Madoff DC, Hicks ME, Abdalla EK, Morris JS, Vauthey JN. Portal vein embolization with polyvinyl alcohol particles and coils in preparation for major liver resection for hepatobiliary malignancy: safety and effectiveness – study in 26 patients. *Radiology*. 2003;227:251-260.
11. Nagino M, Kamiya J, Nishio H, Ebata T, Arai T, Nimura Y. Two hundred forty consecutive portal vein embolizations before extended hepatectomy for biliary cancer: surgical outcome and long-term follow-up. *Ann Surg*. 2006;243:364-372.
12. Nagino M, Kamiya J, Kanai M, et al. Right trisement portal vein embolization for biliary tract carcinoma: technique and clinical utility. *Surgery*. 2000;127:155-160.
13. Baer HU, Dennison AR, Maddern GJ, Blumgart LH. Subtotal hepatectomy: a new procedure based on the inferior right hepatic vein. *Br J Surg*. 1991;78:1221-1222.
14. Hanazaki K, Fujimori Y, Kajikawa S, et al. Mixed hepatocellular carcinoma and cholangiocarcinoma treated by extended left hepatic lobectomy with resection of the right hepatic vein and preservation of the inferior right hepatic vein after hepatic arterial infusion chemotherapy. *Hepatogastroenterology*. 1998;45:812-815.
15. Ozeki Y, Uchiyama T, Katayama M, Sugiyama A, Kokubo M, Matsubara N. Extended left hepatic trisegmentectomy with resection of main right hepatic vein and preservation of middle and inferior right hepatic veins. *Surgery*. 1995;117:715-717.
16. Texler ML, Jamieson GG, Maddern GJ. Left extended hemihepatectomy with preservation of large inferior right hepatic vein: a case report. *HPB Surg*. 1999;11:265-269; discussion 269-270.
17. Yokoi Y, Suzuki S, Baba S, et al. Aggressive hepatectomy for complete remission of metastatic germ cell tumor following chemotherapy: report of a case. *Hepatogastroenterology*. 2003;50:1136-1139.

18. Akgul E, Inal M, Soyupak S, et al. The prevalence and variations of right inferior hepatic veins on contrast enhanced helical CT scanning. *Eur J Radiol.* 2004;52(1): 73-77.
19. Erbay N, Raptopoulos V, Pomfret EA, Kamel IR, Kruskal JB. Living donor liver transplantation in adults: vascular variants important in surgical planning for donors and recipients. *AJR Am J Roentgenol.* 2003;181:109-114.
20. Hribernik M, de Cecchis L, Trotovsek B, Gadzijev EM, Ravnik D. Anatomical variations of the right hepatic veins and their relevance to surgery. *Hepatogastroenterology.* 2003;50:656-660.
21. Kamel IR, Kruskal JB, Warmbrand G, Goldberg SN, Pomfret EA, Raptopoulos V. Accuracy of volumetric measurements after virtual right hepatectomy in potential donors undergoing living adult liver transplantation. *AJR Am J Roentgenol.* 2001;176:483-487.
22. Kim MJ, Choo SW, Do YS, et al. Use of double-occlusion balloon catheter: preoperative portal vein embolization for induction of future remnant liver hypertrophy. *Cardiovasc Intervent Radiol.* 2004;27:16-20.
23. Satake M, Tateishi U, Kobayashi T, Murata S, Kumazaki T. Percutaneous transhepatic portal vein embolization: effectiveness of absolute ethanol infusion with balloon catheter in a pig model. *Acta Radiol.* 2005;46:344-352.
24. Yamakado K, Takeda K, Nishide Y, et al. Portal vein embolization with steel coils and absolute ethanol: a comparative experimental study with canine liver. *Hepatology.* 1995;22: 1812-1818.
25. Denys AL, Abehsera M, Sauvanet A, Sibert A, Belghiti J, Menu Y. Failure of right portal vein ligation to induce left lobe hypertrophy due to intrahepatic portoportal collaterals: successful treatment with portal vein embolization. *AJR Am J Roentgenol.* 1999;173:633-635.
26. Gillams AR, Lees WR. Radiofrequency ablation of lung metastases: factors influencing success. *Eur Radiol.* 2008;18: 672-677.
27. Elias D, Manganas D, Benizri E, et al. The trans-metastasis hepatectomy (through metastases previously ablated with radiofrequency): results of a 13-case study of colorectal cancer. *J Surg Oncol.* 2006;93:8-12.
28. Elias D, De Baere T, Roche A, Mducreux LJ, Lasser P. During liver regeneration following right portal embolization the growth rate of liver metastases is more rapid than that of the liver parenchyma. *Br J Surg.* 1999;86:784-788.
29. Elias D, Santoro R, Ouellet JF, Osmak L, de Baere T, Roche A. Simultaneous percutaneous right portal vein embolization and left liver tumor radiofrequency ablation prior to a major right hepatic resection for bilateral colorectal metastases. *Hepatogastroenterology.* 2004;51:1788-1791.
30. Denys A, Lacombe C, Schneider F, et al. Portal vein embolization with *N*-butyl cyanoacrylate before partial hepatectomy in patients with hepatocellular carcinoma and underlying cirrhosis or advanced fibrosis. *J Vasc Interv Radiol.* 2005;16:1667-1674.

Sequential PVE and TAE for Biliary Tract Cancer and Liver Metastases

25

Yukihiro Yokoyama and Masato Nagino

Abstract

Portal vein embolization (PVE) is a useful tool before major hepatectomy, especially for high-risk patients with chronic liver disease. However, the compensatory hypertrophy of the non-embolized lobe is sometimes insufficient, particularly in patients with severely impaired liver function. In such cases, the addition of transcatheter arterial embolization (TAE) for the segments that underwent PVE could be chosen as one of the options. This procedure induces more atrophy of the embolized lobe and at the same time induces more hypertrophy in the non-embolized lobe, thus extending the indication for liver resection in patients with small remnant liver. However, this technique induces severe parenchymal damage due to hepatic infarction and should be considered a high-risk procedure. Thus, the indication for this technique should be severely restricted, and once it is performed, the patient should be followed up carefully. Further accumulation of data is necessary to determine the indication, the appropriate embolic materials, and the extent of embolization for sequential PVE and TAE.

Keywords

Portal vein embolization • Transcatheter arterial embolization • Liver resection with small remnant liver

The liver receives a dual blood supply from the portal vein and the hepatic artery. The proportion of the portal venous flow is approximately 70–80% in normal livers, whereas that of the hepatic arterial flow is 20–30%. The blood from the portal vein contains abundant nutrition, but the level of oxygen and blood pressure is lower than in the hepatic arterial blood. A dramatic change in hepatic blood flow, especially from the portal venous system, triggers the process of liver regeneration. This process is observed after a specific clinical setting, such as portal vein embolization (PVE).

About 20 years ago, major liver resections for hilar cholangiocarcinoma, hepatocellular carcinoma, or metastatic liver cancer were associated with a high rate of postoperative hepatic failure.[1,2] However, preoperative portal vein embolization (PVE), a procedure developed by Makuuchi et al.[3,4] and Kinoshita et al.[5] in the 1980s, has improved the safety of extensive liver resections. PVE, in general, embolizes the hemihepatic portal vein branch while preserving hepatic arterial

M. Nagino (✉)
Division of Surgical Oncology, Department of Surgery, Nagoya University Graduate School of Medicine, 65 Tsurumai-cho, Showa-ku, Nagoya, Aichi 4668550, Japan
e-mail: nagino@med.nagoya-u.ac.jp

D.C. Madoff et al. (eds.), *Venous Embolization of the Liver*,
DOI 10.1007/978-1-84882-122-4_25, © Springer-Verlag London Limited 2011

flow. In response to a sudden termination of portal venous flow, the hepatic arterial flow increases immediately due to the intrinsic blood flow regulation by the liver, a phenomenon termed the "hepatic arterial buffer response."[6,7] This may preserve the hepatic viability in the embolized lobe, although the total blood flow in the embolized lobe decreases substantially. Consequently, PVE induces atrophy of the embolized lobe and hypertrophy of the non-embolized lobe.

PVE is especially useful for high-risk patients with chronic liver disease.[8] Nevertheless, compensatory hypertrophy of the non-embolized lobe is sometimes insufficient, especially in patients with severely impaired liver function.[9,10] It would be better to choose an additional strategy to improve the outcome of PVE, since otherwise they are unable to receive the operation, even though a curative resection is oncologically possible. One of the options is transcatheter arterial embolization (TAE) for the segments that underwent PVE.[11] This procedure induces more atrophy of the embolized lobe and at the same time induces more hypertrophy in the non-embolized lobe, thus extending the indication for liver resection in patients with small remnant liver. It is also considered a "nonsurgical hepatectomy" since the blood flow to the embolized lobe is almost completely shut down. However, it should be noted that this technique is apparently riskier than PVE alone since it always accompanies severe parenchymal damage due to hepatic infarction. Thus, the indication of this technique should be severely restricted, and, once it is performed, the patient should be followed up carefully. This chapter discusses the indication, technique, usefulness, and potential risk of sequential PVE and TAE before major hepatectomy.

25.1 Dramatic Changes in Hepatic Arterial Flow Following PVE

The hepatic arterial flow changes immediately after PVE due to the hepatic arterial buffer response.[7,12] Experimental studies using rats showed that after the complete ligation of the left portal vein, the left hepatic arterial flow increases by 210% whereas the right hepatic arterial flow decreases by 67%.[13] As a consequence, the total left hepatic flow decreases by 45% whereas the total right hepatic flow increases by 230%. The atrophy rate in the embolized lobe and the hypertrophy rate in the non-embolized lobe linearly correlate to the total blood flow in each lobe.[12,14] Therefore, when the arterial flow in the embolized lobe is further blocked, it ensures that the embolized lobe will achieve more atrophy and the non-embolized lobe will undergo more hypertrophy. The idea of sequential PVE and TAE was proposed with this concept in mind. However, it should be recognized that this procedure results in almost complete blood flow termination and may induce severe parenchymal infarction on the embolized lobe. In contrast to sequential PVE and TAE, TAE before PVE has been shown to be safe and feasible in cases of hepatocellular carcinoma where hepatic functional reserve is insufficient.[15] This procedure is especially useful in cases of hypervascular tumors fed mainly by arterial blood and with a marked arterioportal shunt. Examination of resected specimens after this procedure revealed minimal necrosis of the noncancerous liver but marked necrosis of the tumor. By selecting the arterial branch feeding the tumor, the area of embolization is minimized in this procedure. Moreover, by the time the PVE is performed, embolized materials only remain in the tumor and those in other areas will be washed away. Therefore, subsequent PVE can be performed safely. However, in the case of cholangiocarcinoma or colorectal liver metastasis, it is unrealistic to perform TAE before PVE, because these tumors generally are not fed by the arterial blood flow. Furthermore, in most of the cases of cholangiocarcinoma or colorectal liver metastasis, preoperative PVE results in a sufficient hypertrophy in the non-embolized lobe, and it is not necessary to add TAE to further achieve volume changes.

25.2 Indications and Techniques of Sequential PVE and TAE

Volume changes of the embolized lobe and the non-embolized lobe after PVE are variable, depending on the report.[16] The hypertrophy rate in the non-embolized lobe is approximately 10–20% of the total liver volume, whereas the atrophy rate in the embolized lobe is almost equivalent (~15%) to the hypertrophy rate. Generally, a sufficient volume change is achieved within 14 days after PVE without serious complications. However, in patients with conditions associated with impaired liver regeneration capacity, the hypertrophy rate is severely affected. These conditions include obstructive jaundice,[17-19] severe cirrhosis,[20] diabetes,[21,22] alcoholism,[23,24] malnutrition,[25,26] and others. In these patients, the deteriorating factors should be ameliorated as much as possible before PVE. A longer interval between the embolization and surgery may also be required to achieve sufficient hypertrophy of the future liver remnant.[27] However, even after long periods, some patients still cannot achieve enough hypertrophy of the non-embolized lobe. These patients cannot undergo major hepatectomy due to insufficient future remnant liver volume, even if the tumor is oncologically resectable. The addition of TAE should be considered in such patients.

25.2.1 Indications

The indication for PVE has been discussed in several reports. Ladurner et al.[28] used PVE and reported that the estimated amount of the liver remnant volume was less than or equal to 25% of the total liver volume. Hemming et al.[29] also used PVE with similar results (<25% of the future liver remnant volume). In our institution, we perform PVE for the cases of extended hepatectomy that need a resection of five or more liver segments; i.e., right hepatectomy with caudate lobectomy, right trisegmentectomy, or left trisegmentectomy.[30] PVE is also indicated when a future liver remnant is estimated to be less than 35% of the total liver. The indication of PVE should be changed according to the status of the patients' condition. Elias et al.[31] proposed that the threshold of PVE should be raised to 40% if the patient had undergone multiple courses of chemotherapy. The indication should also be restricted to <40% in patients with chronic liver disease.[8,32] The addition of TAE should be considered when the volume of future liver remnant cannot reach the above-mentioned criteria even after long waiting periods following PVE.

How long should the waiting period be after PVE, before a further step with TAE? After PVE, the process of liver regeneration starts immediately. In a normal liver, PVE can produce a compensatory hypertrophy of the non-embolized lobe within 2 weeks without seriously affecting hepatic function.[27] However, in an abnormal liver (with cirrhosis, hepatitis, alcoholism, etc.), it will take longer. Therefore, the wait should be at least 6 weeks to decide whether further addition of TAE is necessary to improve the outcome of embolization.

Is it possible to perform PVE and TAE simultaneously? The answer is "No." Nakao et al.[33] reported the results of simultaneous PVE and TAE for patients with hepatocellular carcinoma. However, this method is no longer conducted due to a high risk of hepatic abscess and hepatic infarction. A sudden shutdown of dual blood supply from the portal vein and hepatic artery may be too harmful for the liver.

25.2.2 Techniques

25.2.2.1 Embolic Materials

In general, PVE is performed through a transhepatic route using a relatively large size catheter. With this route, any kind of embolic material can be utilized. In contrast, the size of the catheter for TAE is much smaller because it should be inserted through a transarterial route. Then, what kind of embolic material is appropriate for arterial embolization to achieve a sufficient volume change? Nagino et al.[11] used only ethanol in the case of cholangiocarcinoma because it can be injected through a very small-caliber catheter, and it permeates peripherally to destroy the tissue. We should be careful when using this material because it induces severe abdominal pain during injection[34] and always requires intravenous sedative agents during the procedure. Liver abscesses were also observed after using ethanol. In contrast, Gruttadauria et al.[35] used a combination of microspheres (300–500 μm) and Gelfoam sponge or metallic coils for cases of colorectal liver metastasis. In their report, there was no description of posttreatment complications. Therefore, the safety of these materials is unknown. Nonetheless, surgery was eventually performed safely in all cases. Inaba et al.[36] used a combination of lipiodol and Gelfoam sponge in four hepatocellular carcinoma patients who underwent TAE after PVE, and did not experience any posttreatment complications. Fibrin glue has been frequently used as an embolic material for the portal vein.[34,37,38] However, it is not appropriate for the purpose of TAE because a large-caliber catheter is necessary to inject this agent. After any embolic material is used for sequential PVE and TAE, it is very important to observe the patient carefully and to perform examinations frequently to check for the presence of any complication.

25.2.2.2 Extent of Arterial Embolization

Another consideration for the technique of sequential PVE and TAE is the extent of arterial embolization that

Table 25.1 The results of sequential PVE and TAE

Year	2000	2000	2004	2004
Author	Nagino	Nagino	Gruttadauria	Gruttadauria
Age	66	54	62	70
Sex	M	F	M	M
Diagnosis	Hilar bile duct cancer	Hilar bile duct cancer	Colorectal liver metastasis	Colorectal liver metastasis
Liver condition	Alcoholic	Hepatitis C virus infection	Normal	Normal
Volume of the non-embolized lobe (mL)				
Before PVE	485 ↓ (51 days)	643 ↓ (14 days)	379 ↓ (42 days)	302 ↓ (42 days)
After PVE	470 ↓ (71 days)	649 ↓ (55 days)	505 ↓ (63 days)	344 ↓ (63 days)
After TAE	685	789	916	521
Hypertrophy rate (%)				
After PVE	–3.1	0.9	25.0	13.9
After TAE	41.2	22.7	141.7	72.5
Posttreatment complications	Pain, low platelet count	Pain, low platelet count, liver abscess	No description	No description
Embolic materials for PVE	Fibrin glue and iodized oil	Fibrin glue and iodized oil	Microspheres and metallic coils	Microspheres and metallic coils
Embolic materials for TAE	Ethanol	Ethanol	Microspheres and Gelfoam	Microspheres and Gelfoam
Performed surgery	L3 + S1	R2 + S1	ER2	R2

L3 + S1 left trisectionectomy with caudate lobectomy, *R2 + S1* right hepatectomy with caudate lobectomy, *ER2* extended right hepatectomy, *R2* right hepatectomy

will be safe and still achieve a satisfactory effect. Nagino et al.[11] proposed to embolize about 50% of the target hepatic segment, because complete embolization of the arterial supply in segments with no portal venous flow would cause massive necrosis of the hepatic parenchyma. Their report showed that even with 50% embolization, they experienced a severe liver abscess which required interventional drainage after TAE. Therefore, a superselective, extremely careful catheter approach is necessary to access the branch for arterial embolization. There has been no other report that discussed the association between the extent of arterial embolization and post-procedure complications. In this regard, further accumulation of data is necessary.

25.3 Potential Risk

Hepatic infarction following interventional procedures is sometimes fatal.[39] High serum alanine aminotrasferase and aspartate aminotransferase levels are always observed after hepatic infarction. When the remnant liver function is not sufficient, serum total bilirubin levels will also be increased. Other signs of hepatic infarction are high fever, abdominal pain, and fatigue. These signs will usually disappear within 2 weeks. However, when these signs continue, the presence of a liver abscess should be considered, and ultrasonography or CT scans should be performed. In cases of cholangiocarcinoma with biliary stenosis, a bilioenteric stent or percutaneous transhepatic biliary catheter is frequently placed. These catheters can induce an ascending biliary infection (i.e., cholangitis). With this condition, hepatic infarction can lead to fatal hepatic gas gangrene and sepsis. Therefore, for the patient with signs of cholangitis, sequential PVE and TAE should not be performed.

25.4 Case Report of Sequential PVE and TAE

We[38] and others[35] have reported the usefulness of sequential ipsilateral PVE and TAE for patients who did not show sufficient volume increases after PVE. The results are summarized in Table 25.1. Although the indication, the basic condition of the liver, the extent of embolization, and the embolic materials were different between the two reports, all of the patients eventually achieved a sufficient hypertrophy rate of the non-embolized lobe.

We describe here a recent case of hilar cholangiocarcinoma, in which the patient underwent a successful surgery after sequential PVE and TAE. The patient was

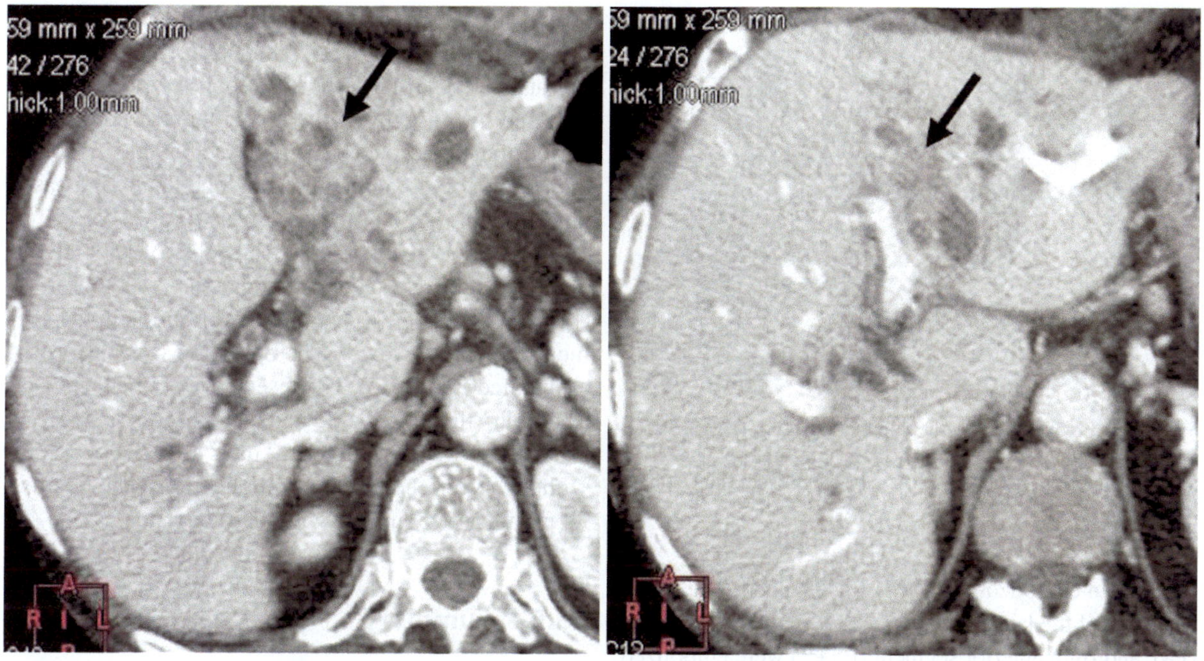

Fig. 25.1 Abdominal computed tomography. A papillary tumor in the intrahepatic bile duct in the lateral lobe was observed (*arrows*)

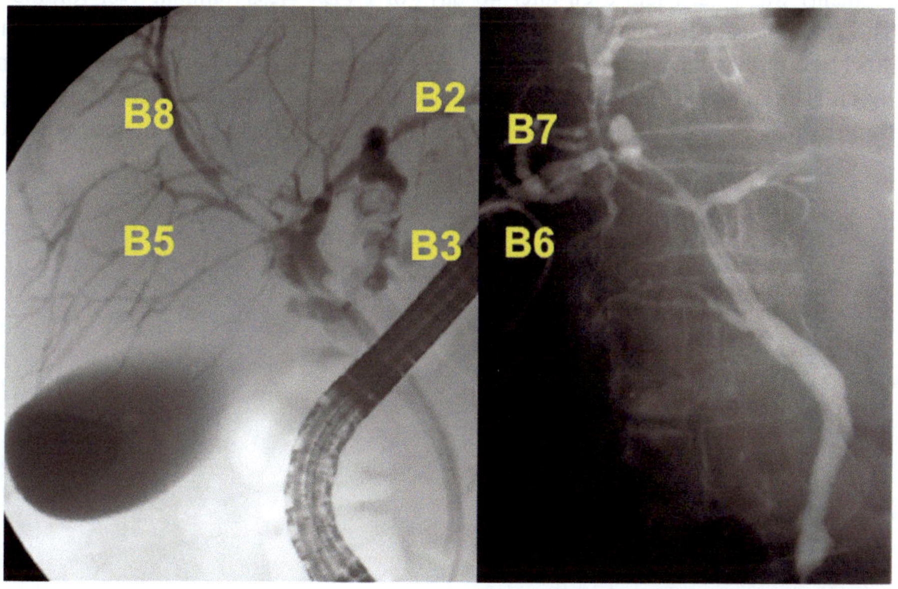

Fig. 25.2 Cholangiography. A papillary tumor in the lateral inferior bile duct (B3) and a stenosis of the right anterior bile duct. The lesion was diagnosed as a bile duct cancer originated from B3 and invaded to the right anterior bile duct (B5, B8). The right posterior bile duct (B6, B7) was free from the tumor

a 73-year-old woman who was initially seen at another institution for an abnormal liver function test. An abdominal ultrasonography revealed a dilatation of the intrahepatic bile duct. After endoscopic retrograde cholangiography (ERC) and percutaneous transhepatic biliary drainage, the patient was referred to our hospital.

Abdominal multidetector computed tomography revealed a papillary tumor in the intrahepatic bile duct in the lateral lobe (arrows) (Fig. 25.1). Cholangiography detected a papillary tumor in the left lateral inferior bile duct (B3) and a stenosis of the right anterior bile duct (Fig. 25.2). The lesion was diagnosed as a bile duct cancer originated from B3 and invaded the right anterior bile duct. Left trisectionectomy, caudate lobectomy, and extrahepatic bile duct resection were necessary to completely remove the tumor. Therefore, a preoperative

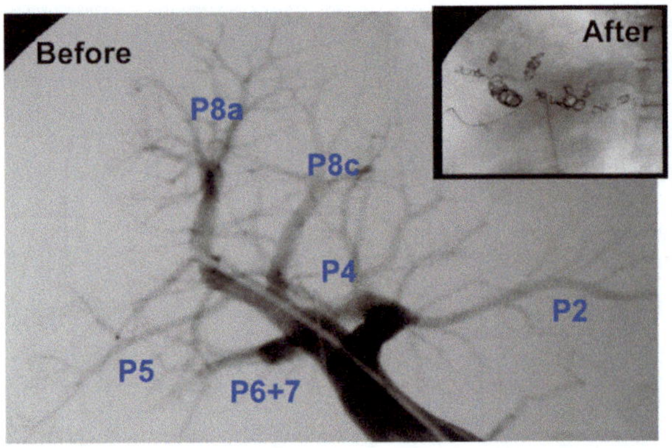

Fig. 25.3 Preoperative portal vein embolization (PVE). Portal branches for the lateral segment (P2+3), medial segment (P4), and right anterior segment (P5+8) were embolized using ethanol and coils

portal vein embolization (PVE) was planned. The portal branches of the lateral segment (P2+3), medial segment (P4), and right anterior segment (P5+8) were embolized using ethanol and coils (Fig. 25.3). However, the hypertrophy response in the non-embolized lobe (the posterior segment) was insufficient even after 40 days of PVE. The volume change in the posterior segment was from 208 (18% of the total liver) to 233 mL (23% of the total liver). Therefore, a sequential TAE was planned and performed on the segments embolized by PVE. Ethanol was injected to the medial segment (S4, 6 mL) and right anterior segment (S8, 3 mL; S5, 3 mL) (Fig. 25.4). TAE was repeated because of insufficient atrophy of the embolized lobe and hypertrophy of the non-embolized lobe. After performing the second TAE (77 days after the first TAE), the volume of the non-embolized lobe finally increased up to 430 mL (43% of the total liver) (Fig. 25.5).

At laparotomy, a marked atrophy of the lateral, medial, and right anterior segments was observed (Fig. 25.6). There was an abscess formation in the segments 3 and 8 (arrows). The operation was performed as planned (Fig. 25.7). The resected specimen revealed a papillary tumor in the B3 and liver abscess (Fig. 25.8). The patient was discharged 27 days after the operation without experiencing any complications and is alive 34 months after surgery without recurrence.

25.5 Summary

Extensive liver resection allows more oncologically safe surgical margins. However, this procedure yields less remnant liver volume and increases the possibility of postoperative liver failure. It is therefore important to obtain enough compensatory hypertrophy in the non-embolized lobe using a technique such as PVE. The rate of hypertrophy is variable, depending on the

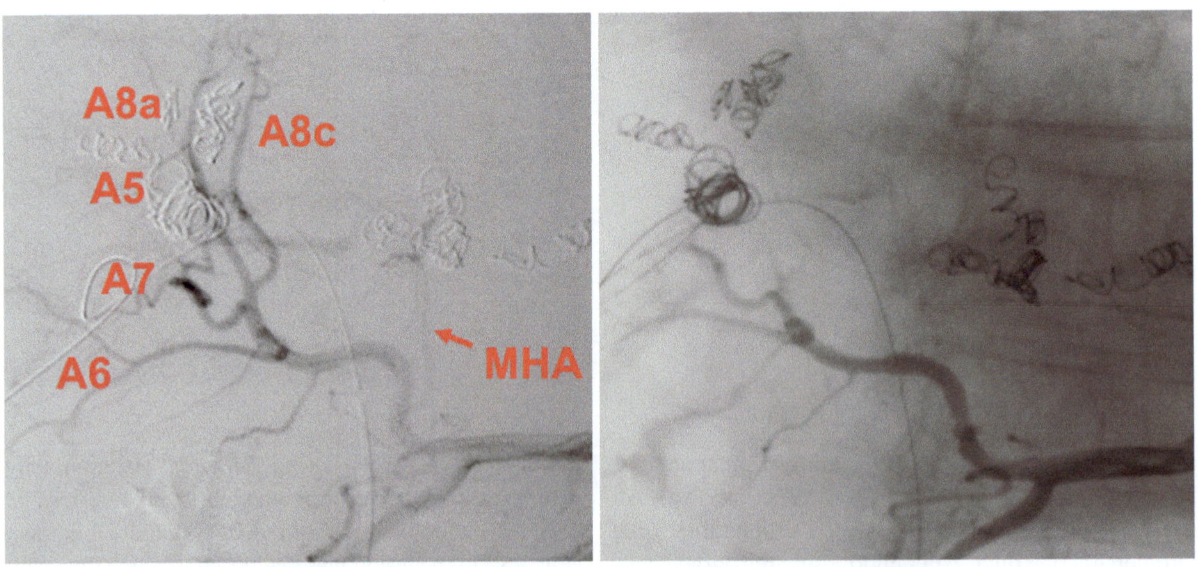

Fig. 25.4 Transcatheter arterial embolization (TAE). Ethanol was injected into the medial segment (S4, 6 mL) and right anterior segment (S8, 3 mL; S5, 3 mL). *MHA* middle hepatic artery (*arrow*)

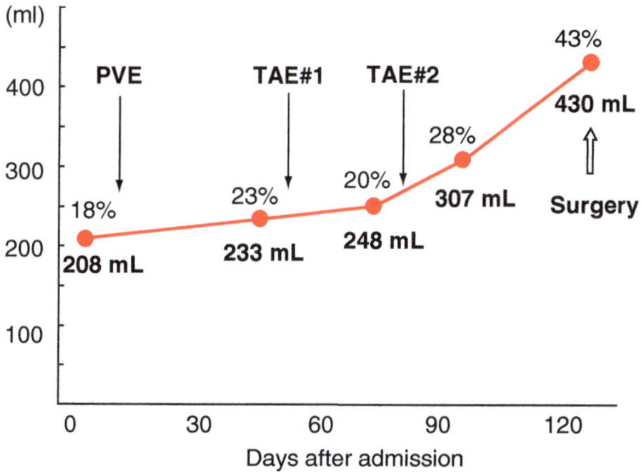

Fig. 25.5 The time course of changes in the volume of the right posterior segment (non-embolized segments). TAE was repeated because of insufficient atrophy of the embolized segments and hypertrophy of the non-embolized segments

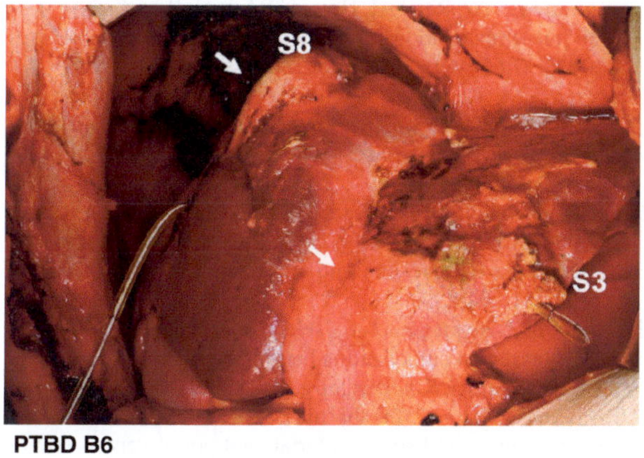

Fig. 25.6 Intraoperative findings. There was a marked atrophy of the lateral, medial, and right anterior segments. There was an abscess formation in the segments 3 and 8 (*arrows*)

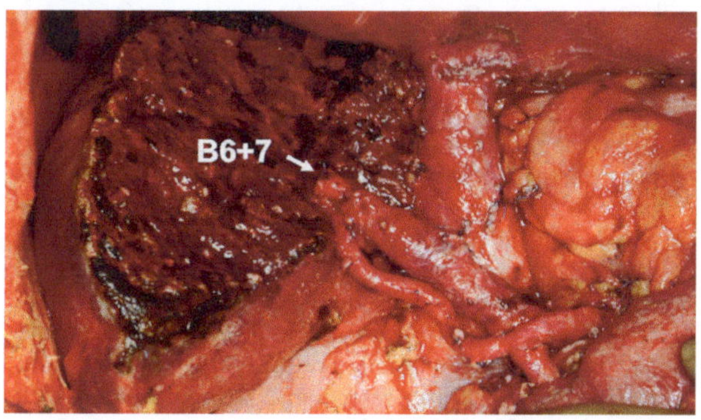

Fig. 25.7 The operation. Left hepatic trisectionectomy, caudate lobectomy, and extrahepatic bile duct resection were performed. The operation time was 10 h and 30 min, and the intraoperative blood loss was 2,330 mL. The stump of bile duct in the segment 6 and 7 (*arrow*)

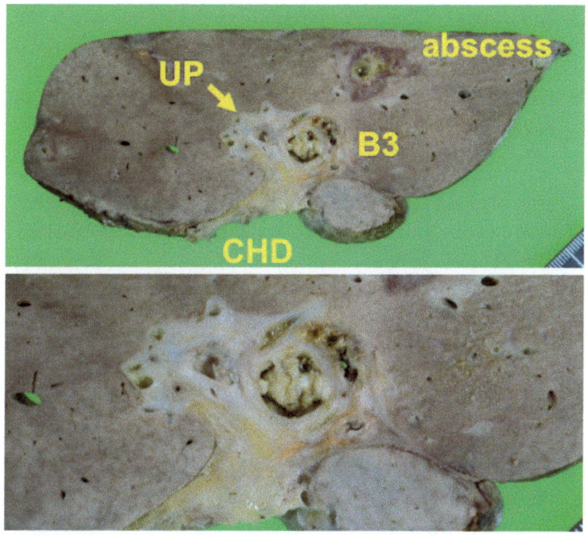

Fig. 25.8 The resected specimen. There was a papillary tumor and an abscess in segment 3. *UP* umbilical portion (*arrow*)

patient; it is usually lower in patients who suffered from chronic liver disease. For these particular patients, performing TAE in addition to PVE is beneficial with regards to the achievement of sufficient hypertrophy rate of the non-embolized lobe. However, the postoperative care should be particularly attentive to potential complications such as high fever, high serum transaminase levels, deterioration of serum total bilirubin levels, and formation of liver abscesses. Because of this high complication rate, sequential PVE, and TAE should be performed only in strictly selected patients. By accumulating further clinical data, the exact indication and the best technique for this procedure should be clarified in the future.

References

1. Blumgart LH, Hadjis NS, Benjamin IS, et al. Surgical approaches to cholangiocarcinoma at confluence of hepatic ducts. *Lancet*. 1984;1:66-70.
2. Nimura Y, Hayakawa N, Kamiya J, et al. Combined portal vein and liver resection for carcinoma of the biliary tract. *Br J Surg*. 1991;78:727-731.
3. Makuuchi M, Thai BL, Takayasu K, et al. Preoperative portal embolization to increase safety of major hepatectomy for hilar bile duct carcinoma: a preliminary report. *Surgery*. 1990;107:521-527.
4. Makuuchi M, Takayasu K, Takuma T, et al. Preoperative transcatheter embolization of the portal venous branch for patients receiving extended lobectomy due to the bile duct carcinoma. *J Jpn Soc Clin Surg*. 1984;45:14-20.

5. Kinoshita H, Sakai K, Hirohashi K, et al. Preoperative portal vein embolization for hepatocellular carcinoma. *World J Surg*. 1986;10:803-808.
6. Lautt WW. Mechanism and role of intrinsic regulation of hepatic arterial blood flow: hepatic arterial buffer response. *Am J Physiol*. 1985;249:G549-G556.
7. Nagino M, Nimura Y, Kamiya J, et al. Immediate increase in arterial blood flow in embolized hepatic segments after portal vein embolization: CT demonstration. *AJR Am J Roentgenol*. 1998;171:1037-1039.
8. Farges O, Belghiti J, Kianmanesh R, et al. Portal vein embolization before right hepatectomy: prospective clinical trial. *Ann Surg*. 2003;237:208-217.
9. Giraudo G, Greget M, Oussoultzoglou E, et al. Preoperative contralateral portal vein embolization before major hepatic resection is a safe and efficient procedure: a large single institution experience. *Surgery*. 2008;143:476-482.
10. Yokoyama Y, Nagino M, Nimura Y. Mechanism of impaired hepatic regeneration in cholestatic liver. *J Hepatobiliary Pancreat Surg*. 2007;14:159-166.
11. Nagino M, Kanai M, Morioka A, et al. Portal and arterial embolization before extensive liver resection in patients with markedly poor functional reserve. *J Vasc Interv Radiol*. 2000;11:1063-1068.
12. Kito Y, Nagino M, Nimura Y. Doppler sonography of hepatic arterial blood flow velocity after percutaneous transhepatic portal vein embolization. *AJR Am J Roentgenol*. 2001;176: 909-912.
13. Rocheleau B, Ethier C, Houle R, et al. Hepatic artery buffer response following left portal vein ligation: its role in liver tissue homeostasis. *Am J Physiol*. 1999;277:G1000-G1007.
14. Goto Y, Nagino M, Nimura Y. Doppler estimation of portal blood flow after percutaneous transhepatic portal vein embolization. *Ann Surg*. 1998;228:209-213.
15. Aoki T, Imamura H, Hasegawa K, et al. Sequential preoperative arterial and portal venous embolizations in patients with hepatocellular carcinoma. *Arch Surg*. 2004;139:766-774.
16. Abdalla EK, Hicks ME, Vauthey JN. Portal vein embolization: rationale, technique and future prospects. *Br J Surg*. 2001;88:165-175.
17. Mizuno S, Nimura Y, Suzuki H, et al. Portal vein branch occlusion induces cell proliferation of cholestatic rat liver. *J Surg Res*. 1996;60:249-257.
18. Suzuki H, Iyomasa S, Nimura Y, et al. Internal biliary drainage, unlike external drainage, does not suppress the regeneration of cholestatic rat liver after partial hepatectomy. *Hepatology*. 1994;20:1318-1322.
19. Tracy TF Jr, Bailey PV, Goerke ME, et al. Cholestasis without cirrhosis alters regulatory liver gene expression and inhibits hepatic regeneration. *Surgery*. 1991;110:176-182; discussion 182–173.
20. Yamanaka N, Okamoto E, Kawamura E, et al. Dynamics of normal and injured human liver regeneration after hepatectomy as assessed on the basis of computed tomography and liver function. *Hepatology*. 1993;18:79-85.
21. Barra R, Hall JC. Liver regeneration in normal and alloxan-induced diabetic rats. *J Exp Zool*. 1977;201:93-99.
22. Imamura H, Shimada R, Kubota M, et al. Preoperative portal vein embolization: an audit of 84 patients. *Hepatology*. 1999; 29:1099-1105.
23. Liatsos GD, Mykoniatis MG, Margeli A, et al. Effect of acute ethanol exposure on hepatic stimulator substance (HSS) levels during liver regeneration: protective function of HSS. *Dig Dis Sci*. 2003;48:1929-1938.
24. Koteish A, Yang S, Lin H, et al. Ethanol induces redox-sensitive cell-cycle inhibitors and inhibits liver regeneration after partial hepatectomy. *Alcohol Clin Exp Res*. 2002;26: 1710-1718.
25. Skullman S, Ihse I, Larsson J. Influence of malnutrition on regeneration and composition of the liver in rats. *Acta Chir Scand*. 1990;156:717-722.
26. Delany HM, John J, Teh EL, et al. Contrasting effects of identical nutrients given parenterally or enterally after 70% hepatectomy. *Am J Surg*. 1994;167:135-143; discussion 143–134.
27. Nagino M, Nimura Y, Kamiya J, et al. Changes in hepatic lobe volume in biliary tract cancer patients after right portal vein embolization. *Hepatology*. 1995;21:434-439.
28. Ladurner R, Brandacher G, Riedl-Huter C, et al. Percutaneous portal vein embolisation in preparation for extended hepatic resection of primary nonresectable liver tumours. *Dig Liver Dis*. 2003;35:716-721.
29. Hemming AW, Reed AI, Howard RJ, et al. Preoperative portal vein embolization for extended hepatectomy. *Ann Surg*. 2003;237:686-691; discussion 691–683.
30. Nagino M, Kamiya J, Nishio H, et al. Two hundred forty consecutive portal vein embolizations before extended hepatectomy for biliary cancer: surgical outcome and long-term follow-up. *Ann Surg*. 2006;243:364-372.
31. Elias D, Ouellet JF, De Baere T, et al. Preoperative selective portal vein embolization before hepatectomy for liver metastases: long-term results and impact on survival. *Surgery*. 2002;131:294-299.
32. Belghiti J. Arguments for a selective approach of preoperative portal vein embolization before major hepatic resection. *J Hepatobiliary Pancreat Surg*. 2004;11:21-24.
33. Nakao N, Miura K, Takahashi H, et al. Hepatocellular carcinoma: combined hepatic, arterial, and portal venous embolization. *Radiology*. 1986;161:303-307.
34. Nagino M, Nimura Y, Hayakawa N. Percutaneous transhepatic portal embolization using newly devised catheters: preliminary report. *World J Surg*. 1993;17:520-524.
35. Gruttadauria S, Luca A, Mandala L, et al. Sequential preoperative ipsilateral portal and arterial embolization in patients with colorectal liver metastases. *World J Surg*. 2006;30: 576-578.
36. Inaba S, Takada T, Amano H, et al. Combination of preoperative embolization of the right portal vein and hepatic artery prior to major hepatectomy in high-risk patients: a preliminary report. *Hepatogastroenterology*. 2000;47:1077-1081.
37. Nagino M, Nimura Y, Kamiya J, et al. Right or left trisegment portal vein embolization before hepatic trisegmentectomy for hilar bile duct carcinoma. *Surgery*. 1995;117:677-681.
38. Nagino M, Nimura Y, Kamiya J, et al. Selective percutaneous transhepatic embolization of the portal vein in preparation for extensive liver resection: the ipsilateral approach. *Radiology*. 1996;200:559-563.
39. Fujiwara H, Kanazawa S, Hiraki T, et al. Hepatic infarction following abdominal interventional procedures. *Acta Med Okayama*. 2004;58:97-106.

Sequential TACE and PVE for Hepatocellular Carcinoma

26

Hiroshi Imamura, Yasuji Seyama, Masatoshi Makuuchi, and Norihiro Kokudo

Abstract

Although hepatic resection is the treatment of choice for large hepatocellular carcinoma (HCC) whenever feasible, it is often precluded by the presence of underlying chronic liver disease. Portal vein embolization (PVE) has been introduced to extend the indications for major hepatic resection to increase the safety of the surgical procedure. Prior to undertaking PVE, the following possibilities should be considered: failure to induce hypertrophy of the nonembolized liver part from underlying fibrosis or cirrhosis, tumor growth acceleration after occlusion of blood flow, and low PVE efficacy due to arterioportal shunts. Sequential transcatheter arterial embolization (TACE) and PVE can be applied to HCC patients to overcome such difficulties. In the literature, as well as our own experience, this double preparation was well tolerated, enhanced the hypertrophy process in the nonembolized liver part, and suppressed tumor growth during the preparation period. Furthermore, PVE also functioned as a preoperative test to select suitable patients for major liver resection. Sequential TACE and PVE are therefore effective preoperative interventions in HCC patients scheduled for major liver resection.

Keywords

Portal vein embolization • Hepatocellular carcinoma • Transcatheter arterial embolization • Liver resection • Sequential transcatheter arterial embolization

Abbreviations

AFP	Alpha-fetoprotein
AST	Aspartate transaminase
ALT	Alanine transaminase
CT	Computed tomography
DCP	Des-γ-carboxy prothrombin
FRL	Future remnant liver
HCC	Hepatocellular carcinoma
ICG-R15	Indocyanine green retention rate at 15 min
PVE	Portal vein embolization

H. Imamura (✉)
Department of Hepatobiliary-Pancreatic Surgery, Juntendo School of Medicine, 2-1-1, Hongo, Bunkyo-ku, Tokyo, 113-8421, Japan
e-mail: himamura-tky@umin.ac.jp

Major liver resection often removes more than 70% of functioning liver parenchyma, leading to an abrupt increase in portal venous pressure and insufficient hepatic functional reserve. The latter is associated with an increased incidence of hepatic dysfunction[1-4] while the former can result in sinusoidal injury which is

D.C. Madoff et al. (eds.), *Venous Embolization of the Liver*,
DOI 10.1007/978-1-84882-122-4_26, © Springer-Verlag London Limited 2011

known as small-for-size graft syndrome in recipients of living donor liver transplantation.[5,6] Both changes can contribute to increased postoperative morbidity and fatal liver failure.

To overcome these issues, portal vein embolization (PVE) has been increasingly applied preoperatively to major liver resection. This aims to induce atrophy of the embolized liver part to be resected, compensatory hypertrophy of the nonembolized future remnant liver (FRL) after hepatectomy, and transient elevation of portal venous pressure in the FRL.[7-9] We first performed this intervention in 1982 for patients with hilar bile duct carcinoma.[10] Due to its technical simplicity and minimal side effects, PVE has become a standard preoperative intervention worldwide, and its indications have been expanded to include patients with hepatocellular carcinoma (HCC).[11-19]

Liver resection remains the mainstay of treatment for HCC, and this is especially true for patients with large HCCs and those with portal venous tumor thrombi, because neither liver transplantation nor ablative therapy can be undertaken in these patients. In addition, segment-oriented anatomical resection is recommended even for small HCCs to prevent postoperative recurrence.[20-23] These considerations inevitably signify that major liver resection is often required in patients with HCC.

On the other hand, transcatheter arterial chemoembolization (TACE) has been widely used for the treatment of patients with unresectable HCC. Because HCC tumors preferentially receive their blood supply from the hepatic artery, occlusion of tumor-feeding arterial branches induces ischemic necrosis in the tumor and enhances the cytotoxicity of the chemotherapeutic agent. Survival benefits were observed in two randomized controlled trials,[24,25] although neoadjuvant TACE in resectable HCC does not appear to improve disease-free survival after resection.[26,27]

26.1 Indications of PVE in Patients with HCC

The ratio of FRL volume to total liver volume, as assessed by computed tomography (CT) volumetric measurement, is used to determine the indication of PVE. The threshold ratio below which PVE is indicated has been arbitrarily determined and varies from 25 to 40% according to respective institutional criteria in patients assumed to have normal underlying liver parenchyma.[12-14,28-30]

However, the situation for HCC is more complex because most HCC patients have impaired liver parenchyma from hepatitis B and/or C virus-associated or alcoholic liver fibrosis/cirrhosis. Major hepatectomy is not indicated for patients who are classified into Child–Turcotte–Pugh grades B and C, so these patients are not potential candidates for PVE. In addition, patients with signs of portal hypertension, i.e., platelet count <100,000/mL, splenomegalies, presence of esophageal varices, and/or port-systemic collateral, are generally not indicated for PVE. A more detailed assessment of liver functional reserve is conducted in the remaining Child-Turcotte-Pugh grade A patients using the indocyanine green retention rate at 15 min (ICG-R15).[31] This is pharmacologically equivalent to the ICG elimination rate constant from the blood to the liver and represents the degree of sinusoidal capillarization, intrahepatic port venous shunting, and alterations of the liver blood flow.[32] The balance between the ratio of FRL volume and ICG-R15 is used to determine the indication of PVE[33] (Fig. 26.1).

26.1.1 Rationale for Conducting Sequential PVE Followed by TACE

While conducting PVE in patients with HCC, several concerns have to be taken into account, and the rationale for combining TACE with PVE lies in overcoming these theoretical drawbacks. First, the regenerative capacity of fibrotic or cirrhotic liver parenchyma is reportedly impaired after hepatectomy or PVE.[13,34-36] This double preparation is carried out with the aim of enhancing hypertrophy of the FRL segments after PVE in chronically injured liver.[11,15]

Second, cessation of the portal flow induces a compensatory increase in the arterial blood flow in the embolized liver part[37,38] and may result in the rapid growth of the tumors after PVE. This concern should not be ignored since the tumor doubling time of HCC[29] is thought to be less than that of hilar bile duct carcinoma, a prototype of slow-growing tumors, and the interval between PVE and liver resection is often prolonged in patients with HCC because of the slow process of liver regeneration.[12] TACE prior to PVE is carried out in order to prevent tumor progression during the interval between the PVE and the planned liver resection.

Finally, HCC is frequently associated with arterioportal shunts, and its incidence is reported to vary from

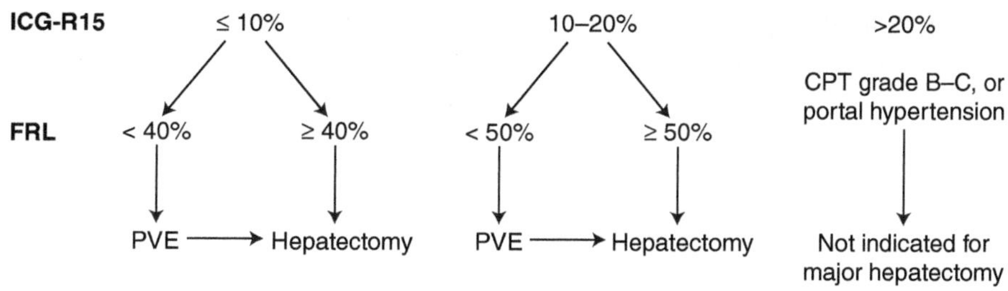

Fig. 26.1 Decision tree to determine the decision of portal vein embolization as a function of volume percent of future remnant liver. *ICG-R15* indocyanine retention rate at 15 min, *FRL* future remnant liver, *PVE* portal vein embolization, *CPT* Child–Turcotte–Pugh classification

4 to 60%.[39-41] These shunts may attenuate the effects of PVE. TACE is conducted for the purpose of strengthening the effect of the PVE by first embolizing any minute arterioportal shunts that may exist.

26.1.2 Sequential TACE and PVE

We first carry out selective TACE for liver segments that bear the HCC tumor(s) (Fig. 26.2a, b).[11,14] Following intra-arterial injection of epirubicin hydrochloride (Farmorubicin; Pharmacai, Tokyo, Japan) and iodized oil (Lipiodol Ultra-Fluide; Andre Guerbet, Aulnay-Soubois, France), the arterial branches of the liver part to be resected are embolized with porous gelatin particles with a diameter of 1–2 mm (Gelpart; Asterals, Tokyo, Japan). In the case of large HCCs, the tumor(s) are often also fed by other arterial branches, such as a branch of segment 4 or the right inferior phrenic artery, and these arterial branches are embolized as well. The latter possibility should always be borne in mind because large HCCs in the right hemiliver, which frequently constitute an indication for PVE, are often adjacent to the diaphragm, which makes the right inferior phrenic artery the major extrahepatic collateral artery. However, this cannot be recognized unless cannulation of the branch is carried out.[42] Finally, iodized oil is administered intra-arterially into the branches of the nonembolized liver part to enable intrahepatic metastases to be detected by subsequent computed tomography.[43] A necroinflammatory reaction usually follows TACE, as reflected by feverish episodes and increased serum aspartate transaminase (AST) and alanine transaminase (ALT) values. Total bilirubin levels also increase mildly. Feverish episodes and deranged biochemical data usually stabilize within 1 week after performing TACE.

The interval between TACE and subsequent PVE varies according to respective institutional criteria. We perform TACE when the patient condition stabilizes, usually 7–10 days after the procedure (Fig. 26.2c).[11] Another report of patients undergoing sequential TACE and PVE described an interval of at least 3 weeks between PVE and TACE.[15] In our previous reports, 5 of 17 patients experienced mild but transient complications after PVE, two of which might be procedure-related, i.e., emergence of transient ascites.

A transhepatic ipsilateral approach under local anesthesia is the procedure of first choice in our institute.[44] When this is impossible due to the presence of tumor(s) in the puncture line, either the transhepatic contralateral approach or transileocolic approach is chosen.[45,46] We use a mixture of 1- to 2-mm-diameter porous gelatin particles, thrombin (Mochida, Tokyo, Japan), diatrizoate sodium meglumine (60% Urografin; Schering AG, Berlin, Germany), coils (Boston Scientific, Tokyo, Japan), and gentamicin as embolization material. Portal venous pressure is measured before and after the procedure, but this measurement is technically impossible in the case of the transhepatic ipsilateral approach.[8]

In some cases, we adopt a modified method for PVE. For example, when segment 6/7 HCC tumor(s) are associated with portal venous thrombi in the common portal branch of segments 6/7, these segments are usually already atrophied because of the decrease in portal flow caused by the tumor thrombi, while segments 5/8 and the left hemiliver show compensatory hypertrophy. Right hepatectomy is indicated and thus PVE to segments 5/8 should be scheduled. In these cases, we perform a percutaneous transhepatic puncture of these portal venous tributaries under ultrasound guidance and directly inject 1–5 mL of absolute ethanol to occlude these tributaries. Occlusion of the portal tributaries after ethanol injection can be confirmed by Doppler

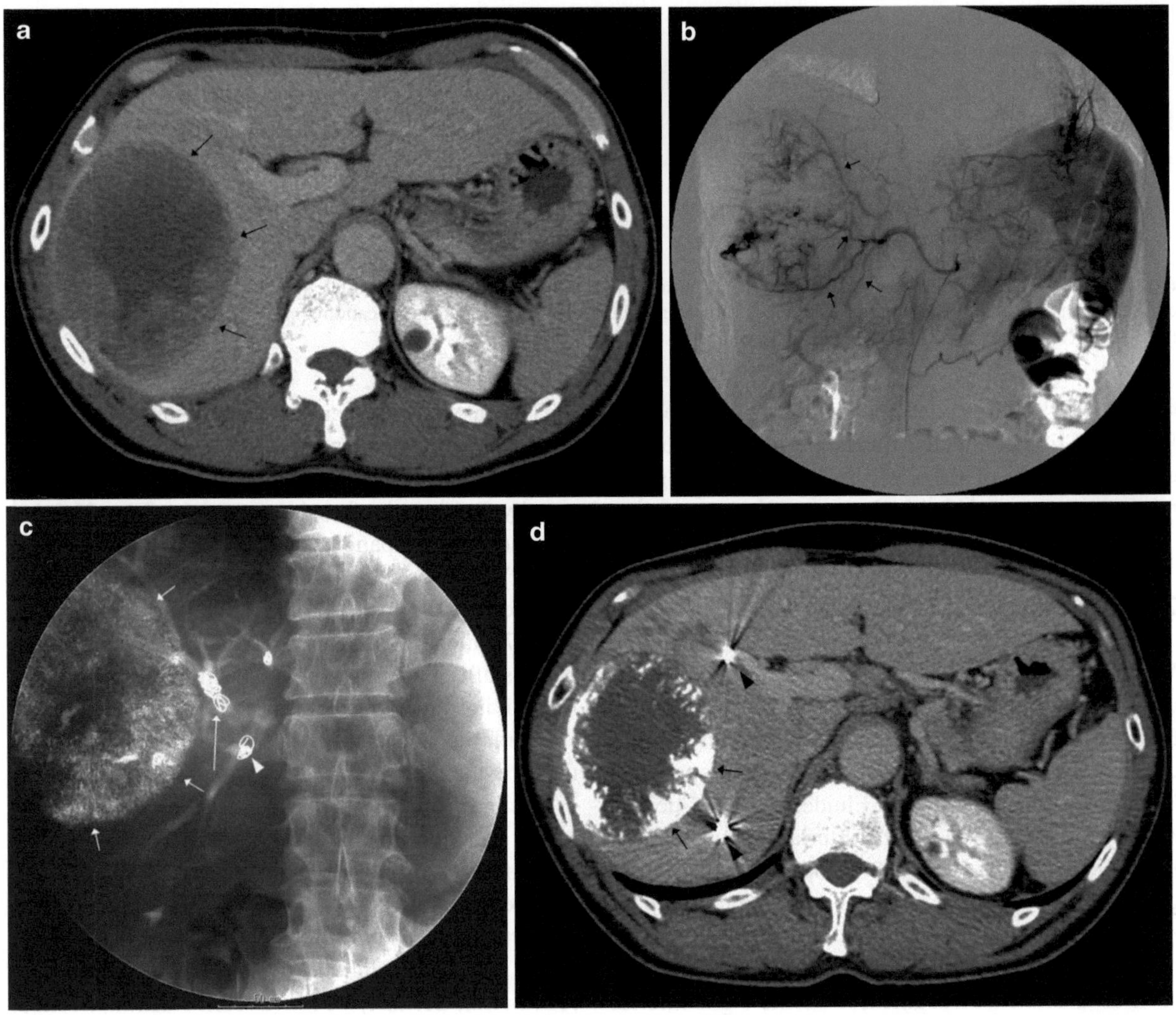

Fig. 26.2 Imaging studies of a 55-year-old male patient with HCC undergoing right hemihepatectomy after sequential TACE and PVE. (**a**) CT scan images before TACE and PVE, portal phase. 10.5×10.0×8.3 cm tumor is located in right hemiliver from right diaphragm to right anterior and posterior portal bifurcation (*arrows*). No portal vein tumor thrombosis was found. Right hemihepatectomy was indicated. ICG-R15 value was 15%, and calculated left liver volume was 40% of the total liver volume. (**b**) Selective TACE images. Tumor was fed by hepatic arterial branches to S5, 6, 7, and 8 (*arrows*). These branches were selectively embolized from right hepatic artery. (**c**) Images of PVE performed 10 days after TACE. Dense accumulation of iodized oil in the tumor was confirmed (*arrows*). PVE was performed through contralateral approach by puncturing a portal venous branch to S3. Portal branches to S5/8 (*long arrow*) and S6/7 (*arrowhead*) were embolized. A portal venous branch to caudate lobe was also embolized. Contrast medium and coils in these branches were visualized after PVE. (**d**) CT scan images 13 days after PVE. Dense accumulation of iodized oil in the tumor (*arrows*) and coils in portal venous branches (*arrowheads*) were visualized. Calculated left liver volume at this time point was 46% of the total liver volume. ICG-R15 value at the corresponding time point was 14%. AFP and DCP values before TACE and after PVE were 3825 ng/mL and 25673 AU/mL (before TACE) and 1457 ng/mL and 144 AU/mL (after TACE and PVE), respectively. (**e**) Finding of the liver surface at operation performed 3 days after confirmation CT scan. The border of liver surface between the embolized right liver and nonembolized left liver was marked by electrocautery (*arrows*). The main tumor in the right liver was recognized from the surface of the liver (*arrowheads*). Intrahepatic metastasis was found intraoperatively in the right liver surface (*long arrow*). (**f**) Finding of the liver after right hepatectomy. (**g**) Finding of the resected right hemiliver. Massive necrosis of the tumor (*arrows*) was observed although viable lesion was also found in the subcapular area (*arrowheads*). No necrosis was found in the nontumorous liver parenchyma. *HCC* hepatocellular carcinoma, *TACE* transcatheter arterial chemoembolization, *ICG-R15* indocyanine green retention rate at 15 min, *PVE* portal vein embolization, *CT* computed tomography, *AFP* alpha-fetoprotein, *DCP* des-γ-carboxy prothrombin

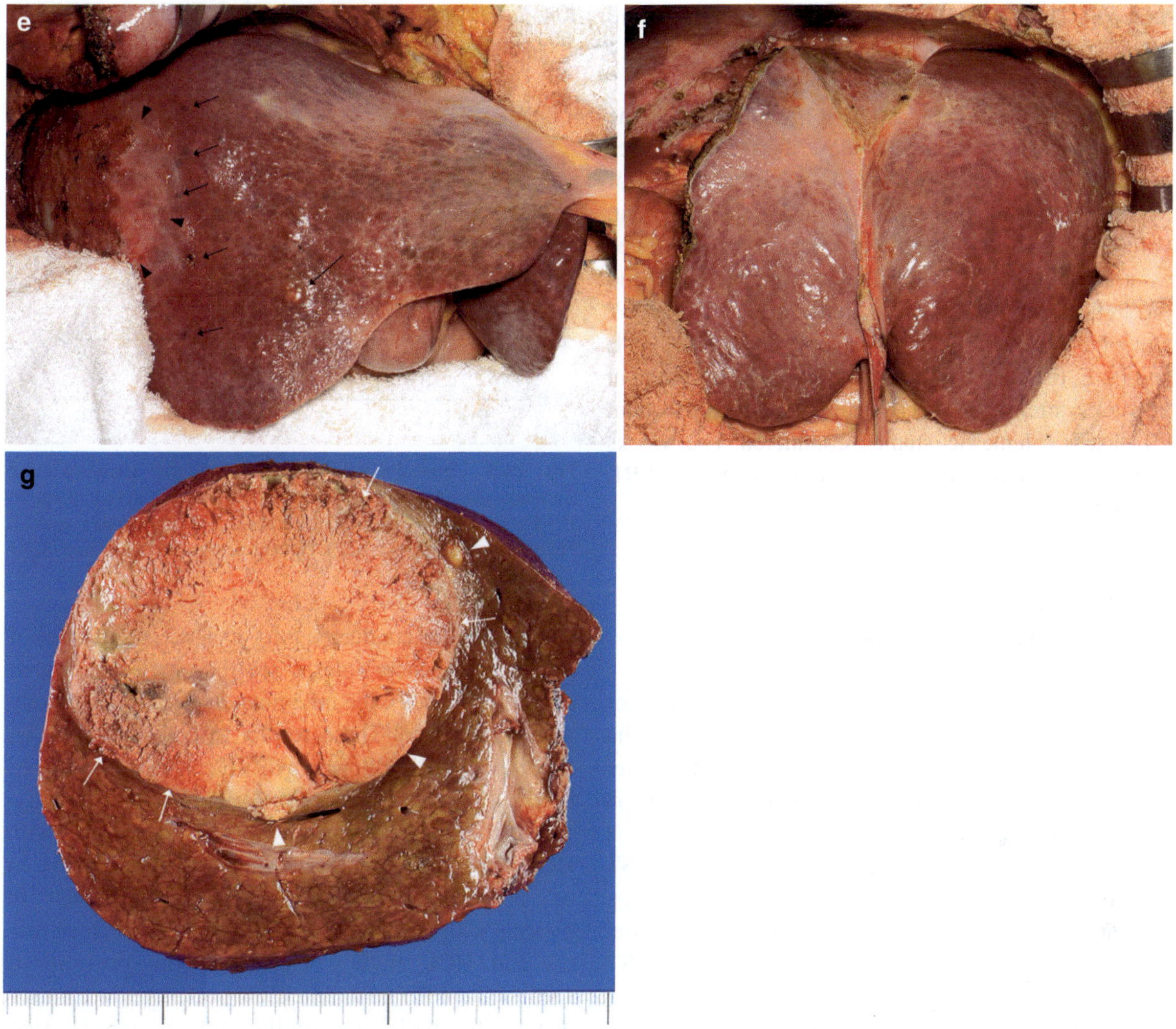

Fig. 26.2 (continued)

ultrasound. However, it should be considered that the effect of PVE in increasing FRL volume is less noticeable the larger the FRL volume prior to PVE.[18,46,47]

26.1.3 Follow-up After Sequential TACE and PVE

We examine portal venous flow in embolized and nonembolized segments every 2–3 days after PVE using Doppler ultrasound. Theoretically, only the hepatic arterial flow can be detected in the embolized segments. Detection of portal venous flow in the corresponding hepatic segments signifies recanalization of the portal vein. We usually inject absolute ethanol into these branches as described earlier.

Triple-phase enhanced CT is conducted 2 weeks after PVE (Fig. 26.2d). In the first phase of CT performed without a contrast medium (Lipiodol-CT), we check for the presence of any tumor nodules in the nonembolized segments.[43] The presence of iodized oil deposition, which is compatible with HCC nodules, indicates a high likelihood of intrahepatic metastasis. In such a case, resection of recognizable tumor nodules may be technically feasible, but this does not signify that curative resectional surgery could be carried out from an oncological point of view.[43] We next recalculate the volumes of embolized and nonembolized segments and the tumor(s). The ICG-R15 value and changes in the serum levels of alpha-fetoprotein (AFP) and des-γ-carboxy prothrombin (DCP) are also reevaluated.

If the FRL volume and ICG-R15 value satisfy the criteria of liver resection as described earlier, liver resection is scheduled (Fig. 26.2e–g). If the degree of hypertrophy of nonembolized segments is insufficient, volumetric changes of the liver segments are followed by a subsequent CT conducted 1–2 weeks later, and the indications for liver resection are reevaluated.[11,14] Out of 54 patients who underwent sequential TACE and PVE, the degree of hypertrophy was insufficient at 2 weeks after PVE in 18 patients, but subsequent CT-based volumetric studies conducted 1–2 weeks later confirmed that the target volume increase in FRL was achieved in 16 of these.

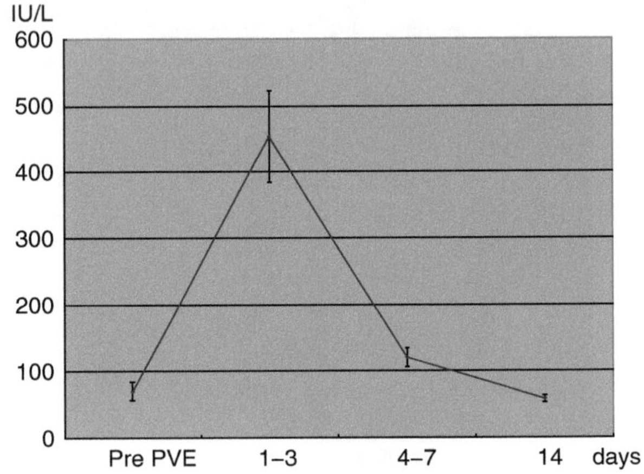

Fig. 26.3 Chronological alterations in the serum alanine transaminase (ALT) in 47 patients after portal vein embolization (PVE) who have undergone preceding transcatheter arterial chemoembolization (TACE). Data are expressed as mean ± SEM

26.1.4 Tolerance of Sequential TACE and PVE and Follow-up

A theoretical drawback of this strategy is the risk of massive infarction of noncancerous liver parenchyma and resultant intolerance of the procedure, such as liver failure and abscess. It has been reported that occlusion of the portal vein alone by PVE does not evoke a necrotic or inflammatory reaction, and that serum AST and ALT levels remain stable after PVE.[46] By contrast, patients undergoing sequential PVE following initial TACE showed a significant elevation of serum AST and ALT, suggesting the occurrence of an inflammatory reaction in the liver parenchyma.[11,15] Nevertheless, this reaction is transient (Fig. 26.3).

Symptoms of the postembolization syndrome that occurs frequently after TACE, such as nausea and feverish episodes, were minimal. The increase in total bilirubin level and decrease in prothrombin time after PVE were mild and transient and comparable to the effect after PVE alone. These findings suggest that the liver functional impairment was minimal and reversible. In addition, examination of resected specimens obtained at the time of the scheduled liver resection revealed that necrosis of the noncancerous liver parenchyma was minimal in most cases while that of HCC tumors was marked (Fig. 26.2g).

The absence of parenchymal necrosis is most likely explained by the recanalization of the hepatic arterial tributaries after TACE, since parenchymal necrosis, albeit partial, was observed in anecdotal cases where repeated TACE was performed after PVE. In addition, when PVE was conducted prior to TACE, as in cases of biliary tract cancer (please see the article by Nagino et al. in this book), the inflammatory reaction is usually more marked.[48,49] These results strongly indicate that sequential TACE followed by PVE can be well tolerated by HCC patients even with underlying liver diseases.

Another concern of applying PVE to patients with HCC is the induction of an overt portal hypertension. In our previous investigations conducted separately in patients with normal livers and those with cirrhotic livers and HCC with a baseline portal pressure of 18.6 ± 4.8 cm H_2O, increments in portal pressure immediately after PVE were similar: 4.9 ± 2.7 mm H_2O vs. 4.1 ± 2.8 cm H_2O, normal livers vs. cirrhotic livers, respectively.[14,50] No information on chronologic changes of portal pressure after PVE is yet available. However, the elevation is thought to be transient, with the pressure gradually returning to baseline within 2–3 weeks as indicated by portal flow velocity (cm/s) changes measured by Doppler ultrasound.[51]

26.2 Efficacy of Sequential TACE and PVE in a Chronically Diseased Liver

The second concern of applying PVE to patients with HCC is whether sufficient hypertrophy of the FRL can be achieved after PVE in a chronically injured liver, and if the process of hypertrophy can be accelerated by the dual embolization of the hepatic artery and portal vein. In a previous study that assessed

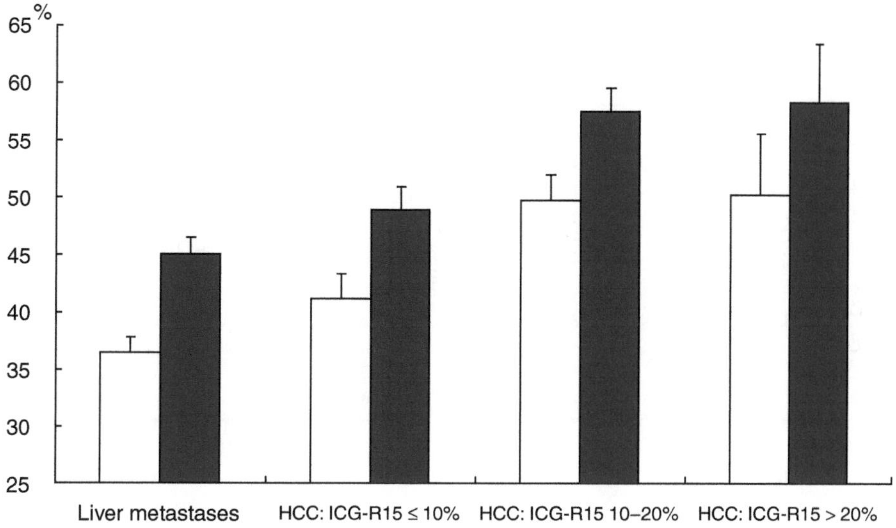

Fig. 26.4 Volumetric change in the future remant liver (FRL) in patients with hepatocellular carcinoma (HCC) after sequential transcatheter arterial chemoembolization (TACE) and portal vein embolization (PVE) ($n=53$). Control data of patients with liver metastases undergoing PVE alone are also shown ($n=40$). HCC ICG-R15≤10% ($n=25$), HCC ICG-R15 10–20% ($n=24$), and HCC ICG-R15>20% ($n=4$). *White columns* indicate values before PVE; *black columns* indicate those after PVE. Data are expressed as mean± SEM. The volumetric gain after PVE (differences in values before and after PVE) in patients with HCC was not statistically significantly different from that in the patients with liver metastases (Dunnett' test). *ICG-R15* indocyanine green retention rate at 15 min. Please note that volume percent of FRL becomes larger with increasing ICG-R15 values because of the indication criteria

volumetric liver regeneration after hepatectomy, the speed of cirrhotic liver regeneration was reduced by approximately 50%, and the level of final regeneration was less than that of normal livers.[36] Likewise, the percent increase of FRL after PVR in patients with chronic liver diseases (9±3%) was less than with normal livers (16±7%).[13]

On the other hand, our early experience revealed that the effect of PVE in inducing hypertrophy in FRL part was strengthened when the procedure was combined with preceding TACE.[16] This finding was further strengthened by Ogata et al.,[15] who reported that in patients with chronic liver diseases, the proportion who showed more than 10% increase of FRL after PVE was much higher when preceding TACE was conducted (12/18:67%) than PVE alone (5/18:28%).

Figure 26.4 depicts the volumetric changes of FRL in patients undergoing right hemiliver PVE. All HCC patients underwent initial TACE before PVE ($n=53$). This group includes anecdotal patients ($n=4$) who underwent PVE despite not satisfying our criteria, i.e., those with an ICG-R15 of >20%. Patients with a normal background liver (control group, $n=40$) underwent PVE alone for metastatic liver tumors are also shown. The degree of hypertrophy of the nonembolized FRL part was of a comparable magnitude, irrespective of ICG-R15 values. This suggests that a similar degree of hypertrophy of the FRL can be expected even in livers with impaired functional reserve when PVE is performed following TACE.

Vetelainen et al.[52] demonstrated that sequential hepatic arterial and portal vein ligation with a 48-h interval in a rat model of hemihepatic portal vein ligation resulted in accelerated hypertrophy in the nonligated lobe, but that the final magnitude of hypertrophy achieved was comparable to that with portal vein ligation alone.

Taking into account all of these issues, it can be concluded that combined use of TACE and PVE accelerates the process of hypertrophy of nonembolized FRL in chronically injured liver but does not modify the extent of hypertrophy finally achieved.

26.2.1 PVE as a Dynamic Preoperative Liver Function Test to Assess the Capacity of Liver Regeneration

Although PVE may induce hypertrophy in nonembolized FRL in chronically injured liver, the capacity of hypertrophy varies between patients. Insufficient

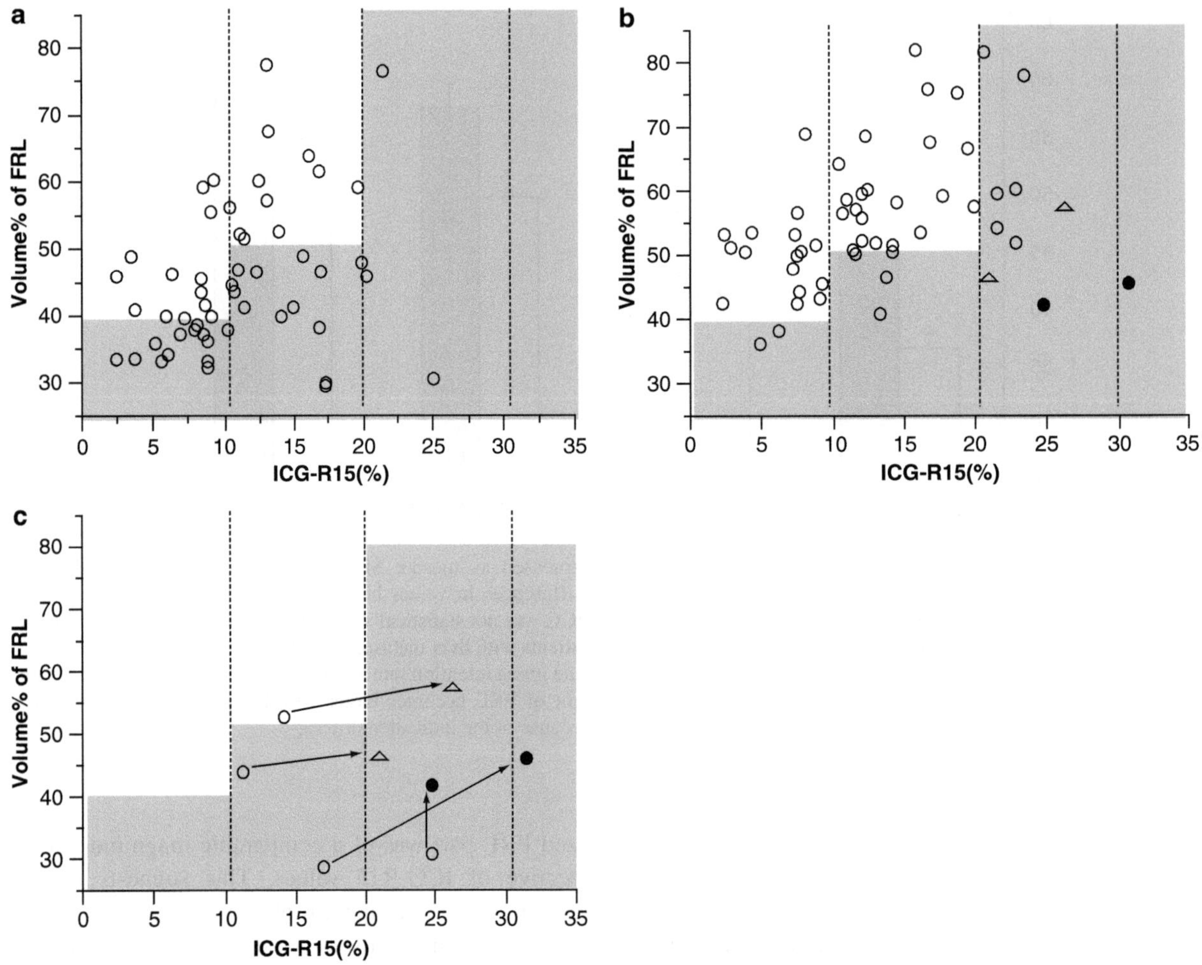

Fig. 26.5 Alterations in future remnant liver volume ratio (volume percent of FRL) and indocyanine green retention rate at 15 min (ICG-R15) in 54 patients undergoing sequential transcatheter arterial chemoembolization (TACE) and portal vein embolization (PVE). (**a**) Values before TACE and PVE. (**b**) Values after TACE and PVE. Using our criteria balancing FRL volume with the extent of liver injury, as evaluated by the ICG-R15 value, major liver resection would be indicated for patients located in the upper left area of this graph (*white zone*). *Clear circles* denote patients who underwent scheduled major liver resection, *clear triangles* denote patients who underwent downscaled liver resection, and *filled circles* denote those in whom liver resection was abandoned. (**c**) Alterations in the volume percent of FRL and ICG-R15 values following TACE and PVE in four patients in whom the scheduled major liver resection was abandoned because of the insufficient liver volumetric increase and/or deterioration in the liver functional reserve

hypertrophy after PVE was reportedly associated with an increased incidence of postoperative complications, mainly due to hepatic dysfunction or insufficiency.[13,15,47,53] On the basis of their experiences, Farges et al.[13] claimed that the failure to increase FRL in fibrotic or cirrhotic patients, despite technically successful PVE, should be considered as an indicator of the inability of the liver to regenerate after hepatectomy and hence contraindicated to major liver resection. Such a dynamic preoperative liver function test to predict outcome after a planned major hepatectomy is also emphasized by Ribero et al.[47]

We carry out a dynamic assessment of the liver following PVE from both volumetric and functional aspects, i.e., measurement of FRL volume and ICG-R15 values (Fig. 26.5a–c). It has been reported that the functional capacity of the total liver and total liver volume remain unaltered after PVE in the normal liver.[54] In 50 of 54 patients who underwent sequential TACE and PVE in our institute, ICG-R15 values after PVE were comparable to those obtained at baseline. Of the 50, scheduled major liver resection was carried out in 46 after confirming a sufficient degree of hypertrophy in the FRL while the operation was abandoned ($n=1$) or modified ($n=3$) because of tumor-related factors in the remaining four patients.

On the other hand, ICG-R15 values deteriorated in 4 of 54 patients even though the degree of volumetric hypertrophy in FRL was acceptable in two of these. Scheduled major liver resection was abandoned and downscaled liver resections (from left trisectoriectomy to extended left hepatectomy, and from extended S6/7 resection to extended S6 resection) were carried out in two patients, and liver resection was entirely abandoned in two patients. The failure of FRL volume to increase and the deterioration of liver functional reserve are most likely ascribed to the development of latent portosystemic collaterals which could not be detected without conducting PVE. These observations are in accordance with previous reports.[13,47]

26.2.2 Outcome Following Liver Resection Conducted After Sequential TACE and PVE

There was no operative mortality in the 51 patients who underwent liver resection following sequential TACE and PVE, including the 46 who underwent major liver resection as scheduled. The median maximum total bilirubin level after major liver resection ($n=46$) was 1.4 (range 0.4–2.8) mg/dL. The 1-, 3-, and 5-year survival values of patients with and without portal venous thrombi who underwent major liver resection after sequential TACE and PVE were 74.1%, 55.6%, and 55.6% ($n=12$) and 84.7%, 64.7%, and 64.7% ($n=34$), respectively.

Although it is generally accepted that sequential TACE and PVE decrease the rate of postoperative complications after major hepatectomy in patients with fibrotic or cirrhotic livers, their effect on long-term patient survival remains unclear. However, two studies reported the results in favor of the use of PVE or combined use of TACE and PVE.[15,53]

26.3 Conclusion

In conclusion, double preparation with initial TACE followed by PVE is an effective preoperative intervention in patients with HCC scheduled for major liver resection. This double preparation is well tolerated and enhances the hypertrophy process of the FRL in patients with chronic liver injury. It also suppresses tumor growth during the preparation period for the resection. Furthermore, PVE functions as a preoperative test to select suitable candidates for major liver resection. The effect of this preparation on long-term outcomes remains to be clarified.

References

1. Schindl MJ, Redhead DN, Fearon KC, et al. The value of residual liver volume as a predictor of hepatic dysfunction and infection after major liver resection. *Gut*. 2005;54: 289-296.
2. Shirabe K, Shimada M, Gion T, et al. Postoperative liver failure after major hepatic resection for hepatocellular carcinoma in the modern era with special reference to remnant liver volume. *J Am Coll Surg*. 1999;188:304-309.
3. Shoup M, Gonen M, D'Angelica M, et al. Volumetric analysis predicts hepatic dysfunction in patients undergoing major liver resection. *J Gastrointest Surg*. 2003;7:325-330.
4. Truant S, Oberlin O, Sergent G, et al. Remnant liver volume to body weight ratio>or=0.5%: a new cut-off to estimate postoperative risks after extended resection in noncirrhotic liver. *J Am Coll Surg*. 2007;204:22-33.
5. Boillot O, Delafosse B, Mechet I. Small-for-size partial liver graft in an adult recipient; a new transplant technique. *Lancet*. 2002;359:406-407.
6. Man K, Fan ST, Lo CM, et al. Graft injury in relation to graft size in right lobe live donor liver transplantation. *Ann Surg*. 2003;237:256-264.
7. Abulkhir A, Limongelli P, Healey AJ, et al. Preoperative portal vein embolization for major liver resection: a meta-analysis. *Ann Surg*. 2008;247:49-57.
8. Imamura H, Takayama T, Makuuchi M. Place of portal vein embolization. In: Blumgart LH, Belghiti J, eds. *Surgery of the Liver, Biliary Tract and Pancreas*. 4th ed. New York: W.B. Saunders; 2006.
9. Makuuchi M, Thai BL, Takayasu K, et al. Preoperative portal embolization to increase safety of major hepatectomy for hilar bile duct carcinoma: a preliminary report. *Surgery*. 1990;107:521-527.
10. Makuuchi M, Takayasu K, Takuma T, et al. Preoperative transcatheter embolization of the portal venous branch for patients receiving extended lobectomy due to the bile duct carcinoma. *J Jpn Surg Assoc*. 1984;45:1558-1564.
11. Aoki T, Imamura H, Hasegawa K, et al. Sequential preoperative arterial and portal venous embolizations in patients with hepatocellular carcinoma. *Arch Surg*. 2004;139:766-774.

12. Azoulay D, Castaing D, Krissat J, et al. Percutaneous portal vein embolization increases the feasibility and safety of major liver resection for hepatocellular carcinoma in injured liver. *Ann Surg*. 2000;232:665-672.
13. Farges O, Belghiti J, Kianmanesh R, et al. Portal vein embolization before right hepatectomy: prospective clinical trial. *Ann Surg*. 2003;237:208-217.
14. Imamura H, Seyama Y, Makuuchi M, et al. Sequential TACE and PVE for HCC: the University of Tokyo experience. *Semin Interv Radiol*. 2008;25:146-154.
15. Ogata S, Belghiti J, Farges O, et al. Sequential arterial and portal vein embolizations before right hepatectomy in patients with cirrhosis and hepatocellular carcinoma. *Br J Surg*. 2006;93:1091-1098.
16. Sugawara Y, Yamamoto J, Higashi H, et al. Preoperative portal embolization in patients with hepatocellular carcinoma. *World J Surg*. 2002;26:105-110.
17. Tanaka H, Hirohashi K, Kubo S, et al. Preoperative portal vein embolization improves prognosis after right hepatectomy for hepatocellular carcinoma in patients with impaired hepatic function. *Br J Surg*. 2000;87:879-882.
18. Yamakado K, Takeda K, Matsumura K, et al. Regeneration of the un-embolized liver parenchyma following portal vein embolization. *J Hepatol*. 1997;27:871-880.
19. Palavecino M, Chun YS, Madoff DC, et al. Major hepatic résection for hepatocellular carcinoma with or without portal vein embolization: perioperative outcome and survival. *Surgery*. 2009;145(4):399-405.
20. Hasegawa K, Kokudo N, Imamura H, et al. Prognostic impact of anatomic resection for hepatocellular carcinoma. *Ann Surg*. 2005;242:252-259.
21. Imamura H, Matsuyama Y, Miyagawa Y, et al. Prognostic significance of anatomical resection and des-γ-carboxy prothrombin in patients with hepatocellular carcinoma. *Br J Surg*. 1999;86:1032-1038.
22. Makuuchi M, Hasegawa H, Yamazaki S. Ultrasonically guided subsegmentectomy. *Surg Gynecol Obstet*. 1985;161: 346-350.
23. Regimbeau JM, Kianmanesh R, Farges O, et al. Extent of liver resection influences the outcome in patients with cirrhosis and small hepatocellular carcinoma. *Surgery*. 2002;131:311-317.
24. Llovet JM, Real MI, Montana X, et al. Arterial embolisation or chemoembolisation versus symptomatic treatment in patients with unresectable hepatocellular carcinoma: a randomised controlled trial. *Lancet*. 2002;18:1734-1739.
25. Lo CM, Ngan H, Tso WK, et al. Randomized controlled trial of transarterial lipiodol chemoembolization for unresectable hepatocellular carcinoma. *Hepatology*. 2002;35: 1164-1171.
26. Chua TC, Liauw W, Saxena A, et al. Systematic review of neoadjuvant transarterial chemoembolization for resectable hepatocellular carcinoma. *Liver Int*. 2010;30:166-174.
27. Zhong C, Guo RP, Li JQ, et al. A randomized controlled trial of hepatectomy with adjuvant transcatheter arterial chemoembolization versus hepatectomy alone for Stage III A hepatocellular carcinoma. *J Cancer Res Clin Oncol*. 2009; 135:1437-1445.
28. Abdalla EK, Barnett CC, Doherty D, et al. Extended hepatectomy in patients with hepatobiliary malignancies with and without preoperative portal vein embolization. *Arch Surg*. 2002;137:675-680; discussion 680–681.
29. Kubota K, Ina H, Okada Y, et al. Growth rate of primary single hepatocellular carcinoma: determining optimal screening interval with contrast enhanced computed tomography. *Dig Dis Sci*. 2003;48:581-586.
30. Kishi Y, Abdalla EK, Chun YS, et al. Three hundred and one consecutive extended right hepatectomies: evaluation of outcome based on systematic liver volumetry. *Ann Surg*. 2009;250:540-548.
31. Imamura H, Seyama Y, Kokudo N, et al. One thousand fifty-six hepatectomies without mortality in 8 years. *Arch Surg*. 2003;138:1198-2106.
32. Imamura H, Sano K, Sugawara Y, et al. Assessment of hepatic reserve for indication of hepatic resection: decision tree incorporating indocyanine green test. *J Hepatobiliary Pancreat Surg*. 2005;12:16-22.
33. Kubota K, Makuuchi M, Kusaka K, et al. Measurement of liver volume and hepatic functional reserve as a guide to decision-making in resectional surgery for hepatic tumors. *Hepatology*. 1997;26:1176-1181.
34. Chen MF, Hwang TL, Hung CF. Human regeneration after major hepatectomy: a study of liver volume by computed tomography. *Ann Surg*. 1991;213:227-229.
35. Nagasue N, Yukaya H, Ogawa Y, et al. Human liver regeneration after major hepatic resection: a study of normal liver and livers with chronic hepatitis and cirrhosis. *Ann Surg*. 1987;206:30-39.
36. Yamanaka N, Okamato E, Kawamura E, et al. Dynamics of normal and injured human liver regeneration after hepatectomy as assessed on the basis of computed tomography and liver function. *Hepatology*. 1993;18:79-85.
37. Lautt WW. Mechanism and role of intrinsic regulation of hepatic arterial blood flow: hepatic arterial buffer response. *Am J Physiol*. 1984;249:G549-G556.
38. Nagino M, Nimura Y, Kamiya J, et al. Immediate increase in arterial blood flow in embolized hepatic segments after portal vein embolization: CT demonstration. *Am J Roentgenol*. 1998;171:1037-1039.
39. Byun JH, Kim TK, Lee CW, et al. Arterioportal shunt: prevalence in small hemangiomas versus that in hepatocellular carcinomas 3 cm or smaller at two-phase helical CT. *Radiology*. 2004;232:354-356.
40. Luo MY, Shan H, Jiang ZB, et al. Capability of multidetector CT to diagnose hepatocellular carcinoma-associated arterio-portal shunt. *World J Gastroenterol*. 2005;11:2666-2669.
41. Ngan H, Peh WC. Arteriovenous shunting in hepatocellular carcinoma: its prevalence and clinical significance. *Clin Radiol*. 1997;52:36-40.
42. Kimura S, Okazaki M, Higashihara H, et al. Analysis of the origin of the right inferior phrenic artery in 178 patients with hepatocellular carcinoma treated by chemoembolization via the right inferior phrenic artery. *Acta Radiol*. 2007;48: 728-733.
43. Nakayama A, Imamura H, Matsuyama Y, et al. Value of lipiodol computed tomography and digital subtraction angiography in the era of helical biphasic computed tomography as preoperative assessment of hepatocellular carcinoma. *Ann Surg*. 2001;234:56-62.
44. Nagino M, Nimura Y, Kamiya J, et al. Selective percutaneous transhepatic embolization of the portal vein in preparation for extensive liver resection: the ipsilateral approach. *Radiology*. 1996;200:559-563.

45. de Baere T, Roche A, Elias D, et al. Preoperative portal vein embolization for extension of hepatectomy indications. *Hepatology*. 1996;24:1386-1391.
46. Imamura H, Shimada R, Kubota M, et al. Preoperative portal vein embolization: an audit of 84 patients. *Hepatology*. 1999;29:1099-1105.
47. Ribero D, Abdalla EK, Madoff DC, et al. Portal vein embolization before major hepatectomy and its effects on regeneration, resectability and outcome. *Br J Surg*. 2007;94:1386-1394.
48. Gruttadauria S, Gridelli B. Sequential preoperative ipsilateral portal and arterial embolization in patients with liver tumors: is it really the best approach? *World J Surg*. 2007;31:2427-2428.
49. Nagino M, Kanai M, Morioka A, et al. Portal and arterial embolization before extensive liver resection in patients with markedly poor functional reserve. *J Vasc Interv Radiol*. 2000;11:1063-1068.
50. Takayama T, Makuuchi M, Kosuge T, et al. Preoperative portal vein embolization. *Ann Surg*. 1997;68:745-750.
51. Goto Y, Nagino M, Nimura Y. Doppler estimation of portal blood flow after percutaneous transhepatic portal vein embolization. *Ann Surg*. 1998;228:209-213.
52. Vetelainen R, Dinant S, van Vliet A, et al. Portal vein ligation is as effective as sequential portal vein and hepatic artery ligation in inducing contralateral liver hypertrophy in a rat model. *J Vasc Interv Radiol*. 2006;17:1181-1188.
53. Wakabayashi H, Ishimura K, Okano K, et al. Application of preoperative portal vein embolization before major hepatic resection in patients with normal or abnormal liver parenchyma. *Surgery*. 2002;131:26-33.
54. Shimada R, Imamura H, Nakayama A, et al. Changes in blood flow and function of the liver after right portal vein embolization. *Arch Surg*. 2002;137:1384-1388.

Part VI

Evidence and the Future

Chemotherapy and Its Effect on Liver Hypertrophy

27

Béatrice Aussilhou and Jacques Belghiti

Abstract

Systemic chemotherapy, which is routinely used before liver resection for colorectal liver metastases (CRLM), can induce parenchymal liver injury, including steatosis, steatohepatitis, and sinusoidal injuries leading to fibrosis. These chemo-induced lesions could decrease the tolerance of liver resection and impair liver regeneration resulting in a higher risk of postoperative complications. We aimed to review in this chapter the occurrence, rate, and consequences of preoperative chemotherapy in patients considered for liver resection of CRLM. We focused on the impact of chemotherapy on liver regeneration considering the need to pursuit oncological treatment in order to prevent tumoral development of CRLM in the future hypertrophied liver. The absence of hypertrophy after portal obstruction remains a contraindication to major liver resection.

Keywords

Systemic chemotherapy • Liver hypertrophy • Liver resection • Portal vein obstruction • Liver insufficiency

Preoperative chemotherapy is increasingly used before liver resection of colorectal liver metastases (CRLM), which remains the unique curative treatment. Optimal chemotherapy, such as FOLFOX (leucovorin, 5-fluorouracil, and oxaliplatin), FOLFIRI (folinic acid, 5-fluorouracil, and irinotecan), and novel targeted agents (humanized monoclonal antibody against vascular endothelial growth factor receptor that inhibits tumor angiogenesis as bevacizumab and an anti-epidermal growth factor receptor as cetuximab) have considerably improved the response rate of CRLM.[1] This medical treatment improves long-term survival, increases the number of patients who become candidates to a curative resection, and gives an important predictive factor for survival when there is a major histological response.[2] Liver surgeons have to face with increasing number of patients, perioperatively treated with chemotherapy, with bilobar CRLM requiring complex liver resection. Future remnant liver (FRL) volume modulation, including preoperative right portal vein embolization (PVE), and the two-stage operative strategy, allows surgeons to perform more extended liver resection. However, the impact of chemotherapy on the non-tumorous liver parenchyma may limit the regenerative capacity of the FRL and the tolerance of these resections.[3] Pathologic findings of the

J. Belghiti (✉)
Department of Hepato-Pancreato-Biliary Surgery and Liver Transplantation, Beaujon Hospital, 100, boulevard du Général Leclerc, 92110 Clichy, France
e-mail: jacques.belghiti@bjn.aphp.fr

D.C. Madoff et al. (eds.), *Venous Embolization of the Liver*,
DOI 10.1007/978-1-84882-122-4_27,

Table 27.1 Liver damages caused by chemotherapy and their impact on postoperative outcome after liver resection

Implicated drugs Liver damages	5 FU and leucovorin	Oxaliplatin	Irinotecan	Targeted therapies	Clinical impact on the postoperative outcome
Steatosis	30–40%	–	–	–	Infectious complications
Steatohepatitis		–	10–20% (higher risk in patients with BMI >25)	–	Liver failure Increased 90-day mortality (15%)
Sinusoidal obstruction syndrome		19–70%	–	–	Liver failure Ascites Increased blood transfusion requirement

non-tumorous liver parenchyma, including steatosis, steatohepatitis, and vascular changes also called "sinusoidal obstruction syndrome" (SOS) could adversely affect regenerative capacity of the liver.[4,5] This review aimed to summarize the impact of chemotherapy on the liver parenchyma regarding its regenerative capacity after partial liver resection or after PVE.

27.1 Hepatotoxicity of Chemotherapy

The types of pathology observed in liver specimens from patients treated with preoperative chemotherapy include steatosis, steatohepatitis, and sinusoidal injuries (Table 27.1). An association between steatosis and chemotherapy was first discovered in patients who received 5-FU,[6,7] but it seems that all the chemotherapy agents used in colorectal cancer appear to be able to induce lesions of steatosis.[8]

Steatohepatitis, including steatosis, lobular inflammation, and ballooning of the hepatocytes was first noted as a complication of chemotherapy in patients treated with irinotecan or oxaliplatin but its association with irinotecan was clearly demonstrated by Vauthey et al.[8] They examined a series of 94 patients treated with FOLFIRI and noted that obese patients had a higher risk for developing irinotecan-induced steatohepatitis. There are controversies concerning prevalence and grading steatosis and steatohepatitis.[9] These variabilities could be related to the high prevalence of steatosis and steatohepatitis in patients with obesity, alcohol consumption, and diabetes.[10,11]

Overall features including vascular changes are called "sinusoidal obstruction syndrome" (SOS). SOS results from damage to endothelial cells lining the sinusoids of the liver. SOS was previously termed veno-occlusive disease which is a well-known complication of the high-dose chemotherapy regimens used in stem cell transplantation. The major liver toxicity of oxaliplatin-based regimen appears to be targeted against the endothelial cells lining the sinusoids with a broader pattern of parenchymal hepatic injury, including centrilobular sinusoidal distension, peliosis, and nodular regenerative hyperplasia (NRH).[4] These lesions of NRH are secondary to obliterative lesions in the portal vein or hepatic sinusoids. Rubbia-Brandt et al. reported an association between oxaliplatin-based regimen and the presence of these vascular changes in 78% of the patients treated with oxaliplatin.[4] The clinical implications of these parenchymal injuries are debated and remain to be fully evaluated.

Fewer data exist about the impact of the targeted therapies on the liver parenchyma. Targeted therapies, which are not clearly responsible of specific parenchymal lesions, seem to have a protective effect against parenchymal changes induced by oxaliplatin.[10] Ribero et al. noted less sinusoidal obstruction after preoperative treatment with bevacizumab in comparison with patients treated with standard chemotherapy in whom the sinusoidal obstruction were more frequent (27% versus 53%).[12]

27.2 Impact of Parenchymal Injuries Induced by Chemotherapy and Its Effects on Liver Hypertrophy After PVO and on Postoperative Outcome After Hepatectomy

Postoperative outcome after liver resection is correlated with the amount of remnant liver and its capacity of regeneration.[13] Liver regeneration is influenced by several factors including extent of resection, age, and hepatotrophic factors in the portal blood.[14-20] Liver regeneration is proportional to the amount of liver resected.[13] On the other hand, the lesser the liver volume was immediately after the operation, the faster the liver regenerated.[21] Starzl et al., in 1975, demonstrated that insulin had an important hepatotrophic influence.[20] This concept could explain the high risk of complications after a concomitant resection of the liver associated with a pancreatoduodenectomy (PD). This surgery including major liver resection and pancreatic resection requires the systematic use of PVE preoperatively.[22] Experimental studies on liver regeneration have postulated that the presence of hepatotrophic pancreatic factors such as glucagon and insulin play a determinant role in hepatic regeneration after liver resection.[23] Moreover, it has been proved recently that platelet derived serotonin, which is activated in the duodenum mediates liver regeneration.[24] The presence of parenchymal changes, i.e., fibrosis, decreases the rate and the rapidity of regeneration.[14] Chemotherapy which alters the non-tumorous parenchyma may influence the tolerance of liver resection. Whether or not chemotherapy may influence liver regeneration after partial resection or after portal vein obstruction remains debated. It is unclear if regeneration can be impaired by the drug itself including novel targeted agents; by the cumulative doses received; by systemic or intra-arterial administration or through histological changes induced by chemotherapy.

There is no consistent data demonstrating that steatosis impairs liver regeneration. Whether or not steatosis increases surgical morbidity remains debated. The impact of steatosis after minor resection is probably negligible. After major resection, patients with severe steatosis (>50–60%) had more postoperative liver dysfunction, infectious complications, and time spent in the intensive care unit.[25]

The presence of steatohepatitis can impair postoperative liver outcome. Fernandez et al. were the first to report post resection liver failure leading to death within 90 days, in a patient who developed severe steatohepatitis following oxaliplatin chemotherapy.[5] These findings suggest that steatohepatitis may result in insufficiency of the remnant liver to regenerate following major hepatic resection, which can lead to liver failure. Vauthey et al. confirmed that steatohepatitis due to irinotecan-based chemotherapy seems to be related to impair liver regeneration which in turn led to liver insufficiency and death after liver resection. They showed that among the 406 patients who were treated for liver metastases, 248 patients (61.1%) received preoperative chemotherapy. Among these latter patients, 92 (22.7%) had parenchymal lesions on the final pathologic analysis of the resected specimen. There were 6 deaths (6.5%) in these 92 patients with hepatic injury in comparison with 5 deaths (1.6%) in 314 patients without hepatic injury. There was no death in the patients who had sinusoidal injury whereas the patients with steatohepatitis had a higher 90-day mortality rate than patients without steatohepatitis (14.7% versus 1.6%, $p=0.001$).[8] However, it should be noted that two smaller surgical series did not show a difference in terms of morbidity or mortality in patients treated preoperatively with chemotherapy including irinotecan-containing regimens.[26,27]

The impact of SOS on liver regeneration was first suggested by Karoui et al. showing that after major liver resection, a moderate and transient liver insufficiency was present in 11% in the group treated with chemotherapy whereas it was nil in the control group.[28] Among the 67 patients included in this study, 45 received preoperative chemotherapy and 22 didn't receive any preoperative treatment. After major hepatic resection, mortality was nil in the two groups within 30 days postoperatively. However, 17 patients of 45 from the group treated with chemotherapy presented postoperative complications whereas there were 3 of 22 in the group without chemotherapy who had postoperative complications ($p=0.003$). The rate of sinusoidal dilatation, which was related to the number of cycles, was 49% of patients in the chemotherapy group whereas it was observed in 25% in the control group ($p=0.005$).[28] Soubrane et al. showed that there was significantly more postoperative liver dysfunction and ascites in patients with severe lesions of SOS compared with patients with moderate lesions of SOS. After 51 major hepatic resections, 26 patients of 38 who had severe lesions of SOS presented postoperative hepatic dysfunction, whereas 3 patients of 13 who had low-grade lesions of SOS had postoperative hepatic dysfunction ($p=0.004$).[29] In the latter study there was no correlation between the dose of administrated chemotherapy before liver resection and severity of SOS. A short interval between the end of chemotherapy and liver resection seemed to be a risk factor of high grade of SOS lesions at the time of surgery. Nakano et al. showed also that sinusoidal damages were associated with an increased morbidity following major liver resection especially a higher risk of postoperative liver insufficiency.[30] Presence of severe sinusoidal obstruction was associated with increased risk of bleeding and blood transfusion by Aloia et al. but not with increased mortality.[31] A large randomized trial from the European Organization for Research and Treatment of Cancer (EORTC), comparing surgical resection alone with perioperative (i.e., chemotherapy before and after surgery) FOLFOX4 chemotherapy showed a higher rate of complications (25% versus 16%) but no difference in mortality.[2] These results suggest that liver damages, in particular vascular changes (SOS), induced by chemotherapy, especially oxaliplatin, seem to cause liver failure due to an impairment of liver regeneration after liver resection.[8] However, the fact that oxaliplatin increases perioperative morbidity following hepatectomy remains controversial. Parikh et al. reported that there was no significant difference in postoperative mortality and morbidity in patients receiving systemic chemotherapy in comparison with those without neoadjuvant chemotherapy.[32] The same results were found by Pawlik et al. showing that in 212 patients treated for liver metastases including 153 who received neoadjuvant chemotherapy, the postoperative complication rate was similar between the no-chemotherapy group (30.5%) and the chemotherapy group (35.3%) ($p=0.79$).[33] They showed the type of chemotherapy predicted distinct hepatic lesions and therefore oxaliplatin was associated with grade 3 sinusoidal dilatation compared with no chemotherapy. The complication rate did not differ based on the type of chemotherapy regimen. Hewes et al. demonstrated no disadvantage related to the use of oxaliplatin in term of the postoperative course, in comparison with patients who had not received oxaliplatin.[34] Mehta et al. noted a nonsignificant trend towards increased biliary complications in patients receiving oxaliplatin.[35] Future studies grading vascular obstruction according to the operative risk would probably clarify the impact of chemotherapy on the post-resection risk. In particular, studies focusing on the presence of NRH in patients considered for major liver resection are required.

In experimental models various antimitotic agents can interfere with liver resection-induced regeneration. The treatment with 5-FU following hepatectomy delayed liver cell division in rats.[36] Di Stefano et al. showed that doxorubicin decreases mitotic index in hepatectomized rats.[37] In their study, Engum et al. evaluating liver regeneration in rats after 70% hepatectomy, showed that (^{3}H-TdR) DNA incorporation was not inhibited by cisplatin.[38]

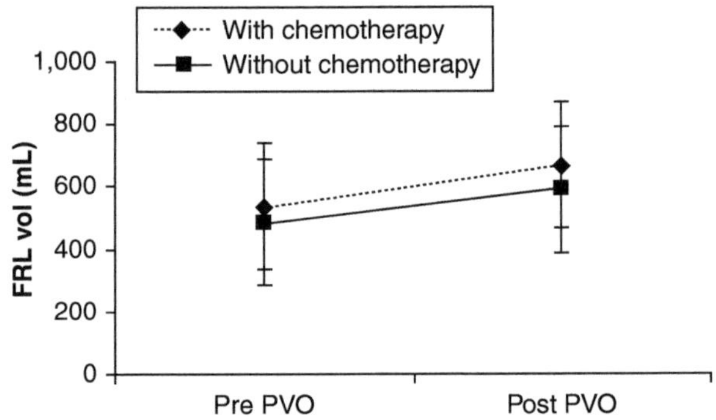

Fig. 27.1 Volume of the future remnant liver (FRL) before and 4–6 weeks after right portal vein obstruction, in patients whose chemotherapy was continued ($n=10$) or interrupted ($n=10$)[41]

The first clinical study showing an impact of chemotherapy on hypertrophy induced by PVE was published in 2006. Beal et al. showed in two small groups of patients that chemotherapy (mainly oxaliplatin-based chemotherapy) administrated in the interval between PVE and hepatectomy impaired liver hypertrophy (89 mL versus 135 mL $p=0.016$).[39] In this latter study, patients without chemotherapy were more likely to have tumor progression between the PVE and the hepatectomy. The authors concluded that peri-procedure chemotherapy did reduce liver hypertrophy following PVE. This intuitive "toxic" effect of chemotherapy on liver regeneration leads many authors to delay for 3–4 weeks both liver resection and PVE in patients who received preoperative chemotherapy.[40] In a retrospective study, we showed that chemotherapy after PV occlusion had no major effect on hypertrophy of the FRL.[41] The comparison of the two groups of patients who had undergone right portal vein obstruction showed that hypertrophy of the FRL was similar in the group in whom chemotherapy was maintained until surgery compared with the group in whom chemotherapy was interrupted at least 1 month prior to portal obstruction (33% vs. 25%) (Fig. 27.1). In addition, the morbidity rate after resection was similar in the two groups (57% in each group). We concluded that continuing chemotherapy while portal vein obstruction is performed did not impair the hypertrophy of the FRL nor the postoperative course after liver resection. This study was confirmed by a similar study from Covey et al.[42] In a subgroup of 43 patients who underwent PVE during neoadjuvant chemotherapy, they showed that after a median wait of 30 ± 2 days after PVE, patients on neoadjuvant chemotherapy experienced a median contralateral (nonembolized) liver

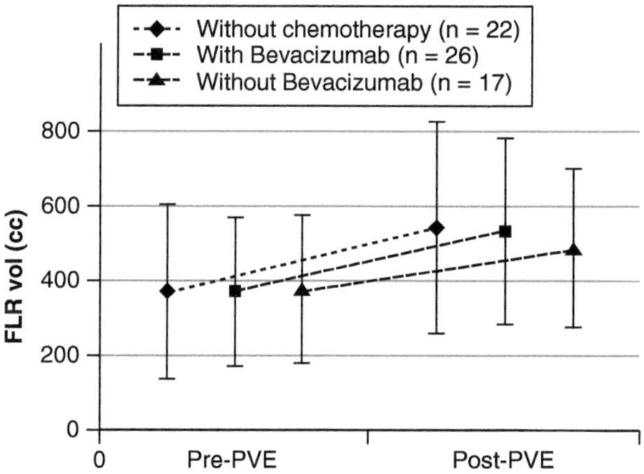

Fig. 27.2 Changes in absolute future liver remnant volume after portal vein embolization in patients without chemotherapy (*solid line*), and with chemotherapy with bevacizumab (*dotted line*), and without bevacizumab (*dashed line*), $p = .35$. Values are mean ± standard deviation[48]

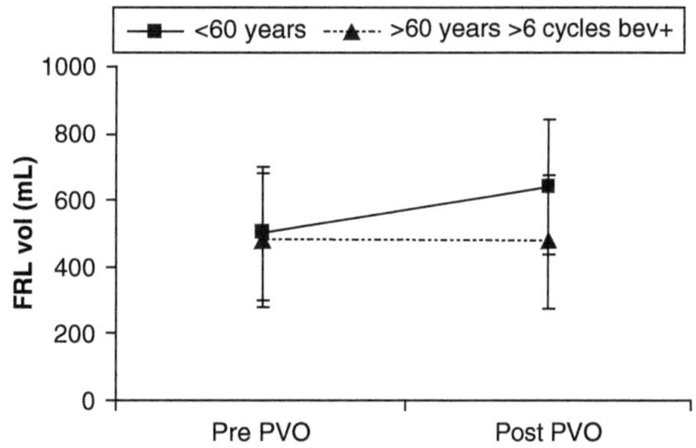

Fig. 27.3 Volume of the future remnant liver (*FRL*) before and after portal vein occlusion (*PVO*) depending on the age of the patients. After PVO, in patients with age ≥60 years who received >6 cycles of bevacizumab (bev+) the hypertrophy rate was significantly lower (0.6 ± 16% *versus* 38 ± 35%, $p < 0.005$) than in patients <60 years who received bevacizumab[49]

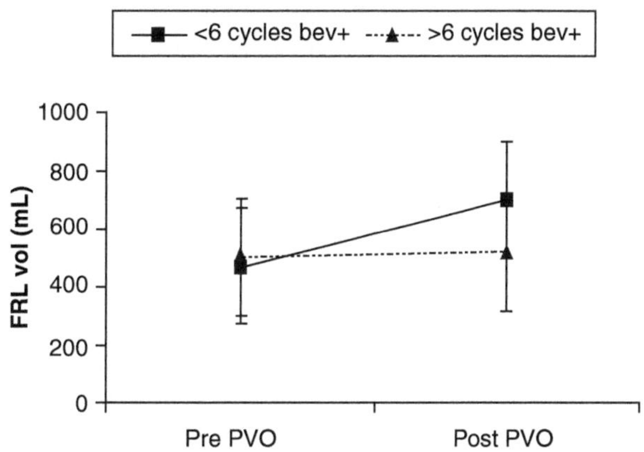

Fig. 27.4 Volume of the future remnant liver (*FRL*) before and after portal vein occlusion (*PVO*) in patients who received bevacizumab (*bev*). In the bev + group, the hypertrophy rate of patients who received <6 cycles was significantly higher than those receiving ≥6 cycles (mean ± SD: 50 ± 15% *versus* 4.7 ± 15%, $p < 0.005$)[49]

growth of 22% compared with 26% for those ($n = 57$) without chemotherapy. More recently, Tanaka et al. confirmed that pre-hepatectomy chemotherapy does not impair liver hypertrophy induced either by PVE or by portal vein ligation.[43]

The impact of targeted therapies on liver regeneration caused a great interest since inhibition of VEGFR-2 can inhibit post-hepatectomy liver regeneration in a murine model and inhibit wound healing in clinical studies.[44] However, the impact of targeted therapies after hepatic resection seems to be limited. The study from Kesmodel et al. comparing 81 patients treated with standard chemotherapy-regimen in association with bevacizumab with 44 patients treated with standard chemotherapy failed to find any difference in morbidity or mortality between the two groups.[45] These results are in accordance with those of two other smaller series raising similar safety of surgery in patients treated with bevacizumab combined with standard chemotherapy.[46,47] Zorzi et al., in a large series of 65 patients including 26 who received bevacizumab, didn't find the negative effect of bevacizumab on liver hypertrophy after PV occlusion.[48] In this retrospective study from 1995 to 2007, FRL hypertrophy was evaluated 2–10 weeks after PVE (Fig. 27.2). In a smaller study, but more recent, we showed a decrease in terms of the degree of hypertrophy after PV occlusion in aged patients (>60 years old) and in those who received more than six cycles of bevacizumab (Figs. 27.3 and 27.4).[49] The hypertrophy rate was significantly lower in the group preoperatively treated with bevacizumab (15%) compared with the hypertrophy rate in the group treated without bevacizumab (40%, $p < 0.05$). Of interest, in this study there was no correlation between the post-chemotherapy parenchymal damages and liver regeneration. In this latter study more patients received more than six cycles and the delay between the end of chemotherapy and PVE was smaller than in the study from Zorzi et al. These methods can explain why they didn't find impaired liver hypertrophy after bevacizumab treatment.

27.3 Conclusion

Surgical resection which remains the unique possibility to obtain a curative treatment for CRLM has been reinforced by perioperative chemotherapy. A great majority of patients in whom extensive liver resection is considered, is routinely treated with numerous cycles of chemotherapy. There are several arguments suggesting that severe histological changes induced by preoperative chemotherapy can impair post resection regeneration. The negative impact of preoperative chemotherapy is enhanced by a large number of chemotherapy cycles, elderly patients, and underlying liver alterations induced by obesity, diabetes, and alcohol consumption. In such risky groups, there are arguments favoring preoperative volume modulation with PV occlusion. PVE which can be routinely and safely performed may have the risk of tumor progression and therefore requires the non interruption of chemotherapy. Chemotherapy has few impacts on preoperative hypertrophy. Providing a delay of 4–6 weeks of interruption is respected before surgery, major procedures can be considered in patients who experienced regeneration after PVE.

References

1. Hurwitz H, Fehrenbacher L, Novotny W, et al. Bevacizumab plus irinotecan, fluorouracil, and leucoverin for metastatic colorectal cancer. *N Engl J Med*. 2004;350:2335-2342.
2. Nordlinger B, Sorbye H, Glimelius B, et al. Perioperative chemotherapy with FOLFOX4 and surgery versus surgery alone for resectable liver metastases from colorectal cancer (EORTC Intergroup trial 40983): a randomised controlled trial. *Lancet*. 2008;371:1007-1016.
3. Zorzi D, Laurent A, Pawlik TM, et al. Chemotherapy-associated hepatotoxicity and surgery for colorectal liver metastases. *Br J Surg*. 2007;94:274-286.
4. Rubbia-Brandt L, Audard V, Sartoretti P, et al. Severe hepatic sinusoidal obstruction associated with oxaliplatin-based chemotherapy in patients with metastatic colorectal cancer. *Ann Oncol*. 2004;15:460-466.
5. Fernandez FG, Ritter J, Goodwin JW, et al. Effect of steatohepatitis associated with irinotecan or oxaliplatin pretreatment on resectability of hepatic colorectal metastases. *J Am Coll Surg*. 2005;200:845-853.
6. Sorensen P, Edal AL, Madsen EL, et al. Reversible hepatic steatosis in patients treated with interferon alfa-2a and 5-fluorouracil. *Cancer*. 1995;75:2592-2596.
7. Moertel CG, Fleming TR, Macdonald JS, et al. Hepatic toxicity associated with fluorouracil plus levamisole adjuvant therapy. *J Clin Oncol*. 1993;11:2386-2390.
8. Vauthey JN, Pawlik TM, Ribero D, et al. Chemotherapy regimen predicts steatohepatitis and an increase in 90-day mortality after surgery for hepatic colorectal metastases. *J Clin Oncol*. 2006;24:2065-2072.
9. Kleiner DE, Brunt ME, Natta MV, et al. Design and validation of a histological scoring system for nonalcoholoc fatty Liver disease. *Hepatology*. 2005;41:1313-1321.
10. Kooby DA, Fong Y, Suriawinata A, et al. Impact of steatosis on perioperative outcome following hepatic resection. *J Gastrointest Surg*. 2003;7:1034-1044.
11. Pathak S, Tang JM, Terlizzo M, et al. Hepatic steatosis, body mass index and long term outcome in patients undergoing hepatectomy for colorectal liver metastases. *Eur J Surg Oncol*. 2010;36:52-57.
12. Ribero D, Wang H, Donadon M, et al. Bevacizumab improves pathologic response and protects against hepatic injury in patients treated with oxaliplatin-based chemotherapy for colorectal liver metastases. *Cancer*. 2007;110:2761-2767.
13. Vauthey JN, Pawlik TM, Abdalla EK, et al. Is extended hepatectomy for hepatobiliary malignancy justified? *Ann Surg*. 2004;239:722-732.
14. Yamanaka N, Okamoto E, Kawamura E, et al. Dynamics of normal and injured human liver regeneration after hepatectomy as assessed on the basis of computed tomography and liver function. *Hepatology*. 1993;18:79-85.
15. Tani M, Tomiya T, Yamada S, et al. Regulating factors of liver regeneration after hepatectomy. *Cancer Chemother Pharmacol*. 1994;33(suppl):29-32.
16. Ogasawara K, Une Y, Nakajima Y, et al. The significance of measuring liver volume using computed tomographic images before and after hepatectomy. *Surg Today*. 1995;25:43-48.
17. Tanaka W, Yamanaka N, Oriyama T, et al. Multivariate analysis of liver regenerative capacity after hepatectomy in humans. *J Hepatobiliary Pancreat Surg*. 1997;4:78-82.
18. Shimada M, Matsumata T, Maeda T, et al. Hepatic regeneration following right lobectomy: estimation of regenerative capacity. *Surg Today*. 1994;24:44-48.
19. Fisher B, Szuch P, Levine M, et al. A portal blood factor as the humoral agent in liver regeneration. *Science*. 1971;171:575-577.
20. Starzl TE, Porter KA, Kashiwagi N, et al. Portal hepatotrophic factors, diabetes mellitus and acute liver atrophy, hypertrophy and regeneration. *Surg Gynecol Obstet*. 1975;141:843-858.
21. Yao AH, Yang Y, Li XC, et al. Hepatic regenerative response in small-sized liver isografts in the rat. *J Surg Res*. 2010;161:328-335.
22. D'Angelica M, Martin RC, Jarnagin WR, et al. Major hepatectomy with simultaneous pancreatectomy for advanced hepatobiliary cancer. *J Am Coll Surg*. 2004;198:570-576.
23. Yokoyama Y, Nagino M, Nimura Y. Mechanism of impaired hepatic regeneration in cholestatic liver. *J Hepatobiliary Pancreat Surg*. 2007;14:159-166.
24. Lesurtel M, Graf R, Aleil B, et al. Platelet derived serotonin mediates liver regeneration. *Science*. 2006;312(5770):104-107.
25. Berhrns KE, Tsiotos GG, DeSouza NF, et al. Hepatic steatosis as a potential risk factor for major hepatic resection. *J Gastrointest Surg*. 1998;2:292-298.
26. Parc Y, Dugué L, Farges O, Hiramatsu K, et al. Preoperative systemic 5-fluorouracil does not increase the risk of liver resection. *Hepatogastroenterology*. 2000;47(36):1703-1705.
27. Yedibela S, Elad L, Wein A, et al. Neoadjuvant chemotherapy does not increase postoperative complication rate after resection of colorectal liver metastases. *Eur J Surg Oncol*. 2005;31:141-146.

28. Karoui M, Penna C, Amin-Hashem M, et al. Influence of preoperative chemotherapy on the risk of major hepatectomy for colorectal liver metastases. *Ann Surg*. 2006;243:1-7.
29. Soubrane O, Brouquet A, Zalinski S, et al. Predicting high grade lesions of sinusoidal obstruction syndrome related to oxaliplatin-based chemotherapy for colorectal liver metastases. *Ann Surg*. 2010;251:454-460.
30. Nakano H, Oussoultzoglou E, Rosso E, et al. Sinusoidal injury increases morbidity after major hepatectomy in patients with colorectal liver metastases receiving preoperative chemotherapy. *Ann Surg*. 2008;247:118-124.
31. Aloia T, Sebagh M, Plasse M, et al. Liver histology and surgical outcomes after preoperative chemotherapy with fluorouracil plus oxaliplatin in colorectal cancer liver metastases. *J Clin Oncol*. 2006;24:4983-4990.
32. Parikh AA, Gentner B, Wu TT, et al. Perioperative complications in patients undergoing major liver resection with or without neoadjuvant chemotherapy. *J Gastrointest Surg*. 2003;7:1082-1088.
33. Pawlik TM, Olino K, Gleisner AL, et al. Preoperative chemotherapy for colorectal liver metastases: impact on hepatic histology and postoperative outcome. *J Gastrointest Surg*. 2007;11:860-868.
34. Hewes JC, Dighe S, Morris RW, et al. Preoperative chemotherapy and the outcome of liver resection for colorectal metastases. *World J Surg*. 2007;31:353-364.
35. Mehta NN, Ravikumar R, Coldham CA, et al. Effect of preoperative chemotherapy on liver resection for colorectal liver metastases. *Eur J Surg Oncol*. 2008;34:782-786.
36. Nagasue N, Kobayashi M, Iwaki A, et al. Effect of 5-fluorouracil on liver regeneration and metabolism after partial hepatectomy in the rat. *Cancer*. 1978;41:435-443.
37. Di Stefano G, Derenzini M, Kratz F, et al. Liver-targeted doxorubicin: effects on rat regenerating hepatocytes. *Liver Int*. 2004;24:246-252.
38. Engum SA, Sidner RA, Miller GA, et al. Early use of cisplatin is safe after partial hepatectomy. *J Pediatr Surg*. 1993;28:411-417.
39. Beal IK, Anthony S, Papadopoulou A, et al. Portal vein embolization prior to hepatic resection for colorectal liver metastases and the effects of periprocedure chemotherapy. *Br J Radiol*. 2006;79:473-478.
40. Wicherts DA, de Haas RJ, Andreani P, et al. Impact of portal vein embolization on long-term survival of patients with primarily unresectable colorectal liver metastases. *Br J Surg*. 2010;97:240-250.
41. Goere D, Farges O, Leporrier J, et al. Chemotherapy does not impair hypertrophy of the left liver after right portal vein obstruction. *J Gastrointest Surg*. 2006;10:365-370.
42. Covey AM, Brown KT, Jarnagin WR, et al. Combined portal vein embolization and neoadjuvant chemotherapy as a treatment strategy for resectable hepatic colorectal metastases. *Ann Surg*. 2008;247:451-455.
43. Tanaka K, Kumamoto T, Matsuyama R, et al. Influence of chemotherapy on liver regeneration induced by portal vein embolization or first hepatectomy of a staged procedure for colorectal liver metastases. *J Gastrointest Surg*. 2010;14:359-368.
44. Van Buren G, Yang A, Dallas N, et al. The effect of molecular therapeutics on liver regeneration in a murine model. *J Clin Oncol*. 2008;26:1836-1842.
45. Kesmodel SB, Ellis LM, Lin E, et al. Preoperative bevacizumab does not significantly increase postoperative complication rates in patients undergoing hepatic surgery for colorectal cancer liver metastases. *J Clin Oncol*. 2008;26:5254-5260.
46. D'Angelica M, Kornprat P, Gonen M, et al. Lack of evidence for increased operative morbidity after hepatectomy with perioperative use of bevacizumab: a matched case-control study. *Ann Surg Oncol*. 2007;14:759-765.
47. Reddy SK, Morse MA, Hurwitz HI, et al. Addition of bevacizumab to irinotecan- and oxaliplatin-based preoperative chemotherapy regimens does not increase morbidity after resection of colorectal liver metastases. *J Am Coll Surg*. 2008;206:96-106.
48. Zorzi D, Chun YS, Madoff DC, Abdalla EK, Vauthey JN. Chemotherapy with bevacizumab does not affect liver regeneration after portal vein embolization in the treatment of colorectal liver metastases. *Ann Surg Oncol*. 2008;15:2765-2772.
49. Aussilhou B, Dokmak S, Faivre S, et al. Preoperative liver hypertrophy induced by portal flow occlusion before major hepatic resection for colorectal metastases can be impaired by bevacizumab. *Ann Surg Oncol*. 2009;16:1553-1559.

Tumor Growth After Portal Vein Embolization

28

Taku Aoki and Norihiro Kokudo

Abstract

Increasing evidence suggests that preoperative PVE itself stimulates tumor growth both in the embolized and nonembolized segments of the liver by altering the blood supply and/or inducing a network of cytokines and growth factors, though the precise mechanism/network has not been fully clarified. This stimulating effect is more obvious in patients with HCC and colorectal liver metastases. Sequential TACE and PVE, two-stage hepatectomy combined with PVE and maintenance chemotherapy after PVE are the currently available strategies to overcome the possible negative effects of PVE on tumor growth without reducing the hypertrophic properties of PVE.

Keywords

Preoperative portal vein embolization • Hepatic resection • Tumor growth after embolization • Embolization and tumor growth

Preoperative portal vein embolization (PVE) is an accepted intervention in patients requiring a major hepatic resection (the resection of three or more Couinaud segments) and in whom the estimated future liver remnant (FLR) is too small to allow a safe resection. First reported by Makuuchi et al.,[1,2] the aim of PVE is to induce the atrophy of the segments to be resected and to induce a compensatory hypertrophy of the nonembolized FLR. Previous reports have documented that PVE has extended the indications for major hepatic resections and has increased the safety of this procedure, even in patients with obstructive jaundice or with underlying chronic liver disease.[3]

N. Kokudo (✉)
Division of Hepato-Biliary-Pancreatic and Transplantation Surgery, Department of Surgery, Graduate School of Medicine, The University of Tokyo, 7-3-1 Hongo, Bunkyo-ku, Tokyo, Japan
e-mail: kokudo-2su@h.u-tokyo.ac.jp

Generally, an interval of 2–4 weeks is required between PVE and resection to enable sufficient hypertrophy of the FLR. During this waiting period, the tumor volume in both the embolized and nonembolized segments is assumed to continue increasing (Figs. 28.1 and 28.2); tumor growth in the nonembolized segments, in particular, may hamper the resectability of the subsequent major hepatectomy. In addition, there is a growing concern that PVE itself may stimulate tumor growth in both the embolized and nonembolized segments. In this chapter, we review the previous reports addressing the effect of PVE on tumor growth.

28.1 Fundamental Speculations on the Effect of PVE on Tumor Growth

Tumor growth after PVE is controlled by three factors: the malignant potential of the tumors, changes in the blood supply after PVE, and changes in cytokines or growth factors after PVE.[4]

D.C. Madoff et al. (eds.), *Venous Embolization of the Liver*,
DOI 10.1007/978-1-84882-122-4_28,

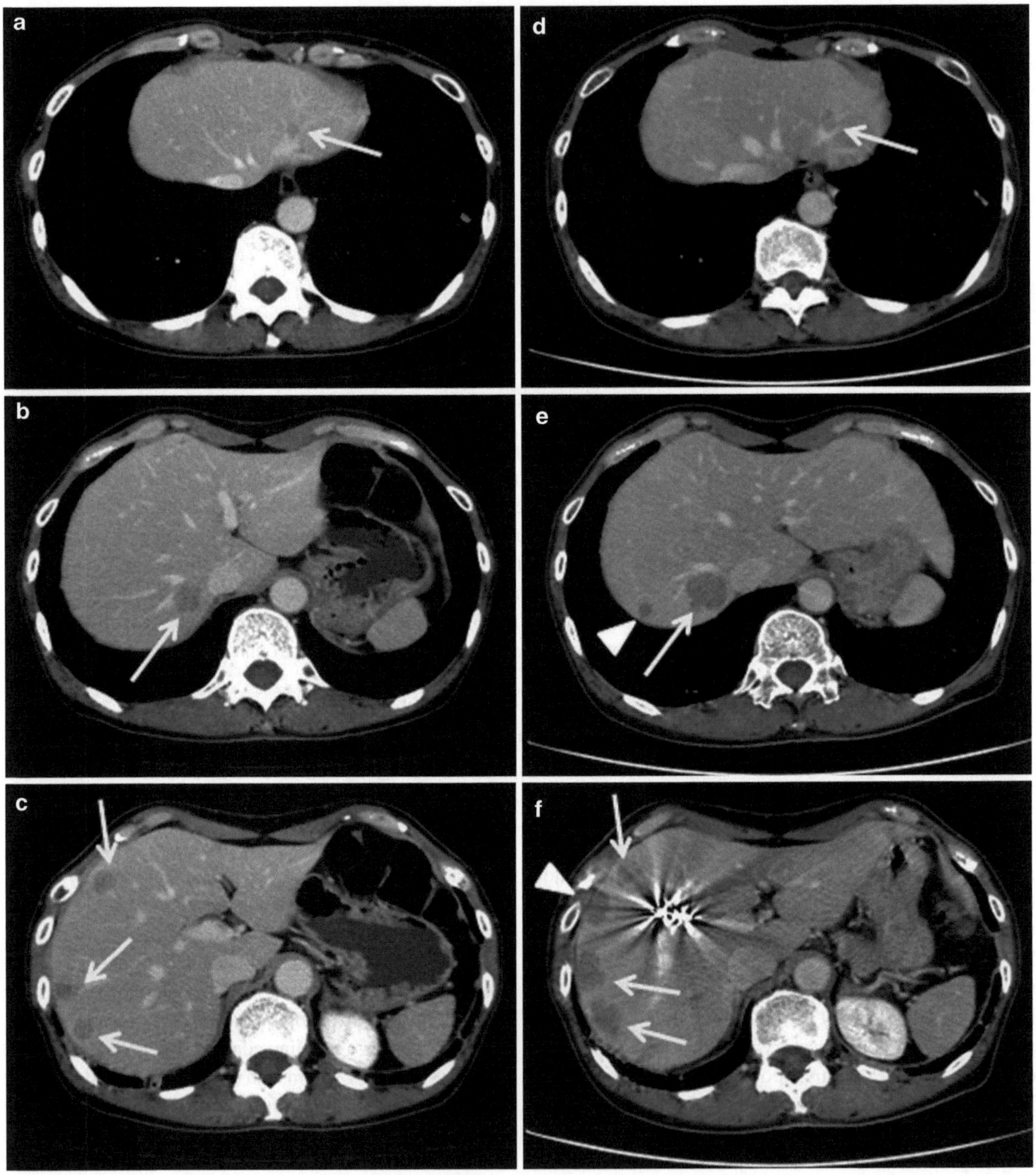

Fig. 28.1 Tumor growth after PVE. CT scans were taken before PVE (**a–c**) and 2 weeks after the PVE (**d–f**). Metastatic tumors showed significant growth in size (*white arrows*) and number (*white arrowheads*) both in the embolized right hemi-liver and nonembolized left hemi-liver. All the tumors were removed by extended right hepatectomy with partial resections, and the patient is alive without recurrecnce 3 years after the operation

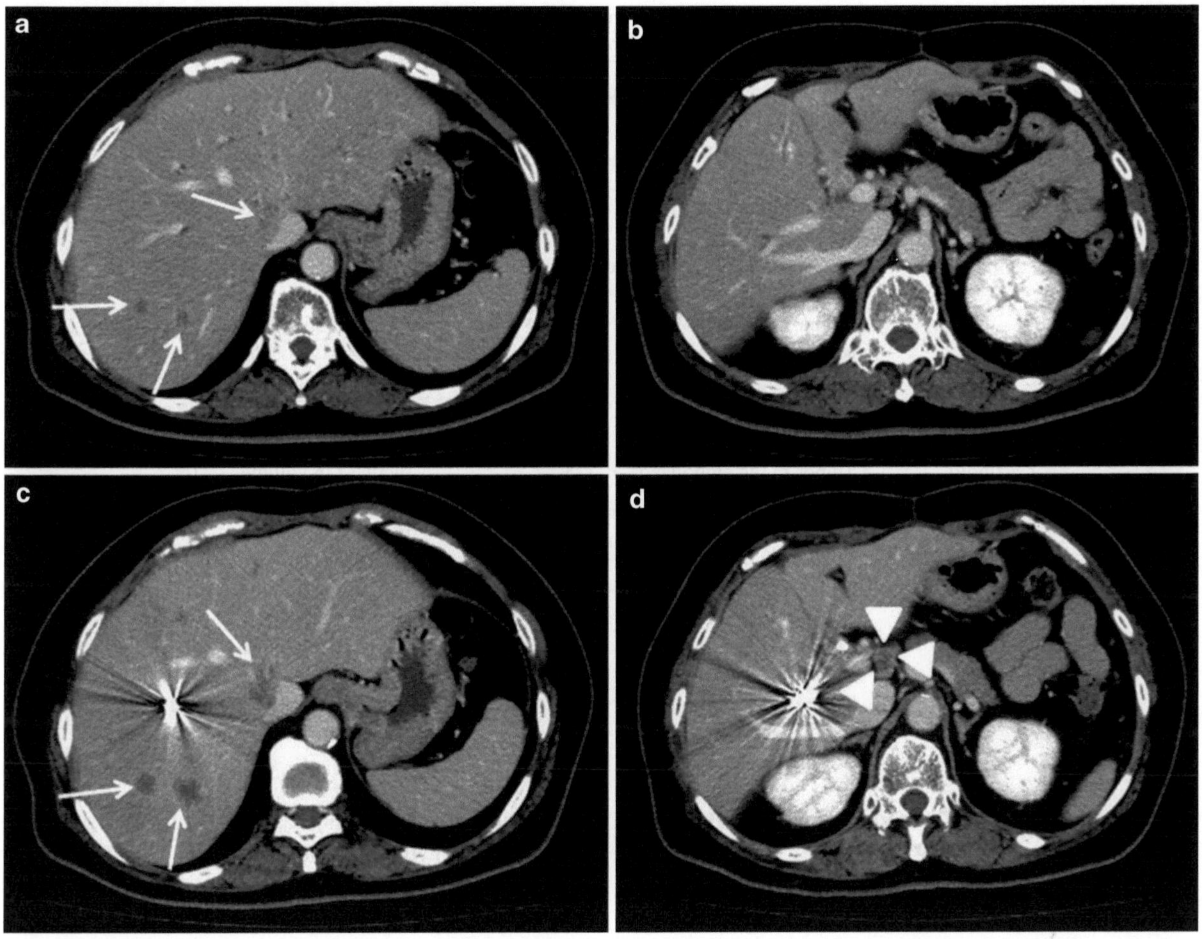

Fig. 28.2 In this case, CT scans taken 2 weeks after the PVE (**c**, **d**) revealed tumor growth in the embolized right h emi-liver (*white arrows*) and lymph nodes metastases in the hepatic hilum (*white arrowheads*) that was not apparent before the PVE (**a**, **b**). The patient underwent systemic chemotherapy, but died 6 months after the PVE due to tumor progression

28.1.1 Changes in Blood Supply After PVE

The liver has a dual blood inflow system, i.e., the portal vein (about 75% of the total hepatic blood flow) and the hepatic artery (about 25% of the total hepatic blood flow). When the hepatic portal blood flow decreases, the total hepatic blood flow is, at least in part, restored by an increase in hepatic arterial blood flow. This regulatory mechanism is known as the hepatic arterial buffer response (HABR).[5,6] This buffer response is maintained, albeit in a blunted manner, even in chronically diseased livers.[7] Actually, the hepatic arterial blood flow in embolized segments has been shown to increase immediately after PVE.[8] Similarly, the portal venous blood flow in the nonembolized segments also increases after PVE. Because the portal vein only passively receives blood flow from the visceral organs, the total portal blood flow remains unchanged before and after PVE.[9] The hepatic arterial blood flow in the nonembolized segments has been reported to be slightly decreased or unchanged after the embolization of the right portal branch.[10]

Because liver tumors are mainly fed by the hepatic artery, the increase in hepatic arterial blood flow induced by HABR may stimulate tumor growth. This theory can explain the accelerated tumor growth in the embolized segments but not in the nonembolized segments, as the arterial flow in the nonembolized segments does not necessarily increase.

Table 28.1 Previous reports describing the influence of PVE on tumor growth

Author	Tumor type	Location	No. of patients	Assessment	Results
Elias et al.[15]	Liver metastases	Tumor in the nonembolized segments	5	Increase in volume	160–1070%
		Liver parenchyma in the nonembolized segments	5	Increase in volume	117–228%
Kokudo et al.[4]	Colorectal metastases	Tumor in the embolized segments	3	Increase in volume	103–106%
		Tumor in the nonembolized segments	3	Increase in volume	105–142%
		Tumor in the embolized segments after PVE	18	Ki-67 labeling index	46.6± 7.2%
		Tumor without PVE	29	Ki-67 labeling index	35.4 ± 12.6%
Barbaro et al.[16]	Colorectal metastases	Tumor in the embolized segments	6	Increase in volume	162–238%
	Cartinoid	Tumor in the embolized segments	3	Increase in volume	0%
Hayashi et al.[17]	HCC	Tumor in the embolized segments	6	Increase in volume before PVE	0.25–3.14 cm^3/day
		Tumor in the embolized segments	6	Increase in volume after PVE	0.71–13.97 cm^3/day
	CCC	Tumor in the embolized segments	2	Increase in volume before PVE	0.22–0.69 cm^3/day
		Tumor in the embolized segments	2	Increase in volume after PVE	0.29–0.69 cm^3/day

28.1.2 Changes in Cytokines or Growth Factors After PVE

The occlusion of portal venous flow is thought to induce the up- and downregulation of numerous cytokines and growth factors, and the process of atrophy/hypertrophy after PVE has been thought to be controlled by the same factors as liver regeneration after a partial hepatectomy[4,11]; however, the complete mechanism responsible for these phenomena remains unclear. Several clinical studies as well as animal experiments have raised a concern that liver regeneration/hypertrophy might promote tumor proliferation, mainly since the growth factors responsible for liver regeneration/hypertrophy had stimulatory effects on tumor cells in vitro. Hepatocyte growth factor (HGF), epidermal growth factor (EGF), transforming growth factor (TGF)-α, tumor necrosis factor (TNF)-α, and interleukin (IL)-6, which are positive regulators of regeneration/hypertrophy, are also candidates for tumor growth–inducing factors after PVE.[12] On the other hand, negative regulators of hepatocyte proliferation, such as TGF-β and IL-1, are strongly expressed in the ligated shrinking lobe in rats.[13] TGF-β works in normal tissue as a tumor suppressor by inhibiting cell proliferation. However, many colorectal carcinomas are resistant to TGF-β-induced growth inhibition, possibly because of the disruption of TGF-β signal transduction; in advanced tumors, TGF-β can even stimulate the proliferation of colon carcinoma cells. Thus, tumor growth may not be inhibited and might even be promoted by negative regulators of liver regeneration/hypertrophy.[4,14]

A recent animal study by Heinrich et al. suggested that the cytokines and growth factors associated with atrophy/hypertrophy after PVE are different from those associated with liver regeneration after a partial hepatectomy: intrahepatic tumor growth was promoted by portal vein ligation, in contrast to its inhibition after a partial hepatectomy. Heinrich et al. also proposed that tumor-derived TGFβ might be the key factor responsible for explaining this difference.[11]

28.1.3 Clinical Findings Regarding Tumor Growth After PVE

To date, four groups have assessed tumor growth after PVE (Table 28.1). A key point of these studies was whether PVE increases the growth rate of the tumor(s)

or the growth rate simply depends on the malignant potential of the tumor(s).

Elias et al.[15] were the first group to report tumor growth after PVE. They assessed the growth rate of the tumor and normal liver parenchyma in the nonembolized segments in five patients with liver metastases and reported that the growth rate of the tumor was more rapid than that of the liver parenchyma. They speculated that the cytokines and growth factors, such as TGF-α, that were induced by PVE stimulated both tumor growth and liver parenchyma hypertrophy to the same degree, suggesting that the natural growth rate of the tumor was enhanced by the additional growth triggered by PVE. However, as the growth rate before PVE was unknown, it was difficult to conclude that PVE further stimulated tumor growth in an additive manner.

Kokudo et al.[4] were the first to report the increased proliferative activity of colorectal liver metastases in embolized segments after PVE. In their study, the Ki-67 labeling index was evaluated in 18 patients with colorectal liver metastases who had undergone hepatic resection after PVE and the results were compared with those for 29 patients who underwent a major hepatic resection without PVE. The authors found that the Ki-67 labeling index of the metastatic lesions was significantly higher in the patients with PVE than in the control patients without PVE. To date, this study is the largest series in which tumor growth after PVE has been studied; however, as the comparison was made between different patient cohorts, the evidence that PVE independently induces tumor growth was circumstantial. Another notable finding of this study was that the disease-free survival period was significantly poorer in the PVE group than in the control group. Although the patients in the PVE group had larger tumors than the control patients, PVE may have enhanced the aggressiveness of the metastatic tumors.

Barbaro et al.[16] also evaluated the tumor volume in embolized segments after PVE. They noted that colorectal liver metastases showed remarkable tumor growth at 1 month after PVE but that metastatic cartinoid tumors did not. Based on these results, they concluded that the increase in tumor volume was correlated with the malignant potential of the tumor, and not with the alteration in hepatic arterial blood flow.

Theoretically, the tumor growth rate after PVE should be compared with that before PVE to determine the direct influence of PVE on tumor growth. Hayashi et al.[17] compared the growth rate of tumors before and after PVE in six patients with hepatocellular carcinoma (HCC) and two patients with cholangiocellular carcinoma (CCC). They found that the tumor growth rate was accelerated by 2.65 times after PVE in the six patients with HCC but that the acceleration rate was only 1.16 in the two patients with CCC. Hayashi's study was the first to demonstrate a PVE-induced increase in tumor growth, compared with the growth rate before PVE, in the same patients.

Accumulating evidence suggests that PVE stimulates tumor growth in addition to the natural volumetric increase that can be expected to occur during the waiting period between PVE and resection. However, the extent of the tumor growth after PVE seems to depend on the tumor type, with HCC and colorectal liver metastases being among the tumors whose tumor growths are significantly enhanced after PVE. Since HCC is a hypervascular tumor and colorectal metastasis is a hypovascular tumor, different mechanisms may induce the growth of these two tumor types after PVE.

28.2 Prevention of Tumor Growth After PVE

Tumor growth after PVE, especially tumor growth in the nonembolized FLR and/or extrahepatic tumor progression, may preclude a curative resection. Previous large series have documented that about 15–20% of patients who underwent PVE did not subsequently undergo hepatic resection because of tumor progression found before or during the laparotomy[18-20]; in the recent meta-analysis, the rate of unresectable tumor progression was 19.3%.[3] To prevent tumor progression during the waiting period after PVE, several strategies have been proposed.

28.2.1 Sequential Transcatheter Arterial Chemoembolization and PVE (Fig. 28.3)

The antitumor effect of transcatheter arterial chemoembolization (TACE) against HCC has been previously reported.[21] TACE is also useful for embolizing the arterio-portal shunts that are frequently found in cirrhotic patients. Thus, the combination of TACE and PVE before planned major hepatic resections may strengthen the effect of PVE while simultaneously preventing

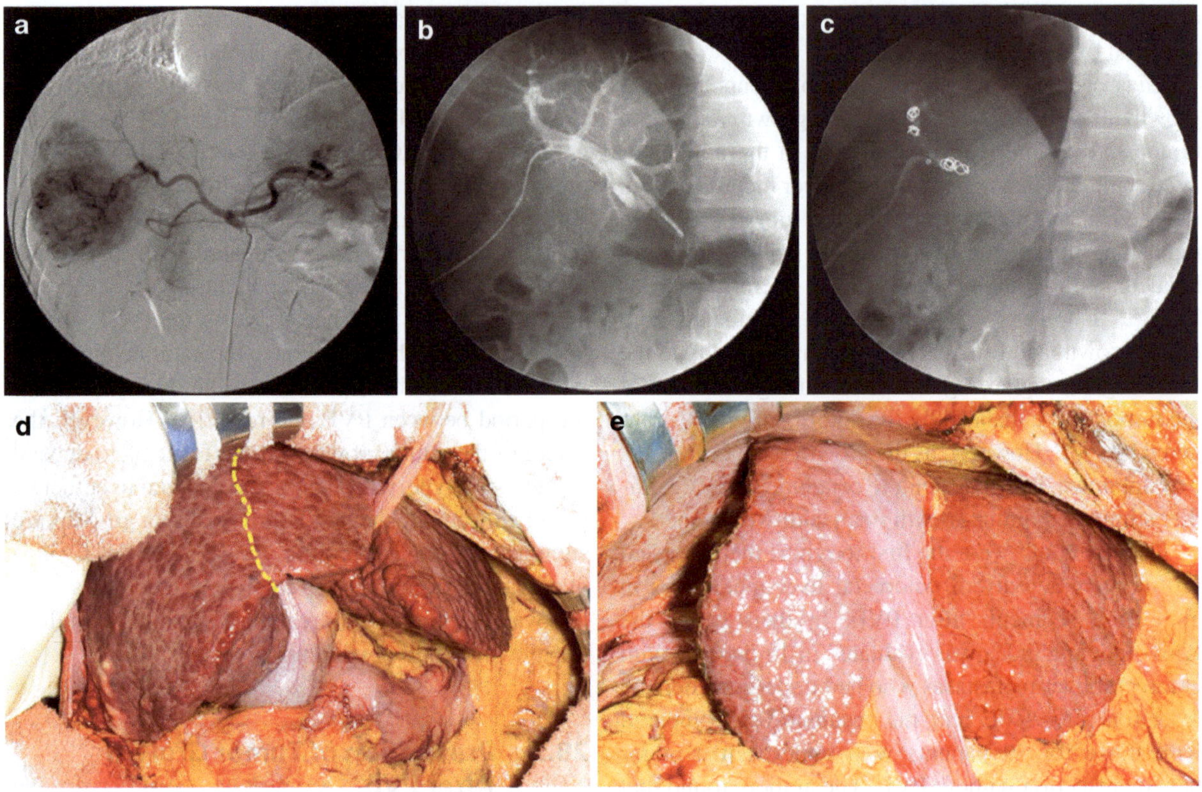

Fig. 28.3 Sequential TACE and PVE for hepatocellular carcinoma. At the first stage, selective TACE was performed (**a**). About 1 week after the TACE, PVE using transhepatic ipsilateral approach was conducted (**b**) and the portal branch in the right hemi-liver was embolized using embolization material and coils (**c**). Two weeks after the PVE, hypertrophy of the left hemi-liver was obtained (**d**), and curative right hemi-hepatectomy was performed without postoperative hepatic insufficiency (**e**). *Yellow dotted line* in the (**d**): Rex-Cantlie line

tumor progression. The authors previously reported the results of sequential preoperative TACE and PVE in 17 patients with HCC.[22] PVE was performed a median of 9 days (range, 4–48 days) after selective TACE of the segments to be resected. Consequently, 16 patients underwent planned hepatic resections a median of 21 days (range, 9–49 days) after PVE. With an interval of about 3 weeks, sufficient hypertrophy of the FLR was attained; meanwhile, tumor progression, as evaluated using the tumor volume, serum alpha-fetoprotein (AFP) level, and plasma des-γ-carboxy prothrombin (DCP) level, was significantly suppressed. In addition, the 5-year overall and disease-free survival rates were 55.6% and 46.7%, respectively; these rates were comparable to previously reported rates for patients with HCC who did not undergo preoperative PVE.

Ogata et al.[23] compared 18 patients who had undergone sequential preoperative TACE and PVE with 18 patients who had had PVE alone. All the patients underwent a right hepatectomy at 4–8 weeks after PVE. They found that the hypertrophy of the FLR was more enhanced in the TACE + PVE group and that the recurrence-free survival period was significantly longer in the TACE + PVE group than in the PVE-alone group. They concluded that a high rate of complete tumor necrosis was induced by sequential TACE and PVE, enabling favorable recurrence-free survival.

Although sequential TACE and PVE is an effective preoperative procedure for hypervascular tumors such as HCC, the possibility of hepatic infarction/necrosis induced by the double occlusion of the arterial and portal venous systems remains a concern. In our experience, a median interval of 9 days between the TACE and PVE procedures resulted in minimal necrotic change in the resected liver parenchyma, although the aspartate aminotransferase (AST) and alanine aminotransferase (ALT) levels were transiently elevated after TACE and PVE.[22]

28.2.2 Combination of Two-Stage Hepatectomy and PVE

As described above, tumor growth in the nonembolized segments after PVE may prevent respectability, leading to unfavorable patient survival. Therefore, tumors located in the nonembolized FLR should ideally be resected before PVE. Jaeck et al.[24] developed a two-stage hepatectomy and PVE strategy for the treatment of multiple and bilobar colorectal metastases. During the first-stage hepatectomy, all the tumors located in the FLR are removed to prevent rapid tumor growth after PVE. PVE is then performed to induce FLR hypertrophy. Finally, a second-stage major hepatic resection is performed to resect the liver metastases in the embolized segments. They reported that this combination procedure was associated with no operative mortalities and a satisfactory morbidity rate (56.0% after the second-stage hepatectomy), in contrast with the high mortality rate after a two-stage hepatectomy without PVE.[25] In addition, the 1- and 3-year survival rates after this combination procedure were 70.0% and 54.4%, respectively; these data are particularly noteworthy considering that these patients initially had unresectable tumors.[26]

28.2.3 Periprocedure Chemotherapy

Recently, an increasing number of patients with colorectal liver metastases are receiving neoadjuvant chemotherapy. Neoadjuvant chemotherapy can reduce the size of metastases that are unresectable rendering them resectable, and postoperative recurrence rates in patients with initially resectable tumors. And in most cases, preoperative chemotherapy does not increase the actual risk of subsequent hepatic resection provided short chemotherapy duration and adequate time interval between the cessation of chemotherapy and surgery are secured.[27,28] However, the liver parenchyma after neoadjuvant chemotherapy using irinotecan is often steatotic, fibrotic, and sometimes cirrhotic; similarly, sinusoidal obstruction syndrome associated with oxaliplatin has also been reported. And some previous reports suggested that such hepatotoxicity resulting from neoadjuvant treatment may result in an adverse clinical outcome.[29,30] Therefore, neoadjuvant chemotherapy is generally discontinued before and after PVE if the procedure is required for a safe major hepatic resection, since chemotherapy is assumed to have an inhibitory effect on the hypertrophy of the nonembolized FLR. Consequently, chemotherapy is usually stopped for several weeks to months, with potential risk of the tumors becoming unresectable. Recently, several groups have evaluated the effect of periprocedure chemotherapy, both on tumor growth and FLR hypertrophy.[31-33]All the groups concluded that hypertrophy of the FLR can occur during chemotherapeutic treatments and that the postoperative course is similar irrespective of the maintenance of chemotherapy after PVE. However, the positive effect of periprocedure chemotherapy on tumor growth was marginal. In a retrospective study by Covey et al.,[33] only 19 out of 43 patients who had received PVE and post-PVE chemotherapy ultimately underwent hepatic resections.

28.3 Conclusions

Increasing evidence suggests that preoperative PVE itself stimulates tumor growth both in the embolized and nonembolized segments of the liver by altering the blood supply and/or inducing a network of cytokines and growth factors, though the precise mechanism/network has not been fully clarified. This stimulating effect is more obvious in patients with HCC and colorectal liver metastases. Sequential TACE and PVE, two-stage hepatectomy combined with PVE and maintenance chemotherapy after PVE, are the currently available strategies to overcome the possible negative effects of PVE on tumor growth without reducing the hypertrophic properties of PVE.

References

1. Makuuchi M, Takayasu K, Takuma T, et al. Preoperative transcatheter embolization of the portal venous branch for patients receiving extended lobectomy due to the bile duct carcinoma. *J Jpn Surg Assoc*. 1984;45:14-20.
2. Makuuchi M, Thai BL, Takayasu K, et al. Preoperative portal embolization to increase safety of major hepatectomy for hilar bile duct carcinoma: a preliminary report. *Surgery*. 1990;107:521-527.
3. Abulkhir A, Limongelli P, Healy AJ, et al. Preoperative portal vein embolization for major liver resection: a meta-analysis. *Ann Surg*. 2008;247:49-57.
4. Kokudo N, Tada K, Seki M, et al. Proliferative activity of intrahepatic colorectal metastases after preoperative hemihepatic portal vein embolization. *Hepatology*. 2001;34: 267-272.

5. Lautt WW. Role and control of the hepatic artery. In: Lautt WW, ed. *Hepatic Circulation in Health and Disease*. New York: Raven; 1981:203-226.
6. Lautt WW. Mechanism and role of intrinsic regulation of hepatic arterial blood flow: hepatic arterial buffer response. *Am J Physiol*. 1985;249:G549-G556.
7. Aoki T, Imamura H, Kaneko J, et al. Intraoperative direct measurement of hepatic arterial buffer response in patients with or without cirrhosis. *Liver Transpl*. 2005;11:684-691.
8. Nagino M, Nimura Y, Kamiya J, et al. Immediate increase in arterial blood flow in embolized hepatic segments after portal vein embolization: CT demonstration. *Am J Roentgenol*. 1998;171:1037-1039.
9. Denys AL, Abehsera M, Leloutre B, et al. Intrahepatic hemodynamics changes following portal vein embolization: a prospective Doppler study. *Eur Radiol*. 2000;10:1703-1707.
10. Kito Y, Nagino M, Nimura Y. Doppler sonography of hepatic arterial blood flow velocity after percutaneous transhepatic portal vein embolization. *Am J Roentgenol*. 2001;176:909-912.
11. Heinrich S, Jochum W, Graf R, et al. Portal vein ligation and partial hepatectomy differently influence growth of intrahepatic metastasis and liver regeneration in mice. *J Hepatol*. 2006;45:35-42.
12. Christophi C, Harun N, Fifis T. Liver regeneration and tumor stimulation – a review of cytokines and angiogenic factors. *J Gastrointest Surg*. 2008;12:966-980.
13. Uemura T, Miyazaki M, Hirai R, et al. Different expression of positive and negative regulators of hepatocyte growth in growing and shrinking hepatic lobes after portal vein branch ligation in rats. *Int J Mol Med*. 2000;5:173-179.
14. de Graaf W, van den Esschert JW, van Lienden KP, et al. Induction of tumor growth after preoperative portal vein embolization: Is it a real problem? *Ann Surg Oncol*. 2009;16:423-430.
15. Elias D, de Baere T, Roche A, et al. During liver regeneration following right portal embolization the growth rate of liver metastases is more rapid than that of the liver parenchyma. *Br J Surg*. 1999;86:784-788.
16. Barbaro B, Di Stasi C, Nuzzo G, et al. Preoperative right portal vein embolization in patients with metastatic liver disease: metastatic liver volumes after RPVE. *Acta Radiol*. 2003;44:98-102.
17. Hayashi S, Baba Y, Ueno K, et al. Acceleration of primary liver tumor growth rate in embolized hepatic lobe after portal vein embolization. *Acta Radiol*. 2007;48:721-727.
18. Imamura H, Shimada R, Kubota M, et al. Preoperative portal vein embolization: an audit of 84 patients. *Hepatology*. 1999;29:1099-1105.
19. Hemming AW, Reed AI, Howard RJ, et al. Preoperative portal vein embolization for extended hepatectomy. *Ann Surg*. 2003;237:686-693.
20. Ribero D, Abdalla EK, Madoff DC, et al. Portal vein embolization before major hepatectomy and its effects on regeneration, respectability and outcome. *Br J Surg*. 2007;94:1386-1394.
21. Llovet JM, Bruix J. Systematic review of randomized trials for unresectable hepatocellular carcinoma: chemoembolization improves survival. *Hepatology*. 2003;37:429-442.
22. Aoki T, Imamura H, Hasegawa K, et al. Sequential preoperative arterial and portal venous embolizations in patients with hepatocellular carcinoma. *Arch Surg*. 2004;139:766-774.
23. Ogata S, Belghiti J, Farges O, et al. Sequential arterial and portal vein embolizations before right hepatectomy in patients with cirrhosis and hepatocellular carcinoma. *Br J Surg*. 2006;93:1091-1098.
24. Jaeck D, Bachellier P, Nakano H, et al. One or two-stage hepatectomy combined with portal vein embolization for initially nonresectable colorectal liver metastases. *Am J Surg*. 2003;185:222-230.
25. Adam R, Laurent A, Azoulay D, et al. Two-stage hepatectomy: a planned strategy to treat irresectable liver tumors. *Ann Surg*. 2000;232:777-785.
26. Jaeck D, Oussoultzoglou E, Rosso E, et al. A two-stage hepatectomy procedure combined with portal vein embolization to achieve curative resection for initially unresectable multiple and bilobar colorectal liver metastases. *Ann Surg*. 2004;240:1037-1051.
27. Abdalla EK, Vauthey JN. Chemotherapy prior to hepatic resection for colorectal liver metastases: Helpful until harmful? *Dig Surg*. 2008;25:421-429.
28. Chun YS, Laurent A, Maru D, et al. Management of chemotherapy-associated hepatotoxicity in colorectal liver metastases. *Lancet Oncol*. 2009;10:278-286.
29. Karoui M, Penna C, Amin-Hashem M, et al. Influence of preoperative chemotherapy on the risk of major hepatectomy for colorectal liver metastases. *Ann Surg*. 2006;243:1-7.
30. Zorzi D, Laurent A, Pawlik TM, et al. Chemotherapy-associated hepatotoxicity and surgery for colorectal liver metastases. *Br J Surg*. 2007;94:274-286.
31. Beal IK, Anthony S, Papadopoulou A, et al. Portal vein embolisation prior to hepatic resection for colorectal liver metastases and the effect of periprocedure chemotherapy. *Br J Radiol*. 2006;79:473-478.
32. Goere D, Farges O, Leporrrier J, et al. Chemotherapy does not impair hypertrophy of the left liver after right portal vein obstruction. *J Gastrointest Surg*. 2006;10:365-370.
33. Covey AM, Brown KT, Jarnagin WR, et al. Combined portal vein embolization and neoadjuvant chemotherapy as a treatment strategy for resectable hepatic colorectal metastases. *Ann Surg*. 2008;247:451-455.

Enhancing Hepatic Regeneration with Stem Cells and Portal Vein Embolization

29

Günter Fürst, Jan Schulte am Esch, and Wolfram T. Knoefel

Abstract

In patients scheduled for extended right hemihepatectomy, portal venous embolization (PVE) as an isolated modality may fail to induce an adequate hepatic volume response within a reasonable period of time. In particular, patients with very small future liver remnant volumes, compromised hepatic parenchyma or comorbidity, and impaired liver regeneration capacity may be initially considered unsuitable for resection. Hematopoietic and mesenchymal stem cells are promising candidates for cell-based approaches for the treatment of liver diseases. Possible stem cell interactions with the liver include stimulation of endogenous hepatocyte proliferation, transdifferentiation to hepatocytes, fusion of stem cells and hepatocytes, antifibrotic and immunomodulatory effects. In a new concept, autologous hematopoietic CD133+ stem cells are used to augment left lateral liver volume prior to extended liver resection. PVE was used as a strong proliferation stimulus to the nonembolized liver segments. Significantly increased hepatic growth rates and reduction of waiting time from PVE to resection surgery were found compared to a control group. No complications or side effects linked to the stem cell treatment were observed. Clinical follow-up revealed no significant differences in tumor-free survival times and recurrence rates. A randomized trial will be performed to validate the findings and to clarify if stem cells are a powerful adjunct to PVE in patients supposed to respond inadequately to PVE alone.

Keywords

Adult bone marrow stem cells • Liver regeneration • Portal vein embolization • AC133 antigen • Somatic cell therapy • Clinical trials • Clinical stem cell transplantation

Abbreviations

BM	Bone marrow
BMSC	Bone marrow stem cell
CD	Cluster of differentiation
CP	Child–Pugh
CT	Computed tomography
CXCR4	CXC-receptor-4
EGF	Epidermal growth factor
FACS	Fluorescence assorted cell sorting
FGF	Fibroblast growth factor
FLRV	Future liver remnant volume
G-CSF	Granulocyte-colony-stimulating factor

G. Fürst (✉)
Department of Diagnostic and Interventional Radiology, University Hospital and Heinrich-Heine-University of Düsseldorf, Moorenstrasse 5, 40225 Düsseldorf, Germany
e-mail: fuerst@med.uni-duesseldorf.de

D.C. Madoff et al. (eds.), *Venous Embolization of the Liver*,
DOI 10.1007/978-1-84882-122-4_29, © Springer-Verlag London Limited 2011

HGF	Hepatocyte growth factor
HSC	Hematopoietic stem cells
IGF	Insulin-like growth factor
INR	International normalized ratio
LPC	Liver progenitor cell
MELD	Model for end-stage liver disease
MMP	Matrix metalloproteinase
MSC	Mesenchymal stem cell
PI	Propidium iodide
PVE	Portal vein embolization
SC	Stem cell
SCF	Stem cell factor
SDF-1	Stroma-derived factor-1
TACE	Transcatheter arterial chemoembolization
TLV	Total liver volume

29.1 Clinical Scenario

Complete resection of hepatic tumors remains the first choice for curative treatment in patients with primary or secondary hepatobiliary malignancy. In up to 45% of patients, extended hepatectomy (more than five segments) is necessary to achieve margin negative resection. Until now the minimal hepatic volume required to support postoperative liver function has not been clearly defined. However, it is generally accepted that patients with an anticipated future liver remnant volume (FLRV) below 25% of the total liver volume (TLV) have an increased risk of postoperative morbidity and mortality.[1-4] In these patients, the concept of preoperative expansion of the left-lateral FLRV (segments II and III), utilizing selective portal venous embolization (PVE) of contralateral liver segments I and IV to VIII, is increasingly performed as a safe and effective concept to provide a proliferation stimulus.[4,5]

High regeneration rates up to 20 mL/day, and relative volume gains of more than 30% have been reported for patients without cirrhosis or diabetes prior to standard right hepatectomy.[6,7] However, patients eligible for extended liver resection frequently suffer from large and fast progressing liver lesions limiting the waiting time after PVE to reach an adequate left lateral liver mass. Time to surgery may be unacceptably long (observed to be up to 150 days), particularly if the left lateral liver segments determining the FLRV are small and quality of hepatic parenchyma is limited by cirrhosis, fibrosis, severe steatosis, or hepatotoxic chemotherapy.[5] These patients, in particular, may be initially considered unsuitable for resection due to lack of sufficient remaining normal parenchyma.

A growing body of evidence suggesting that extrahepatic stem cells (SCs) like hematopoietic and mesenchymal progenitor cells participate in the concert of liver regeneration led us to investigate whether SCs may be helpful to further accelerate liver augmentation after PVE.[8-11]

29.2 Liver Stem Cell Populations

The liver has a tremendous regenerative capacity to respond to cell loss secondary to chemical or surgical liver injury. Several groups have developed experimental models of liver injury to activate and augment specific cell populations. A detailed review of cell responses in injury models has been recently given by Walkup and Gerber.[12]

It has been hypothesized that three levels of cells in the hepatic lineage are involved in the response to injury: (1) mature hepatocytes, (2) intrahepatic progenitor cells (LPC), and (3) extrahepatic liver stem cells, which may derive from circulating hematopoietic stem cells or bone marrow stem cells.

29.2.1 Hepatocytes

The mature hepatocyte proliferates after normal tissue renewal, less severe liver damage, and partial hepatectomy. Also, hepatocyte replication proved to be responsible for augmentation of the future liver remnant following PVE. In an experimental study, Duncan et al.[13] used bromodeoxyuridine for visualization of mitotic cells in pigs, revealing a maximum of 14% of hepatocytes at replication 7 days after PVE.

Due to the extensive self-maintaining capacity of adult hepatocytes, it has been proposed to perceive hepatocytes as unipotent committed "stem cells" that are normally quiescent; however, they can be activated to differentiate along a hepatocytic lineage on demand.[14]

29.2.2 Intrahepatic Liver Progenitor Cells

Research during the last decade has indicated that liver progenitor cells (LPC) are an important alternative source of cells for liver regeneration. This intrahepatic stem cell population can take over liver regeneration when hepatocyte replication fails. Especially in scenarios of higher levels of hepatocytic damage, this pathway may play a significant role.[15] These cells have been also identified as a cellular precursor to hepatocellular carcinoma. The terms "LPC" and "oval cells" are used interchangeably by some authors, whereas others reserve oval cells only for LPC observed in rodents.[16,17] The description "oval" cells is due to the large nucleus-to-cytoplasma ratio and ovoid shaped morphology in cross section.[18] Although the location of oval cells has been a subject of controversy, it is generally accepted that they are placed near the portal triad, adjacent to the terminal ducts of the biliary tree. In contrast to hepatocytes, LPCs can be regarded as bipotent precursors, capable to differentiate into the two hepatic lineages and expressing markers in common with bile duct cells, fetal, and adult hepatocytes such as albumin[19,20], alpha-fetoprotein[19-21], and cytokeratin markers (CK17 and CK19).[22,23]

29.2.3 Extrahepatic Adult Stem Cells

Stem cells can be defined as cells that are clonogenic, self-renewing, and capable of differentiating into multiple cell lineages. Two types of adult extrahepatic stem cells, hematopoietic (HSC) and mesenchymal stem cells (MSC), are found predominantly in the bone marrow.

Hematopoietic BMSCs (HSC) have been intensively investigated as a potential source of liver stem cells participating in hepatic regeneration.[24,25] It has been postulated that HSCs are able to transdifferentiate into both hepatocytes and bile duct cells.[26-31] BM-derived hepatocytes may populate the regenerating liver due to transdifferentiation without fusion.[31,32] Also, conversion to liver cells via cellular fusion (bone marrow cell with hepatocyte) was reported.[33,34] HSCs as source for intrahepatic oval cells (LPC) were hypothesized as another way to support liver regeneration.[24] It was also suggested that oval cells can express the hematopoietic stem cell markers CD34+,[35,36] Thy-1,[37] and c-kit.[38] However, a growing body of work suggests that LPCs are an independent stem cell population, distinct from HSCs.[39]

MSCs can also be derived from BM and give rise to hepatocyte-like progeny positive for mRNA albumin expression.[40] Very recently, BM-derived MSCs were demonstrated to rescue experimental liver failure and offer a potentially alternative therapy to organ transplantation.[41] However, the most dominant axis of this stem cell population seems to be transdifferentiation to a myofibroblast cell population and it is questionable whether MSCs contribute to hepatocyte regeneration at all.[42]

BMSCs have been demonstrated to contribute to the non-parenchymal cells within the liver such as neutrophils, lymphocytes, and other inflammatory cells and may play a role in the immunoregulation of the liver. Others hypothesized that BMSCs may serve as a source for the replacement of endothelial cells and may provide factors required for efficient healing of the damaged liver.[43]

Two basic hypotheses discuss how extrahepatic BMSCs may contribute to the regeneration of the damaged liver subsequent to therapeutic application. (A) The concept of adding hepatocytes and hepatocyte precursors to the regenerating liver to reconstitute the local body of primary liver cells.[44-47] (B) The theory of remodeling the local regenerating capacity to optimize the extensive self-renewing potential via direct and/or humoral interaction or horizontal gene transfer with (to) liver-based actors and infrastructure in hepatic healing processes.[43,48,49] Although both phenomena may occur, hypothesis B would explain a relevant part of the contradiction that BM was demonstrated to participate in extensive forms of liver regeneration,[26,50] but the tractable number of events of BMSC homing as primary liver cells subsequent to regeneration of the damaged liver was clinically observed to be rare.[51,52] Whether BMSC contributes to regeneration indirectly by coordinating the local regeneration process or directly by transdifferentiation to (modified) hepatocytes (formed by transdifferentiation or fusion) remains unclear and needs to be further evaluated. Both may occur simultaneously, which would open the question whether such two modalities of BMSC homing to the liver act independently or as an alliance in hepatic regeneration.

29.2.4 Stem Cell Homing, Proliferation, and Differentiation

The damaged liver is known to express chemokines and possible chemotactants, such as stroma-derived factor-1 (SDF-1), stem cell factor (SCF), hepatic growth factor (HGF), interleukin-8 (IL-8), and others, discussed to participate in the concert of SC homing from extrahepatic sources to the liver.[53-56] Hepatic engraftment from extrahepatic progenitor cells is accelerated in cases of liver damage if contrasted with non-injured liver tissue.[57] It was demonstrated that the injured liver does express increased levels of SDF-1, attracting CD133+ BMSCs, that are positive for the SDF-1 receptor CXCR4. CD133+ BMSCs are likely to follow an SDF-1 gradient, get mobilized into peripheral blood, and subsequently take part in hepatic regeneration.[58] In vitro results suggest that the SDF-1-CXCR4 and HGF-c-met axes as well as epidermal growth factor (EGF), fibroblast growth factor (FGF), insulin-like growth factor (IGF), and matrix metalloproteinases (MMP) may be involved in recruitment of expanded MSCs to damaged tissues.[59,60] Cholestatic serum promoted the differentiation of beta-2-microglobulin-negative/Thy-1(+) BMSCs into mature hepatocytes metabolizing ammonia into urea depending on a yet nondescript humoral signal.[61] A wide range of factors were recently identified by transcriptome profiling (including cytokines, chemokines and growth factors, cell differentiation and proliferation regulation factors plus proteolysis and peptidolysis genes) and demonstrated to be upregulated in rat livers subsequent to common bile duct ligation.[62] However, further studies are required to better understand the roles of these genes involved in regulation of BMSC recruiting, repopulation, and engraftment in regenerating livers.

29.3 Own Experimental Data

Experimental data indicate that stem cells contribute to liver regeneration after partial hepatectomy in mice.[11] In humans, mobilization of peripheral, hematopoietic, autologous CD34+ stem cells have been demonstrated to be 10-fold higher after liver resection than after liver sparing abdominal surgery.[63] Also, substantial increases of CD133+ and CD14+ mononucleated cells were observed after partial loss of liver tissue subsequent to hepatectomy, but not after other major abdominal surgery.[64] In that same study, CD133+ cells demonstrated the capacity to differentiate into a hepatic lineage.

In an own unpublished study, we investigated peripheral mobilization of CD133+ and CD34+ cells in the early course of clinical hepatic resection using FACS-analyses in 26 patients. CT-volumetry preoperatively and 24 h following resection was utilized to determine the exact extent of liver-volume loss. Patients with resection volume less than 30% (group 1) of the preoperative total liver volume were contrasted to those patients with a resection extent of 30–65% (group 2) concerning CD133+ and CD34+ progenitor cells in peripheral blood: Both cell types demonstrated significant increases compared to the preoperative baseline. CD133+ cells presented a significantly more pronounced increase in group 2 patients compared to group 1 peaking on day 2 after resection with a more than fivefold rise in cell count. CD 34+ cell mobilization was comparable but less pronounced in both groups. Thus, we demonstrated for the first time a correlation of loss of liver parenchyma and the level of peripheral stem cell mobilization. Consequently, CD133+ cells seem to play a dominant role in that respect if contrasted to CD34+ cells supporting CD133 as a selection marker for therapeutic BMSC applications. In a small sample of patients, cytofluorometric analysis revealed a more than 2.5-fold elevation of peripheral CD133+ and CD34+ cells as compared to preinterventional cell counts following PVE. These data may suggest that BMSCs are also involved in promoting liver regeneration after PVE.

Only little is known about factors released in the course of liver resection that have an impact on SC-mobilization, homing to the liver, and differentiation of SCs. We[53] and others[65] demonstrated SCF to be upregulated subsequent to liver resection in patients' serum in the early course of partial hepatectomy. The extent of expression correlated with the extent of parenchymal loss. However, detailed analyses of factors in patient serum subsequent to liver resection and their impact on HSC like CD133+BMSC are required to gain more understanding of the participation of stem cells in liver repair in order to develop tools to improve stem cell-based therapy.

29.4 Stem Cell Treatment in Chronic Liver Disease

Experimental data have encouraged a fast growing number of clinical trials. In cardiologic literature, there are now many studies with controlled and often double-blinded trials using BMSCs therapeutically to promote recovery of the left ventricular systolic function in patients with myocardial infarction. They show variable success. In contrast, clinical trials using BMSCs to treat patients with liver disease are still mostly uncontrolled and small-scale feasibility and safety studies. Most of the trials investigated whether these procedures led to clinical benefit in patients with chronic liver disease. Serum albumin level, bilirubin level, international normalized ratio (INR), Child–Pugh (CP), and/or model for end-stage liver disease (MELD) score or other scores were measured at baseline and after various follow-up periods.

To date, there are several published clinical studies.[66-74] A critical review has been recently given by Houlihan DD and Newsome PN.[75] The results of this review are summarized in the following: In one study, mobilization of BMSCs with granulocyte-colony-stimulating factor (G-CSF) was used in patients with chronic liver disease. Results were encouraging in so far as the CP score improved by two points or more in four of eight patients, whereas deteriorated in one patient and remained unchanged in the remaining three patients.[66]

In a second type of trials, autologous bone marrow cells were collected and administered either into a peripheral vein or the hepatic artery.[67-71] Patients with established cirrhosis or decompensated cirrhosis enlisted on a waiting list for liver transplantation were enrolled. With the exception of one study, that was prematurely terminated after the death of two of the patients,[68] all studies revealed benefits with respect to the evaluated parameters.

A third category of trials investigated effects of collection (±ex vivo manipulation) and re-infusion of mobilized bone marrow cells.[72-74] In a preliminary uncontrolled study in five patients with liver insufficiency, Gordon et al.[72] showed a transient improvement in serum bilirubin and albumin levels after portal vein or hepatic artery infusion of autologous CD34+ BMSCs. In one patient, complete resolution of ascites was observed. Outcomes of these patients were published recently indicating a trend toward reduced serum bilirubin and increased albumin levels.[73] Unsorted peripheral blood stem cells collected after G-CSF application were used to treat two patients with decompensated alcoholic cirrhosis by Yannaki et al.[74] Improvements in CP and MELD scores were observed in both patients. Also, serum concentrations of interleukin-6 and soluble tumor necrosis factor-α-receptor, known to be correlated with the outcome in alcoholic cirrhosis, decreased.

Although these trials provide encouraging results in the treatment of patients with chronic liver disease, the proof that BMSCs robustly induce in vivo organ regeneration is still lacking. Randomized, controlled, and double-blinded stem cell trials are needed to confirm these data. Also, in none of the trials so far has colonization or engraftment of transplanted cells been demonstrated in the recipient liver.

29.5 Stem Cells to Stimulate Hepatic Regeneration

Given that growing evidence suggesting the existence of a BM-hepatic axis, we used autologous CD133+ BMSC to stimulate the liver's regeneration capacity in patients scheduled for extended right hemihepatectomy (Figs. 29.1–29.4).[76,77] Until now, ten patients with large central malignancies of the liver scheduled for extended right hepatectomy underwent PVE and intraportal administration of CD133+ BMSCs. Ten patients underwent PVE alone and served as a control group. Patients in both groups were characterized by a FLRV of less than 25% of the total liver volume (TLV) minus tumor volume, except one patient with liver cirrhosis. In the stem cell group, PVE as an isolated technique was questionably sufficient to induce adequate proliferation of the left lateral liver segments within a reasonable time. A panel of criteria was used indicating compromised hepatic parenchyma or comorbidity, possibly impairing liver regeneration capacity,[78] including liver cirrhosis (CP score A) in two patients, fibrosis following chronic replicating hepatitis, severe liver steatosis and prior hepatotoxic chemotherapy in (each) one patient. Other patients showed unusual low basal volume of segments II and III (two patients) and fast progressing liver lesions (one patient). In two patients, limited volume response following PVE was expected due to tumor-associated thrombosis of one sectoral portal branch or several segmental portal branches presumably exhausting the proliferation capacity of the left lateral liver. None of the control patients had comparable hepatic comorbidities.

29.5.1 PVE Procedure

We used PVE of liver segments I and IV–VIII as a strong proliferation stimulus to the nonembolized left lateral segments II and III, to which CD133+ BMSCs were applied. The techniques of PVE are described in detail in Chaps. 15–17. Until now, a transileocolic portal venous

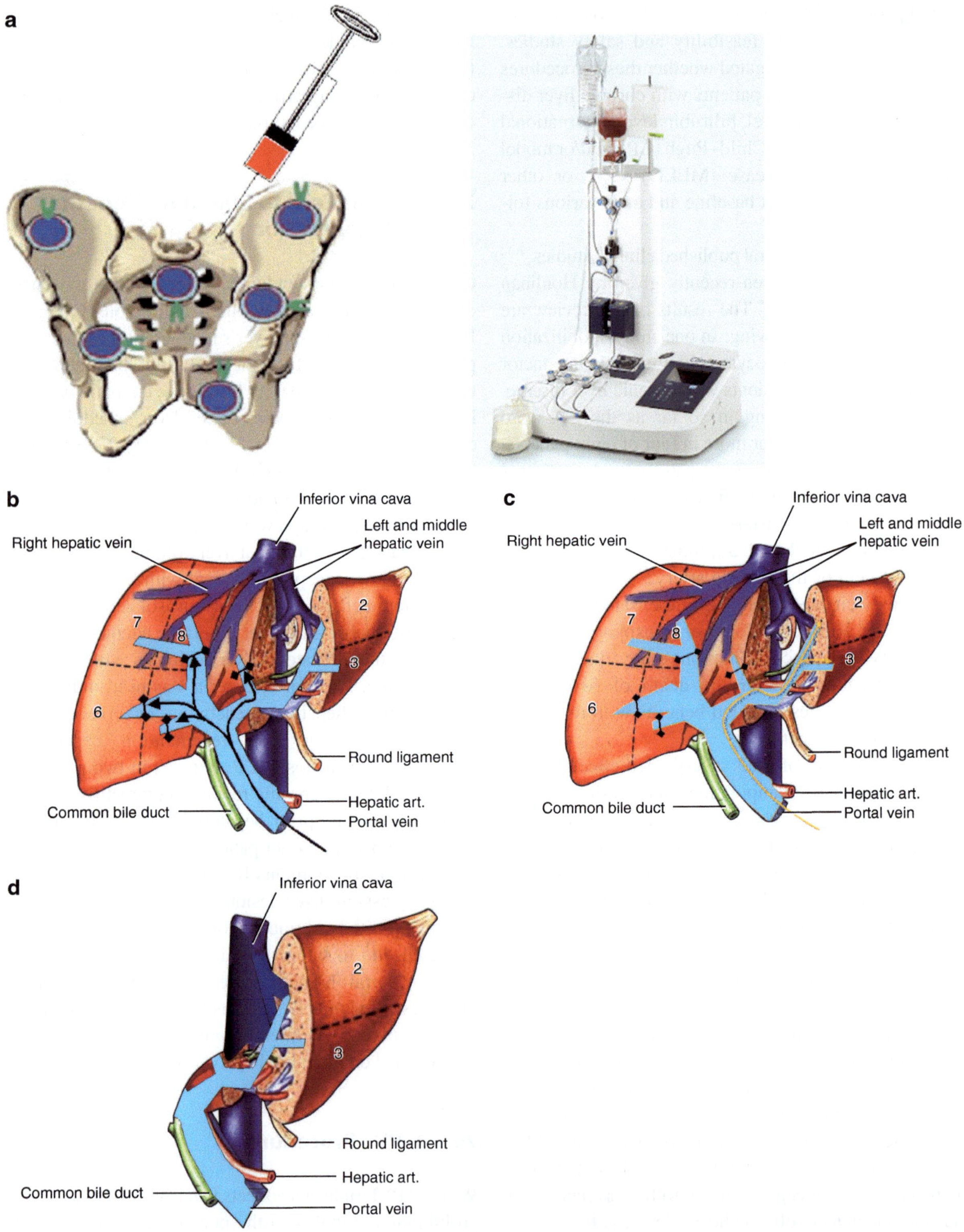

Fig. 29.1 Concept of PVE and portal application of BMSCs: (**a**) autologous bone marrow is aspirated and processed by a GMP-grade cell-selection unit to enrich for CD 133+ cells, (**b**) PVE of liver segments I and IV–VIII, (**c**) selective readministration of selected cells to the non-occluded portal branches of liver segments II and III. The whole procedure from harvesting bone marrow until readministration is performed in a closed system, (**d**) extended right hepatectomy with resection of segments I and IV–VIII about 3 weeks later

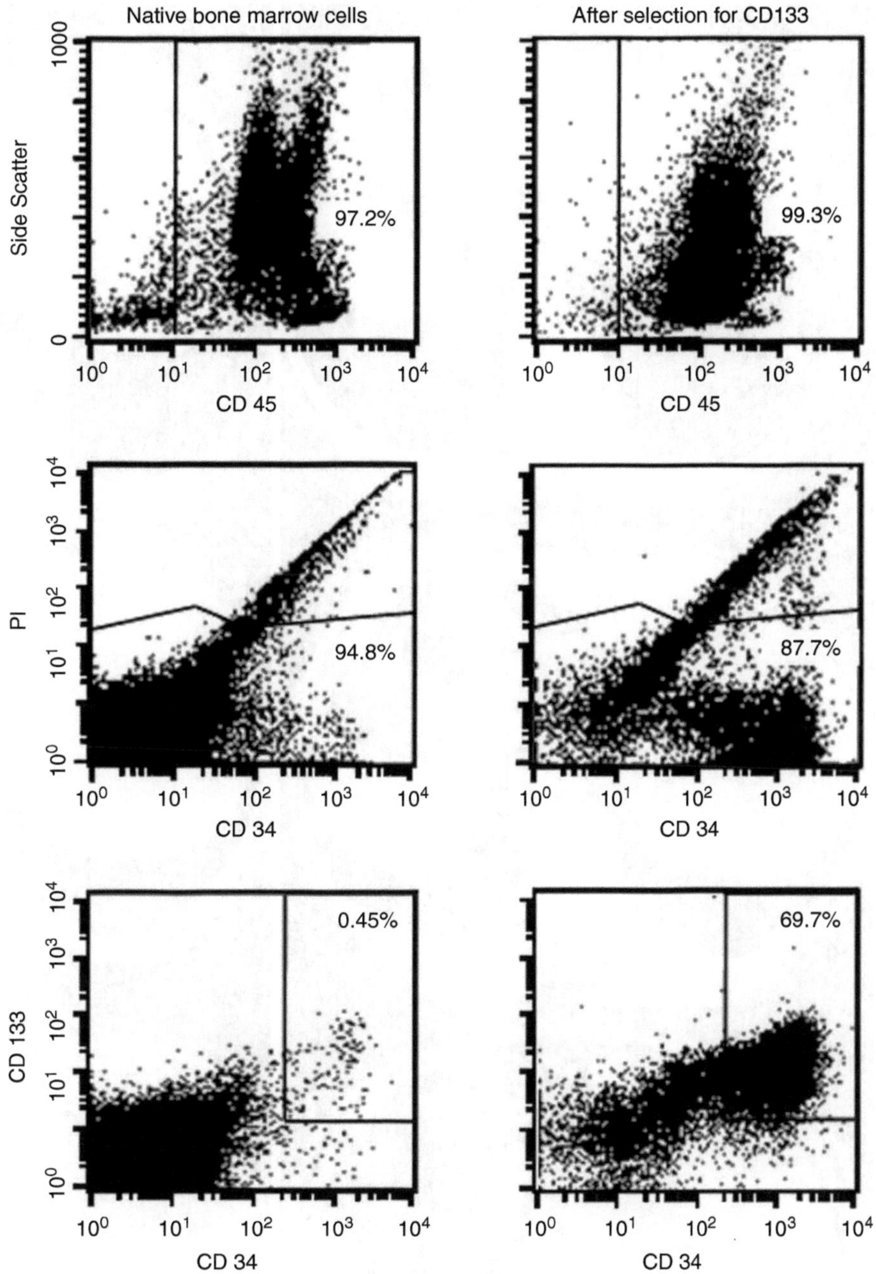

Fig. 29.2 Representative cytofluorometric analyses of applied CD133+BMSCs. Aliquots of unselected bone marrow (*left panels*) harvested from patients and the re-administered positive fractions after enrichment for stem cell marker CD133 (*right panels*) were analyzed by FACS. Upper panels demonstrate the concentration of leucocytes detected by anti-CD45 antibodies. DNA-stain propidium iodide (P1) was employed to assess rate of cell viability (*middle panels*). Utilizing anti-CD133 and anti-CD34 antibodies the concentration for CD133+ cells was evaluated (*lower panels*) (From Schulte am Esch et al.,[76] with permission)

access with direct cannulation has been used in all of our patients scheduled for SC application. This approach with general anesthesia was preferred to the percutaneous approach, because safe catheter placement and harvesting of bone marrow could be performed during the same intervention. However, the portal system can be accessed alternatively by using a percutaneous transhepatic approach from the right or left side under fluoroscopic and ultrasonographic guidance. Until recently, we used small polyvinyl alcohol particles ranging from 300 to 500 μm (Contour; Boston Scientific/Target Vascular, Freemont, CA, USA) first to occlude the distal smaller portal branches for embolization of segments V–VIII. PVE was performed until stasis or near-stasis was achieved. Subsequently, a 1:2 cyanoacrylate-to-iodinized oil mixture (Braun, Tuttlingen, Germany; Guerbet, Roissy, France) was used to obtain complete occlusion of these segments. We have now switched over to a 1:3

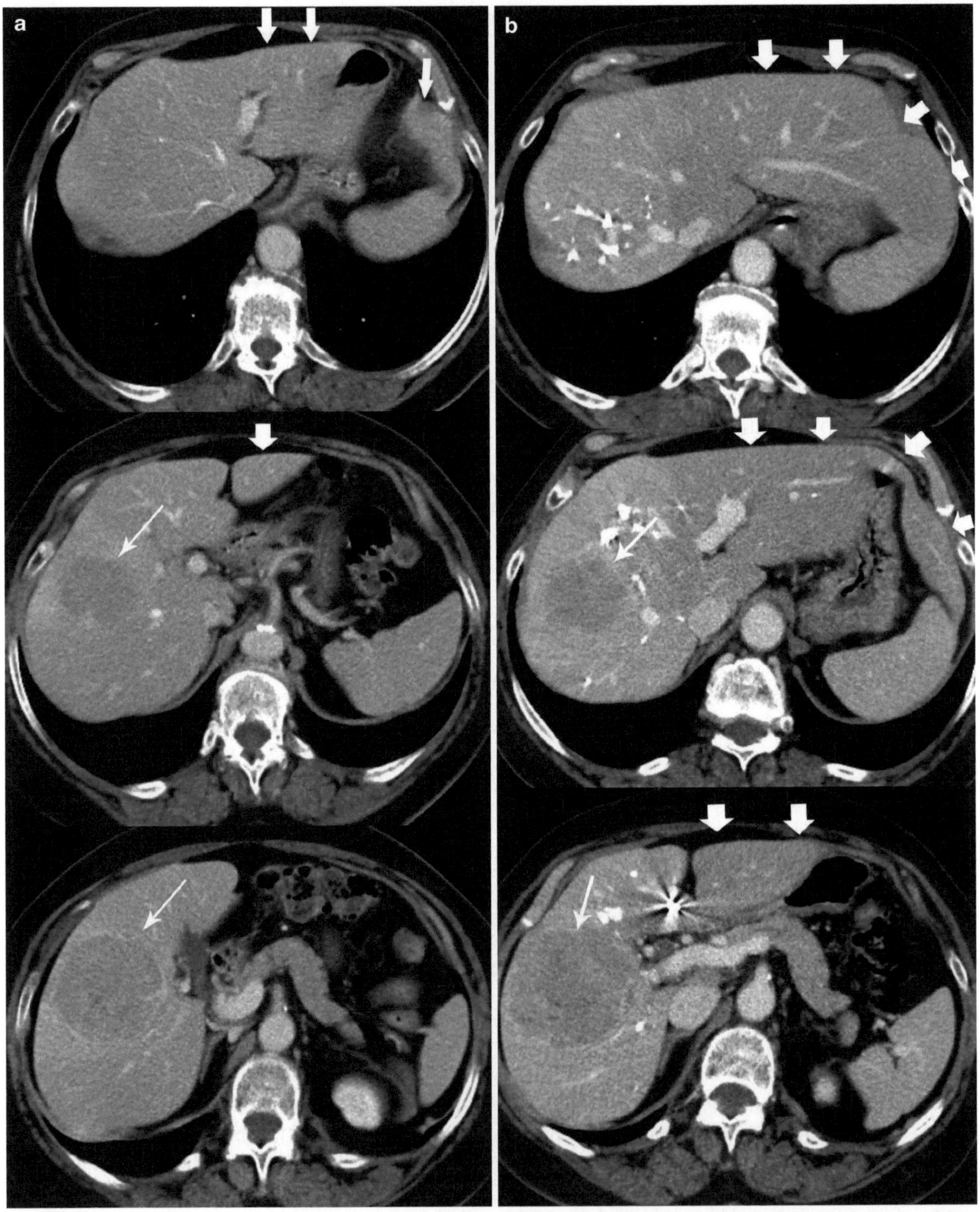

Fig. 29.3 Transverse CT scans from helical CT data sets of a patient with hepatocellular carcinoma (*long arrows*) obtained (**a**) before, (**b**) 14 days after, and (**c**) 12, 18 and 36 months after PVE and intraportal CD133+ BMSC application. (**a**) Preinterventional CT volumetry revealed TLV of 1,317 mL, tumor volume of 177 mL, FLRV of 217 mL (*short arrows*), and relative FLRV of 19%. (**b**) Post-interventional CT volumetry yielded marked augmentation of left lateral liver segments (*short arrows*), indicated by an absolute gain in FLRV of 223 mL, and hepatic daily gain rate of 15.9 mL/day. (**c**) Follow-up CT examinations revealed postoperative TLV of 1,100 mL 12 months after PVE (*upper panel*), a small focus of hypervascularized recurrent tumor (*long arrow*) 18 months after PVE (*middle panel*), and no hepatic relapse after successful tumor resection 36 months after PVE (below)

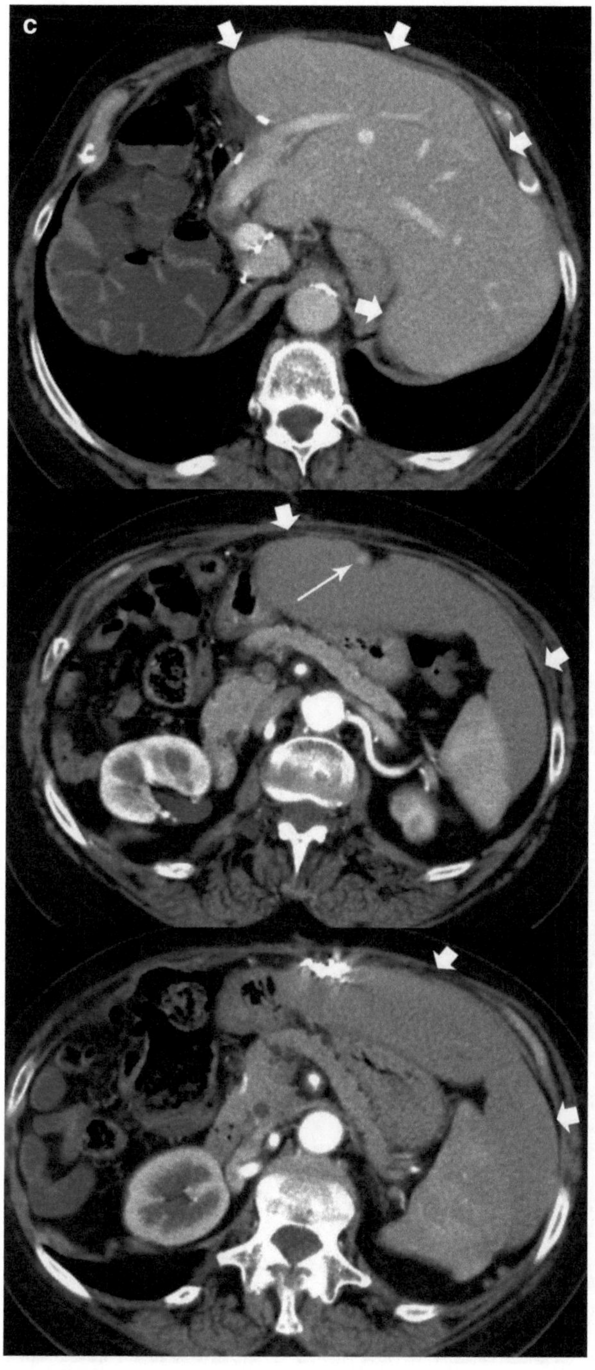

Fig. 29.3 (continued)

cyanoacrylate-to-iodinized oil mixture for PVE of the right liver lobe and normally abstain from microparticles. In contrast, polyvinyl alcohol particles and microcoils (Platinum Microcoils; Target Therapeutics) are preferred to embolize segments I and IV.

29.5.2 Preparation, Characterization, and Application of BMSCs

The procedure of harvesting bone marrow for readministration of selected cells was performed in a closed system and general anesthesia. Autologous bone marrow aspirated from the posterior iliac crest was drawn in heparin-coated syringes. BM cells were prepared simultaneously with PVE. The cell suspension was first filtered to remove bone spicule and was then processed by using a good manufacturing practice-grade cell-suspension unit (ClinMACS; Miltenyi Biotech, Bergisch-Gladbach, Germany) to immunomagnetically enrich CD133+ cells as previously described.[79] The protocol is certified by competent authorities (Paul Ehrlich Institute). Like CD34, CD133 is a highly conserved antigen (5-transmembrane glycoprotein) expressed on hematopoietic stem cells with unknown function. Compared to CD34, CD133 is a more pluripotent stem cell marker, that is believed to represent a more stem cell–enriched subpopulation of CD34+ cells.

After approximately 2½h, the mononuclear cells were ready for intrahepatic application. Cells were resuspended in a phosphate-buffered solution. Aliquots from the bone marrow aspirate and the injected cell fraction were collected for cytofluorometric analyses (Fig. 29.2). The number of mononuclear cells was determined by using a cell counter. In our recent study, aspirated total BM volumes ranged between 60 mL and 440 mL, the CD133+ purity of cells for application was between 12% and 94%, and the absolute number of CD133+ cells varied between 2.4 and 12.3 × 10 million.[77]

For readministration of the cell suspension, a 5-F cobra catheter was introduced into the non-occluded left lateral portal vein system under fluoroscopic guidance. The time needed for the entire procedure ranged between 3.5 h and 5.5 h. No special medication was required after BMSC administration.

Even though the optimal technique for SC application has not been defined (peripheral venous or hepatic arterial application is alternatively possible), we hypothesized that the direct portal administration of high concentrations of CD133+ BMSCs may ease the homing to the target segments II and III. The rationale for this application mode was supported by a study in which a high percentage of first-pass entrapment of BMSCs to the liver when applied to the portal vein was reported.[80] In the same study, it was suggested that

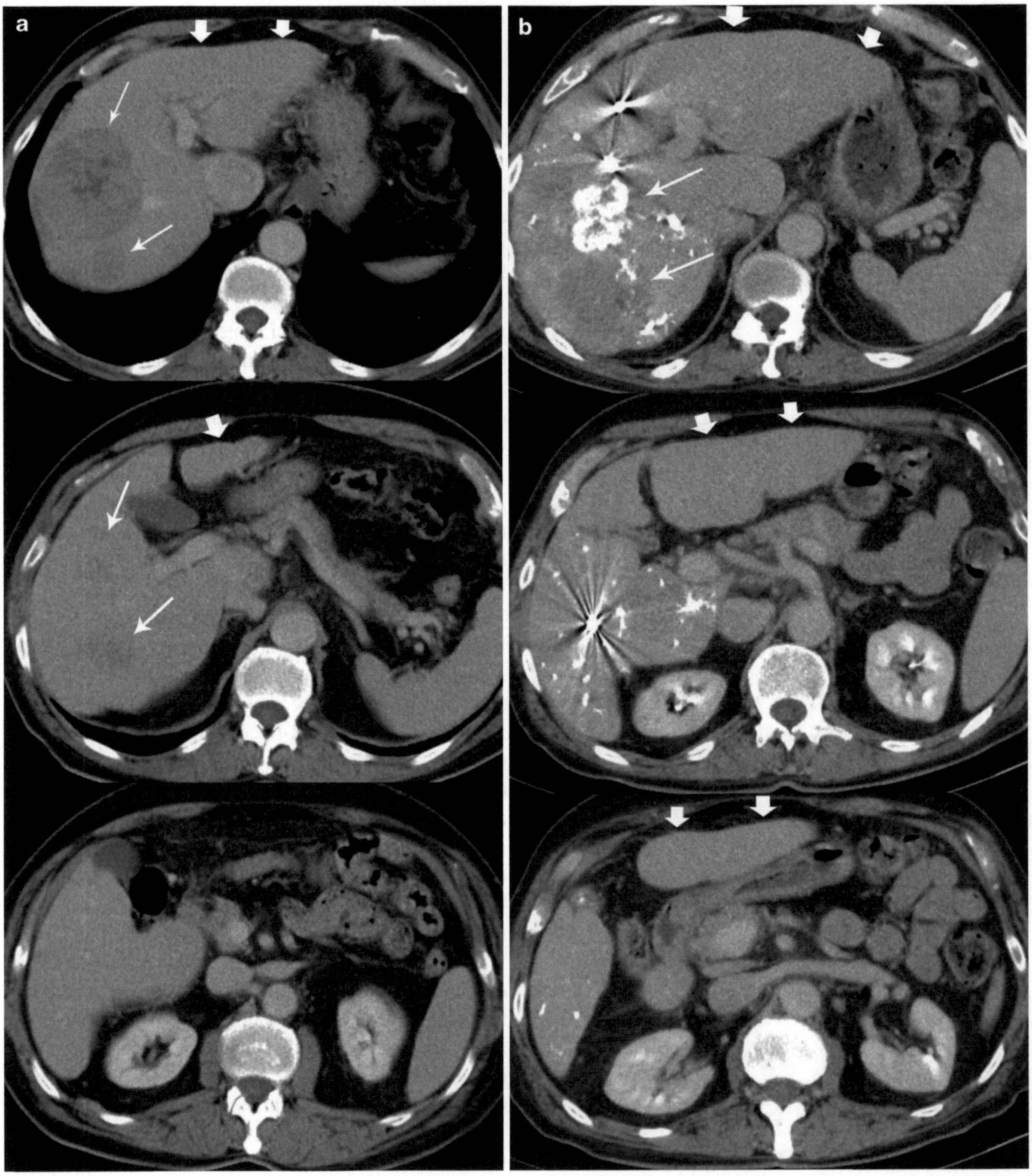

Fig. 29.4 Transverse CT scans from helical CT data sets of a patient with hepatocellular carcinoma (*long arrows*) and liver cirrhosis (Child–Pugh A) obtained (**a**) before, and (**b**) 14 days after PVE and intraportal CD133+ BMSC application. This patient had also undergone TACE 1 week before PVE. (**a**) Preinterventional CT volumetry revealed TLV of 1,790 mL, tumor volume of 341 mL, FLRV of 297 mL (*short arrows*), and relative FLRV of 20.5%. (**b**) Post-interventional CT volumetry yielded marked hypertrophy of left lateral liver segments (*short arrows*), indicated by an absolute gain in FLRV of 263 mL, and hepatic daily gain rate of 18.8 mL/day

interaction of stem cells with stromal cells in the liver is a crucial step for successful engraftment.

29.5.3 Volumetric Assessments

All patients underwent helical computed tomography (CT) to estimate liver volumes prior to PVE, 2 weeks after PVE, and then in 1–2 weeks intervals to determine the degree of induced hypertrophy until FLRV was adequate for extended right hepatectomy. CT examinations were performed using multisection CT scanners. Transverse scans were obtained in the portal venous phase to measure the TLV, the FLRV (segments II and III), and the intrahepatic tumor volume. Currently, measurements are performed manually with respect to the hepatic segmentation on the basis of the distribution of the portal pedicles and the location of the hepatic veins (Couinaud classification system).

29.5.4 Clinical Results

In our series, we found a twofold higher mean daily hepatic growth rate in patients treated with PVE and BMSCs compared with patients who underwent PVE alone (10.8 mL/day vs. 5.2 mL/day; $p<0.05$). Also, the relative and absolute volume gains were significantly higher in the patients treated with BMSCs (70.8% vs. 41.3% and 178 mL vs. 118 mL; $p<0.05$). The increased proliferation rate resulted in a significant reduction of the waiting time from PVE to resection surgery (46 days vs. 30 days; $p<0.05$). No complications or side effects linked to the BMSC-treatment were observed. Solely, minimal transient elevations of the routinely assessed markers (total bilirubin level, INR, and aspartate aminotransferase and alanine aminotransferase levels) normalized to their preinterventional levels 4 or 5 days after PVE, which indicated no lasting effect on liver metabolism, hepatic synthesis capacity, and hepatocellular integrity.

Markers of liver function in the early course after partial hepatectomy served as an indicator for the quality of liver tissue grown subsequent to PVE. These data demonstrated the functional quality of liver parenchyma, that grew faster subsequent to additional CD133+ BMSC-treatment, to be comparable to hepatic tissue that proliferated more slowly after PVE without CD133+ BMSC application.[81,82] Mean hospital stays were comparable in both groups (30 days in the stem cell group vs. 35 days in the control group), whereas intensive care stays were longer in the stem cell group (13 days vs. 6 days). The latter observation is possibly explained by the higher comorbidity rate in this group. Given a median follow-up of 30 months, tumor-free survival times, hepatic and non-hepatic recurrence rates were almost identical in both groups.

The currently available data suggest that the concept of PVE with CD133+ BMSC administration to the liver bears the potential to accelerate and augment the proliferation of the FLRV more than does PVE alone. The modality seems to be safe and suitable in preparation for extensive liver resection. In particular, CD133+ stem cells may be a powerful adjunct to PVE in patients with very small left lateral segments, limited quality of hepatic parenchyma, and a large and fast-progressing tumor mass.

29.5.5 Mechanisms and Possible Adverse Reactions

In our study, we were able to show that FLRV is significantly higher in patients after administration of CD133+ cells subsequent to PVE than in patients without stem cell application. Although we neither investigated the fate of the injected adult stem cells nor the mechanisms causative for the enforced liver regeneration, it is conceivable that a variety of mechanisms may be involved. Current evidence suggests that transdifferentiation and fusion of BMSCs do not play a predominant in the repopulation of the hepatic parenchyma, whereas the concept of paracrine effects on endogenous hepatocytes is gaining support. Antifibrotic effects are unlikely to play a significant role in the setting of our study and are rather attributed to MSCs.[75] However, in cirrhotic livers, hepatocytes are reported to have reduced proliferative capacity, either secondary to the inhibitory effect of adjacent collagen or replicative senescence after many rounds of injury and repair.[83-86] In this scenario, stem cells have been hypothesized not only to increase the intrinsic ability of hepatocytes to replicate by release of trophic factors, but also to facilitate the degradation of scar tissue, thereby removing the block to proliferation. It is unclear whether an antifibrotic stem cell effect may have contributed to liver augmentation in two of our patients with liver cirrhosis (CP score A) and hepatocellular carcinoma who presented substantial relative and absolute FLRV gains (Fig. 29.4).

On the other hand, there is evidence that BM can also give rise to fibrogenic cells (hepatic stellate cells and myofibroblasts). Although BM-derived myofibroblasts originated largely from the BM's MSCs in murine models, the development of progressive liver fibrosis represents a concern regarding long-term safety of stem cell administration.[87,88]

The question of whether hepatocellular carcinoma may arise from transdifferentiation of SCs or dedifferentiation of mature cells remains controversial.[89,90] Consequently, the development or progression of tumor following stem cell therapy cannot be excluded as another long-term adverse effect. Tumor progression has also been reported as a possible adverse effect of preoperative PVE. However, clinical evidence concerning a direct increase in tumor growth resulting from PVE is not proven until this day.[91]

29.6 Conclusions

Early clinical experience with a novel concept to promote liver regeneration in patients scheduled for extended right liver resection demonstrated a significant increase in proliferation rates of the left lateral segments subsequent to application of CD133+ BMSCs and PVE. As these results are limited by the small number of patients and the lack of a randomized reference group, a controlled trial is needed to validate the findings in a larger group of patients. Also, experimental investigations are required to gain further insight in faith and mechanisms of CD133+ BMSCs applied to promote physiological liver regeneration processes. Beyond the surgical treatment of oncological patients with the indication for extensive partial hepatectomy, the findings derived from these studies may have an impact on therapeutic promotion of organ regeneration following other scenarios of acute and chronic liver damage.

References

1. Brancatisano R, Isla A, Habib N. Is radical hepatic surgery safe? *Am J Surg*. 1998;175:161-163.
2. Bozetti F, Gennari L, Regalia E, et al. Morbidity and mortality after surgical resection of liver tumors: analysis of 229 cases. *Hepatogastroenterology*. 1992;39:237-241.
3. Cunningham JD, Fong Y, Shriver C, et al. One hundred consecutive hepatic resections: blood loss, transfusion, and operative technique. *Arch Surg*. 1994;129:1050-1056.
4. Hemming AW, Reed AI, Howard RJ, et al. Preoperative portal embolization for extended hepatectomy. *Ann Surg*. 2003;237:686-691.
5. Broering DC, Hillert C, Krupski G, et al. Portal vein embolization vs. portal vein ligation for induction of hypertrophy of the future remnant. *J Gastrointest Surg*. 2002;6:905-913.
6. Lee KC, Kinoshita H, Hirohashi K, et al. Extension of surgical indications for hepatocellular carcinoma by portal vein embolization. *World J Surg*. 1993;17:109-115.
7. de Baire T, Roche A, Elias D, et al. Preoperative portal vein embolization for extension of hepatectomy indications. *Hepatology*. 1996;24:1386-1391.
8. Oyagi S, Hirose M, Kojima M, et al. Therapeutic effect of transplanting HGF-treated bone marrow mesenchymal cells into CCl4-injured rats. *J Hepatol*. 2006;44:42-48.
9. Zhao DC, Lei JX, Chen R, et al. Bone marrow-derived mesenchymal stem cells protect against experimental liver fibrosis in rats. *World J Gastroenterol*. 2005;11:3431-3440.
10. Yannaki E, Athanasiou E, Xagorari A, et al. G-CSF-primed hematopoietic stem cells or G-CSF per se accelerate recovery and improve survival after liver injury, predominantly by promoting endogenous repair programs. *Exp Hematol*. 2005;33:108-119.
11. Fujii H, Hirose T, Oe S, et al. Contribution of bone marrow cells to liver regeneration after partial hepatectomy in mice. *J Hepatol*. 2002;36:653-659.
12. Walkup MH, Gerber DA. Hepatic stem cells: in search of. *Stem Cells*. 2006;24:1833-1840.
13. Duncan JR, Hicks ME, Cai SR, et al. Embolization of portal vein branches induces hepatocyte replication in swine: a potential step in hepatic gene therapy. *Radiology*. 1999;210:467-477.
14. Potten CS, Loeffler M. Stem cells: attributes, cycles, spirals, pifalls and uncertainties: lessons for and from the crypt. *Development*. 1990;110:1001-1020.
15. Alison MR, Golding M, Sarraf CE. Liver stem cells: when the going gets tough they get going. *Int J Exp Pathol*. 1997;78:365-381.
16. Knight B, Matthews VB, Olynyk JK, Yeoh GC. Jekyll and Hyde: evolving perspectives on the function and potential of the adult liver progenitor (oval) cell. *Bioessays*. 2005;27:1192-1202.
17. Roskams TA, Theise ND, Balabaud C, et al. Nomenclature of the finer branches of the biliary tree: canals, ductules, and ductular reactions in human livers. *Hepatology*. 2004;39:1739-1745.
18. Farber E. Similarities in the sequence of early histological changes induced in the liver of the rat by ethionine, 2-acetyamino-fluorene, and 3′-methyl-4-dimethylaminoazobenzene. *Cancer Res*. 1956;16:142-148.
19. Shinozuka H, Lombardi B, Sell S, Iammarino RM. Early histological and functional alterations of ethionine liver carcinogenesis in rats fed a choline-deficient diet. *Cancer Res*. 1978;38:1092-1098.
20. Sell S. Distribution of alpha-fetoprotein- and albumin-containing cells in the livers of Fischer rats fed four cycles of N-2-fluorenylacetamide. *Cancer Res*. 1978;38:3107-3113.
21. Omori M, Evarts RP, Omori N, et al. Expression of alpha-fetoprotein and stem cell factor/c-kit system in bile duct ligated young rats. *Hepatology*. 1997;25:1115-1122.
22. Golding M, Sarraf CE, Lalani EN, et al. Oval cell differentiation into hepatocytes in the acetylaminofluorene-treated regenerating rat liver. *Hepatology*. 1995;22:1243-1253.

23. Sarraf CE, Lalani EN, Golding M, et al. Cell behaviour in the acetylaminofluorene-treated regenerating rat liver: light and electron microscopic observations. *Am J Pathol.* 1994; 145:1114-1126.
24. Petersen BE, Bowen WC, Patrene KD, et al. Bone marrow as a potential source of hepatic oval cells. *Science.* 1999; 284:1168-1170.
25. Alison MR, Poulsom R, Jeffery R, et al. Hepatocytes from non-hepatic adult stem cells. *Nature.* 2000;406:257.
26. Theise ND, Badve S, Saxena R, et al. Derivation of hepatocytes from bone marrow cells in mice after radiation-induced myeloablation. *Hepatology.* 2000;31:235-240.
27. Lagasse E, Connors H, Al-Dhalimy M, et al. Purified hematopoietic stem cells can differentiate into hepatocytes in vivo. *Nat Med.* 2000;6:1229-1234.
28. Crosby HA, Kelly DA, Strain AJ. Human hepatic stem-like cells isolated using c-kit or CD34 can differentiate into biliary epithelium. *Gastroenterology.* 2001;120:534-544.
29. Körbling M, Katz RL, Khanna A, et al. Hepatocytes and epithelial cells of donor origin in recipients of peripheral-blood stem cells. *N Engl J Med.* 2002;346:738-746.
30. Schwartz RE, Reyes M, Koodie L, et al. Multipotent adult progenitor cells from bone marrow differentiate into functional hepatocyte-like cells. *J Clin Invest.* 2002;109:1291-1302.
31. Newsome PN, Johannessen I, Boyle S, et al. Human cord blood-derived cells can differentiate into hepatocytes in the mouse liver with no evidence of cellular fusion. *Gastroenterology.* 2003;124:1891-1900.
32. Jang YY, Collector MI, Baylin SB, et al. Hematopoietic stem cells convert into liver cells within days without fusion. *Nat Cell Biol.* 2004;6:532-539.
33. Wang X, Willenbring H, Akkari Y, et al. Cell fusion is the principal source of bone-marrow-derived hepatocytes. *Nature.* 2003;422:897-901.
34. Vassilopoulos G, Wang PR, Russell DW. Transplanted bone marrow regenerates liver by cell fusion. *Nature.* 2003;422: 901-904.
35. Blakolmer K, Jaskiewicz K, Dunsford HA, Robson SC. Hematopoietic stem cell markers are expressed by ductal plate and bile duct cells in developing human liver. *Hepatology.* 1995;21:1510-1516.
36. Lemmer ER, Shephard EG, Blakolmer K, et al. Isolation from human fetal liver cells coexpressing CD34 haematopoietic stem cell and CAM 5.2 pancytokeratin markers. *J Hepatol.* 1998;29:450-454.
37. Fiegel HC, Park JJ, Lioznov MV, et al. Characterization of cell types during rat liver development. *Hepatology.* 2003;37: 148-154.
38. Monga SP, Tang Y, Candotti F, et al. Expansion of hepatic and hematopoietic stem cells utilizing mouse embryonic liver explants. *Cell Transplant.* 2001;10:81-89.
39. Nierhoff D, Ogawa A, Oertel M, et al. Purification and characterization of mouse fetal liver epithelial cells with high in vivo repopulation capacity. *Hepatology.* 2005;42:130-139.
40. Sato Y, Araki H, Kato J, et al. Human mesenchymal stem cells xenografted directly to rat liver are differentiated into human hepatocytes without fusion. *Blood.* 2005;106:756-763.
41. Kuo TK, Hung SP, Chuang CH, et al. Stem cell therapy for liver disease: parameters governing the success of using bone marrow mesenchymal stem cells. *Gastroenterology.* 2008;134:2111-2121.
42. Kallis YN, Alison MR, Forbes SJ. Bone marrow stem cells and liver disease. *Gut.* 2007;56:716-724.
43. Grompe M. The role of bone marrow stem cells in liver regeneration. *Semin Liver Dis.* 2003;23:363-372.
44. Fiegel HC, Lange C, Kneser U, et al. Fetal and adult liver stem cells for liver regeneration and tissue engineering. *J Cell Mol Med.* 2006;10:577-587.
45. Almeida-Porada G, Porada CD, Chamberlain J, et al. Formation of human hepatocytes by human hematopoietic stem cells in sheep. *Blood.* 2004;104:2582-2590.
46. Okumoto K, Saito T, Haga H, et al. Characteristics of rat bone marrow cells differentiated into a liver cell lineage and dynamics of the transplanted cells in the injured liver. *J Gastroenterol.* 2006;41:62-69.
47. Thorgeirsson SS, Grisham JW. Hematopoietic cells as hepatocyte stem cells: a critical review of the evidence. *Hepatology.* 2006;43:2-8.
48. Forbes SJ. Stem cell therapy for chronic liver disease—choosing the right tools for the job. *Gut.* 2008;57:153-155.
49. Brulport M, Schormann W, Bauer A, et al. Fate of extrahepatic human stem and precursor cells after transplantation into mouse livers. *Hepatology.* 2007;46:861-870.
50. Theise ND, Krause DS. Bone marrow to liver: the blood of Prometheus. *Semin Cell Dev Biol.* 2002;13:411-417.
51. Fausto N, Campbell JS. The role of hepatocytes and oval cells in liver regeneration and repopulation. *Mech Dev.* 2003;120:117-130.
52. Cantz T, Sharma AD, Jochheim-Richter A, et al. Reevaluation of bone marrow-derived cells as a source for hepatocyte regeneration. *Cell Transplant.* 2004;13:659-666.
53. Krieg A, Schmelzle M, Schulte am Esch J, et al. Stem cell factor levels do increase in patients subsequent to hepatectomy with the extend of parenchymal loss. *Transplant Proc.* 2006;38:3556-3558.
54. Kollet O, Shivtiel S, Chen YQ, et al. HGF, SDF-1, and MMP-9 are involved in stress-induced human CD34+ stem cell recruitment to the liver. *J Clin Invest.* 2003;112: 160-169.
55. Hatch HM, Zheng D, Jorgensen ML, et al. SDF-1alpha/CXCR4: a mechanism for hepatic oval cell activation and bone marrow stem cell recruitment to the injured liver of rats. *Cloning Stem Cells.* 2002;4:339-351.
56. Dalakas E, Newsome PN, Harrison DJ, Plevris JN. Hematopoietic stem cell trafficking in liver injury. *FASEB J.* 2005;19:1225-1231.
57. Wang X, Ge S, McNamara G, et al. Albumin-expressing hepatocyte-like cells develop in the livers of immune-deficient mice that received transplants of highly purified human hematopoietic stem cells. *Blood.* 2003;101:4201-4208.
58. Ratajczak MZ, Kucia M, Reca R, et al. Stem cell plasticity revisited: CXCR4-positive cells expressing mRNA for early muscle, liver and neural cells 'hide out' in the bone marrow. *Leukemia.* 2004;18:29-40.
59. Lange C, Bruns H, Kluth D, et al. Hepatocytic differentiation of mesenchymal stem cells in cocultures with fetal liver cells. *World J Gastroenterol.* 2006;12:2394-2397.
60. Son BR, Marquez-Curtis LA, Kucia M, et al. Migration of bone marrow and cord blood mesenchymal stem cells in vitro is regulated by stromal-derived factor-1-CXCR4 and hepatocyte growth factor-c-met axes and involves matrix metalloproteinases. *Stem Cells.* 2006;24:1254-1264.
61. Avital I, Inderbitzin D, Aoki T, et al. Isolation, characterization, and transplantation of bone marrow-derived hepatocyte stem cells. *Biochem Biophys Res Commun.* 2001;288: 156-164.

62. Xu J, Deng X, Demetriou AA, et al. Factors released from cholestatic rat livers possibly involved in inducing bone marrow hepatic stem cell priming. *Stem Cells Dev*. 2008;17:143-155.
63. De Silvestro G, Vicarioto M, Donadel C, et al. Mobilization of peripheral blood hematopoietic stem cells following liver resection surgery. *Hepatogastroenterology*. 2004;51:805-810.
64. Gehling UM, Willems M, Dandri M, et al. Partial hepatectomy induces mobilization of a unique population of haematopoietic progenitor cells in human healthy liver donors. *J Hepatol*. 2005;43:845-853.
65. Baccarani U, De Stasio G, Adani GL, et al. Implication of stem cell factor in human liver regeneration after transplantation and resection. *Growth Factors*. 2006;24:107-110.
66. Gaia S, Smedile A, Omedè P, et al. Feasibility and safety of G-CSF administration to induce bone marrow-derived cells mobilization in patients with end stage liver disease. *J Hepatol*. 2006;45:13-19.
67. Terai S, Ishikawa T, Omori K, et al. Improved liver function in patients with liver cirrhosis after autologous bone marrow cell infusion therapy. *Stem Cells*. 2006;24:2292-2298.
68. Mohamadnejad M, Namiri M, Bagheri M, et al. Phase 1 human trial of autologous bone marrow-hematopoietic stem cell transplantation in patients with decompensated liver cirrhosis. *World J Gastroenterol*. 2007;28:3359-3363.
69. Mohamadnejad M, Alimoghaddam K, Mohyeddin-Bonab M, et al. Phase 1 trial of autologous bone marrow mesenchymal stem cell transplantation in patients with decompensated cirrhosis. *Arch Iran Med*. 2007;10:459-466.
70. Lyra AC, Soares MB, da Silva LF, et al. Feasibility and safety of autologous bone marrow mononuclear cell transplantation in patients with advanced chronic liver disease. *World J Gastroenterol*. 2007;13:1067-1073.
71. Lyra AC, Soares MB, da Silva LF, et al. A pilot randomised controlled study used to evaluate efficacy of bone marrow mononuclear cells transplantation in patients with advanced chronic liver disease (abstr). *Hepatology*. 2007;46(Suppl 1): 271A.
72. Gordon MY, Levicar N, Pai M, et al. Characterization and clinical application of human CD34+ stem/progenitor cell populations mobilized into the blood by granulocyte colony-stimulating factor. *Stem Cells*. 2006;24:1822-1830.
73. Levicar N, Pai M, Habib NA, et al. Long-term clinical results of autologous infusion of mobilized adult bone marrow derived CD34+ cells in patients with chronic liver disease. *Cell Prolif*. 2008;41:115-125.
74. Yannaki E, Anagnostopoulos A, Kapetanos D, et al. Lasting amelioration in the clinical course of decompensated alcoholic cirrhosis with boost infusions of mobilized peripheral blood stem cells. *Exp Hematol*. 2006;34:1583-1587.
75. Houlihan DD, Newsome PN. Critical review of clinical trials of bone marrow stem cells in liver disease. *Gastroenterology*. 2008;135:438-450.
76. Schulte am Esch J 2nd, Knoefel WT, Klein M, et al. Portal application of autologous CD133+ bone marrow cells to the liver: a novel concept to support hepatic regeneration. *Stem Cells*. 2005;23:463-470.
77. Fürst G, Schulte am Esch J, Poll LW, et al. Portal vein embolization and application of autologous CD133+ bone marrow stem cells for liver regeneration: initial experience. *Radiology*. 2006;243:171-179.
78. Nagasue N, Yukaya H, Ogawa Y, et al. Human liver regeneration after major hepatic resection: a study of normal liver and livers with chronic hepatitis and cirrhosis. *Ann Surg*. 1987;206:30-39.
79. Ghodsizad A, Klein HM, Borowski A, et al. Intraoperative isolation and processing of BM-derived stem cells. *Cytotherapy*. 2004;6:523-526.
80. Fan TX, Hisha H, Jin TN, et al. Successful allogeneic bone marrow transplantation (BMT) by injection of bone marrow cells via portal vein: stromal cells as BMT-facilitating cells. *Stem Cells*. 2001;19:144-150.
81. Fürst G, Knoefel WT, Fritz LB et al. Portal vein embolization and autologous CD133+ bone marrow stem cells for liver regeneration: early clinical results. Paper presented at: Radiological Society of North America 92nd Scientific Assembly and Annual Meeting; November 26–December 1, 2006; Chicago, IL. p. 385
82. Schulte am Esch J, Schmelzle M, Fürst G et al. Infusion of CD133+ bone marrow derived stem cells after selective portal embolization enhances functional hepatic reserves after extended right hepatectomy. A retrospective single center study. Ann Surg. 2011: in press.
83. Körbling M, Estrov Z. Adult stem cells for tissue repair – A new therapeutic concept? *N Engl J Med*. 2003;349: 570-582.
84. Fassett JT, Tolbot D, Nelsen CJ, et al. The role of collagen structure in mitogen stimulation of ERK, cyclin D1 expression, and G1-S progression in rat hepatocytes. *J Biol Chem*. 2003;278:31691-31700.
85. Fassett JT, Tolbot D, Hansen LK. Type I collagen structure regulates cell morphology and EGF signaling in primary rat hepatocytes through cAMP-dependent protein kinase A. *Mol Biol Cell*. 2006;17:345-356.
86. Trak-Smayra V, Contreras J, Dondero F, et al. Role of replicative senescence in the progression of fibrosis in hepatitis C virus (HCV) recurrence after liver transplantation. *Transplantation*. 2004;77:1755-1760.
87. Russo FP, Alison MR, Bigger BW, et al. The bone marrow functionally contributes to liver fibrosis. *Gastroenterology*. 2006;130:1807-1821.
88. Kisseleva T, Uchinami H, Feirt N, et al. Bone marrow-derived fibrocytes participate in pathogenesis of liver fibrosis. *J Hepatol*. 2006;45:429-438.
89. Wu XZ, Chen D. Origin of hepatocellular carcinoma: role of stem cells. *J Gastroenterol Hepatol*. 2006;21:1093-1098.
90. Dumble ML, Croager EJ, Yeoh GC, Quail EA. Generation and characterization of p53 null transformed hepatic progenitor cells: oval cells give rise to hepatocellular carcinoma. *Carcinogenesis*. 2002;23:435-445.
91. De Graaf W, van den Esschert JW, van Lienden KP, van Gulik TM. Induction of tumor growth after portal vein embolization: Is it a real problem? *Ann Surg Oncol*. 2009;16(2):423-430.

Portal Vein Embolization Prior to Major Hepatectomy: The Evidence

30

Eddie K. Abdalla

Abstract

Portal vein embolization (PVE) is increasingly used to increase the volume and function of the liver that will remain after resection of large and multiple liver tumors. This chapter examines the strong, extensive evidence supporting the use of preoperative PVE prior to major hepatic resection based on analysis of the future liver remnant (FLR), or liver that will remain after resection. Specifically, data demonstrate that liver function is linked both to FLR volume and to the quality of the underlying liver (from normal to diseased to cirrhotic liver along a continuum). The safe limits of resection are defined based on these factors derived from objective studies which reveal the safe limits of resection and the indications for preoperative PVE. Adequate FLR volume in patients with normal liver has been determined to be 20% of the standardized total liver volume, or TLV; in patients with diseased liver, 30% of the TLV; and in patients with (well compensated) cirrhosis, 40% of the TLV. Important evidence demonstrates that PVE can be used to convert a patient with an inadequate FLR to a patient with an FLR sufficient to ensure safe surgery and adequate post-resection liver function, and demonstrates that the hypertrophic response or degree of hypertrophy of the FLR after PVE predicts post-resection liver function. Finally, evidence suggests that a prospective, randomized trial to test the utility of PVE is neither feasible nor necessary based on currently available data.

Keywords

Portal vein embolization • Hepatectomy and portal vein embolization • Liver volume • Evidence for portal vein embolization before hepatectomy

Major hepatectomy is increasingly used to treat benign and malignant tumors of the liver. Major technical complications and fatal liver failure are rare; however, as the limits of resection are tested and extended hepatectomy is used to remove larger and larger proportions of liver parenchyma, complications resulting from cholestasis and impaired synthetic function contribute to morbidity and prolonged recovery in some patients.[1,2]

It is now recognized that recovery from major hepatic resection hinges less on what has been removed (the resected liver) and more on what remains after

E.K. Abdalla
Department of Surgical Oncology, The University of Texas M.D. Anderson Cancer Center, 1400 Holcombe Boulevard, Unit 444, Houston, TX, USA
e-mail: eabdalla@mdanderson.org

D.C. Madoff et al. (eds.), *Venous Embolization of the Liver*,
DOI 10.1007/978-1-84882-122-4_30,

resection (the future liver remnant [FLR]). Patients with an adequate FLR recover from major hepatic resection rapidly, even in the event of a complication. In contrast, patients with an inadequate FLR may develop no surgical complications whatsoever but progressively become jaundiced (even with relatively normal prothrombin time) and eventually die of liver failure (typically within 90 days after surgery). Patients with a marginal FLR are vulnerable to a cascade of problems if a surgical complication occurs – if such patients develop pneumonia or a perihepatic collection, they may suffer a prolonged, complicated postoperative course and recovery or succumb to multiple organ failure. These problems can occur both in patients with normal livers and in those with diseased livers when the FLR volume is marginal or inadequate.[1,3,4]

It is also now recognized that not only the size of the remnant liver but also the quality of the underlying liver affects outcomes after resection, that is, in a patient with a normal liver, a smaller FLR might support normal functional recovery, whereas in a patient with a diseased liver (e.g., a cirrhotic liver), a larger FLR is necessary to ensure adequate liver function.

Portal vein embolization (PVE) has been proposed[5] and is increasingly used[1,6] prior to major hepatic resection in patients with normal and diseased underlying liver parenchyma to induce hypertrophy and to enhance the function of the FLR, when the preoperative judgment is made that resection would leave an FLR inadequate to support posthepatectomy liver function. PVE was first used by Kinoshita et al.[7] not to induce liver hypertrophy but to prevent tumor extension of hepatocellular carcinoma. In the context of major hepatectomy, PVE has been proposed to shift liver function from the embolized liver (the liver to be resected) to the nonembolized liver (the FLR).

The premise of this book is that PVE is useful and that it works – that appropriate preoperative application of PVE can prevent postoperative liver dysfunction. But where is the evidence that PVE should be used to induce hypertrophy of the FLR prior to resection and that such hypertrophy prevents postoperative complications associated with an inadequate FLR?

This chapter examines the strong, extensive evidence supporting the use of preoperative PVE performed prior to major hepatic resection. The discussion is organized around several specific questions:

1. Is liver function linked to liver volume?
2. Is there a limit to the extent of resection that can be performed safely, i.e., is there truly a remnant that is functionally too small to support post-resection liver function? If so, what is that limit?
3. Can PVE convert a patient with an inadequate FLR into a patient with an FLR adequate to ensure post-resection liver function?
4. Should a prospective, randomized trial be proposed to assess the value of PVE? If so, in what population?

30.1 Is Liver Function Linked to Liver Volume?

There is substantial evidence that liver function is linked to liver volume in patients undergoing liver resection, and there is little evidence to refute this connection.

The concept that liver function and liver volume are linked is intuitive. Certainly, it is inarguable that liver volume of zero (the anhepatic state) is not compatible with prolonged life. Reports of recovery following more than 1 to 2 days in the anhepatic state are anecdotal, and such recovery can occur only when liver volume is restored, i.e., when liver transplantation is accomplished.[8]

The concept that sufficient volume of liver must remain after resection to ensure patient survival is not new – Bismuth taught this "reglée" of liver surgery more than 25 years ago.[9] Ample evidence supports this contention.

30.1.1 Liver Volume Is Related to Patient Size

Liver volume is clearly related to patient size.[10] In fact, liver volume and body surface area (BSA) are related in a linear fashion[11] – larger patients have larger livers; smaller patients, smaller livers. The correlation between patient size and liver volume is tighter in small, thin patients and children[12] than in larger, obese patients,[13] but the linear relationship holds true in all patient subgroups. There are at least 12 publications in the literature describing the important relationship between patient size and liver volume (the 12 references are found in the meta-analysis from Johnson et al.[10]).

30.1.2 Evidence from Liver Transplantation: Importance of the Graft Volume

As living-donor liver transplantation evolved, interest in the relationship between liver volume and patient size grew because of the observations that the graft volume, as measured on computed tomography (CT) volumetry, was a critical factor in liver transplantation[14,15] and that the graft volume is related to liver function after transplantation.[16-18] There was a need to understand the minimum volume of liver needed to support post-transplantation liver function in both the donor and the transplant recipient.

Recognition of the "small-for-size" syndrome – i.e., inadequate volume of the liver graft leading to poor function of the perfectly normal graft suffering only from the transplantation-related insults (resection from the donor, cold ischemia, warm reperfusion, and importantly, support of 100% of portal flow in a relatively small graft) – focused attention on the need for accurate assessment of graft volume in the donor and accurate assessment of the liver function/volume needs of the recipient. It was found that the most accurate predictor of the graft function after living-donor liver transplantation was graft volume.[15-18]

Further, the recognition that patient size predicted liver-volume needs led to the development of formulas to estimate the recipient's total liver volume (TLV) from BSA or body weight and also led to the use of the graft-volume-to-recipient's-body-weight ratio (graft volume ÷ body weight) to determine what graft volume would be adequate.[12] Numerous studies have shown that a graft-volume-to-recipient's-body-weight ratio of 0.8 is the minimum needed to ensure adequate liver function after transplantation. Body weight and BSA can be used with equal efficacy in this setting.[19]

30.1.3 Evidence from Extensive Hepatic Resection: Importance of the FLR Volume

As extensive hepatectomy was increasingly performed and some patients suffered post-resection complications resembling small-for-size syndrome in liver transplantation (poor liver function including cholestasis, ascites, and peripheral edema),[1,2] the significance of FLR volume emerged,[1] and interest in the liver function–liver volume relationship grew in the field of resective surgery.

Initially, confusion existed regarding the safe extent of surgery, which was variously described as resection of anywhere from 40% to 65% of the liver.[20-24] (Safe extent of resection is discussed in detail in the following section.) Confusion regarding the safe extent of surgery was most likely related to differences in methods of assessing the FLR volume before surgery and differences in anesthetic technique, resection technique, and postoperative care. Today, whereas anesthetic technique, resection technique, and postoperative care have largely been optimized, a lack of standardization persists with respect to the method of volumetric assessment of the FLR prior to resection. As the method of measuring FLR volume can influence the results of studies on the liver volume–liver function relationship, the various methods of FLR volume measurement will be briefly discussed here.

In resective surgery, Vauthey et al.[25] advanced a standardized method of calculating the FLR. With this method, TLV was calculated on the basis of BSA (initially according to the formula of Urata,[12] but later improved based on a newer, more accurate formula described below). TLV calculated in this manner is referred to as "standardized TLV" because the TLV is standardized to BSA. Specifically, CT is used to measure the FLR (since the FLR is normal and CT volumetry is accurate to within ±5% in the measurement of normal liver parenchyma[23,26]), and the FLR volume is expressed as a percentage of the TLV such that standardized TLV = (FLR volume from CT) ÷ (TLV from formula). FLR volume calculated in this manner – on the basis of the standardized TLV – is referred to as "standardized FLR volume." The method of Vauthey et al. for calculating FLR volume had the advantages of an objectively determined denominator (TLV based on BSA) and a simple and easy to understand description of FLR volume. Further, future measurements of the FLR volume can be standardized to the same denominator to allow accurate comparison of FLR volume before and after interventions.

Using this method of calculating FLR volume, Vauthey et al. demonstrated that major complications after hepatic resection correlated not with the volume of liver resected but with the standardized FLR volume. They demonstrated that results of postoperative liver function tests, including tests of prothrombin time and bilirubin level, were related to FLR volume and that global indicators of recovery, including length of intensive care unit stay, number and severity of complications, and length of hospital stay, were inversely proportional to FLR volume.[25]

An alternative method of FLR volumetry has also been used in patients undergoing resection.[14] With this method, as with the method of Vauthey et al., CT is used for FLR volume measurement; however, whereas with the method of Vauthey et al. TLV is calculated on the basis of BSA, with this alternative method, TLV and liver tumor volumes are measured directly by CT, and a "corrected TLV" is calculated by subtracting the measured tumor volumes from the measured TLV. This alternative method can introduce significant error into both pre- and post-PVE volume determinations because (1) the liver is diseased (either contains tumors or, in the case of cirrhosis, may be enlarged or shrunken), (2) additive measurement error occurs because of the standard error in liver volume determination combined with the standard error in tumor volume determinations, and (3) different TLV denominators are used to calculate FLR volume before and after PVE because the actual TLV changes after PVE. Further, the lack of standardization of TLV to patient size using body weight or BSA reduces the value of the FLR volume calculation and fails to recognize the significance of the liver volume–patient size correlation.[27]

Subsequent evidence supported the findings of Vauthey et al.'s initial study. An analysis of patients with normal underlying liver who underwent hepatic resection of similar extent (all underwent extended right hepatectomy) showed that complication rates related directly to FLR volume calculated on the basis of the standardized TLV.[28] Specifically, patients with FLR volume >20% of the standardized TLV had a complication rate of 13%, compared to 50% in patients with FLR volume ≤20% of the standardized TLV (Fig. 30.1). Recently, data regarding 301 consecutive extended right hepatectomies were reported from our institution.[27] This study demonstrated a clear correlation between postoperative liver insufficiency and FLR volume calculated on the basis of the standardized TLV. In this study, not only were complications studied but "liver insufficiency" was also objectively defined on the basis of validated data[3] and was specifically studied with respect to FLR volume. Finally, direct comparison of patients with small (≤20% of TLV), intermediate (20.1–30% of TLV), and large (≥30% of TLV) FLR volumes demonstrated increased risk for liver insufficiency and postoperative death in patients with small FLR volumes (discussed in detail below).[27]

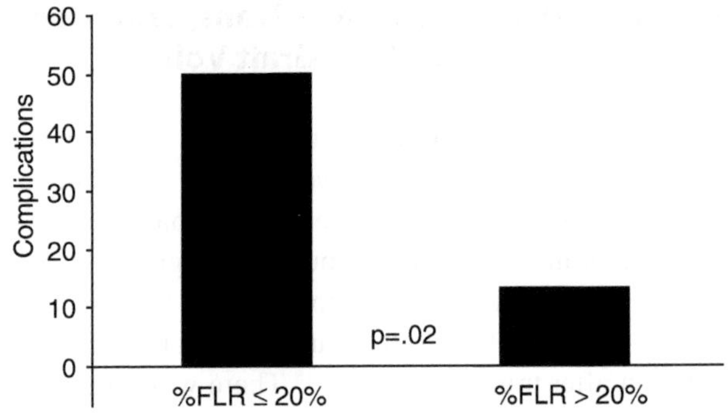

Fig. 30.1 Complication rate stratified by standardized FLR volume (%FLR) in patients with normal underlying liver. Fifty percent of patients with FLR≤20% experienced complications, compared to only 15% of those with %FLR>20% (p=0.02) (Adapted from Abdalla et al.,[28] with permission)

Data in cirrhotic patients undergoing major hepatectomy further substantiate a correlation between liver volume and liver function. Kubota et al.[20] demonstrated that cirrhotic patients with normal preoperative liver function who underwent major hepatectomy developed hyperbilirubinemia when FLR volumes were small but did not develop hyperbilirubinemia when FLR volumes were large (>40% of TLV). Shirabe and Shimada took this line of inquiry one step further, in a subsequent study of cirrhotic patients who had undergone right hepatectomy.[4] They demonstrated that patients who died of liver failure had significantly smaller FLR volumes than patients who did not die of liver failure ($p<0.008$). Further, using standardized liver volumetry (FLR volume standardized to BSA), they demonstrated that the incidence of liver failure in patients with an FLR volume of<250 mL/m² BSA was 38% versus 0% in patients with an FLR volume>250 mL/m² ($p<0.001$).[4]

Little evidence exists to refute these findings of an association between FLR volume and liver function in patients undergoing major hepatectomy. A single large study suggested that extended right hepatectomy can be performed without risk for liver failure,[29] but liver failure and liver insufficiency are not defined in the study report and no data on FLR volume are provided, which makes it impossible to establish any link between liver volume and liver function in that study. All deaths reported were said to occur before 90 days postoperatively, and the authors reported that no out-of-hospital deaths occurred.[30] No published experience with extensive liver resection corroborates these findings, which remain to be validated.

Other data have been cited to suggest that volume resected, not FLR volume, is of interest. Analysis of these well-done studies, however, shows that they do not address the question at hand, i.e., whether liver volume and function are linked. First, a report of a huge institutional series of hepatic resections[31] including all resections performed at the institution, both major and minor resections, is often cited, but does not actually provide a basis to assess risk associated with extensive resection with minimal remnant liver volume. In another important series of major hepatic resections,[32] the authors reported a low (6%) in-hospital mortality rate, but the study did not examine the outcome based on FLR volume so that no conclusions can be drawn regarding the relationship between liver volume and liver function. Subsequently, however, centers of excellence, such as the one from which these reports emanated, reassessed their former assertion that resection extent predicts outcome[33] and, on re-analysis of their own data using volumetry, found that outcome after resection was linked not to resection extent but rather to FLR volume.[34] Thus, evidence is substantial supporting the volume-function link pertaining to liver resection.

30.2 FLR Volume: How Small Is Too Small?

Given that liver volume and liver function are linked and that an inadequate FLR volume increases the risk of complications of liver resection, a logical next question is "What is the minimum safe FLR volume for hepatic resection?"

As stated in the Introduction, liver function is affected by the presence and degree of underlying liver disease.[35] Thus, the minimum safe FLR volume is also affected by underlying liver disease. For patients with normal liver, several different limits have been proposed for the minimum safe FLR volume, ranging from a high of 30% of TLV[36-38] to a low of 20% of TLV.[1,27,35,39] For patients with well-compensated cirrhosis, most reports suggest that an FLR volume of 40% of TLV is required for safe major hepatectomy (Fig. 30.2).[4,20,35]

In the setting of living-donor liver transplantation, the minimum safe graft volume is less controversial

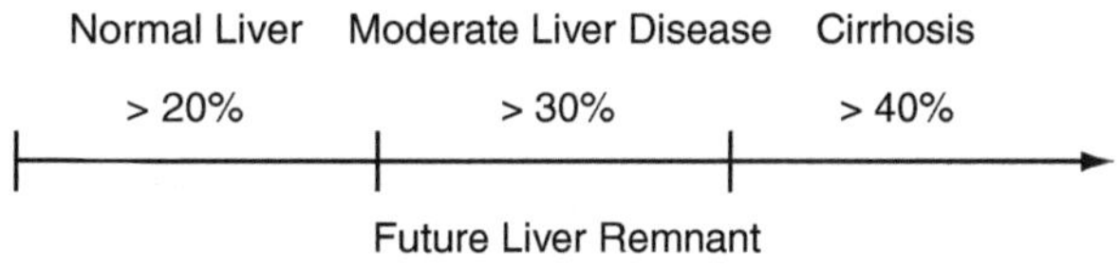

Fig. 30.2 Minimum FLR volume needed for safe hepatic resection in patients with normal liver, intermediate liver disease, or cirrhotic liver (Adapted from Zorzi et al.,[40] with permission)

and is generally agreed to be approximately 0.8 mL/kg body weight (approximately 40% of the standardized TLV).[15-18]

30.2.1 Normal Liver

Most of the data on the minimum safe FLR volume after hepatic resection come from patients with normal or relatively normal underlying liver parenchyma.

30.2.1.1 Arbitrary Cutoff: 30% of TLV

Many authors use an arbitrarily determined cutoff for safe resection: an FLR volume of 30% of TLV.[36-38] Thus, there are no particular studies or data to support this volume limit – it is simply stated and used by the referenced authors.

30.2.1.2 European Studies: Approximately 25% of TLV

A report from Italy of an objective analysis of the relationship between FLR volume and outcome included the conclusion that the safe limit for the FLR volume is 25–30% of TLV. However, this analysis included no patient with an FLR volume<25% of TLV.[41] Since no patient with a smaller FLR volume was included, it cannot necessarily be concluded that 25% of TLV is the minimum safe FLR volume.

Schindl et al.[42] from the United Kingdom published a well-done analysis of outcome after liver resection based on FLR volume. They used defined measures of hepatic dysfunction (including total serum bilirubin level, prothrombin time, serum lactate level, and encephalopathy grade[43]) and postoperative infection as end points and found that postoperative hepatic dysfunction correlated directly with FLR volume (Fig. 30.3). Using receiver operating characteristic curve analysis, they defined the minimum safe FLR volume to be 26.6% of TLV.[42] Further, they found that 73% of patients with severe hepatic dysfunction developed infection, compared

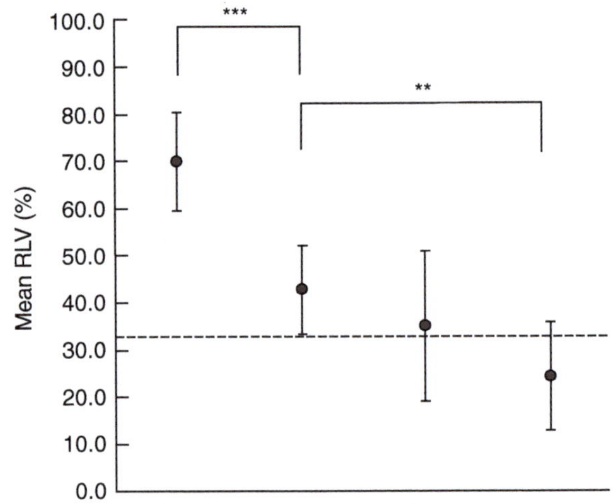

Hepatic dysfunction	No	Mild	Moderate	Severe
n	27	42	22	13
Mean %RLV	69.9	42.9	35.3	24.5
SD	22.6	15.4	15.3	6.0

Fig. 30.3 Mean relative residual liver volume (%RLV, commonly referred to as FLR volume or %FLR) following liver resection. There was a continuum of liver dysfunction based on FLR volume – severe liver dysfunction was seen in patients with very small FLR volume, and no dysfunction was seen in patients with large FLR volume (Adapted from Schindl et al.,[42] with permission)

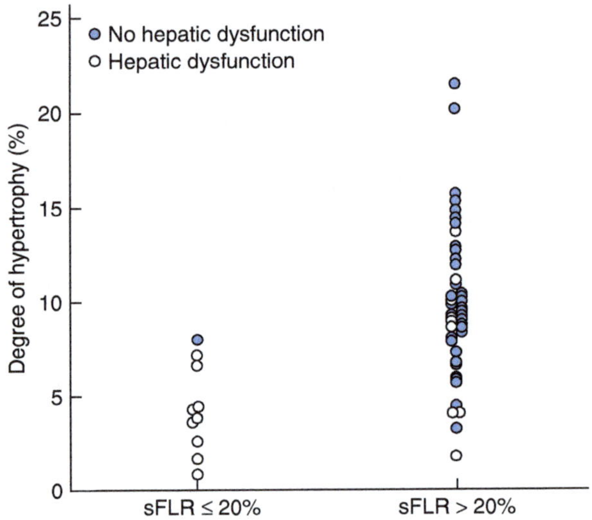

Fig. 30.4 Scatter plot of the incidence of hepatic dysfunction according to degree of hypertrophy, stratified by standardized FLR volume (sFLR or %FLR). Incidence of liver dysfunction was extremely low in patients with FLR>20% and degree of hypertrophy>5% (Adapted from Ribero et al.,[45] with permission)

to only 18% of patients without severe hepatic dysfunction ($p=0.030$). In multivariate analysis, FLR volume<26.6% and high BMI>30 kg/m^2 predicted hepatic dysfunction. CT volumetry was used, but the TLV was measured directly by CT rather than being calculated on the basis of BSA, which introduced the problems described above with nonstandardized liver volumes and may have resulted in a higher minimum safe FLR volume than would have resulted from the use of standardized TLV. These authors also found that high BMI predicted liver dysfunction, an important finding that was later corroborated in other studies.[27]

30.2.1.3 Current Standard: 20% of TLV

An early study from our institution found a minimum safe FLR volume of 25% of the standardized TLV in patients who underwent extended right hepatectomy.[44] This study used standardized TLV calculated using the Urata formula.[12] We subsequently found that the Urata formula underestimated the TLV for western patients, and we developed a more accurate formula following analysis of a large population of patients from the Americas and Western Europe.[13]

This new Vauthey formula was subsequently found in meta-analysis to be the most accurate, least biased formula for estimation of TLV.[10] Using the new formula in a study of the relationship between outcome after extended right hepatectomy and standardized FLR volume in patients with FLR volumes as small as 11% of TLV,[28] we showed that 50% of patients with an FLR volume≤20% of TLV suffered complications versus only 13% of patients with an FLR volume>20% of TLV. This study suggested a new, smaller cutoff and was likely more accurate because of the use of a more accurate TLV to which the FLR was standardized (i.e., TLV calculated from an appropriate formula) and because this study, unlike the aforementioned studies from Italy and the United Kingdom, included patients with very small FLR volumes.

Two large follow-up studies confirmed the 20% FLR limit for patients with normal liver.[27,45] The first[27,45] used established definitions for hepatic dysfunction[34,44] and hepatic insufficiency[44] and used receiver operating characteristic analysis to assess the volume limit for safe resection in a series of 112 patients who underwent major or extended hepatectomy at one institution between 1995 and 2006 (Fig. 30.4) These authors used systematic standardized liver volumetry and demonstrated that overall, major and liver-related complications, hepatic dysfunction or insufficiency, hospital

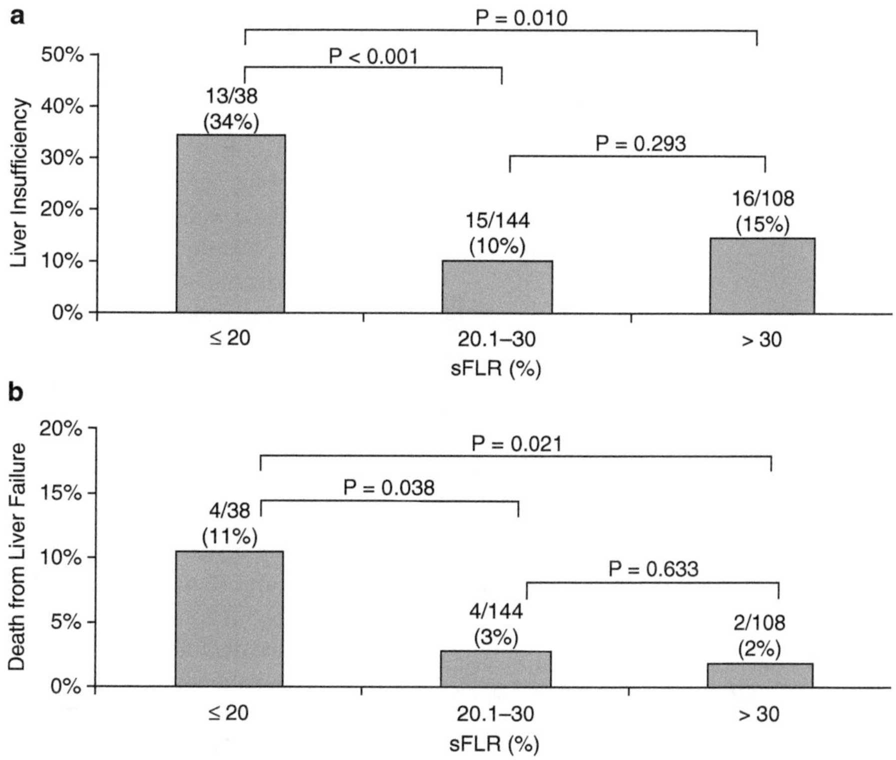

Fig. 30.5 Incidence of postoperative liver insufficiency (**a**) and death due to liver failure (**b**) according to preoperative standardized FLR volume [sFLR (%)]. These data show that patients with sFLR (%) 20.1–30% have no more liver insufficiency or death than those with sFLR (%) >30% (Adapted from Kishi et al.,[27] with permission)

stay, and 90-day mortality rate were significantly greater in patients with a standardized FLR of <20% of TLV compared to those with greater FLR volumes. The second study[27] was an analysis of 301 patients who underwent extended right hepatectomy, again using standardized volumetry and an objective, established definition of liver insufficiency: a postoperative bilirubin level reaching 7 mg/dL.[3] Importantly, this study examined outcomes in patients with standardized FLR volume ≤20% of TLV, 20.1–30% of TLV, or >30% of TLV and showed that liver insufficiency and death from liver failure were no more common in patients with FLR volume 20.1–30% of TLV than in patients with FLR volume >30% of TLV (Fig. 30.5). However, the group with FLR volume ≤20% of TLV experienced an increased risk of liver insufficiency and death from liver failure ($p < 0.05$).

Thus, the minimum safe FLR volume in patients with normal liver was established as >20% of the standardized TLV. This limit was published in 2006 in the consensus statement made following a consensus conference on hepatic colorectal metastases sponsored by the American Hepato-Pancreato-Biliary Association and cosponsored by the Society for Surgery of the Alimentary Tract, Society of Surgical Oncology, GI Symposium Steering Committee, and The University of Texas M. D. Anderson Cancer Center.[35]

30.2.2 Diseased Liver

There have been no studies on the minimum safe FLR volume for patients with liver disease except in patients with well-compensated cirrhosis. The first study in such patients, from Kubota et al.,[20] examined outcome following hepatic resection in cirrhotic patients and found that those with FLR volume >40% of TLV experienced normal evolution of postoperative liver functions and no mortality. No patients in this study had liver insufficiency postoperatively; therefore, it is possible that a lower limit could have been defined, but certainly this study established FLR volume ≥40% of TLV as a starting point.

A subsequent examination of 80 patients with cirrhosis who underwent major resection focused on seven patients (8.8%) who died of liver failure postoperatively.[4] None of the seven died as a result of a technical complication rather, they died of pure liver failure

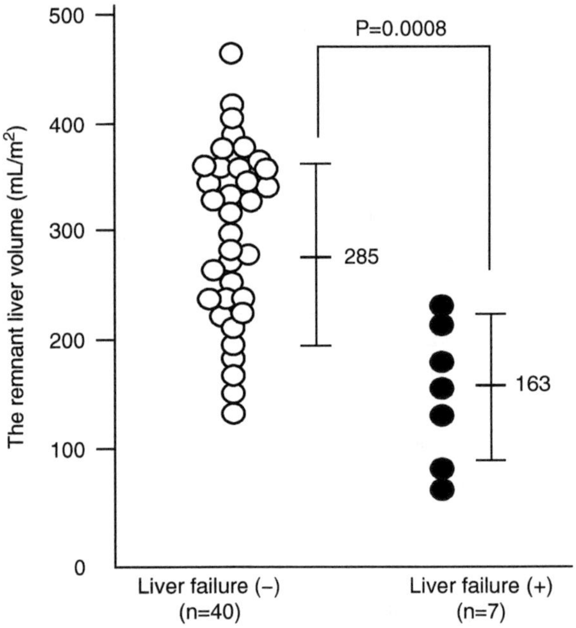

Fig. 30.6 Complication rate stratified by standardized FLR volume standardized to body surface area in cirrhotic patients who underwent right hepatectomy. Mean FLR volume in patients who died of liver failure (163 mL/m^2) was significantly smaller than that (285 L/m^2) in patients who did not die of liver failure (p=0.0008). No patient with FLR volume more than 250 mL/m^2 died of liver failure (Adapted from Shirabe et al.,[4] with permission)

or its consequences. Further, analysis of potential risk factors for death (including age, gender, preoperative liver function, and indocyanine green retention [ICG-R]) in the 47 patients who underwent right lobectomy, a group that included all seven patients who died of liver failure after surgery, revealed no preoperative factor that predicted death except for standardized FLR volume.[4] Mean FLR volume was 163 mL/m^2 BSA in patients who died of liver failure versus 285 mL/m^2 in patients without liver failure (p=0.0008) (Fig. 30.6). No patient with an FLR volume>250 mL/m^2 died. In addition, over half of the patients who died also had diabetes mellitus (which has been shown to impact the kinetics and degree of liver hypertrophy). Thus, FLR volume proved again to be a predictor of liver failure and death after liver resection. This study, which used "standardized" volumetry (FLR÷BSA), suggested a minimum safe FLR volume of 250 mL/m^2, which corresponds to about 40% of TLV.

There are limited data suggesting that ICG-R can be used in addition to liver volume to select cirrhotic patients for resection. One study suggests that the FLR volume should be at least 40% of TLV in patients with ICG-R<10%,[46] and another study suggests that the FLR volume should be at least 60% of TLV in patients with ICG-R of 10–20%.[47] However, the limited availability of the agent (ICG dye) and lack of supportive data preclude widespread use of ICG-R for this purpose.

Worthy of note are two recent studies specifically in patients with cirrhosis and hepatocellular carcinoma who underwent right hepatectomy.[47,48] Both examine outcomes following a sequence of transarterial chemoembolization (TACE) to treat the liver tumor, followed at an interval (usually 2 weeks) by right PVE. The first, from Aoki et al.,[47] demonstrated an average of 22% hypertrophy of the FLR following TACE+PVE. No patient experienced posthepatectomy liver failure, and the 5-year overall and disease-free survival rates after curative resection were 55.6% and 46.7%, respectively. The second, from Ogata et al.,[48] found similar results and demonstrated that no deaths post resection occurred in patients with FLR hypertrophy>10%, and all deaths occurred in patients with FLR hypertrophy<10%. Further, the latter study, which compared PVE alone to TACE+PVE, demonstrated a greater proportion (67%) of patients experienced>10% hypertrophy with TACE+PVE versus PVE alone (28% experienced>10% FLR hypertrophy). Oncologic results in the Ogata study were similar to Aoki et al., and the pathologic complete necrosis rate in the resected patients was impressive, with TACE+PVE (83%) compared to PVE alone (6%) providing an oncologic basis to consider the combined embolization approach. These studies not only provide evidence that PVE is of significant clinical utility in patients with cirrhosis, but also suggest that TACE+PVE might be an approach which should be considered in the future.

30.3 Can PVE Increase FLR Volume?

Given that liver volume and liver function are linked and that the minimum safe FLR volume for resection is 20% of TLV in patients with normal liver and 40% of TLV in patients with cirrhosis, a logical next question is, "Can PVE increase the volume of the FLR?"

More than 75 studies published in peer-reviewed journals have demonstrated that the FLR volume increases after PVE performed prior to major hepatectomy.[6] A recent meta-analysis of 1,088 patients who underwent PVE for a variety of indications across a spectrum of normal to cirrhotic liver revealed that the FLR volume increased following PVE in every study.[6] The overall morbidity rate for PVE was 2.2% and no deaths due to PVE were reported. Eighty-five percent of patients underwent resection after PVE, and the incidence of transient liver failure following resection was only 2.5%; the mortality rate from liver failure was 0.8%.[6]

This meta-analysis demonstrates that PVE does increase FLR volume and that resection after PVE is safe. In addition, both the incidence of liver failure and the incidence of death due to liver failure in this meta-analysis were dramatically less than the corresponding rates for major and extended resection in series in which patients did not undergo preoperative PVE.

30.4 Does Increased FLR Volume After PVE Mean Increased Liver Function?

Three objective pieces of data that demonstrated a shift in liver function from the embolized liver to the FLR after PVE deserve comment.[49-51] The first study examined ICG excretion, liver volume, and bile volume in the FLR before and after PVE.[51] The amount of ICG excreted by the left lobe (FLR) as a proportion of total ICG excretion increased by 20.1%, and the volume of the left lobe as a proportion of TLV increased by 8.3%, indicating an actual shift in liver function to the nonembolized liver after PVE. In fact, the shift in function was greater than the shift in volume.

The second study examined liver volume and function using CT and technetium-99 m-galactosyl human serum albumin scintigraphy before and after PVE[22] and confirmed both a volume and a function shift to the nonembolized lobe after PVE. Of note, no patients with an FLR volume>40% of TLV experienced postoperative liver failure, whereas patients with an FLR volume<34% of TLV did experience liver failure. Also of note was that patients without liver failure experienced significant increase in FLR volume after PVE, whereas patients with liver failure did not.

The case report demonstrated an actual shift in bile flow to the FLR after PVE.[50] In this study, percutaneous transhepatic catheters in the embolized and nonembolized sectors of the liver allowed measurement of bile flow and bile concentration before and after embolization. Before PVE, the FLR (36% of TLV measured by CT volumetry) provided 72% of bile clearance. Jaundice persisted despite complete drainage of the liver. Following PVE, the FLR volume increased 23%, but bile clearance in the FLR increased by 84-fold and the jaundice cleared. Resection was subsequently completed. Thus, overall liver function improved after PVE, and there was an objective shift in liver function to the nonembolized liver following PVE.[50]

30.5 Can PVE Convert a High-Risk (Low-FLR-Volume) Patient to a Low-Risk (Adequate-FLR-Volume) Patient?

A landmark study reported in 2009[30] (described in some detail in the section "Current standard: 20% of TLV" above) showed that PVE can allow patients with an initial FLR volume≤20% of TLV to experience a postoperative course similar to that of patients with a larger initial FLR volume and that the true cutoff for safe surgery is 20%, not 30%. In this study, 301 consecutive patients underwent right hepatectomy extended to all or part of segment 4 (extended right hepatectomy). Known risk factors for liver insufficiency including FLR volume, incidences of liver insufficiency, and death from liver failure were studied. Patients were divided into three groups: those with FLR volume≤20% of TLV at the time of resection, those with FLR volume 20.1–30% of TLV, and those with FLR volume>30% of TLV. Liver insufficiency was defined as a postoperative bilirubin level reaching 7 mg/dL, as previously described.[3] Multivariate analysis revealed that BMI>25 kg/m^2, intraoperative blood transfusion, and FLR≤20% of TLV independently predicted postoperative liver insufficiency (odds ratio 2.18, CI, 1.34–7.54). Further, patients with a pre-PVE FLR volume≤20% of TLV who underwent PVE and experienced FLR growth to>20% of TLV had a postoperative course similar to that of patients with FLR volume>20% of TLV without PVE. These patients post-PVE did not have a postoperative course similar to patients operated with an FLR≤20%. This strongly suggests that the risk profile was effectively decreased in this high-risk population.

A prospective study demonstrated that PVE has no benefit in patients with normal liver and an adequate

FLR volume.[52] Specifically, patients undergoing right hepatectomy were alternately allocated to PVE versus no PVE. This study is misunderstood and misquoted as demonstrating that PVE is not indicated in patients with normal liver. In fact, the study showed that PVE is not indicated in patients with normal liver with an FLR volume>30%. As would be expected, PVE did not reduce the incidence of postoperative complications compared to no PVE in this group of patients without indication for PVE. Restated, this evidence is valuable and supports the contention that PVE is not indicated for patients with FLR volume≥30% of TLV. This study does not, however, demonstrate that patients with normal liver do not need PVE, as patients at risk for inadequate FLR volume after resection were not studied. Analysis of segmental liver volumes demonstrates that the vast majority of patients without tumor-related volume shift in the liver have a left liver volume≥30% of TLV.[53]

The same study[52] demonstrated that PVE is beneficial before right hepatectomy in patients with cirrhosis. Postoperative complications, duration of intensive care unit stay, and duration of hospital stay were significantly decreased in cirrhotic patients who underwent right hepatectomy after PVE versus those who underwent right hepatectomy without PVE. Patients with cirrhosis who underwent PVE had a mean FLR of 35% of TLV – an indication for PVE in cirrhotic patients according to the work of Kubota et al.[20], as described above. Thus, it is not surprising that this aspect of the study demonstrated a benefit of PVE compared to no PVE (cirrhotic patients without PVE had a mean FLR of 39% of TLV). The proportion of patients with one or more complications and the incidences of pulmonary complications, ascites, and liver failure were lower in the PVE group (all $p<0.05$). These authors did reinforce the initial finding of Hirai et al.[49] that FLR hypertrophy in response to PVE is prognostic. Specifically, the patient who died in the PVE arm did not experience hypertrophy in response to PVE.

We recently examined our experience with major hepatectomy for hepatocellular carcinoma.[54] Twenty-one patients who underwent major hepatectomy after PVE were compared to 33 patients who underwent hepatectomy without PVE. Overall complication rates were similar between the groups, but the major complication rate in the non-PVE group was 35% versus only 10% in the PVE group ($p=0.028$), and there were no perioperative deaths in the PVE group versus six deaths (18%) in the non-PVE group ($p=0.038$). In five patients, postoperative death was related to liver insufficiency leading to multiorgan failure; the sixth patient died with multiorgan dysfunction including renal failure. It is interesting that the two patients in the non-PVE group who underwent preoperative volumetry did not experience complications. Importantly, oncologic outcomes were equivalent between patients with and without PVE.

30.6 Should a Prospective, Randomized Trial Be Conducted to Assess the Value of PVE?

Some authors have proposed a prospective, randomized trial to increase the strength of the evidence that PVE is useful. If so, based on current evidence, how would such a study be designed?

30.6.1 Patients with Normal Liver

Among patients with normal liver, the evidence presented herein demonstrates the following:

1. In a prospective, alternate allocation study,[52] PVE provided no benefit in patients with FLR volume>30% of TLV.
2. At least three studies have demonstrated that resection with FLR volume≤20% of TLV is not safe,[27,28,45] and those authors who propose a minimum safe FLR volume of 30% of TLV[36-38] agree by definition that FLR volume≤20% of TLV is inadequate.
3. The postoperative course in patients with FLR volume 20.1–30% of TLV is no different from that in patients with FLR volume>30% of TLV.[27]
4. The risk associated with PVE itself is low but not nil.[6,55]
5. Oncologic outcomes are equivalent with and without PVE.[37,56-59]

Given these principles, it would be unethical to randomize patients with FLR volume≤20% of TLV to no PVE, as the risk for complications, liver insufficiency, and liver failure is established in this group. Further, it would be unethical to randomize patients with FLR volume>20% of TLV to PVE because the lack of value of PVE in this group is established. Thus, no randomized trial of PVE versus no PVE can be readily devised for patients with normal liver.

30.6.2 Patients with Cirrhosis

Among patients with cirrhosis, the evidence demonstrates the following:

1. Retrospective studies have established that resection in patients with well-compensated cirrhosis with FLR volume>40% of TLV is safe.[4,20] Risk for death in patients with a larger FLR is very low in properly selected cirrhotic patients.[60-62] High risk of death from liver failure is established in patients with cirrhosis and FLR volume<40% of TLV.[4,20,63,64]
2. A prospective, alternate allocation study showed that in cirrhotic patients with FLR volume≤40% of TLV, PVE was associated with a substantial decrease in postoperative complications compared to the rate of complications in patients without PVE.[52]
3. Retrospective study showed that major hepatectomy after PVE in cirrhosis was associated with markedly fewer major complications and no death compared to increased major complications and death in similar patients without PVE.[54]
4. Oncologic outcomes are equivalent following resection with and without PVE.[54]
5. Hypertrophy of the FLR may be greater and oncologic outcomes may be superior with the combination of transarterial chemoembolization and PVE compared to PVE alone.[46,47]
6. The risk associated with PVE, though low, is higher in cirrhotic patients than in patients with normal liver.[6,55]

Sufficient data exist to demonstrate that the safe cutoff for resection in patients with well-compensated cirrhosis is FLR volume of 40% of TLV. The group of patients with FLR volume<40% of TLV is at very high risk and cannot be denied PVE in a randomized study. Risk is too low in patients with FLR volume>40% of TLV to make a study valuable – sample size would likely be prohibitive and the question of little clinical interest in this population. Trying to define a larger FLR group that might benefit from PVE using ICG-R or other methods is not of major interest. In the cirrhotic population with hepatocellular carcinoma, a comparison of transarterial chemoembolization plus PVE versus PVE alone in patients with FLR volume<40% of TLV may be of interest, though such a study would not be a study of PVE versus no PVE. Formulating a trial around an oncologic question rather than a volume question regarding PVE in cirrhosis would be equally difficult. Considering the small volume of major resections performed worldwide for cirrhotic patients with hepatocellular carcinoma, it would be difficult to ensure adequate power for such a trial.

30.6.3 Intermediate Liver Disease

If no good randomized study of PVE can be designed for patients with normal liver or with cirrhosis, then might patients with intermediate degrees of liver injury (e.g., from extensive chemotherapy) be the best subjects for prospective study?

Great care would have to be exercised in the development of a trial for patients with "intermediate" liver disease. Selection criteria for such gray-zone patients would have to be well defined but clinically relevant. Patients with known risk (very small FLR volume) could not be randomized to no PVE, whereas patients with low risk (e.g., FLR volume≥40% of TLV) would not be appropriately randomized to PVE. Allocating all patients with liver disease from "prolonged" chemotherapy is vague, variable, and poorly defined. A trial in patients with cholangiocarcinoma ("intermediate" liver injury from biliary obstruction) would be faced with the problem of small patient numbers, and excellent outcomes following PVE are already established in this group.[65]

A highly innovative study, such as a study of PVE with or without infusion of growth factors or stem cells into the remnant liver, may be the area of greatest interest for a prospective study of PVE. The utility of PVE is clearly established, such that there appears to be relatively little potential gain from randomized trials studying PVE versus no PVE. Rather, future studies should investigate methods to build on the clearly established benefit of PVE in selected populations.

30.7 Conclusion

In summary, given the current level of evidence, the following statement, originally made in 2001, appears to remain true today: "A randomized trial cannot be recommended to test the efficacy of PVE, for it would be unethical to deny the benefit of the technique and safer resection to patients who are otherwise poor candidates for resection based on inadequate liver size or function".[1]

References

1. Abdalla EK, Hicks ME, Vauthey JN. Portal vein embolization: rationale, technique and future prospects. *Br J Surg*. 2001;88:165-175.
2. Cunningham JD, Fong Y, Shriver C, Melendez J, Marx WL, Blumgart LH. One hundred consecutive hepatic resections. Blood loss, transfusion, and operative technique. *Arch Surg*. 1994;129:1050-1056.
3. Mullen JT, Ribero D, Reddy SK, et al. Hepatic insufficiency and mortality in 1,059 noncirrhotic patients undergoing major hepatectomy. *J Am Coll Surg*. 2007;204:854-862; discussion 862–854.
4. Shirabe K, Shimada M, Gion T, et al. Postoperative liver failure after major hepatic resection for hepatocellular carcinoma in the modern era with special reference to remnant liver volume. *J Am Coll Surg*. 1999;188:304-309.
5. Makuuchi M, Thai BL, Takayasu K, et al. Preoperative portal embolization to increase safety of major hepatectomy for hilar bile duct carcinoma: a preliminary report. *Surgery*. 1990;107:521-527.
6. Abulkhir A, Limongelli P, Healey AJ, et al. Preoperative portal vein embolization for major liver resection: a meta-analysis. *Ann Surg*. 2008;247:49-57.
7. Kinoshita H, Sakai K, Hirohashi K, Igawa S, Yamasaki O, Kubo S. Preoperative portal vein embolization for hepatocellular carcinoma. *World J Surg*. 1986;10:803-808.
8. Detry O, De Roover A, Delwaide J, et al. 60 h of anhepatic state without neurologic deficit. *Transpl Int*. 2006;19:769.
9. Bismuth H, Houssin D, Castaing D. Major and minor segmentectomies "reglees" in liver surgery. *World J Surg*. 1982;6:10-24.
10. Johnson TN, Tucker GT, Tanner MS, Rostami-Hodjegan A. Changes in liver volume from birth to adulthood: a meta-analysis. *Liver Transpl*. 2005;11:1481-1493.
11. DeLand FH, North WA. Relationship between liver size and body size. *Radiology*. 1968;91:1195-1198.
12. Urata K, Kawasaki S, Matsunami H, et al. Calculation of child and adult standard liver volume for liver transplantation. *Hepatology*. 1995;21:1317-1321.
13. Vauthey JN, Abdalla EK, Doherty DA, et al. Body surface area and body weight predict total liver volume in Western adults. *Liver Transpl*. 2002;8:233-240.
14. Kawasaki S, Makuuchi M, Matsunami H, et al. Preoperative measurement of segmental liver volume of donors for living related liver transplantation. *Hepatology*. 1993;18:1115-1120.
15. Kiuchi T, Kasahara M, Uryuhara K, et al. Impact of graft size mismatching on graft prognosis in liver transplantation from living donors. *Transplantation*. 1999;67:321-327.
16. Kiuchi T, Tanaka K, Ito T, et al. Small-for-size graft in living donor liver transplantation: How far should we go? *Liver Transpl*. 2003;9:S29-S35.
17. Man K, Fan ST, Lo CM, et al. Graft injury in relation to graft size in right lobe live donor liver transplantation: a study of hepatic sinusoidal injury in correlation with portal hemodynamics and intragraft gene expression. *Ann Surg*. 2003;237:256-264.
18. Soejima Y, Shimada M, Suehiro T, et al. Outcome analysis in adult-to-adult living donor liver transplantation using the left lobe. *Liver Transpl*. 2003;9:581-586.
19. Chun YS, Ribero D, Abdalla EK, et al. Comparison of two methods of future liver remnant volume measurement. *J Gastrointest Surg*. 2008;12:123-128.
20. Kubota K, Makuuchi M, Kusaka K, et al. Measurement of liver volume and hepatic functional reserve as a guide to decision-making in resectional surgery for hepatic tumors. *Hepatology*. 1997;26:1176-1181.
21. Monaco AP, Hallgrimsson J, McDermott WV Jr. Multiple adenoma (hamartoma) of the liver treated by subtotal (90 percent) resection: morphological and functional studies of regeneration. *Ann Surg*. 1964;159:513-519.
22. Nagasue N, Yukaya H, Ogawa Y, Kohno H, Nakamura T. Human liver regeneration after major hepatic resection. A study of normal liver and livers with chronic hepatitis and cirrhosis. *Ann Surg*. 1987;206:30-39.
23. Soyer P, Roche A, Elias D, Levesque M. Hepatic metastases from colorectal cancer: influence of hepatic volumetric analysis on surgical decision making. *Radiology*. 1992;184:695-697.
24. Starzl TE, Putnam CW, Groth CG, Corman JL, Taubman J. Alopecia, ascites, and incomplete regeneration after 85 to 90 per cent liver resection. *Am J Surg*. 1975;129:587-590.
25. Vauthey JN, Chaoui A, Do KA, et al. Standardized measurement of the future liver remnant prior to extended liver resection: methodology and clinical associations. *Surgery*. 2000;127:512-519.
26. Heymsfield SB, Fulenwider T, Nordlinger B, Barlow R, Sones P, Kutner M. Accurate measurement of liver, kidney, and spleen volume and mass by computerized axial tomography. *Ann Intern Med*. 1979;90:185-187.
27. Kishi Y, Abdalla EK, Chun YS, et al. Three hundred and one consecutive extended right hepatectomies: evaluation of outcome based on systematic liver volumetry. *Ann Surg*. 2009;250:540-548.
28. Abdalla EK, Barnett CC, Doherty D, Curley SA, Vauthey JN. Extended hepatectomy in patients with hepatobiliary malignancies with and without preoperative portal vein embolization. *Arch Surg*. 2002;137:675-680; discussion 680–671.
29. Halazun KJ, Al-Mukhtar A, Aldouri A, et al. Right hepatic trisectionectomy for hepatobiliary diseases: results and an appraisal of its current role. *Ann Surg*. 2007;246:1065-1074.
30. Lodge J. Author reply. *Ann Surg*. 2008;248:139-140.
31. Bennett JJ, Blumgart LH. Assessment of hepatic reserve prior to hepatic resection. *J Hepatobiliary Pancreat Surg*. 2005;12:10-15.
32. Melendez J, Ferri E, Zwillman M, et al. Extended hepatic resection: a 6-year retrospective study of risk factors for perioperative mortality. *J Am Coll Surg*. 2001;192:47-53.
33. Jarnagin WR, Gonen M, Fong Y, et al. Improvement in perioperative outcome after hepatic resection: analysis of 1,803 consecutive cases over the past decade. *Ann Surg*. 2002;236:397-406; discussion 406–397.
34. Shoup M, Gonen M, D'Angelica M, et al. Volumetric analysis predicts hepatic dysfunction in patients undergoing major liver resection. *J Gastrointest Surg*. 2003;7:325-330.
35. Abdalla EK, Adam R, Bilchik AJ, Jaeck D, Vauthey JN, Mahvi D. Improving resectability of hepatic colorectal metastases: expert consensus statement. *Ann Surg Oncol*. 2006;13:1271-1280.
36. Adam R, Lucidi V, Bismuth H. Hepatic colorectal metastases: methods of improving resectability. *Surg Clin North Am*. 2004;84:659-671.

37. Oussoultzoglou E, Bachellier P, Rosso E, et al. Right portal vein embolization before right hepatectomy for unilobar colorectal liver metastases reduces the intrahepatic recurrence rate. *Ann Surg*. 2006;244:71-79.
38. Wicherts DA, de Haas RJ, Adam R. Bringing unresectable liver disease to resection with curative intent. *Eur J Surg Oncol*. 2007;33(Suppl 2):S42-S51.
39. Ribero D, Curley SA, Imamura H, et al. Selection for resection of hepatocellular carcinoma and surgical strategy: indications for resection, evaluation of liver function, portal vein embolization, and resection. *Ann Surg Oncol*. 2008;15:986-992.
40. Zorzi D, Laurent A, Pawlik TM, et al. Chemotherapy-associated hepatotoxiciy and surgery for colorectal liver metastases. *Br J Surg*. 2007;94:274-286.
41. Capussotti L, Muratore A, Ferrero A, Anselmetti GC, Corgnier A, Regge D. Extension of right portal vein embolization to segment IV portal branches. *Arch Surg*. 2005;140:1100-1103.
42. Schindl MJ, Redhead DN, Fearon KC, Garden OJ, Wigmore SJ. The value of residual liver volume as a predictor of hepatic dysfunction and infection after major liver resection. *Gut*. 2005;54:289-296.
43. Ferenci P, Lockwood A, Mullen K, Tarter R, Weissenborn K, Blei AT. Hepatic encephalopathy—definition, nomenclature, diagnosis, and quantification: final report of the working party at the 11th World Congresses of Gastroenterology, Vienna, 1998. *Hepatology*. 2002;35:716-721.
44. Vauthey JN, Pawlik TM, Abdalla EK, et al. Is extended hepatectomy for hepatobiliary malignancy justified? *Ann Surg*. 2004;239:722-730; discussion 730–722.
45. Ribero D, Abdalla EK, Madoff DC, Donadon M, Loyer EM, Vauthey JN. Portal vein embolization before major hepatectomy and its effects on regeneration, resectability and outcome. *Br J Surg*. 2007;94:1386-1394.
46. Wakabayashi H, Ishimura K, Okano K, et al. Application of preoperative portal vein embolization before major hepatic resection in patients with normal or abnormal liver parenchyma. *Surgery*. 2002;131:26-33.
47. Aoki T, Imamura H, Hasegawa K, et al. Sequential preoperative arterial and portal venous embolizations in patients with hepatocellular carcinoma. *Arch Surg*. 2004;139:766-774.
48. Ogata S, Belghiti J, Farges O, Varma D, Sibert A, Vilgrain V. Sequential arterial and portal vein embolizations before right hepatectomy in patients with cirrhosis and hepatocellular carcinoma. *Br J Surg*. 2006;93:1091-1098.
49. Hirai I, Kimura W, Fuse A, Suto K, Urayama M. Evaluation of preoperative portal embolization for safe hepatectomy, with special reference to assessment of nonembolized lobe function with 99mTc-GSA SPECT scintigraphy. *Surgery*. 2003;133:495-506.
50. Ijichi M, Makuuchi M, Imamura H, Takayama T. Portal embolization relieves persistent jaundice after complete biliary drainage. *Surgery*. 2001;130:116-118.
51. Uesaka K, Nimura Y, Nagino M. Changes in hepatic lobar function after right portal vein embolization. An appraisal by biliary indocyanine green excretion. *Ann Surg*. 1996;223:77-83.
52. Farges O, Belghiti J, Kianmanesh R, et al. Portal vein embolization before right hepatectomy: prospective clinical trial. *Ann Surg*. 2003;237:208-217.
53. Abdalla EK, Denys A, Chevalier P, Nemr RA, Vauthey JN. Total and segmental liver volume variations: implications for liver surgery. *Surgery*. 2004;135:404-410.
54. Palavecino M, Chun YS, Madoff DC, et al. Major hepatic resection for hepatocellular carcinoma with or without portal vein embolization: perioperative outcome and survival. *Surgery*. 2009;145:399-405.
55. Madoff DC, Abdalla EK, Vauthey JN. Portal vein embolization in preparation for major hepatic resection: evolution of a new standard of care. *J Vasc Interv Radiol*. 2005;16:779-790.
56. Azoulay D, Castaing D, Smail A, et al. Resection of nonresectable liver metastases from colorectal cancer after percutaneous portal vein embolization. *Ann Surg*. 2000;231:480-486.
57. Chun YS, Vauthey JN, Ribero D, et al. Systemic chemotherapy and two-stage hepatectomy for extensive bilateral colorectal liver metastases: perioperative safety and survival. *J Gastrointest Surg*. 2007;11:1498-1504; discussion 1504–1495.
58. Elias D, Ouellet JF, De Baere T, Lasser P, Roche A. Preoperative selective portal vein embolization before hepatectomy for liver metastases: long-term results and impact on survival. *Surgery*. 2002;131:294-299.
59. Jaeck D, Oussoultzoglou E, Rosso E, Greget M, Weber JC, Bachellier P. A two-stage hepatectomy procedure combined with portal vein embolization to achieve curative resection for initially unresectable multiple and bilobar colorectal liver metastases. *Ann Surg*. 2004;240:1037-1049; discussion 1049–1051.
60. Imamura H, Seyama Y, Kokudo N, et al. One thousand fifty-six hepatectomies without mortality in 8 years. *Arch Surg*. 2003;138:1198-1206; discussion 1206.
61. Miyagawa S, Makuuchi M, Kawasaki S, Kakazu T. Criteria for safe hepatic resection. *Am J Surg*. 1995;169:589-594.
62. Torzilli G, Makuuchi M, Inoue K, et al. No-mortality liver resection for hepatocellular carcinoma in cirrhotic and noncirrhotic patients: Is there a way? A prospective analysis of our approach. *Arch Surg*. 1999;134:984-992.
63. Tanabe G, Sakamoto M, Akazawa K, et al. Intraoperative risk factors associated with hepatic resection. *Br J Surg*. 1995;82:1262-1265.
64. Tjandra JJ, Fan ST, Wong J. Peri-operative mortality in hepatic resection. *Aust N Z J Surg*. 1991;61:201-206.
65. Nagino M, Kamiya J, Nishio H, Ebata T, Arai T, Nimura Y. Two hundred forty consecutive portal vein embolizations before extended hepatectomy for biliary cancer: surgical outcome and long-term follow-up. *Ann Surg*. 2006;243:364-372.

Future Perspectives

31

Yuji Nimura

Abstract

Portal vein embolization (PVE) has been widely used to increase safety of major hepatectomy for patients with hepatobiliary malignancies, and advantages of PVE have been reported. Although procedure-related morbidity is quite low, further technical development is necessary to reduce complications and to estimate the functional and volumetric changes of the hepatic lobe after PVE. Moreover, the indication and selection criteria of patients with underlying liver disease (i.e., cirrhosis, cholestasis, or normal liver with metastases) should be clarified more precisely. Clinical and basic studies on liver regeneration after PVE will contribute toward the future development of extended liver surgery for hepatobiliary malignancies.

Keywords

Portal vein embolization • Hepatobiliary surgery • Hepatectomy • Hepatocellular carcinoma

Portal vein embolization (PVE) made a large contribution toward the recent progress of hepatobiliary surgery since Makuuchi and Kinoshita have reported their clinical practices of this technique[1-3] and a lot of reports not only on clinical issues but also on basic researches have been published. In this chapter, future perspectives of this technique are presented.

Y. Nimura
Aichi Cancer Center, 1-1 Kanokoden, Chikusa-ku, Nagoya 464-8681, Japan
e-mail: ynimura@aichi-cc.jp

31.1 Technical Developments

PVE was first performed intraoperatively via the ileocolic vein,[1] and percutaneous transhepatic portal vein embolization was developed[2] and has been used in most worldwide centers. Moreover, an ipsilateral approach[4-7] has been considered more preferable than a contralateral approach[2] to prevent unexpected portal thrombosis in the future remnant liver (FRL), and the procedure became to be safer.

As of now, there has only been a small number of complications of unexpected portal vein thrombosis beyond the portal bifurcation and/or in the FRL; however, further technical developments are needed to

D.C. Madoff et al. (eds.), *Venous Embolization of the Liver*,
DOI 10.1007/978-1-84882-122-4_31, © Springer-Verlag London Limited 2011

prevent minor but serious complications. Sequential portal vein and hepatic artery embolization have been reported as another technical development to increase the volume of the small FRL and to decrease the postoperative risk of impaired functional liver resection.[8-10] This procedure was applied for patients with HCC or cholangiocarcinoma developed in chronic liver disease. The estimated functional reserve of the FRL was poor or those with colorectal liver metastases, and the FRL volume was quite small. As the major item of concern involved liver abscess with or without fatal sepsis developed after this procedure, safer technical developments and reappraisal of the indication of this procedure are needed.

Contrary to those reports, sequential arterial and portal embolizations before right hepatectomy were carried out to improve the rate of hypertrophy of the FRL in patients with liver cirrhosis and hepatocellular carcinoma (HCC). Selective transcatheter arterial chemoembolization (TACE) preceded PVE by 3–4 weeks, and this procedure was safer than the sequential portal and arterial embolization and increased further the rate of hypertrophy of the FRL and led to a high rate of complete tumor necrosis associated with longer recurrence-free survival.[11] As this procedure might have prevented intrahepatic metastasis of HCC via the portal blood flow, more clinical studies are expected to clarify the interesting results of this study. Moreover, sequential preoperative ipsilateral hepatic vein embolization after PVE was developed and clinically applied to induce further liver regeneration in patients with limited liver enlargement after PVE alone. The right hepatic vein was embolized with multiple coils after insertion of vena cava filters or vascular plugs after right PVE. This ideal procedure was safe and accelerated liver regeneration even in chronic liver diseases by inducing more apoptosis in the embolized liver area than PVE alone.[12] Further technical development is expected to simplify this complex procedure.

31.2 Specific Substances for Portal Vein Embolization

Different embolic materials have been used for PVE. Gelatin sponge powder or particles with or without coils had been commonly used for transcatheter arterial embolization and also applied to PVE with varying degree of success.[1,3,13-17] Recanalization was a main problem of this substance, but was less frequently encountered after PVE using fibrin glue with iodized oil.[4-7] Ethanolamine oleate, *N*-butyl cyanoacrylate, and pure ethanol are considered as the most effective embolic materials to induce greater liver atrophy/hypertrophy due to their strong local chemical reaction to the vessel wall: phlebitis which develops complete intravascular thrombosis of the portal vein. However, this strong chemical reaction also induces extravascular inflammation: periphlebitis with extravascular fibrosis which disturbs surgeons to dissect the hepatic hilus and to skeletonize the portal bifurcation.[17-23]

Further clinical study is necessary to decrease recanalization and to obtain complete PVE. On the other hand, every effort should be made to eliminate adverse effect of PVE, for example, unexpected migration of embolic material toward the FRL must be prevented.[5,18,24] Moreover, it is necessary to clarify the preferable kind and adequate volume of embolic materials in each sectional or segmental portal branch to minimize perivascular fibrosis.

31.3 Reappraisal of Indication of Portal Vein Embolization

Although PVE has been carried out safely and the reported morbidity rates of this procedure have been low, serious complication of transient liver failure developed after PVE in patients with chronic liver disease.[25] However, careful estimation of FRL function alleviated the contraindication of PVE for patients with chronic liver disease, which increased the safety and resectability of HCC in injured liver with a benefit in prolonged survival.[26] Another important issue is PVE for normal liver with liver metastases. The postoperative course of patients with normal liver who underwent PVE before right hepatectomy was similar to those with immediate surgery.[27] Although PVE reduces intrahepatic recurrence rate after right hepatectomy for patients with unilobar colorectal liver metastasis,[28] the growth rate of liver metastasis in the FRL is increased after PVE.[29-32] Further, the long-term survival is reduced, and disease recurrence is enhanced by PVE.[30,33] However, preoperative chemotherapy does not impair liver regeneration after PVE, and liver resection can be preformed safely in patients treated with preoperative chemotherapy before PVE.[34] Therefore, suitable patients with colorectal liver metastases should be carefully selected for preoperative chemotherapy followed by PVE.

31.4 Summary

Clinical advantages of PVE have already been reported, and hepatobiliary surgeons have adopted PVE as a useful preoperative measure in preparation of patients undergoing major hepatectomy for hepatobiliary malignancies. However, further clinical studies are necessary to increase the safety of this procedure, to develop more effective embolic materials, and to refine the methods for evaluating volumetric and functional changes of the hepatic lobe after PVE. Although a randomized controlled trial to evaluate the real value of PVE is difficult, prospective clinical studies should be done to define the indication and selection criteria of patients with underlying liver diseases (i.e., cirrhosis, cholestasis, or normal liver with metastasis).[35]

References

1. Makuuchi M, Takayasu Y, et al. Intrahepatic portal vein embolization before hepatectomy for bile duct cancer. *J Jpn Surg Assoc*. 1984;45:1558-1564 (in Japanese).
2. Kinoshita H, Sakai K, et al. Preoperative portal vein embolization for hepatocellular carcinoma. *World J Surg*. 1986;10:803-808.
3. Makuuchi M, Le Thai B, et al. Preoperative portal embolization to increase safety of major hepatectomy for hilar bile duct carcinoma: a preliminary report. *Surgery*. 1990;107:521-527.
4. Nagino M, Nimura Y, Hayakawa N, et al. Percutaneous transhepatic portal embolization using newly devised catheters: preliminary report. *World J Surg*. 1993;17:520-524.
5. Nagino M, Nimura Y, Kamiya J, et al. Selective percutaneous transhepatic embolization of the portal vein in preparation for extensive liver resection: the ipsilateral approach. *Radiology*. 1996;200:559-563.
6. Nagino M, Kamiya J, Kanai M, et al. Right trisegment portal vein embolization for biliary tract carcinoma: technique and clinical utility. *Surgery*. 2000;127:155-160.
7. Nagino M, Nimura Y, Kamiya J, et al. Right or left trisegment portal vein embolization before hepatic trisegmentectomy for hilar bile duct carcinoma. *Surgery*. 1995;117:677-681.
8. Takada T, Ammori BJ, et al. Combined preoperative embolization of the right portal vein and hepatic artery for hepatic resection in a high-risk patient. *Am J Roentgenol*. 1999; 173:165-167.
9. Nagino M, Kanai M, Morioka A, et al. Portal and arterial embolization before extensive liver resection in patients with markedly poor functional reserve. *J Vasc Interv Radiol*. 2000;11:1063-1068.
10. Gruttadauria S, Luca A, et al. Sequential preoperative ipsilateral portal and arterial embolization in patients with colorectal liver metastases. *World J Surg*. 2006;30: 576-578.
11. Ogata S, Belghiti J, et al. Sequential arterial and portal vein embolizations before right hepatectomy in patients with cirrhosis and hepatocellular carcinoma. *Br J Surg*. 2006;93: 1091-1098.
12. Hwang S, Lee SG, et al. Sequential preoperative ipsilateral hepatic vein embolization after portal vein embolization to induce further liver regeneration in patients with hepatobiliary malignancy. *Ann Surg*. 2009;249:608-616.
13. Imamura H, Shimada R, et al. Preoperative portal vein embolization: an audit of 84 patients. *Hepatology*. 1999; 29:1099-1105.
14. Kakizawa H, Toyota N, et al. Preoperative portal vein embolization with a mixture of gelatin sponge and iodized oil: efficacy and safety. *Acta Radiol*. 2006;47:1022-1028.
15. Huang JY, Yang WZ, et al. Portal vein embolization induces compensatory hypertrophy of remnant liver. *World J Gastroenterol*. 2006;12:408-414.
16. Tsuda M, Kurihara N, et al. Ipsilateral percutaneous transhepatic portal vein embolization with gelatin sponge particles and coils in preparation for extended right hepatectomy for hilar cholangiocarcinoma. *J Vasc Interv Radiol*. 2006;17:989-994.
17. de Baere T, Roche A, et al. Preoperative portal vein embolization for extension of hepatectomy indications. *Hepatology*. 1996;24:1386-1391.
18. Madoff DC, Hicks ME, et al. Portal vein embolization with polyvinyl alcohol particles and coils in preparation for major liver resection for hepatobiliary malignancy: safety and effectiveness – study in 26 patients. *Radiology*. 2003;227: 251-260.
19. Ko GY, Sung KB, et al. Preoperative portal vein embolization with a new liquid embolic agent. *Radiology*. 2003;227: 407-413.
20. Covey AM, Tuorto S, et al. Safety and efficacy of preoperative portal vein embolization with polyvinyl alcohol in 58 patients with liver metastases. *Am J Roentgenol*. 2005;85:1620-1626.
21. Tarazov PG, Granov DA, et al. Preoperative portal vein embolization for liver malignancies. *Hepatogastroenterology*. 2006;53:566-570.
22. de Baere T, Denys A, et al. Comparison of four embolic materials for portal vein embolization: experimental study in pigs. *Eur Radiol*. 2009;19:1435-1442.
23. Bent CL, Low D, et al. Portal vein embolization using a nitinol plug (Amplatzer vascular plug) in combination with histoacryl glue and iodinized oil: adequate hypertrophy with a reduced risk of nontarget embolization. *Cardiovasc Intervent Radiol*. 2009;32:471-477.
24. Di Stefano DR, de Baere T, et al. Preoperative percutaneous portal vein embolization: evaluation of adverse events in 188 patients. *Radiology*. 2005;234:625-630.
25. Ribero D, Curley SA, et al. Selection for resection of hepatocellular carcinoma and surgical strategy: indications for resection, evaluation of liver function, portal vein embolization, and resection. *Ann Surg Oncol*. 2008;15:986-992.
26. Azoulay D, Castaing D, et al. Percutaneous portal vein embolization increases the feasibility and safety of major liver resection for hepatocellular carcinoma in injured liver. *Ann Surg*. 2000;232:665-672.

27. Farges O, Belghiti J, et al. Portal vein embolization before right hepatectomy: prospective clinical trial. *Ann Surg*. 2003;237:208-217.
28. Oussoultzoglou E, Bachellier P, et al. Right portal vein embolization before right hepatectomy for unilobar colorectal liver metastases reduces the intrahepatic recurrence rate. *Ann Surg*. 2006;244:71-79.
29. Elias D, De Baere T, et al. During liver regeneration following right portal embolization the growth rate of liver metastases is more rapid than that of the liver parenchyma. *Br J Surg*. 1999;86:784-788.
30. Kokudo N, Tada K, et al. Proliferative activity of intrahepatic colorectal metastases after preoperative hemihepatic portal vein embolization. *Hepatology*. 2001;34:267-272.
31. Pamecha V, Levene A, et al. Effect of portal vein embolisation on the growth rate of colorectal liver metastases. *Br J Cancer*. 2009;100:617-622.
32. Mueller L, Hillert C, et al. Major hepatectomy for colorectal metastases: Is preoperative portal occlusion an oncological risk factor? *Ann Surg Oncol*. 2008;15:1908-1917.
33. Pamecha V, Glantzounis G, et al. Long-term survival and disease recurrence following portal vein embolisation prior to major hepatectomy for colorectal metastases. *Ann Surg Oncol*. 2009;16:1202-1207.
34. Zorzi D, Chun YS, et al. Chemotherapy with bevacizumab does not affect liver regeneration after portal vein embolization in the treatment of colorectal liver metastases. *Ann Surg Oncol*. 2008;15:2765-2772.
35. Abdalla EK, Hicks ME, Vauthey JN. Portal vein embolization: rationale, technique and future prospects. *Br J Surg*. 2001;88:165-175.

Index

D.C. Madoff et al. (eds.), *Venous Embolization of the Liver*,
DOI 10.1007/ 978-1-84882-122-4, © Springer-Verlag London Limited 2011

R

MIX
Papier aus verantwortungsvollen Quellen
Paper from responsible sources
FSC® C105338
FSC
www.fsc.org

If you have any concerns about our products,
you can contact us on
ProductSafety@springernature.com

In case Publisher is established outside the EU,
the EU authorized representative is:
Springer Nature Customer Service Center GmbH
Europaplatz 3, 69115 Heidelberg, Germany

Printed by Libri Plureos GmbH
in Hamburg, Germany